T0325370

CANCER AND AGING HANDBOOK

CANCER AND AGING HANDBOOK
RESEARCH AND PRACTICE

Edited by

Keith M. Bellizzi, PhD, MPH
Associate Professor
Human Development and Family Studies
Center for Public Health and Health Policy
University of Connecticut
Storrs, CT, USA

Margot Ann Gosney, MD, FRCP
Director
Clinical Health Sciences
University of Reading
Reading, UK

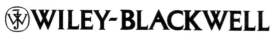

A JOHN WILEY & SONS, INC., PUBLICATION

Published by John Wiley & Sons, Inc., Hoboken, New Jersey
Published simultaneously in Canada

Wiley-Blackwell is an imprint of John Wiley & Sons, formed by the merger of Wiley's global Scientific, Technical, and Medical business with Blackwell Publishing.

For general information on our other products and services or for technical support, please contact our Customer Care Department within the United States at 877-762-2974, outside the United States at 317-572-3993 or fax 317- 572-4002.

Wiley also publishes its books in a variety of electronic formats. Some content that appears in print may not be available in electronic formats. For more information about Wiley products, visit our web site at www.wiley.com.

Library of Congress Cataloging-in-Publication Data:

Cancer and aging handbook / [edited by] Keith M. Bellizzi, Margot Ann Gosney.
    p. ; cm.
  Includes bibliographical references.
  Summary: "First multidisciplinary book available that examines the cancer and aging interface. Include specific points about how cancer and aging interrelate to guide training, research, and intervention"–Provided by publisher.
  ISBN 978-0-470-87442-4 (hardback)
  I. Bellizzi, Keith M., II. Gosney, Margot Ann.
  [DNLM: 1. Neoplasms–prevention & control. 2. Aged. 3. Aging–physiology. 4. Neoplasms–therapy. QZ 200]

  616.99′4–dc23

2012027799

Printed in the United States of America

10 9 8 7 6 5 4 3 2 1

■ CONTENTS

PART III   CANCER SCREENING GUIDELINES FOR OLDER ADULTS

PART IV   CANCER TREATMENT

PART V   COMMON CANCERS IN THE ELDERLY

You may open the window
And fail to see the fields and the river;
Even if you are not blind
You may be unable to enjoy the view of trees and flowers!

These verses of Fernando Pessoa are engraved on his monumental tomb in the Lisboa cathedral. They crystallize more eloquently than any scientific paper the urgency to study geriatric oncology. Diversity is a hallmark of aging. Individuals of the same chronologic age may differ substantially in life expectancy and tolerance of stress. When it comes to older individuals, the art of medicine consists in identifying those patients who are more likely to benefit from an aggressive treatment and those that are more likely to be harmed by it. In addition, the goals of treatment may change from patient to patient according to one's physical stamina and one's lifetime priorities. To a large extent, the management of an older individual is a social issue, involving the home caregiver and all the persons connected with the caregiver. It behooves the practitioner to ensure that the caregiver is appropriate for the patient's need and that caregiving does not disrupt the caregiver's family life.

The management of older individuals, including older cancer patients, involves a wisdom developed over a lifetime, thanks to time-consuming listening and painstaking collection and interpretation of clinical details. Only a practitioner willing to invest the time necessary to these endeavors will be able to provide safe and effective care to the older patient. In the management of older individuals with cancer, the practitioner needs to feel comfortable with uncertainty; to enjoy being creative in novel situations; to think outside the box; and to enrich with his/her own experience the dictates of medical textbooks, treatment guidelines, and clinical pathways. The best source of clinical evidence, the randomized clinical trials, are not very helpful for personalized care, because they cannot encompass the variety of conditions encountered in older individuals. A prominent geriatrician from the UK has defined evidence-based medicine as "evidence-biased medicine" [1], as the controlled conditions of clinical trials are rarely, if ever, reproducible in the practice arena.

There are other reasons for studying geriatric oncology beside the uniqueness of each cancer patient. They include the biological interactions of aging and cancer. Aging is a risk factor for carcinogenesis. This statement is confirmed by the association of smoking cessation with an epidemic of lung cancer in the elderly (people who no longer die of a coronary attack live long enough to develop lung cancer) [2] and that age is a risk factor for chemotherapy-induced acute myelogenous leukemia [3]. Also, the behavior of neoplasias may change with aging. For example, the prevalence of adverse prognostic factors increases with the age of patients with acute myelogenous leukemia [4], whereas breast cancer may become more indolent in the elderly [5]. The tumor host interactions represent a fascinating and largely unknown subject.

The problems of geriatric oncology are becoming everyday problems in the practice of oncology, given the rapid expansion of the aging population [6]. By the year 2000 50% of all malignancies occurred in the 12% of the population aged 65 and over; by the year 2030 it is predicted that individuals 65 and over will account for 20% of the population and 70% of all cancers in the United States [6]. This book, which gathers the contributions of some of the world's best known experts in the field, could not be more timely.

Perhaps more than any other field of medicine, geriatric oncology is rapidly evolving. Nobody will be able to provide a final word, during our lifetimes, at least. This book should be considered as an important foundation supporting both the practitioner of oncology and the clinical and basic investigators in the area. It is necessary, every so often, to summarize where we are and to decide where we should be going. By providing such a beacon, the book will have fulfilled this goal.

In one of his first novels, Love and Pedagogy, Miguel de Unamuno stated: "The truth is the worst of all lies." This paradox certainly applies to a medicine carved in stone rather than lived as an ongoing journey and a fascinating adventure. This book provides a current guide to practitioners and scientists involved in the journey.

LODOVICO BALDUCCI

REFERENCES

1. Evans GG. Evidence based and evidence-biased medicine. *Age Ageing* 1995;**24**:461–463.
2. Peto J. The lung cancer incidence falls in ex-smokers: misconception 2. *Br J Cancer* 2011;**104**:389.
3. Lyman GH, Dale DC, Wolff DA, et al. Acute myeloid leukemia or myelodysplastic syndrome in randomized controlled clinical trials of cancer chemotherapy with granulocyte colony stimulating factor. A systematic review. *J Clin Oncol* 2010;**28**:2914–2924.
4. Lugar SM. Treating the elderly patients with acute myelogenous leukemia. *Am Soc Hematol Educ Program* 2010;62–69.
5. Spazzapan S, Crivellari D, Bedard P, et al. Therapeutic management of breast cancer in the elderly. *Expert Opin Pharmacother* 2011;**12**:945–960.
6. Balducci L, Ershler WB. Cancer and aging: A nexus at several levels. *Natl Rev Cancer* 2005;**5**:655–662

Since the 1980s there has been an unprecedented increase in the attention being paid to the topic of cancer and aging. This is reflected by a 2007 Institute of Medicine workshop on cancer in the elderly and several special journal issues on this topic [1–3]. This response is the direct result of three converging forces: the aging of the population, the age-sensitive nature of cancer, and innovations in medical care. The confluence of these factors represents a significant public health challenge for the future. This challenge is further complicated by a potential shortage of oncologists, geriatricians, and nurses due to the projected exponential increase in incidence and prevalence of cancer in older adults coupled with a reduction in healthcare professionals entering into these fields [4,5].

These trends provide both challenges and opportunities. A central challenge is building the evidence base from epidemiologic, clinical trial, and behavioral research focusing on care for older adults across the cancer care continuum. Unfortunately the science of cancer care in the elderly population lags far behind what is known in children and other adults with cancer. Therefore, much of what is being practiced is extrapolated from studies of younger cohorts or based on clinical judgment. Another challenge is our capacity to respond to the complex healthcare needs of older adults given the projected shortages of geriatric/gerontology-trained healthcare workers. We believe that the answer to this question is multifaceted and will require thinking "outside the box" to (1) test new models of cancer care: (2) encourage new physicians to pursue geriatric fellowships: (3) provide broader geriatric and gerontology training for primary-care physicians and nurses: and (4) foster research and clinical collaboration among geriatricians, gerontologists, adult oncologists, and behavioral scientists. This latter endeavor is important as each of these disciplines contributes different perspectives, all essential to providing quality care to the growing population of older adults.

With challenges come opportunities. As we age, we become more heterogeneous in terms of physical and psychosocial health as a result of our previous lifestyles, environmental exposure, and genetic composition. Cancer care for older adults will likely be based on individualized approaches that account for this heterogeneity as well as the needs and preferences of the individual. This will likely require a paradigm shift from population-based medical care and healthcare to patient-centered care, which, we believe, will ultimately result in the highest-quality and most cost-effective care.

This multidisciplinary book was written by some of the most prominent international experts in the field of cancer and aging. The chapters in this book provide a synthesis of findings from current epidemiologic, behavioral, and clinical trial research across the entire continuum of cancer care, from prevention and screening, to treatment and survivorship, to end-of-life care. This book also includes a section on emerging issues in cancer care for older adults, including chapters focusing on caregivers, comprehensive geriatric assessment, the economic cost of treating older adults with cancer, and finally a discussion of multidisciplinary models of care. For some topics in this book, the evidence is still nascent, and the authors were challenged to provide recommendations for future research in these areas. In doing so, they raise some interesting questions about the complex issues facing older adults before, during, or after the diagnosis of cancer.

We believe that this book will demonstrate that the answer to addressing one of the biggest public health challenges of our time does not rest within any one discipline and that a broader knowledge and multidisciplinary approach is required to care for older adults at risk for, or living with, cancer. Our hope is that this information will be useful for healthcare providers, medical students, public health professionals, and policymakers who care for, or make policies that pertain to, the health of older adults.

KEITH M. BELLIZZI
MARGOT A. GOSNEY

REFERENCES

1. Institute of Medicine. *Cancer in Elderly People: Workshop Proceedings*, Washington, DC, 2007.

2. Lichtman SM, Balducci L, Aapro M. Geriatric oncology: A field coming of age. *J Clin Oncol* 2007;**25**:1821–1823.

3. Bellizzi KM, Mustian KM, Bowen DJ, Resnick B, Miller SM. Aging in the context of cancer prevention and control: Perspectives from behavioral medicine. *Cancer* 2008;**113**:3479–3483.

4. Erikson C, Salsberg E, Forte G, Bruinooge S, Goldstein M. Future supply and demand for oncologists: challenges to assuring access to oncology services. *Journal of Oncology Practice*. 2007;**3**(2):79–86.

5. Association of Directors of Geriatric Academic Programs. Geriatric medicine: A clinical imperative for an aging population, Part I. *Ann Long-Term Care* 2005;**13**:18–22.

Matti S. Aapro, MD, Dean, Multidisciplinary Oncology Institute, Clinique de Genolier, Switzerland

Angela Marie Abbatecola, MD, PhD, Italian National Research Center on Aging (INRCA), Scientific, Direction, Ancona 60100, Italy

Darrell E. Anderson, The Scientific Consulting Group, Gaithersburg, MD 20878

Riccardo A. Audisio, MD, FRCS, Honorary Professor, University of Liverpool; Consultant Surgical Oncologist, St. Helens Teaching Hospital, Marshalls Cross Road, Merseyside, UK

Lodovico Balducci, MD, Program Leader, Senior Adult Oncology Program, H. Lee Moffitt Cancer Center & Research Institute, 12902 Magnolia Dr., Tampa, FL 33612

Keith M. Bellizzi, PhD, MPH, Associate Professor, Department of Human Development and Family Studies, Center for Public Health and Health Policy. University of Connecticut, Storrs, CT 06269

Laura Biganzoli, MD, "Sandro Pitigliani" Medical Oncology Unit, Department of Oncology, Hospital of Prato, Istituto Toscano Tumori, Prato, Italy

Thomas O. Blank, PhD, Professor, Human Development and Family Studies, University of Connecticut, Storrs, CT 06269.

Manpreet K. Boparai, PharmD, CGP, BCACP, Department of Pharmacy, Memorial Sloan-Kettering Cancer Center, New York, NY 10065

Karen Bowman, Research Associate Professor, Department of Sociology, Case Western Reserve University, Cleveland OH 44106

Kerri M. Clough-Gorr, DSc, MPH, Section of Geriatrics, Boston University Medical Center, Robinson Building, Boston, MA 02118; Institute of Social and Preventive Medicine (ISPM), University of Bern, CH3012 Bern, Switzerland; National Institute for Cancer Epidemiology and Registration (NICER) Institute of Social and Preventive Medicine (ISPM), University of Zürich, CH3001 Zürich, Switzerland

Harvey Jay Cohen, MD, Walter Kempner Professor of Medicine and Director, Center for the Study of Aging, Duke University Medical Center, Durham, NC 27706

Nessa Coyle, NP, PhD, Department of Medicine, Memorial Sloan-Kettering Cancer Center, New York, NY 10065

Gary T. Deimling, PhD, Professor, Deptartment of Sociology and Director, Cancer Survivors Research Program, Case Western Reserve University, Cleveland, OH 44106

Konstantin H. Dragnev, MD, Hematology/Oncology Section, Norris Cotton Cancer Center, Dartmouth–Hitchcock Medical Center, Lebanon, NH 03756

Jean-Pierre Droz, MD, PhD, Geriatric Oncology Program, Department of Medical Oncology, Leon Berard Cancer Center, Claude Bernard Lyon 1 University, Lyon, France

Barbara K. Dunn, MD, PhD, Medical Officer, Division of Cancer Prevention, National Cancer Institute, National Institutes of Health, Bethesda, MD 20892

Barbara Ercole, MD, Department of Urology, School of Medicine, University of Texas, Health Science Center, San Antonio, TX 78229

William B. Ershler, MD, Division of Hematology/Oncology, Institute for Advanced Studies in Aging, Gaithersburg, MD 20877

Martine Extermann, MD, PhD, Senior Adult Oncology Program, Lee Moffitt Cancer Center & Research Institute, 12902 Magnolia Dr., Tampa, FL 33612

Claire Falandry, MD, PhD, Geriatrics Unit, Lyon University Hospices Civils de Lyon, Pierre-Bénite, France

Richard Fortinsky, PhD, Professor of Medicine, Physicians Health Services Chair in Geriatrics and Gerontology, UConn Center on Aging, University of Connecticut Health Center, Farmington, CT 06030

Gilles Freyer, MD, PhD, Medical Oncology Department, Lyon University Hospices Civils de Lyon, Pierre-Bénite, France

Barbara A. Given, PhD, RN, FAAN, Associate Dean of Research, College of Nursing, Michigan State University, East Lansing, MI 48823

Charles W. Given, PhD, Professor, Deptartment of Family Medicine, College of Human Medicine, Michigan State University, East Lansing, MI 48823

Paul Glare, MD, Chief, Pain and Palliative Care Service, Department, of Medicine, Memorial Sloan-Kettering Cancer Center, New York, NY 10065

Margot Ann Gosney, MD, FRCP, Director, Clinical Health Sciences, University of Reading, Reading, UK

Peter Greenwald, MD, PhD, Associate Director for Prevention Office of the Director National Cancer Institute, National Institutes of Health, Bethesda, MD 20892

Ernest T. Hawk, MD, MPH, Boone Pickens Distinguished Chair for Early Prevention of Cancer, Division of Cancer Prevention and Population Sciences, The University of Texas MD Anderson Cancer Center, Houston, TX 77030

Boaz Kahana, Professor, Deptartment of Psychology, Cleveland State University, Cleveland, OH 44115

Beatriz Korc-Grodzicki, MD, PhD. Chief of the Geriatrics Service, Department of Medicine, Memorial Sloan-Kettering Cancer Center, New York, NY 10065

George A. Kuchel, MD, Professor of Medicine, Citicorp Chair in Geriatrics & Gerontology; Director, UConn Center on Aging; Chief, Division of Geriatric Medicine, University of Connecticut Health Center, Farmington, CT 06030

Ian Kunkler, FRCR, Edinburgh Cancer Centre, University of Edinburgh, Western General Hospital, Edinburgh, UK

Diane E. Meier, MD, Director, Center of Advance Palliative Care, Vice Chair for Public Policy, Department of Geriatrics and Palliative Care, Mount Sinai School of Medicine, New York, NY 10029

Anthony B. Miller, MD, Dalla Lana School of Public Health, University of Toronto, Toronto, Ontario, Canada M5S IA1

Lopa Mishra, MD, Chair, Department of Gastroenterology, Hepatology and Nutrition, The University of Texas MD Anderson Cancer Center, Houston, TX 77030

Nicolas Mottet, MD, PhD, Service d'Urologie, Clinique Mutualiste de la Loire, San Saint-Etienne, Saint Priest en Jarez, France

Hyman B. Muss, MD, Professor of Medicine, University of North Carolina at Chapel Hill; Director of Geriatric Oncology, Lineberger Comprehensive Cancer Center, Chapel Hill, NC 27599

Heidi D. Nelson, MD, MPH, Departments of Medical Informatics and Clinical Epidemiology and Medicine, Oregon Health & Science University; Providence Cancer Center, Providence Health and Services, Portland, OR 97201

Jeanne F. Noe, PharmD, Protocol Development Associate, Lineberger Comprehensive Cancer Center, University of North Carolina at Chapel Hill, Chapel Hill, NC 27599

Catherine Oakman, MD, "Sandro Pitigliani" Medical Oncology Unit, Department of Oncology, Hospital of Prato, Istituto Toscano Tumori, Prato, Italy

Demetris Papamichael, MB, FRCP, Bank of Cyprus Oncology Centre, Nicosia, Cyprus

Kush K. Patel, Virginia Commonwealth University, Richmond, VA 23284

Sherri L. Patterson, University of Texas MD Anderson Cancer Center, Houston, TX 77030

Eric Pujade-Lauraine, MD, PhD, Department of Oncology, Université Paris Descartes, Paris, France

Catherine Quarini, MD, Department of Psychiatry, Warneford Hospital, Headington, Oxford, UK

Malcolm Walter Ronald Reed, Academic Unit of Surgical Oncology, Head of Department of Oncology, University of Sheffield, Royal Hallamshire Hospital, Glossop, UK

Lazzaro Repetto, MD, PhD, Italian National Research Center on Aging (INRCA), Research Hospital of Rome, Oncology Department, Rome, Italy

Thompson Gordon Robinson, BMedSci, MD, FRCP, Departments of Ageing and Stroke Medicine and Cardiovascular Sciences, University Hospitals of Leicester NHS Trust, Leicester, UK

Julie Robison, PhD, Associate Professor, UConn Center on Aging, University of Connecticut Health Center, Farmington, CT 06030

Paula R. Sherwood, PhD, RN, CNRN, FAAN, Professor, Vice Chair of Research, Department of Acute and Tertiary Care, School of Nursing, University of Pittsburgh, Pittsburgh, PA 15260

Ya-Chen Tina Shih, PhD, Associate Professor, Section of Hospital Medicine, Department of Medicine; Director, Program in Economics of Cancer, University of Chicago, Chicago, IL 60637

Samira Shojaee, MD, Pulmonary/Critical Care Medicine, Norris Cotton Cancer Center, Dartmouth–Hitchcock Medical Center, Lebanon, NH 03756

Rebecca A. Silliman, MD, PhD, Section of Geriatrics, Boston University Medical Center, Boston, MA 02118

Benjamin D. Smith MD, Assistant Professor, Department of Radiation Oncology, Division of Radiation Oncology, The University of Texas MD Anderson Cancer Center, Houston, TX 77025

Cardinale Smith, MD, Assistant Professor, Division of Hematology/Medical Oncology and Department of Geriatrics and Palliative Medicine, Mount Sinai School of Medicine, New York, NY 10029

Catherine Terret, MD, PhD, Geriatric Oncology Program, Department of Medical Oncology, Leon Berard Cancer Center, Claude Bernard Lyon 1 University, Lyon, France

Mya Thein, MD, Hematology/Immunology Unit, Translational Research Section, Clinical Research Branch, Intramural Research Program, National Institute on Aging, Baltimore, MD, 21225

Ian M. Thompson, Jr, MD, Director, Cancer Therapy and Research Center, The University of Texas, Health Science Center, San Antonio, TX 78229

Gabriel Tinoco, MD, Department of Internal Medicine, Harbor Hospital, Baltimore, MD 21225

Kathleen Tschantz Unroe, MD, Division of Geriatric Medicine and Center for the Aging, Duke University Medical Center, Durham, NC 27705

Ulrich Wedding, MD, Department of Internal Medicine/Palliative Care, Universitätsklinikum Jena, Erlanger Allee 101, 07747 Jena, Germany

Hans Wildiers MD, PhD, Department of General Medical Oncology/Multidisciplinary Breast Centre, University Hospitals Leuven, Leuven, Belgium

Lynda Wyld, Academic Unit of Surgical Oncology, University of Sheffield, Royal Hallamshire Hospital, Glossop, UK

PART I

CANCER AND AGING IN CONTEXT

CHAPTER 1

Epidemiology of Cancer in the Older-Aged Person

LODOVICO BALDUCCI

Senior Adult Oncology Program, H. Lee Moffitt Cancer Center & Research Institute, Tampa, FL

1.1 INTRODUCTION

Age is a risk factor for most cancers. In the United States 50% of all malignancies occur in men and women over the age of 65, which represents 12% of the population. With the current growth rate of the older population, it is estimated that 70% of all cancers will occur in the elderly by the year 2030 [1,2]. This finding is a call to face incoming cancer epidemics in a population that has been grossly understudied. As in other fields of geriatrics [3], clinical epidemiology will have a critical role in determining the best cancer care in older heterogeneous adults.

In this chapter we will examine how clinical epidemiology may help us to gain insight into the biology and the management of cancer in the older person. In closing we will explore new epidemiological approaches to determine benefits and risk of cancer treatment in older individuals.

1.2 AGE AND CANCER BIOLOGY

Clinical epidemiology helps us understand the interaction of aging with carcinogenesis and tumor behavior. The study of the incidence of cancer in advanced age may shed light on age-related factors that favor cancer development. Likewise, comparison of the natural history of cancer in younger and older individuals indicates that some cancers may become more aggressive and others more indolent with aging.

1.2.1 Aging and Carcinogenesis

The increased incidence of cancer in the older person may be due to three not necessarily mutually exclusive mechanisms. These include duration of carcinogenesis, increased susceptibility of older tissues to environmental carcinogens, and changes in body environment (chronic inflammation, increased resistance to insulin) [4].

Cancer and Aging Handbook: Research and Practice, First Edition. Edited by Keith M. Bellizzi and Margot A. Gosney.
© 2012 Wiley-Blackwell. Published 2012 by John Wiley & Sons, Inc.

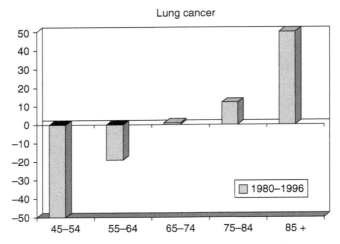

Figure 1.1   Changes in lung-cancer-related mortality [5].

The changing epidemiology of lung cancer supports the fact that aging is associated with cancer because carcinogenesis is a time-consuming process. As of 2005 the median age of lung cancer was around 71 years, up from 55 years in the mid-1970s [5]. This shift is arguably due to smoking cessation that is associated with a rapid decline in cardiovascular mortality. Ex-smokers now do live long enough to develop lung cancer [6,7]. Indeed, ex-smokers or never smokers account for an increasing proportion of newly diagnosed lung cancer [8]. Figure 1.1 summarizes the age-related changes in lung cancer mortality over a 20-year period.

A number of experimental studies have shown that some older tissues are primed to the action of environmental carcinogens and are more likely to undergo malignant transformation than younger tissues when exposed to the same dose of carcinogens [4]. Clinical epidemiology suggests that this is the case in older humans as well for the following reasons:

- The incidence of some cancers, such as prostate and colon cancer, increases more rapidly with age. This finding suggests that older tissues are more susceptible to environmental carcinogens. In support of this theory, the rate of malignant transformation of adenomatous polyps becomes more rapid with the age of the patient [2].

- Since the 1970s there has been a dramatic increase in the incidence of certain tumors, such as non-Hodgkin's lymphoma and malignant brain tumors in older individuals [9,10]. This finding suggests the possibility that older people develop cancer more quickly than younger ones when exposed to new environmental carcinogens.

- Age is a risk factor for the development of myelodysplasia and acute myelogenous leukemia after anthracycline-based adjuvant chemotherapy of breast cancer or after treatment for lymphoma [11,12].

- In a more recent longitudinal study of the population of Bruneck, Italy, individuals with shortest leukocyte telomeres had more than a threefold increase in the risk of cancer with respect to those with the longest telomeres [13]. According to a number of studies, summarized in Reference 14, telomere length is a mirror of the functional age of a person.

There is no convincing epidemiologic evidence supporting the association of cancer with changes in body environment, including immune-senescence, endocrine senescence, and proliferative senescence of fibroblasts. This possibility is suggested by the increased incidence of lymphatic tumors in presence of immune suppression and increased incidence of colon cancer in the presence of obesity [15].

Epidemiology has also produced some hypothesis-generating information related to the prevention of cancer in older individuals. This includes reduced incidence of cancer of the large bowel with regular use of aspirin [16] and reduced incidence of breast cancer in patients treated with selective estrogen receptor modulators (SERMs) or aromatase inhibitors for the adjuvant treatment of breast cancer.

1.2.2 Aging and Tumor Behavior

The clinical behavior of some tumors changes with the age of the patient (Table 1.1) [17]. The table highlights two important facts, emerging from clinical epidemiology:

1. Contrary to common belief, some neoplasms become more aggressive and more lethal with aging.
2. The change in tumor behavior involves at least three mechanisms: intrinsic cellular changes and changes in the tumor host and in the treatment received. If one tries to compare the growth of the cancer to that of a plant, the changes in growth rate depend on the seed, the soil, and the gardener.

It has always been known that age is a poor prognostic factor for acute myelogenous leukemia (AML), due to changes in the biology of the disease, which include higher prevalence of multidrug resistance, of unfavorable cytogenetics, and of NPM1 unmutated and flt3 mutated tumors [18]. At least in part, these changes may be explained by the fact that AML in older patients is preceded by myelodysplasia, a disease that affects the early hematopoietic progenitors.

Age is a poor prognostic factor for both aggressive and indolent non-Hodgkin's lymphomas [19]. Increased circulating concentrations of interleukin 6 (IL6), a powerful

TABLE 1.1 Clinical Behavior of Tumors Change with Age

Cancer	Clinical Behavior in the Aged	Mechanism
Acute myelogenous leukemia	More resistant to treatment	Increased prevalence of unfavorable genomic changes and of resistance to chemotherapy
Non-Hodgkin's lymphoma	Age is a poor prognostic factor	Increased circulating concentrations of interleukin 6 and increased risk of undertreatment
Breast cancer	More indolent	Increased prevalence of hormone-receptor-rich tumors; endocrine senescence
Ovarian cancer	More lethal	Unknown
Malignant brain tumors	More lethal	Increased prevalence of unfavorable genomic changes

stimulator of lymphocyte replication, may, in part, explain, this finding [20]. In the case of large cell lymphomas, clinical epidemiology suggests another important possibility: inadequate doses of chemotherapy. A systematic review demonstrated that individuals 60 and older had the same outcome as did younger adults if they received the same dose intensity of chemotherapy [21]. The review does not address the important question as to whether the undertreatment of the aged was justified by comorbidity and poor functional reserve, but it underlines the possibility that undertreatment may be responsible for some of the age-related prognostic changes in cancer, such as decreased survival in patients 60 and over with large cell lymphoma.

It is well established that metastatic breast cancer is associated with a more indolent course in older women, which include higher prevalence of bone and skin metastases in lieu of visceral and brain metastases. This finding may be due to increased prevalence of well-differentiated, hormone-receptor-rich tumors, endocrine senescence that disfavor the growth of hormone sensitive cancer, and availability of several forms of endocrine treatment [22]. Nevertheless, despite a more indolent course, breast cancer is still a lethal disease in older women and should be treated aggressively. Also, not all breast cancers in older women are indolent. Even in the oldest ages at least 20% of tumors are hormone receptor poor and very aggressive. Age is a risk factor for early death in glyoblastoma multiformis and malignant astrocytoma [9].

Epidemiological observations have identified important age-related differences in tumor behavior that have led to the discovery of underlying molecular or physiologic mechanisms. In addition, clinical epidemiology has revealed that inadequate treatment might have been responsible for poorer outcomes among older patients.

1.2.3 Age and Clinical Presentation of Cancer

Heterogeneity in terms of function and life expectancy is a hallmark of aging [23,24]. The practitioner managing older patients is faced with a number of issues, including whether (1) cancer screening and cancer treatment may reduce cancer-related mortality in patients with limited life expectancy and (2) older individuals are able to tolerate aggressive cancer treatment. Clinical epidemiology has given important insights into these issues.

A number of older studies summarized in Goodwin et al. [25] demonstrate that the majority of cancers were diagnosed at a more advanced stage in older compared with younger adults. The reasons for delayed diagnosis are poorly understood and may involve decreased awareness of early symptoms of cancer in the aging population and their providers. It is possible that symptoms such as pain, constipation, malaise, or weight loss be mistakenly ascribed to preexisting diseases or even to age itself. Another potential cause of delayed diagnosis is limited access to healthcare. One reversible cause of delayed diagnosis is reduced utilization of effective screening interventions such as mammography or colonoscopy by older individuals [26]. Disturbingly, lack of physician recommendations might have been the major cause of underutilization of these life-saving procedures by the elderly. Thus, public and professional education may reduce the cancer-related mortality of older individuals.

Multiple Malignancies As aging is a risk factor for cancer, it should not be unexpected for older cancer patients to present with more than one malignant disease. Excluding non-melanomatous skin cancer, approximately 20% of cancer patients 70 and older have more than one neoplasm in their lifetime [27]. This association may be explained by several factors, such as:

- The phenomenon of *field carcinogenesis*, which explains how patients who experience a previous cancer are susceptible to a second neoplasm in the same organ, as all cells of that organ have been exposed to the same carcinogen
- More frequent clinical monitoring of individuals with previous history of cancer (e.g., frequent utilization of CT scans or MRI may explain the association between lymphoma and renal cell carcinoma)
- Carcinogenic effects of previous cancer treatment, including chemotherapy-induced AML in patients who received adjuvant chemotherapy from previous cancers [11,12].
- Increased prevalence of indolent malignancies, including prostate cancer and chronic lymphocytic leukemia in older individuals

At present there is no evidence of a special genetic profile that renders certain older individuals more susceptible to multiple neoplasms requiring more intense monitoring. Also, a history of multiple neoplasms does not appear to increase the risk of an older patient to die of cancer [27].

1.2.4 Clinical Profile of the Older Cancer Patient

At least three studies have explored function and comorbidity of older cancer patients and have revealed that 70% of individuals over 70 years of age reported dependence in one or more instrumental activities of daily living (IADL) and that significant comorbidity was present in 40–90% of patients [28–30]. The prevalence of memory disorders, malnutrition, and dependence in one or more basic activity of daily living was present in as many as 20% of patients [28–30]. These studies revealed that the majority of older cancer patients needed some assistance in receiving and managing cancer treatment. When compared with an age-matched population without cancer, older cancer patients appeared to be in better health, but with reduced number of comorbid conditions and reduced prevalence of functional dependence. The impression that cancer may be a disease of "healthy elderly" is reinforced by the low prevalence of neoplastic diseases among patients living in institutions [31]. Thus, clinical epidemiology suggests that the majority of older individuals with cancer may benefit from cancer treatment if they have adequate medical and social support.

A study in 2000 was particularly provocative as it showed that women 80 and older diagnosed with breast cancer have a longer life expectancy than do women of the same age without breast cancer, according to SEER data [32]. These data may be misleading, however, because in the majority of the patients with breast cancer, the cancer was diagnosed at mammography. It is reasonable to expect that only the healthiest octogenarians might have been chosen to undergo mammography.

1.2.5 Age and Cancer Management

Diversity is a hallmark of the aged population [23,24]. The influence and the interactions of comorbidity, polypharmacy, geriatric syndromes, and social support on cancer diagnosis and outcome are best studied in large databases where this information is prospectively collected. So far the main source of information related to the prevention and treatment of cancer in older people has been the Surveillance, Epidemiology, and End Results (SEER) program. SEER is the US National Cancer Institute–funded cancer registry representing four main geographic areas of the United States and includes information on cancer in approximately 21% of the US population [32]. When coupled with the Medicare data, SEER allows us to study the benefits and risks of cancer treatment in individuals 65 and older.

Indeed, SEER has been the source of important, albeit inadequate, information. Through SEER we have learned that

- Women aged 70–79 had a twofold reduction in breast cancer mortality if they underwent at least two mammographic examinations [33–35]. The benefit was present even in women with moderate comorbidity [35].
- Androgen deprivation in older men was associated with increased risk of bone fractures when the treatment was protracted longer than one year [36]. Androgen deprivation was also associated with increased risk of diabetes and myocardial infarction.
- Age was a risk factor for chemotherapy-induced acute leukemia, and this effect was enhanced by the use of hemopoietic growth factors [11,12].
- Age was a risk factor for anthracycline-induced chronic cardiomyopathy [37].

In other areas, however, the information provided by SEER has been inconclusive, as is the issue of whether cancer chemotherapy is a cause of dementia in older breast cancer patients [38,39]. The main limitation of the SEER data is the absence of information related to the function, severity of comorbidity, cognition, social support, and geriatric syndromes. This information is crucial to the advancement of geriatric oncology for several reasons: (1) function, comorbidity, and geriatric syndromes determine the so-called active life expectancy that is as important as survival and disease-free survival as treatment outcome in the older population [17]; (2) this information predicts the risk of mortality of older individuals [23,24]; and (3) a number of more recent and yet largely unpublished studies showed that function, cognition, comorbidity, risk of falls, and other geriatric syndromes may be used to predict the risk of complications from cancer treatment in older individuals [40,41]. Only by collecting a host of pretreatment information may we be able to fine-tune our predictions and decide for which patients cancer treatment may be beneficial or detrimental. New tumor registries, including the Endhoven registry in the Netheralands, have made a concerted effort to collect this prospective information.

1.3 CONCLUSIONS

Clinical epidemiology has a unique role in the study of older cancer patients. In the case of carcinogenesis and cancer behavior, clinical epidemiology has been the dictionary allowing us to translate bench findings into clinical data. It has demonstrated that older individuals are more susceptible to carcinogens than younger ones, and that the clinical behavior of cancer changes with age, due to a combination of "seed and soil" factors.

From a clinical standpoint, clinical epidemiology has demonstrated that older cancer patients are generally healthier than older individuals without cancer, and that age is a risk factor for delayed diagnosis and undertreatment of cancer. Clinical epidemiology is the best available approach to establish whether cancer treatment benefit older patients in terms of active life expectancy and which age-related factors may influence the treatment toxicity and the disease outcome. For this purpose it is important to have a prospective collection of data related to function, comorbidity, geriatric syndromes, and social support.

REFERENCES

1. Smith BD, Smith GL, Hurria A, et al. Future of cancer incidence in the United States: Burdens upon an aging, changing nation. *J Clin Oncol* 2009;**27**(17):2758.

2. Yancik R, Ries LA. Cancer in the older person. An international issue in an aging world. *Semin Oncol* 2004;**31**(2):128–136.

3. Olshansky SJ, Goldman DP, Zheng Y, et al. Aging in America in the twenty-first century: Demographic forecasts from the MacArthur Foundation Research Network on an Aging Society. *Milbank Q* 2009;**87**(4):842–862.

4. Balducci L, Ershler WB. Cancer and aging: A nexus at several levels. *Nat Rev Cancer* 2005;**5**:655–662

5. Edwards BK, Brown ML, Wingo PA, et al. Annual report to the nation on the status of cancer, 1975–2002, featuring population-based trends in cancer treatment. *J Natl Cancer Inst* 2005;**97**(19):1407–1427.

6. Crispo A, Brennan P, Jöckel KH, et al. The cumulative risk of lung cancer among current, ex- and never-smokers in European men. *Br J Cancer* 2004;**91**(7):1280–1286.

7. Freedman DA, Navidi WC. Ex-smokers and the multistage model for lung cancer. *Epidemiology* 1990;**1**(1):21–29.

8. Hecht SS, Kassie F, Hatsukami DK. Chemoprevention of lung carcinogenesis in addicted smokers and ex-smokers. *Nat Rev Cancer* 2009;**9**(7):476–488.

9. Hoffman S, Propp JM, McCarthy BJ. Temporal trends in incidence of primary brain tumors in the United States, 1985–1999. *Neurol Oncol* 2006;**8**(1):27–37.

10. Han YY, Dinse GE, Umbach DM, et al. Age-period-cohort analysis of cancers not related to tobacco, screening, or HIV: Sex and race differences. *Cancer Causes Control* 2010;**21**(8):1227–1236.

11. Lyman GH, Dale DC, Wolff DA, et al. Acute myeloid leukemia or myelodysplastic syndrome in randomized controlled clinical trials of cancer chemotherapy with granulocyte colony-stimulating factor: A systematic review. *J Clin Oncol* 2010;**28**(17):2914–2924.

12. Gruschkus SK, Lairson D, Dunn JK, et al. Use of white blood cell growth factors and risk of acute myeloid leukemia or myelodysplastic syndrome among elderly patients with non-Hodgkin lymphoma. *Cancer* 2010;**115**:5279–5289.

13. Willeit P, Willeit J, Mayr A, et al. Telomere length and risk of incident cancer and cancer mortality. *JAMA* 2010;**304**(1):69–75.

14. Houben JM, Giltay EJ, Rius-Ottenheim N, et al. Telomere length and mortality in elderly men: The Zutphen elderly study. *J Gerontol A Biol Sci Med Sci* 2011;**66**:38–44.

15. Pais R, Silaghi H, Silaghi AC. Metabolic syndrome and risk of colorectal cancer. *World J Gastroenterol* 2009;**15**(41):5141–5148.

16. Rothwell PM, Wilson M, Elwin CE, et al: Long-term effect of aspirin on colorectal cancer incidence and mortality: 20-year follow-up of five randomised trials. *Lancet* 2011;**377**:31–41.

17. Carreca I, Balducci L. Cancer chemotherapy in the older cancer patient. *Urol Oncol* 2009;**27**(6):633–642.

18. Roellig C; Thiede C; Gramatzky M, et al: A novel prognostic model in elderly patients with acute myeloid leukemia. Results of 909 patients entered into the prospective AML 96 trial. *Blood* 2010;**116**:971–978.

19. Troch M, Wöhrer S, Raderer M. Assessment of the prognostic indices IPI and FLIPI in patients with mucosa-associated lymphoid tissue lymphoma. *Anticancer Res* 2010;**30**(2):635–639.

20. Duletić-Nacinović A, Sever-Prebelić M, Stifter S. Interleukin-6 in patients with aggressive and indolent non-Hodgkin's lymphoma: A predictor of prognosis? *Clin Oncol (R Coll Radiol)*. 2006;**18**(4):367–368.

21. Lee KW, Kim DY, Yun T, et al. Doxorubicin-based chemotherapy for diffuse large B-cell lymphoma in elderly patients: Comparison of treatment outcomes between young and elderly patients and the significance of doxorubicin dosage. *Cancer* 2003;**98**(12):2651–2656.

22. Carlson RW, Moench S, Hurria A, et al. NCCN task force report: Breast cancer in the older woman. *J Natl Comprehen Cancer Netw* 2008;**6** (Suppl 4):S1–S25.

23. Lee SJ, Lindquist K, Segal MR, et al. Development and validation of a prognostic index for 4-year mortality in older adults. *JAMA* 2006;**295**(7):801–808.

24. Carey EC, Covinsky KE, Lui LY, et al. Prediction of mortality in community-living frail elderly people with long-term care needs. *J Am Geriatr Soc* 2008;**56**(1):68–75.

25. Goodwin JS, Osborne C. Factors affecting the diagnosis and treatment of older patients with cancer. In Balducci L, Lyman GH, Ershler WB, Extermann M, eds. *Comprehensive Geriatric Oncology*, Taylor & Francis, London, 2004, pp 56–66.

26. Terret C, Castel-Kremer E, Albrand G, et al. Effects of comorbidity on screening and early diagnosis of cancer in elderly people. *Lancet Oncol* 2009;**10**(1):80–87 (review).

27. Luciani A, Balducci L. Multiple primary malignancies. *Semin Oncol* 2004;**31**(2):264–273.

28. Extermann M, Overcash J, Lyman GH, et al. Comorbidity and functional status are independent in older cancer patients. *J Clin Oncol* 1998;**16**:1582–1587.

29. Repetto L, Fratino L, Audisio RA, et al. Comprehensive geriatric assessment adds information to the eastern cooperative group performance status in elderly cancer patients. An Italian group for geriatric oncology study. *J Clin Oncol* 2002;**20**:494–502.

30. Ingram SS, Seo PH, Martell RE, et al. Comprehensive assessment of the elderly cancer patient: The feasibility of self-report methodology. *J Clin Oncol* 2002;**20**:770–775.

31. Ferrell BA. Care of cancer patients in nursing homes. Oncology 1992;**6**(2 Suppl):141–145.

32. Diab SG, Elledge RM, Clark GM. Tumor characteristics and clinical outcome of elderly women with breast cancer. *J Natl Cancer Inst* 2000;**92**:550–556.

33. Mccarthy EP, Burns RB, Freund KM, et al. Mammography use, breast cancer stage at diagnosis, and survival among older women. *J Am Geriatr Soc* 2000;**48**:1226–1233.

34. Randolph WM, Goodwin JS, Mahnken JD, et al. Regular mammography use is associated with elimination of age-related disparities in size and stage of breast cancer at diagnosis. *Ann Intern Med* 2002;**137**:783–790.

35. McPherson CP, Swenson KK, Lee MW. The effects of mammographic detection and comorbidity on the survival of older women with breast cancer. *J Am Geriatr Soc* 2002;**50**:1061–1068.

36. Saylor PJ, Keating NL, Smith MR. Prostate cancer survivorship: Prevention and treatment of the adverse effects of androgen deprivation therapy. *J Gen Intern Med* 2009;**24**(Suppl 2):S389–S394.

37. Pinder MC, Duan Z, Goodwin JS, et al. Congestive heart failure in older women treated with adjuvant anthracycline chemotherapy for breast cancer. *J Clin Oncal* 2007;**25**:3808–3815.

38. Heck JE, Albert SM, Franco R, Gorin SS. Patterns of dementia diagnosis in surveillance, epidemiology, and end results breast cancer survivors who use chemotherapy. *J Am Geriatr Soc* 2008;**56**(9):1687–1692.

39. Baxter NN, Durham SB, Phillips KA, Habermann EB, Virning BA. Risk of dementia in older breast cancer survivors: A population-based cohort study of the association with adjuvant chemotherapy. *J Am Geriatr Soc* 2009;**57**(3):403–411.

40. Pace Participants: Shall we operate? Preoperative assessment in elderly cancer patients (PACE) can help. A SIOG surgical task force prospective study. *Crit Rev Oncol Hematol* 2008;**65**:156–163.

41. Extermann M, Hurria A. Comprehensive geriatric assessment for older patients with cancer. *J Clin Oncol* 2007;**25**(14):1824–1831.

CHAPTER 2

Biological Aspects of Aging and Cancer

GABRIEL TINOCO

Department of Internal Medicine, Harbor Hospital, Baltimore, MD

MYA THEIN

Hematology/Immunology Unit, National Institute on Aging, Baltimore, MD

WILLIAM B. ERSHLER

Division of Hematology/Oncology, Institute for Advanced Studies in Aging, Gaithersburg, MD

2.1 INTRODUCTION

Cancer incidence increases with each decade of adult life [1,2], and with the current public interest and emphasis on both healthcare and aging, there is an expanding interest in geriatric oncology [3–11]. In addition to the clinical and policy issues relevant to the dramatic increase in the number of older patients with cancer, there remain the very important questions of why and how aging predisposes to cancer. Understanding this association may provide fundamental clues to the biological underpinnings of both processes. In this chapter we attempt to establish a framework around themes in aging biology that are relevant to the development and progression of cancer.

2.2 NORMAL AGING

It is a central gerontologic principle that aging is not a disease. The gradual functional declines that accompany normal aging have been well characterized in the literature (see Ref. 12 for a review), but under normal circumstances do not account for symptoms of disease. For example, kidney function declines with age [13]. and, in fact, has proved to be a useful biological marker of aging (see discussion below). Yet, clinical consequences of this change in renal function, in the absence of a disease or the exposure to an exogenous nephrotoxic agent, are not observed. Similarly, bone marrow changes with age. Although there are stem cell changes reported with age (see below), hematopoietic function is basically intact. For example, even when bone marrow is donated from a 65-year-old person to an human leukocyte antigen (HLA)-matched

Cancer and Aging Handbook: Research and Practice, First Edition. Edited by Keith M. Bellizzi and Margot A. Gosney.
© 2012 Wiley-Blackwell. Published 2012 by John Wiley & Sons, Inc.

younger recipient, the transferred marrow supports hematopoiesis for the life of the recipient, a finding that confirms similar studies in laboratory animals [14].

Unlike the commonly held notion that stem cell compartments diminish in either number or function with age ultimately resulting in an inability to meet homeostatic demands, age-related hematopoietic stem cell (HSC) changes appear to be an exception, at least for murine species in which this issue has been most directly addressed. Early work demonstrated that marrow serially transplanted could reconstitute hematopoietic function for an estimated 15–20 lifespans [15]. Furthermore, the capacity for old marrow to reconstitute proved superior to that of young marrow [16]. Subsequently, a number of investigators using a variety of techniques have concluded that HSC concentration in old mice is approximately twice that found in young mice [17–20]. Some evidence suggests that the intrinsic function of HSC changes somewhat with age, most notably with a shift in lineage potential from lymphoid to myeloid development. This may contribute to an observed relative increase in neutrophils and decrease in lymphocytes in the peripheral blood of older people [21].

Although marrow stem cell numbers are preserved, the proliferative potential of progenitor cells is less [14,18]. In addition, erythropoietin responses are blunted with advancing age even in the absence of clinical disease [22,23], and low levels of anemia are commonly observed in otherwise healthy older people [22–24]. The diminished bone marrow reserve is also of clinical importance in considering cytotoxic chemotherapy for myelotoxicity is clearly greater in older cancer patients [25–27].

Distinct changes in measurable immune functions have been described with age, reviewed elsewhere [28], but the clinical consequences of these are minimal or even nonexistent in the absence of disease (see discussion below). Whether these changes contribute to a heightened susceptibility to infection remains a subject of debate.

Thus, aging is not a disease, but the consequences of aging may render an individual susceptible to disease. For example, there are age-associated changes described in immune functions and, although not of sufficient magnitude to pose primary problems, these alterations may render an individual susceptible to reactivation of tuberculosis [29,30] or herpes zoster [31] and less capable of responding to influenza vaccine with protective titers of antibody [32,33]. The immune decline, however, is not of sufficient magnitude or duration to account for the increased incidence of cancer in old people [34]. In fact, findings in experimental animals, have led some researchers to postulate that immune senescence may contribute to the observed reduced tumor growth and spread in a variety of tumors (discussed below).

2.2.1 Life Expectancy, Lifespan, and Maximum Survival

From the perspective of those who study aging, there is an important distinction made between median (life expectancy) and maximum lifespan. Over the past several decades, with the advent of modern sanitation, refrigeration, and other public health measures including vaccination and antibiotics, there has been a dramatic increase in median survival [35]. Early deaths have been diminished and more individuals are reaching old age. In the United States today, life expectancy for bot genders approaches 80 years [36]. Median survival is what concerns public health officials and healthcare providers, but for those studying the biology of aging, it is maximum survival that is the focus of greatest attention. Significantly, it has been estimated that if atherosclerosis and cancer were eliminated from the population as a cause of death, about 10 years would be added to the average human lifespan, yet there would be no change in maximum lifespan [37].

The oldest human being alive today (i.e., early 2012) is approximately 120 years old. What is intriguing is that the record has remained stable, unchanged by the public health initiatives mentioned above. In fact, some more recent data indicate that the maximum survival is actually declining in the United States [38,39]. In the laboratory, similar limits have been established for a variety of species. Drosophila, free of predators, can live for 30 days, whereas C57BL/6 mice maintained in a laboratory environment on a healthy diet ad libitum may survive for 40 months. What is interesting is that, unlike the public health initiatives in humans, experimental interventions in lower species have been associated with a prolongation of maximum survival. In drosophila, for example, transgenic offspring producing extra copies of the free-radical scavenging enzymes superoxide dismutase and catalase survived about 33% longer than controls [40]. However, there has been some criticism of this work, based on the claim that the controls were unusually shortlived. In mammalian species, the only experimental intervention that characteristically prolongs maximum survival is the restriction of caloric intake. In fact, dietary restriction (DR) has become a common experimental paradigm exploited in the investigation of primary processes of aging [41].

2.2.2 Cellular versus Organismal Aging

There has been much written about cellular senescence and the events that lead up to cell death [42,43]. After a finite number of divisions, normal somatic cells invariably enter a state of irreversibly arrested growth, a process termed *replicative senescence* [44]. In fact, it has been proposed that escape from the regulators of senescence is the antecedent of malignant transformation. However, the role of replicative senescence as an explanation of organismal aging remains the subject of vigorous debate. The controversy relates, in part, to the fact that certain organisms (e.g., drosophila, *Caenorhabditis elegans*) undergo an aging process, yet all of their adult cells are postreplicative.

What is clear is that the loss of proliferative capacity of human cells in culture is intrinsic to the cells and not dependent on environmental factors or even culture conditions [44]. Unless transformation occurs, cells age with each successive division. The number of divisions turns out to be more important than the actual amount of time passed. Thus, cells held in a quiescent state for months, when allowed back into a proliferative environment, will continue to undergo approximately the same number of divisions as those that were allowed to proliferate without a quiescent period [45].

The question remains whether this *in vitro* phenomenon is relevant to animal aging. One theory is that fibroblasts cultured from samples of old skin undergo fewer cycles of replication than those from young [46]. Furthermore, when various species are compared, replicative potential is directly and significantly related to lifespan [47]. An unusual β-galactosidase with activity peaks at pH 6 has proved to be a useful biomarker of *in vitro* senescence because it is expressed by senescent but not presenescent or quiescent fibroblasts [48]. This particular β-galactosidase isoform was found to have the predicted pattern of expression in skin from young and old donors with measurably increased levels in dermal fibroblasts and epidermal keratinocytes with advancing age [48]. The nature of the expression of this *in vivo* biomarker of aging in other tissues will be important to discern.

TABLE 2.1 Theories of Aging

Intrinsic stochastic	Somatic mutation; intrinsic mutagenesis; impaired DNA repair; error catastrophe
Extrinsic stochastic	Ionizing radiation; free-radical damage
Genetically determined	Neuroendocrine; immune

2.3 THEORIES OF AGING

Providing a rational, unifying explanation for the aging process has been the subject of a great number of theoretical expositions. Yet, no single proposal suffices to account for the complexities observed (Table 2.1). The fact that genetic controls are involved seems obvious when one considers that lifespan is highly species-specific. For example, mice generally live for about 30 months and humans about 90 years. However, the aging phenomenon is not necessarily a direct consequence of primary DNA sequence. For example, mice and bats have 0.25% difference in their primary DNA sequence, but bats live for 25 years, 10 times longer than mice. Thus, regulation of gene expression seems likely to be the source of species longevity differences.

Although there is considerable intraspecies (within-species) variation in longevity, this variability is much lower with inbred strains or among monozygotic twins, than with dizygotic twins or nontwin siblings. Also, various genetically determined syndromes have remarkable (albeit incomplete) features of accelerated aging. These include Hutchison–Guilford syndrome (early-onset progeria), Werner's syndrome (adult-onset progeria), and Down's syndrome [49]. Although no progeria syndrome manifests a complete phenotype of advanced age, identification of the genes responsible for these particular syndromes is beginning to pay dividends by providing clues to the molecular mechanisms involved in the aging process. For example, Werner's syndrome is now known to be caused by mutations in a single gene on chromosome 8 that encodes a protein containing a helicase domain [50,51]. Similarly, a mutation in the lamin A (LMNA) gene localized to chromosome 1 has been demonstrated to be the cause of the Hutchison-Guilford syndrome [52]. The future functional characterization of these specific proteins will, no doubt, increase our level of understanding of the aging process (Table 2.2). Examination of aging in yeast has also been informative with regard to the genetic controls of aging. These single-cell organisms follow the replicative limits of mammalian cells, and it has been observed that *lifespan* is related to silencing large chromosomal regions. Mutations in these silencing genes lead to increased longevity [53]. Thus, if there are certain genes that regulate normal aging, or at least are associated with the development of an aged phenotype, it stands to reason that acquired damage to those genes might influence the rate of aging. Over the years several theories have been proposed that relate to this supposition. In general, they hypothesize a random or stochastic accumulation of damage to either DNA or protein that eventually leads to dysfunctional cells, cell death and subsequent organ dysfunction, and ultimately organism death. Prominent among these is the *somatic mutation* theory [54], which predicts that genetic damage from background radiation, for example, accumulates and produces mutations and results in functional decline. A variety of refinements have been suggested to this theory invoking the importance of mutational interactions [55], transposable elements [56], and changes in DNA methylation status [57].

TABLE 2.2 Progeria-Related Disorders

Disorder	Age of Onset	Common Clinical Manifestations	Molecular Defects	Cancer-Prone?
Werner's syndrome	Adolescence	Short stature	Abnormal helicase; abnormal gene expression	Yes, particularly tumors of mesenchymal origin and leukemias
Cockayne's syndrome	First year of life	Photosensitivity; neurodegeneration; short stature	Defective gene repair; abnormal helicase; abnormal gene expression	—
Hutchinson–Gilford syndrome	First year of life	Short stature	Abnormal gene expression	—
Rothmund–Thomson syndrome	Neonatal period	Short stature; neurodegeneration	Abnormal overall DNA repair; increased sensitivity to X-ray and UV light	Yes, particularly osteogenic sarcomas and squamous cell carcinomas
Wiedermann–Rautenstrauch syndrome	Neonatal period	Short stature; neurodegeneration	Abnormal gene expression	—

A related hypothesis is Burnet's *intrinsic mutagenesis* theory [58], which proposes that spontaneous or endogenous mutations occur at different rates in different species and that this accounts for the variability observed in lifespan. Closely related to this notion is the *DNA repair* theory [59], which initially generated great excitement about as it was found that longlived animals had demonstrably greater DNA repair mechanisms than did shorterlived species [59], However, longitudinal studies within a species have not revealed a consistent decline in repair mechanisms with age. This, of course, does not rule out the possibility that repair of certain specific and critical DNA lesions are altered with advancing age. We now understand that there are multiple DNA repair mechanisms, including base excision repair, transcription-coupled repair, and most recently, even DNA repair mechanisms based in mitochondria. Disorders involving one or a subset of repair mechanisms could lead to accumulation of DNA damage and dysfunction.

In yet another intrinsic/stochastic model, the *error catastrophe* theory proposed by Orgel [60], it is suggested that random errors in protein synthesis occur and when the proteins involved are those responsible for DNA or RNA synthesis, there is resultant DNA damage and the consequences thereof to daughter cells. Although this model has appeal, there has been no reported evidence for impaired or inaccurate protein synthesis machinery with advancing age. However, a protein that has proved central in the process of cellular aging is telomerase. This critical enzyme comprises protein plus an RNA template and is necessary for maintaining telomere length and cell replicative potential. As cells senesce *in vitro*, telomerase activity declines, telomeres shorten, and ultimately replicative potential is lost [61–63].

Evidence that exogenous factors are involved in the acquisition of age-associated damage to DNA and protein is derived from a number of observations, many of which are circumstantial or correlative, but nonetheless provocative. It now appears that the accumulation of abnormal protein within senescent cells, as predicted by the *error catastrophe* theory, actually reflects posttranslational events, such as oxidation or glycation and resultant crosslinking. There is theoretic appeal to the concept that key proteins, such as collagen or other extracellular matrix proteins and DNA, become dysfunctional with age as a result of the impairment produced by these crosslinks [64].

One mechanism producing crosslinks is the nonenzymatic reaction of glucose with the amino groups of proteins (glycation). Presumably, glycation would occur more readily in the presence of higher serum levels of glucose; thus, this theory fits well with the observed, age-associated dysregulation of glucose metabolism and prevalent hyperglycemia in geriatric populations. Of course, this also points out its deficiency as a unifying mechanism, as there is no question that individuals with well-maintained glucose levels throughout there lifespan will still be subject to acquired changes typical of aging.

Another mechanism responsible for crosslinking is the damage produced by free radicals, and this forms the basis of the *free-radical hypothesis* initially proposed by Harman [65,66]. This theory suggests that aging is the result of DNA and protein damage (e.g., mutagenesis or crosslinking) by atoms or molecules that contain unpaired electrons (free radicals). These highly reactive species are produced as byproducts of a variety of metabolic processes and are normally inhibited by intrinsic cellular antioxidant defense mechanisms. If free-radical generation increases with age, or if the defense mechanisms that scavenge free radicals (e.g., glutathione) or repair free-radical damage decline, the accumulated free-radical damage may account for altered DNA and protein function. Evidence to support this widely held notion is incomplete. It is known that free-radical generation in mammals correlates inversely with longevity [67] and, similarly, that the level of free-radical-inhibiting enzymes, such as superoxide dismutase, are higher in those species with longer lifespans [68]. However, efforts at enhancing antioxidant mechanisms with dietary vitamin E have resulted in only a modest enhancement of median survival in mice and no effect on maximum lifespan [69].

More recently, there has been much attention focused on mitochondrial function in the context of free-radical damage because the bulk of oxidative metabolism and the production of reactive-oxygen species occurs in these organelles. Although mitochondrial DNA codes for antioxidant enzymes in addition to enzymes involved in energy production, it is currently believed that energy production declines with age, due to mitochondrial DNA damage by those reactive products. Indeed, mitochondrial damage increases with age in experimental models [70–72], and the shortened survival of knockout mice deficient in mitochondrial antioxidant enzymes has supported the potential importance of this mechanism [73].

The most compelling data to date in support of the free-radical hypothesis come from the experiments of Orr and Sohal in which transgenic drosophila producing enhanced levels of superoxide dismutase and catalase had a maximum survival 33% greater than controls [40]. Furthermore, it is known that flies produce high levels of free radicals associated with their impressive metabolic requirements, and that survival is enhanced dramatically when the ability to fly is experimentally hindered [74]. However, the generalizability of these findings has been questioned. Some have criticized the transgenic drosophila experiment, claiming that the controls were rather shortlived. Furthermore, transgenic mice overexpressing free-radical scavenging enzymes have produced very modest effects on lifespan [75]. Thus, the conclusion that augmentation of free-radical scavenging mechanisms increases longevity cannot be considered an established fact.

A different perspective suggests very good evidence implicating a nonrandom, perhaps genetically regulated endogenous mechanism involved in aging. For example, the *neuroendocrine* theory suggests that the decrements in neuronal and associated hormonal function are central to aging. It has been suggested that age-associated decline of hypothalamic–pituitary–adrenal axis function results in a physiological cascade, leading ultimately to the "frail" phenotype. This hypothesis is appealing because it is well established that this neuroendocrine axis regulates much of development and also the involution of ovarian and testicular function. Furthermore, age-associated declines in growth hormone and related factors [76], dehydroepiandrosterone [77], and secondary sex steroids [78] have been implicated in age-associated impairment, including a reduction in lean body mass and bone density. Furthermore, pharmacological reconstitution using these or related hormones has met with some success at reversing age-associated functional decline [78,79].

2.4 AGING AND CANCER

Aging is associated with molecular, cellular, and physiological changes that influence carcinogenesis and cancer growth. Multicellular organisms contain actively growing (mitotic) and mature (postmitotic, i.e., unable to divide) cells. The mitotic cells are susceptible to hyperproliferative disease, most prominently cancer [80]. This is because renewable tissues are generally repaired and replenished by cell proliferation, an early and essential step in the development of cancer. Also, DNA replication greatly increases the probability of acquiring, fixing, and propagating somatic mutations, a major driving force behind malignant transformation. This danger is offset by the coevolution of tumor suppressor mechanisms [81].

2.4.1 Molecular Aspects of Both Cancer and Aging

Although several theories have been proposed, none suffice to account for the complexities of aging. Lifespan is finite and varies generally from species to species and much less so within species. Mice live, on average, 2.5 years, monkeys 30 years, and humans about 90. Among species, larger animals generally live longer than do smaller ones, but within species (e.g., dogs) smaller animals are likely to live longer. It is clear that aging is not entirely explained by DNA sequence. For example, mice and bats have only 0.25% difference in their primary DNA sequence, but bats live for 25 years, 10 times longer than mice. A commonly held notion is that regulation of gene expression accounts for longevity difference between species.

It is now clearly established that certain specific genes can alter lifespan, at least in lower animals, but whether these same genes regulate "aging" is still in question. For example, transgenic drosophila expressing increased copies of the free-radical scavenging enzymes, superoxide dismutase and catalase, live, on average, a third longer than the appropriate controls. In even lower species [40] (e.g., yeast and nematodes), the identification of specific genes that influence lifespan [82,83] has led to the optimistic impression that analogous genes in higher organisms will lead to greater insight into the aging process. Yet, the identification and functional analysis of analogous genes in humans remain elusive.

If certain genes regulate normal aging, or at least are associated with the aging phenotype, it stands to reason that acquired damage to those genes might influence the rate of aging. It has been proposed that a random or stochastic accumulation of damage to DNA or protein eventually leads to dysfunctional cells, cell death and subsequent organ dysfunction, and ultimately organism death.

Tumor suppressor genes can be classified into two broad categories: caretakers and gatekeepers [84]. *Caretaker* tumor suppressor genes prevent cancer by protecting the genome from mutations. They do this generally by preventing DNA damage and/or optimizing DNA repair. In addition to preventing cancers, genes that help maintain genomic integrity also prevent or retard the development of other phenotypes and age-related pathologies [85]. These caretaker tumor suppressor genes are in essence longevity assurance genes.

Gatekeeper tumor suppressor genes, in contrast, prevent cancer by acting on the intact cells—specifically, mitotic cells that are at risk for neoplastic transformation. Gatekeepers can virtually eliminate potential cancer cells by inducing programmed cell death (apoptosis). Alternatively, they can prevent potential cancer cells from proliferating by inducing permanent withdrawal from the cell cycle (cellular senescence). Although little is known about how cells choose between apoptotic and senescence responses, both responses are crucial for suppressing cancer [86,87]. By inducing cellular quiescence or death, gatekeeper genes may, themselves, be causally related to age-acquired functional decline and even longevity [88].

The process of apoptosis could eventually deplete nonrenewable tissues of irreplaceable postmitotic cells and renewable tissue of stem cells. The senescence response could similarly deplete tissue of proliferating or stem cell pools. In addition, senescent cells may have lost sufficient metabolic activity and thereby disrupt normal tissue function as they accumulate [89,90].

Actively dividing cells undergo many divisions before reaching a stable postmitotic state (replicative senescence). It was discovered that proliferating cells reach this state because of repeated DNA replication causes shortening of the end pieces of chromosomes (telomeres) and eventually malfunction [91]. Telomeres are the DNA sequence and proteins that cap the ends of linear chromosomes and prevent their fusion by cellular DNA repair processes. Because functional telomeres maintain the integrity and stability of the genome, they suppress the development of cancer. Cells that fail to age and proliferate despite dysfunctional telomeres develop chromosomal aberrations, which may result in malignant transformation [92]. Thus, cellular senescence ensures that cells with dysfunctional telomeres are permanently withdrawn from the cell cycle, rendering them incapable of forming a tumor.

Many kinds of oncogenic stressful stimuli can also induce cellular senescence. These include certain types of DNA damage, including DNA breaks and oxidative lesions caused by environmental insults, genetic defects, or endogenous processes [85,93]. These can also lead to senescence in response to epigenetic changes within chromatin or those caused by pharmacological agents or altered expression of proteins that modify DNA or histones [94–96]. Such changes can alter the expression of protooncogenes or tumor suppressor genes and are a frequent occurrence among malignant tumors. Thus the senescence response prevents the growth of cells that experience any one of an assortment of potentially oncogenic stimuli.

Although diverse stimuli can induce a senescence response, they appear to converge on one or both of the two pathways that establish and maintain the senescence growth arrest. These pathways are governed by the gatekeeper tumor suppressor proteins p53 and pRB [89,97,98]. Dysfunctional telomere activates many components of p53-mediated damage response, and the senescence response to dysfunctional telomeres requires the integrity of p53 pathway [99,100]. Also overexpressed ras may trigger a p53-dependent damage response by producing high levels of DNA damaging reactive-oxygen species (ROS) [100–102]. However, oncogenic ras can also induce p16, an activator of the pRB pathways, which provides a second barrier to the proliferation of potentially oncogenic cells. There is an emerging consensus that senescence occurs through one pathway or the other, with the p53 pathway mediating senescence due primarily to telomere dysfunction and DNA damage and p16/pRB pathway mediating senescence due primarily to oncogenes, chromatin disruption, and various stresses. It is difficult to determine the extent to which the senescent states are induced by the ep53 and pRB pathways are distinct or similar. In addition, depending on the tissue and species of origin, cells may differ in both their senescent phenotype and the relative importance of the p53 or pRB pathways for the senescence response [103–105].

How might senescent cells promote aging phenotypes or age-related pathology? Because tissues have a fairly constant number of cells, the accumulation of nondividing senescent cells may compromise tissue renewal or repair. In addition, of the genes that are upreguated by the senescence response, many encode secreted proteins that can alter tissue structure and function [106–108]. Both possibilities are viable, but at present, evidence for the latter possibility is stronger.

Factors secreted by senescent cells vary by cell type. Senescent fibroblasts secrete high levels of matrix metalloproteinases, epithelial growth factors, and inflammatory cytokines [109]. In many ways the secretory phenotype of the senescent fibroblast resembles that of fibroblasts undergoing the wound response, which entails the local remodeling of tissue structure [110]. The wound response also entails local inflammation, a common feature in aging tissue and a proposed initiating or causative factor in a number of age-related diseases [111]. Apparent in wounds are cells that resemble cancer-associated fibroblasts. These cells are components of the so-called reactive stroma, which facilitate the progression of epithelial cancers [112,113]. Thus senescent cells might contribute to aging and age-related pathology by stimulating chronic tissue remodeling and/or local inflammation, which might compromise tissue structure and function. In addition, senescent cells may stimulate the proliferation of cells that harbor preneoplastic mutations. More recent findings suggest that senescent fibroblasts can disrupt the functional and morphological differentiation of epithelial cells, at least in three-dimensional cultures of mammary epithelial cells [114]. In these models, senescent fibroblasts perturbed alveolar morphogenesis and reduced milk protein expression by normal mammary epithelial cells. They also stimulated aberrant branching morphogenesis by normal breast epithelial cells, owing in large measure to their secretion of a specific matrix metalloproteinase (MMP3). This finding suggests that senescent stromal cells might promote the development of hyper plastic epithelial lesions *in vivo*. In addition, apparently normal tissue may harbor cells with oncogenic mutations, and the incidence of mutant cells increases with age [115,116]. Further, many cells with oncogenic mutations are held in check by the tissue microenvironment [113]. Thus, it is possible that change in the microenvironment caused by the senescent cells can fuel the growth and progression to malignancy. Indeed, there is mounting evidence that senescent fibroblasts create a local tissue environment that promotes the growth of initiated or preneoplastic epithelial cells, both in culture and *in vivo* [117–119].

A more speculative, but potentially important, consequence of cellular senescence may be its impact on stem cells. Embryonic stem cells, whether human or rodent, express high level of telomerase and thus are considered resistant to replicative senescence [120,121]. However, mammalian adult stem cells or progenitor cells do not proliferate indefinitely [122–125]. The ability of stem cells to undergo senescence and apoptosis appears to be an important mechanism for preventing cancer [126,127]. These changes may negatively influence stem cells in a number of ways. A primary consequence would be an absolute depletion of progenitor cell numbers. Additionally, the presence of senescent cells (i.e, the stem cells themselves or surrounding progeny) could disrupt the proliferative microenvironment, which might further influence proliferation, differentiation, and/or mobilization of the remaining resident stem cells.

Accordingly, it is currently believed that cellular senescence is controlled by the p53 and pRB tumor suppressor proteins in a complex process that, when functioning properly, has the added effect of restricting cancer cell development. Nonetheless, senescent cells acquire phenotypic changes that contribute to aging of the organism and a predisposition to certain age-related diseases, including late-life cancer. Thus, the senescent response may be antagonistically pleotropic, promoting early-life survival by curtailing the development of cancer but eventually limiting longevity as dysfunctional senescent cells accumulate. [128]

2.4.2 Aging and Carcinogenesis

The age-associated increase in incidence of cancer may be accounted for by three mechanisms: duration of exposure to carcinogenic factors, increased susceptibility of aging cells to carcinogens (seed effect), and microenvironmental conditions favoring tumor development (soil effect).

Carcinogenesis is a multistage process involving serial alterations of cellular genes. These include oncogenes and antiproliferative genes (antioncogenes), which modulate cell proliferation and genes that prevent apoptosis. The multistage nature of carcinogenesis has been shown in experimental models with strong circumstantial support in human cancers. For example, for the case of colorectal cancer, Vogelstein et al described a sequence of genetic alterations leading from normal mucosal epithelium to invasive carcinoma [129]. One step, the loss of the familial adenomatous polyposis (FAP) gene on the fifth chromosome, is associated with hyperproliferation of the mucosal cells and formation of adenomatous polyps. Additional changes in the expression of the p53 gene on chromosome 18 and the DCC gene on chromosome 17 may lead to a more malignant phenotype. Likewise, in the case of brain tumors, loss of a portion of the seventeenth chromosome (17p) is seen in malignancy of all grades, whereas loss of chromosome 10 and of the genes encoding interferon receptors was found only in glioblastoma multiforme [130]. These changes may provide the genetic basis for the transformation from indolent to more aggressive disease. Sequential genetic changes leading to more aggressive neoplasms have been reported for many other diseases, including breast, cervical, renal, and lung cancer [131–137].

The interpretation of carcinogenesis as a multistage process presents at least two non–mutually exclusive explanations for the increasing incidence of cancer with age. The first and simplest is that the tissues of an older person will have had greater time to accumulate a series of stochastic "hits" to the relevant DNA and/or protein. Accordingly, the cancers more prevalent among the aged, such as prostate, colon, or breast cancer, are those involving a greater number of steps. In contrast, this hypothesis would predict that tumors more common in young people (lymphoma, leukemia, neuroblastoma, etc.) would require fewer steps in the progression from normal to the malignant state.

The second hypothesis holds that age itself is a risk factor for cancer because the process of aging involves genetic events similar to those occurring early in carcinogenesis. Thus, the number of cells that would be susceptible to the effects of late-stage carcinogens increases with age. Both experimental findings and clinical evidence support this theory. Cytogenetic and molecular changes observed in early carcinogenesis are also seen in cells maintained in long-term culture. These changes include formation of DNA adducts, DNA hypomethylation, chromosomal breakage, and translocation [138,139]. Also, the accumulation of iron commonly observed in some aging cells may cause oncogene activation and antioncogene suppression [138,140]. The likelihood of neoplastic transformation after exposure to late-stage carcinogens is higher in tissues from older animals than in those of younger animals, both in tissue culture and in cross-transplant experiments [141–144].

Epidemiologic data for some cancers suggest that the susceptibility to late-stage carcinogens increases with age [145]. The comparison between the incidence of melanoma and of squamous cell carcinoma (SCC) of the skin is particularly illustrative [146,147]. In the United States, whereas the incidence of melanoma plateaus at age 45 for women and 61 for men, the incidence of SCC continues to rise even beyond age 85. This is what might be predicted if there were more steps in the generation of SCC than in melanoma. However, the increased number of steps is not the total explanation because the incidence of SCC increases logarithmically with age [146], suggesting either an association of longevity with a genetic predisposition to SCC or an increased susceptibility with age to late-stage carcinogens. It should be underscored that both basic and clinical data suggest that there is an increased susceptibility and that it may be tissue- and organ-specific. For example, skin epithelium, and liver and lymphoid tissues, but not nervous or muscular tissues, show increased susceptibility to late-stage carcinogens in older rodents [148,149]. Similarly, the incidence of melanoma and mesothelioma in humans demonstrates an age-related plateau, suggesting that these tissues are not more susceptible to late-stage carcinogens [145–147].

Other age-related factors that may increase cancer risk include age-impaired DNA repair mechanisms and decreased carcinogen catabolism [149,150]. It has been proposed that these lead to an accelerated carcinogenic process with more rapid generation of cells susceptible to late-stage carcinogens (promoters) [151].

2.4.3 Immune Senescence and Cancer

There is a commonly held notion that immune senescence is in some way related to the observed increased rate of cancer with advancing age. However, despite the appeal of such an hypothesis, scientific support has been limited and the topic remains controversial. It is difficult to deny that profoundly immunodeficient animals or humans are subject to a more frequent occurrence of malignant disease, and it would stand to reason that others with less severe immunodeficiency would also be subject to greater malignancy, perhaps less dramatically so. However, the malignancies associated with profound immunodeficiency (e.g., with AIDS or after organ transplantation) are usually lymphomas, Kaposi's sarcoma, or leukemia and not the more common malignancies of geriatric populations (lung, breast, colon, and prostate cancers). Accordingly, it is fair to say that the question of the influence of age-acquired immunodeficiency on the incidence of cancer is unresolved.

2.4.4 Explanations for Changes in Tumor Progression Observed with Advanced Age

There has been a long-held but incompletely documented clinical notion that cancers in older people are less aggressive. However, epidemiologic data from tumor registries or large clinical trials have not been supportive of this notion. This may be because this type of data is confounded by special problems common to geriatric populations (e.g., comorbidity, "polypharmacy," physician or family bias regarding diagnosis and treatment in older patients, and age-associated life stresses), and these factors may counter any primary influence that aging might have on tumor aggressiveness. However, there is experimental support for the contention that there is reduced tumor aggressiveness with age. Data obtained from laboratory animals with a wide range of tumors under highlycontrolled circumstances show slower tumor growth, fewer experimental metastases, and longer survival in old mice [152–155].

What accounts for the age-associated changes observed in these experimental systems? One explanation derives from the understanding that the tumors, although histologically quite similar, may be biologically very different in older patients (seed effect). For example, breast cancer cells from older patients are more likely to contain estrogen receptors, and leukemic cells have particular cytogenetic abnormalities in elderly patients. Each of these associations has prognostic significance. Furthermore, there is the issue of the *timeline* artifact (Fig. 2.1) that implies that old patients (more so than young) may develop slow-growing tumors on the basis of time required to develop such slow tumors. This is, of course, consistent with the multistep hypothesis discussed above.

It is probable that certain factors that influence tumor growth change with age. With this in mind, various endocrine, nutritional, wound-healing, and angiogenesis factors have been explored. For some tumors, age-associated changes in these factors have been correlated with reduced tumor growth [152,153,155–160]. However, several early observations led to the seemingly paradoxical conclusion that immune senescence accounted for a large component of the observed reduced tumor growth with age. For example, B16 melanoma grew less well in congenitally immunodeficient mice [161] and in young mice rendered T-cell-deficient [155]. Furthermore, when young, thymectomized, lethally irradiated mice received bone marrow or splenocytes from old donor mice, tumor growth was less than when the spleen or bone marrow was from young donor mice [155,157].

It is believed that competent immune cells provide factors that augment tumor growth under certain circumstances. If a tumor is only weakly antigenic, nonspecific growth stimulatory factors provided by lymphocytes or monocytes may actually counteract the inhibitory forces provided by those same cells (because of the lack of tumor

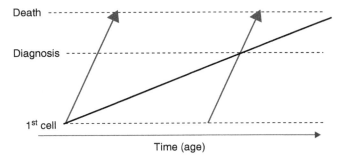

Figure 2.1 One explanation for varying tumor aggressiveness with age. Rates of tumor proliferation may play a role in the apparent slower growth of tumors. For example, if two tumors, one rapidly growing and one slowly, growing, both arise at the same stage of life, the form tumor would present clinically at a younger age. This model might explain why tumors arising in younger patients tend to be more aggressive, and why there is such significant heterogeneity in tumor characteristics (e.g., aggressiveness) in older individuals.

antigen). In this situation immunodeficiency does not render a host more susceptible to aggressive tumor growth and spread. In fact, immunodeficiency renders a host more resistant because those cells are less likely to provide the nonspecific stimulatory factors. This hypothesis is akin to the immune enhancement theory promoted several decades ago by Prehn and Lappe [162]. Briefly stated in the context of cancer and aging, the positive growth, angiogenic, and other tumorstimulatory signals produced nonspecifically by cells considered part of the immune system will be produced less by cells from old animals. In other words, the "soil" is less fertile for aggressive tumor growth.

2.5 CONCLUSIONS

It has been claimed that all medical oncologists, with the exception of those who restrict their practice to pediatric patients, are *geriatric oncologists*. This claim, of course, arose because the average age of cancer is in excess of 65 years and the median age of most common adult tumors approaches 70 years. Yet, without an appreciation, if not understanding, of the physiological changes associated with aging, a physician might overlook important modifiable changes that could influence the malignant characteristics of a tumor or its treatment. From a more basic scientific perspective, the explosion of information regarding mechanisms responsible for cancer development and growth has resulted in expanded understanding of the molecular and cellular processes of aging. These include the controls of cellular proliferation, mechanisms of DNA repair, and programmed cell death. Yet there remain striking voids in our understanding of the aging process. What has become clear is that aging and cancer involve many of the same pathways and, like the clinical oncologist who recognizes that he/she is also a geriatrician, basic scientists in cancer research are becoming increasingly familiar with the molecular and cellular biology of aging. This is a good thing!

REFERENCES

1. Doll R, Peto R. The causes of cancer: Quantitative estimates of avoidable risks of cancer in the United States today. *J Natl Cancer Inst* 1981;**66**(6):1191–1308.

2. Edwards BK, Howe HL, Ries LA, et al. Annual report to the nation on the status of cancer, 1973–1999, featuring implications of age and aging on U.S. cancer burden. *Cancer* 2002;**94**(10):2766–2792.

3. Balducci L, Ershler WB. Cancer and ageing: A nexus at several levels. *Nat Rev Cancer* 2005;**5**(8):655–662.

4. Denduluri N, Ershler WB. Aging biology and cancer. *Semin Oncol* 2004;**31**(2):137–148.

5. Extermann M, Meyer J, McGinnis M, et al. A comprehensive geriatric intervention detects multiple problems in older breast cancer patients. *Crit Rev Oncol Hematol* 2004;**49**(1):69–75.

6. Finkel T, Serrano M, Blasco MA. The common biology of cancer and ageing. *Nature* 2007;**448**(7155):767–774.

7. Irminger-Finger I. Science of cancer and aging. *J Clin Oncol* 2007;**25**(14):1844–1851.

8. Yancik R, Ries LA. Cancer in older persons: An international issue in an aging world. *Semin Oncol* 2004;**31**(2):128–136.

9. Calabresi P, Rosso R, Yancik R, Balducci L. Priorities in geriatric oncology—conference summary. *Cancer Control* 1995;**2**(2 Suppl 1):47.

10. Yancik R, Ries LA. Aging and cancer in America. Demographic and epidemiologic perspectives. *Hematol Oncol Clin North Am* 2000;**14**(1):17–23.

11. Yancik R, Ganz PA, Varricchio CG, Conley B. Perspectives on comorbidity and cancer in older patients: Approaches to expand the knowledge base. *J Clin Oncol* 2001;**19**(4):1147–1151.

12. Duthie EH. Physiology of aging: Relevance to symptoms, perceptions and treatment tolerance. In Balducci L, Lyman GH, Ershler WB, eds. *Comprehensive Geriatric Oncology*, Amsterdam, Harwood Academic, 1998, pp. 247–262.

13. Lindeman RD. Overview: Renal physiology and pathophysiology of aging. *Am J Kidney Dis* 1990;**16**(4):275–282.

14. Harrison DE. Proliferative capacity of erythropoietic stem cell lines and aging: An overview. *Mech Ageing Devel* 1979;**9**(5–6):409–426.

15. Harrison DE, Astle CM. Loss of stem cell repopulating ability upon transplantation. Effects of donor age, cell number, and transplantation procedure. *J Exp Med* 1982;**156**(6):1767–1779.

16. Harrison DE. Long-term erythropoietic repopulating ability of old, young, and fetal stem cells. *J Exp Med* 1983;**157**(5):1496–1504.

17. de Haan G, Van Zant G. Dynamic changes in mouse hematopoietic stem cell numbers during aging. *Blood* 1999;**93**(10):3294–3301.

18. Harrison DE, Astle CM, Stone M. Numbers and functions of transplantable primitive immunohematopoietic stem cells. Effects of age. *J Immunol* 1989;**142**(11):3833–3840.

19. Liang Y, Van Zant G, Szilvassy SJ. Effects of aging on the homing and engraftment of murine hematopoietic stem and progenitor cells. *Blood* 2005;**106**(4):1479–1487.

20. Sudo K, Ema H, Morita Y, Nakauchi H. Age-associated characteristics of murine hematopoietic stem cells. *J Exp Med* 2000;**192**(9):1273–1280.

21. Leng SX, Hung W, Cappola AR, Yu Q, Xue Q-L, Fried LP. White blood cell counts, insulinlike growth factor-1 levels, and frailty in community-dwelling older women. *J Gerontol A Biol Sci Med Sci* 2009;**64A**(4):499–502.

22. Artz AS, Fergusson D, Drinka PJ, et al. Mechanisms of unexplained anemia in the nursing home. *J Am Geriatr Soc* 2004;**52**(3):423–427.

23. Makipour S, Kanapuru B, Ershler WB. Unexplained anemia in the elderly. *Semin Hematol* 2008;**45**(4):250–254.

24. Izaks GJ, Westendorp RG, Knook DL. The definition of anemia in older persons. *JAMA.* 1999;**281**(18):1714–1717.

25. Balducci L. Aging, frailty, and chemotherapy. *Cancer Control* 2007;**14**(1):7–12.

26. Balducci L, Corcoran MB. Antineoplastic chemotherapy of the older cancer patient. *Hematol Oncol Clin North Am* 2000;**14**(1):193–212, x–xi.

27. Balducci L, Extermann M. Cancer chemotherapy in the older patient: What the medical oncologist needs to know. *Cancer* 1997;**80**(7):1317–1322.

28. Grubeck-Loebenstein B, Wick G. The aging of the immune system. *Adv Immunol* 2002;**80**:243–284.

29. Dubrow EL. Reactivation of tuberculosis: A problem of aging. *J Am Geriatr Soc* 1976;**24**(11):481–487.

30. Nagami PH, Yoshikawa TT. Tuberculosis in the geriatric patient. *J Am Geriatr Soc* 1983;**31**(6):356–363.

31. Schmader K. Herpes zoster in the elderly: Issues related to geriatrics. *Clin Infect Dis* 1999;**28**(4):736–739.

32. Hilleman MR. Realities and enigmas of human viral influenza: Pathogenesis, epidemiology and control. *Vaccine* 2002;**20**(25–26):3068–3087.

33. Powers DC, Sears SD, Murphy BR, Thumar B, Clements ML. Systemic and local antibody responses in elderly subjects given live or inactivated influenza A virus vaccines. *J Clin Microbiol* 1989;**27**(12):2666–2671.

34. Kaesberg PR, Ershler WB. The importance of immunesenescence in the incidence and malignant properties of cancer in hosts of advanced age. *J Gerontol* 1989;**44**(6):63–66.

35. Christensen K, Vaupel JW. Determinants of longevity: Genetic, environmental and medical factors. *J Intern Med* 1996;**240**(6):333–341.

36. Arias E. United States life tables, 2004. *Natl Vital Stat Rep* 2007;**56**(9):1–39.

37. Mackenbach JP, Kunst AE, Lautenbach H, Oei YB, Bijlsma F. Gains in life expectancy after elimination of major causes of death: Revised estimates taking into account the effect of competing causes. *J Epidemiol Community Health* 1999;**53**(1):32–37.

38. Hirsch HR. Can an improved environment cause maximum lifespan to decrease? Comments on lifespan criteria and longitudinal Gompertzian analysis. *Exp Gerontol* 1994;**29**(2):119–137.

39. Riggs JE. Longitudinal Gompertzian analysis of stroke mortality in the U.S., 1951–1986: Declining stroke mortality is the natural consequence of competitive deterministic mortality dynamics. *Mech Ageing Devel* 1990;**55**(3):235–243.

40. Orr WC, Sohal RS. Extension of life-span by overexpression of superoxide dismutase and catalase in Drosophila melanogaster. *Science* 1994;**263**(5150):1128–1130.

41. Roth GS, Ingram DK, Joseph JA. Nutritional interventions in aging and age-associated diseases. *Ann NY Acad Sci* 2007;**1114**:369–371.

42. Cristofalo VJ. Overview of biological mechanism of aging. *Annu Rev Gerontol Geriatr* 1990;**10**:1–22.

43. Cristofalo VJ, Gerhard GS, Pignolo RJ. Molecular biology of aging. *Surg Clin North Am* 1994;**74**(1):1–21.

44. Hayflick L. The limited *in vitro* lifetime of human diploid cell strains. *Exp Cell Res* 1965;**37**:614–636.

45. Cristofalo VJ. Cell culture aging: Insights for cell aging *in vivo*? *Aging* (Milano). 1999;**11**(1):1–3.

46. Schneider EL, Mitsui Y. The relationship between *in vitro* cellular aging and *in vivo* human age. *Proc Natl Acad Sci USA* 1976;**73**(10):3584–3588.

47. Rohme D. Evidence for a relationship between longevity of mammalian species and life spans of normal fibroblasts *in vitro* and erythrocytes *in vivo*. *Proc Natl Acad Sci USA* 1981;**78**(8):5009–5013.

48. Dimri GP, Lee X, Basile G, et al. A biomarker that identifies senescent human cells in culture and in aging skin *in vivo*. *Proc Natl Acad Sci USA* 1995;**92**(20):9363–9367.

49. Martin GM. The genetics of aging. *Hosp Pract* (Official ed.) 1997;**32**(2):47–50, 55–56, 59–61 passim.

50. Yu CE, Oshima J, Fu YH, et al. Positional cloning of the Werner's syndrome gene. *Science* 1996;**272**(5259):258–262.

51. Yu CE, Oshima J, Wijsman EM, et al. Mutations in the consensus helicase domains of the Werner syndrome gene. Werner's Syndrome Collaborative Group. *Am J Hum Genet* 1997;**60**(2):330–341.

52. Eriksson M, Brown WT, Gordon LB, et al. Recurrent de novo point mutations in lamin A cause Hutchinson-Gilford progeria syndrome. *Nature* 2003;**423**(6937):293–298.

53. Kaeberlein M, Andalis AA, Liszt GB, Fink GR, Guarente L. Saccharomyces cerevisiae SSD1-V confers longevity by a Sir2p-independent mechanism. *Genetics* 2004;**166**(4): 1661–1672.

54. Szilard L. On the nature of the aging process. *Proc Natl Acad Sci USA* 1959;**45**(1):30–45.

55. Morley AA. Is ageing the result of dominant and co-dominant mutations? *J Theor Biol* 1982;**98**(3):469–474.

56. Cummings DJ. Mitochondrial DNA in Podospora anserina. A molecular approach to cellular senescence. *Monogr Devel Biol* 1984;**17**:254–66.

57. Fairweather DS, Fox M, Margison GP. The *in vitro* lifespan of MRC-5 cells is shortened by 5-azacytidine-induced demethylation. *Exp Cell Res* 1987;**168**(1):153–159.

58. Burnet M. *Intrinsic Mutagenesis: A Genetic Approach for Aging*, Wiley, New York, 1974.

59. Hart RW, Setlow RB. Correlation between deoxyribonucleic acid excision-repair and life-span in a number of mammalian species. *Proc Natl Acad Sci USA* 1974;**71**(6):2169–2173.

60. Orgel LE. The maintenance of the accuracy of protein synthesis and its relevance to ageing. *Proc Natl Acad Sci USA* 1963;**49**:517–521.

61. Allsopp RC, Chang E, Kashefi-Aazam M, et al. Telomere shortening is associated with cell division *in vitro* and *in vivo*. *Exp Cell Res* 1995;**220**(1):194–200.

62. Allsopp RC, Morin GB, DePinho R, Harley CB, Weissman IL. Telomerase is required to slow telomere shortening and extend replicative lifespan of HSCs during serial transplantation. *Blood* 2003;**102**(2):517–520.

63. Allsopp RC, Vaziri H, Patterson C, et al. Telomere length predicts replicative capacity of human fibroblasts. *Proc Natl Acad Sci USA* 1992;**89**(21):10114–10118.

64. Bjorksten J. Cross linkage and the aging process. In Rothstein M, ed. *Theoretical Aspects of Aging*, Academic Press, New York, 1974, p. 43.

65. Harman D. Aging: A theory based on free radical and radiation chemistry. *J Gerontol* 1956;**11**(3):298–300.

66. Harman D. The aging process. *Proc Natl Acad Sci USA* 1981;**78**(11):7124–7128.

67. Sohal RS, Svensson I, Sohal BH, Brunk UT. Superoxide anion radical production in different animal species. *Mech Ageing Devel* 1989;**49**(2):129–135.

68. Sohal RS, Sohal BH, Brunk UT. Relationship between antioxidant defenses and longevity in different mammalian species. *Mech Ageing Devel* 1990;**53**(3):217–227.

69. Sohal RS, Weindruch R. Oxidative stress, caloric restriction, and aging. *Science* 1996; **273**(5271):59–63.

70. Lee CM, Chung SS, Kaczkowski JM, Weindruch R, Aiken JM. Multiple mitochondrial DNA deletions associated with age in skeletal muscle of rhesus monkeys. *J Gerontol* 1993;**48**(6):B201–B205.

71. Melov S, Shoffner JM, Kaufman A, Wallace DC. Marked increase in the number and variety of mitochondrial DNA rearrangements in aging human skeletal muscle. *Nucleic Acids Res*. 1995;**23**(20):4122–6.

72. Schwarze SR, Lee CM, Chung SS, Roecker EB, Weindruch R, Aiken JM. High levels of mitochondrial DNA deletions in skeletal muscle of old rhesus monkeys. *Mech Ageing Devel* 1995;**83**(2):91–101.

73. Li Y, Huang TT, Carlson EJ, et al. Dilated cardiomyopathy and neonatal lethality in mutant mice lacking manganese superoxide dismutase. *Nat Genet* 1995;**11**(4):376–381.

74. Sohal RS. Hydrogen peroxide production by mitochondria may be a biomarker of aging. *Mech Ageing Devel* 1991;**60**(2):189–98.

75. Epstein CJ, Avraham KB, Lovett M, et al. Transgenic mice with increased Cu/Zn-superoxide dismutase activity: animal model of dosage effects in Down syndrome. *Proc Natl Acad Sci USA* 1987;**84**(22):8044–8048.

76. Harris TB, Kiel D, Roubenoff R, et al. Association of insulin-like growth factor-I with body composition, weight history, and past health behaviors in the very old: The Framingham Heart Study. *J Am Geriatr Soc* 1997;**45**(2):133–139.

77. Birkenhager-Gillesse EG, Derksen J, Lagaay AM. Dehydroepiandrosterone sulphate (DHEAS) in the oldest old, aged 85 and over. *Ann NY Acad Sci* 1994;**719**:543–552.

78. Rudman D, Drinka PJ, Wilson CR, et al. Relations of endogenous anabolic hormones and physical activity to bone mineral density and lean body mass in elderly men. *Clin Endocrinol* (Oxford) 1994;**40**(5):653–661.

79. Hobbs CJ, Plymate SR, Rosen CJ, Adler RA. Testosterone administration increases insulin-like growth factor-I levels in normal men. *J Clin Endocrinol Metab* 1993;**77**(3):776–779.

80. Hanahan D, Weinberg RA. The hallmarks of cancer. *Cell* 2000;**100**(1):57–70.

81. Campisi J. Senescent cells, tumor suppression, and organismal aging: Good citizens, bad neighbors. *Cell* 2005;**120**(4):513–522.

82. Murakami S, Johnson TE. A genetic pathway conferring life extension and resistance to UV stress in Caenorhabditis elegans. *Genetics* 1996;**143**(3):1207–1218.

83. Sun J, Kale SP, Childress AM, Pinswasdi C, Jazwinski SM. Divergent roles of RAS1 and RAS2 in yeast longevity. *J Biol Chem* 1994;**269**(28):18638–18645.

84. Kinzler KW, Vogelstein B. Cancer-susceptibility genes. Gatekeepers and caretakers. *Nature* 1997;**386**(6627):761–763.

85. Hasty P, Campisi J, Hoeijmakers J, van Steeg H, Vijg J. Aging and genome maintenance: lessons from the mouse? *Science* 2003;**299**(5611):1355–1359.

86. Campisi J. Cellular senescence as a tumor-suppressor mechanism. *Trends Cell Biol* 2001;**11**(11):S27–S31.

87. Green DR, Evan GI. A matter of life and death. *Cancer Cell* 2002;**1**(1):19–30.

88. Campisi J. Cellular senescence and apoptosis: How cellular responses might influence aging phenotypes. *Exp Gerontol* 2003;**38**(1–2):5–11.

89. Campisi J. Cancer and ageing: Rival demons? *Nat Rev Cancer* 2003;**3**(5):339–349.

90. Kirkwood TB, Austad SN. Why do we age? *Nature* 2000;**408**(6809):233–238.

91. Shay JW, Wright WE. Hayflick, his limit, and cellular ageing. *Nat Rev Mol Cell Biol* 2000;**1**(1):72–76.

92. Artandi SE, Chang S, Lee SL, et al. Telomere dysfunction promotes non-reciprocal translocations and epithelial cancers in mice. *Nature* 2000;**406**(6796):641–645.

93. Samper E, Nicholls DG, Melov S. Mitochondrial oxidative stress causes chromosomal instability of mouse embryonic fibroblasts. *Aging Cell* 2003;**2**(5):277–285.

94. Bandyopadhyay D, Medrano EE. The emerging role of epigenetics in cellular and organismal aging. *Exp Gerontol* 2003;**38**(11–12):1299–1307.

95. Narita M, Lowe SW. Executing cell senescence. *Cell Cycle* 2004;**3**(3):244–246.

96. Neumeister P, Albanese C, Balent B, Greally J, Pestell RG. Senescence and epigenetic dysregulation in cancer. *Int J Biochem Cell Biol* 2002;**34**(11):1475–1490.

97. Bringold F, Serrano M. Tumor suppressors and oncogenes in cellular senescence. *Exp Gerontol* 2000;**35**(3):317–329.

98. Lundberg AS, Hahn WC, Gupta P, Weinberg RA. Genes involved in senescence and immortalization. *Curr Opin Cell Biol* 2000;**12**(6):705–709.

99. Itahana K, Dimri G, Campisi J. Regulation of cellular senescence by p53. *Eur J Biochem* 2001;**268**(10):2784–2791.

100. Serrano M, Lin AW, McCurrach ME, Beach D, Lowe SW. Oncogenic ras provokes premature cell senescence associated with accumulation of p53 and p16INK4a. *Cell* 1997;**88**(5):593–602.

101. Ferbeyre G, de Stanchina E, Querido E, Baptiste N, Prives C, Lowe SW. PML is induced by oncogenic ras and promotes premature senescence. *Genes Devel* 2000;**14**(16):2015–2027.

102. Pearson M, Carbone R, Sebastiani C, et al. PML regulates p53 acetylation and premature senescence induced by oncogenic Ras. *Nature* 2000;**406**(6792):207–210.

103. Ben-Porath I, Weinberg RA. When cells get stressed: An integrative view of cellular senescence. *J Clin Invest* 2004;**113**(1):8–13.

104. Collins CJ, Sedivy JM. Involvement of the INK4a/Arf gene locus in senescence. *Aging Cell* 2003;**2**(3):145–50.

105. Wright WE, Shay JW. Historical claims and current interpretations of replicative aging. *Nat Biotechnol* 2002;**20**(7):682–688.

106. Chang BD, Watanabe K, Broude EV, et al. Effects of p21Waf1/Cip1/Sdi1 on cellular gene expression: Implications for carcinogenesis, senescence, and age-related diseases. *Proc Natl Acad Sci USA* 2000;**97**(8):4291–4296.

107. Shelton DN, Chang E, Whittier PS, Choi D, Funk WD. Microarray analysis of replicative senescence. *Curr Biol*. 1999;**9**(17):939–945.

108. Zhang H, Pan KH, Cohen SN. Senescence-specific gene expression fingerprints reveal cell-type-dependent physical clustering of up-regulated chromosomal loci. *Proc Natl Acad Sci USA* 2003;**100**(6):3251–3256.

109. Krtolica A, Campisi J. Cancer and aging: A model for the cancer promoting effects of the aging stroma. *Int J Biochem Cell Biol* 2002;**34**(11):1401–1414.

110. Grinnell F. Fibroblast biology in three-dimensional collagen matrices. *Trends Cell Biol* 2003;**13**(5):264–269.

111. Longo VD, Finch CE. Evolutionary medicine: From dwarf model systems to healthy centenarians? *Science* 2003;**299**(5611):1342–1346.

112. Olumi AF, Grossfeld GD, Hayward SW, Carroll PR, Tlsty TD, Cunha GR. Carcinoma-associated fibroblasts direct tumor progression of initiated human prostatic epithelium. *Cancer Res* 1999;**59**(19):5002–5011.

113. Park CC, Bissell MJ, Barcellos-Hoff MH. The influence of the microenvironment on the malignant phenotype. *Mol Med Today* 2000;**6**(8):324–329.

114. Parrinello S, Coppe JP, Krtolica A, Campisi J. Stromal-epithelial interactions in aging and cancer: Senescent fibroblasts alter epithelial cell differentiation. *J Cell Sci*. 2005;**118**(Pt 3):485–96.

115. Dolle ME, Snyder WK, Dunson DB, Vijg J. Mutational fingerprints of aging. *Nucleic Acids Res* 2002;**30**(2):545–549.

116. Jonason AS, Kunala S, Price GJ, et al. Frequent clones of p53-mutated keratinocytes in normal human skin. *Proc Natl Acad Sci USA* 1996;**93**(24):14025–14029.

117. Dilley TK, Bowden GT, Chen QM. Novel mechanisms of sublethal oxidant toxicity: Induction of premature senescence in human fibroblasts confers tumor promoter activity. *Exp Cell Res* 2003;**290**(1):38–48.

118. Krtolica A, Parrinello S, Lockett S, Desprez PY, Campisi J. Senescent fibroblasts promote epithelial cell growth and tumorigenesis: A link between cancer and aging. *Proc Natl Acad Sci USA* 2001;**98**(21):12072–7.

119. Roninson IB. Oncogenic functions of tumour suppressor p21(Waf1/Cip1/Sdi1): Association with cell senescence and tumour-promoting activities of stromal fibroblasts. *Cancer Lett* 2002;**179**(1):1–14.

120. Miura T, Mattson MP, Rao MS. Cellular lifespan and senescence signaling in embryonic stem cells. *Aging Cell* 2004;**3**(6):333–343.

121. Odorico JS, Kaufman DS, Thomson JA. Multilineage differentiation from human embryonic stem cell lines. *Stem Cells* 2001;**19**(3):193–204.

122. Chen J. Senescence and functional failure in hematopoietic stem cells. *Exp Hematol* 2004;**32**(11):1025–1032.

123. Geiger H, Van Zant G. The aging of lympho-hematopoietic stem cells. *Nat Immunol* 2002;**3**(4):329–333.

124. Park IK, Morrison SJ, Clarke MF. Bmi1, stem cells, and senescence regulation. *J Clin Invest* 2004;**113**(2):175–179.

125. Villa A, Navarro-Galve B, Bueno C, Franco S, Blasco MA, Martinez-Serrano A. Long-term molecular and cellular stability of human neural stem cell lines. *Exp Cell Res* 2004;**294**(2):559–570.

126. Boulanger CA, Smith GH. Reducing mammary cancer risk through premature stem cell senescence. *Oncogene* 2001;**20**(18):2264–2272.

127. Serakinci N, Guldberg P, Burns JS, et al. Adult human mesenchymal stem cell as a target for neoplastic transformation. *Oncogene* 2004;**23**(29):5095–5098.

128. Campisi J. Aging, tumor suppression and cancer: High wire-act! *Mech Ageing Devel* 2005;**126**(1):51–58.

129. Vogelstein B, Fearon ER, Hamilton SR, et al. Genetic alterations during colorectal-tumor development. *N Engl J Med* 1988;**319**(9):525–532.

130. James CD, Carlbom E, Dumanski JP, et al. Clonal genomic alterations in glioma malignancy stages. *Cancer Res* 1988;**48**(19):5546–5551.

131. Aoyagi Y, Yokose T, Minami Y, et al. Accumulation of losses of heterozygosity and multistep carcinogenesis in pulmonary adenocarcinoma. *Cancer Res* 2001;**61**(21):7950–7954.

132. Boyle P, Leake R. Progress in understanding breast cancer: Epidemiological and biological interactions. *Breast Cancer Res Treat* 1988;**11**(2):91–112.

133. Carney DN, Byrne A. Etoposide in the treatment of elderly/poor-prognosis patients with small-cell lung cancer. *Cancer Chemother Pharmacol* 1994;**34**(Suppl):S96–S100.

134. Correa P. Molecular and biochemical methods in cancer epidemiology and prevention: The path between the laboratory and the population. AACR special conference in cancer research. *Cancer Epidemiol Biomark Prevent* 1993;**2**(1):85–88.

135. el-Azouzi M, Chung RY, Farmer GE, et al. Loss of distinct regions on the short arm of chromosome 17 associated with tumorigenesis of human astrocytomas. *Proc Natl Acad Sci USA* 1989;**86**(18):7186–7190.

136. Harris JR, Lippman ME, Veronesi U, Willett W. Breast cancer (1). *N Engl J Med* 1992;**327**(5):319–328.

137. Linehan WM, Gnarra JR, Lerman MI, Latif F, Zbar B. Genetic basis of renal cell cancer. *Import. Adv Oncol* 1993:47–70.

138. Anisimov VN. Age as a factor of risk in multistage carcinogenesis. In Balducci L, Lyman, GH, Ershler WB, Extermann M, eds. *Geriatric Oncolgy*, Lippincott, Philadelphia, 1992, pp. 53–60.

139. Franco EL. Prognostic value of human papillomavirus in the survival of cervical cancer patients: An overview of the evidence. *Cancer Epidemiol Biomark Prev* 1992;**1**(6): 499–504.

140. Stevens RG, Jones DY, Micozzi MS, Taylor PR. Body iron stores and the risk of cancer. *N Engl J Med* 1988;**319**(16):1047–1052.

141. Anisimov VN, Zhukovskaya NV, Loktionov AS, Vasilyeva IA, Kaminskaya EV, Vakhtin YB. Influence of host age on lung colony forming capacity of injected rat rhabdomyosarcoma cells. *Cancer Lett* 1988;**40**(1):77–82.

142. Anisimov VN, Loktionov AS, Khavinson VK, Morozov VG. Effect of low-molecular-weight factors of thymus and pineal gland on life span and spontaneous tumour development in female mice of different age. *Mech Ageing Devel* 1989;**49**(3):245–257.

143. Ward JM, Lynch P, Riggs C. Rapid development of hepatocellular neoplasms in aging male C3H/HeNCr mice given phenobarbital. *Cancer Lett* 1988;**39**(1):9–18.

144. Yong LC, Brown CC, Schatzkin A, et al. Intake of vitamins E, C, and A and risk of lung cancer. The NHANES I epidemiologic followup study. First National Health and Nutrition Examination Survey. *Am J Epidemiol* 1997;**146**(3):231–243.

145. Kaldor JM, Day NE. Interpretation of epidemiological studies in the context of the multistage model of carcinogenesis. In Barrett JC, ed. *Carcinogenesis* MoE, vol. 2, CRC Press, Boca Raton, FL, 1987, pp. 21–57.

146. Glass AG, Hoover RN. The emerging epidemic of melanoma and squamous cell skin cancer. *JAMA* 1989;**262**(15):2097–2100.

147. Tantranond P, Balducci L, Karam F, et al. Alternative management of cutaneous squamous cell carcinoma in an elderly man: report of a case and review of the literature. *J Am Geriatr Soc* 1992;**40**(5):510–512.

148. Himes CL. Elderly Americans. *Popul Bull*. 2002;**56**(4):3–42.

149. Matoha MF, Cosgrove JW, Atak JR, et al. Selective elevation of the c-myc transcript levels in the liver of the aging Fischer 344 rat. *Biochem Biophys Res Commun* 1987;**147**:1–7.

150. Bohr VA, Evans MK, Fornace AJ Jr. DNA repair and its pathogenetic implications. *Lab Invest* 1989;**61**(2):143–161.

151. Randerath K, Reddy MV, Disher RM. Age- and tissue-related DNA modifications in untreated rats: Detection by 32P-postlabeling assay and possible significance for spontaneous tumor induction and aging. *Carcinogenesis* 1986;**7**(9):1615–1617.

152. Ershler WB, Berman E, Moore AL. Slower B16 melanoma growth but greater pulmonary colonization in calorie-restricted mice. *J Natl Cancer Inst* 1986;**76**(1):81–85.

153. Ershler WB, Gamelli RL, Moore AL, Hacker MP, Blow AJ. Experimental tumors and aging: local factors that may account for the observed age advantage in the B16 murine melanoma model. *Exp Gerontol* 1984;**19**(6):367–376.

154. Ershler WB, Stewart JA, Hacker MP, Moore AL, Tindle BH. B16 murine melanoma and aging: slower growth and longer survival in old mice. *J Natl Cancer Inst* 1984;**72**(1): 161–164.

155. Tsuda T, Kim YT, Siskind GW, et al. Role of the thymus and T-cells in slow growth of B16 melanoma in old mice. *Cancer Res* 1987;**47**(12):3097–3100.

156. Ershler WB. The change in aggressiveness of neoplasms with age. *Geriatrics* 1987;**42**(1): 99–103.

157. Ershler WB, Moore AL, Shore H, Gamelli RL. Transfer of age-associated restrained tumor growth in mice by old-to-young bone marrow transplantation. *Cancer Res* 1984;**44**(12Pt 1): 5677–5680.

158. Hadar EJ, Ershler WB, Kreisle RA, Ho SP, Volk MJ, Klopp RG. Lymphocyte-induced angiogenesis factor is produced by L3T4+ murine T lymphocytes, and its production declines with age. *Cancer Immunol Immunother* 1988;**26**(1):31–34.

159. Kreisle RA, Stebler BA, Ershler WB. Effect of host age on tumor-associated angiogenesis in mice. *J Natl Cancer Inst* 1990;**82**(1):44–47.

160. Simon SR, Ershler WB. Hormonal influences on growth of B16 murine melanoma. *J Natl Cancer Inst* 1985;**74**(5):1085–1088.

161. Fidler IJ, Gersten DM, Riggs CW. Relationship of host immune status to tumor cell arrest, distribution, and survival in experimental metastasis. *Cancer* 1977;**40**(1):46–55.

162. Prehn RT, Lappe MA. An immunostimulation theory of tumor development. *Transplant Rev* 1971;**7**:26–54.

CHAPTER 3

Physiological, Psychological, and Social Aspects of Aging

GEORGE A. KUCHEL, JULIE ROBISON, and RICHARD FORTINSKY

University of Connecticut Health Center, Farmington, CT

3.1 INTRODUCTION AND BACKGROUND

Cancer is increasingly viewed as a disease of old age since 60% of all newly diagnosed cancers and 70% of all cancer deaths occur in individuals who are 65 years and older [1]. Moreover, it has been estimated that the total US cancer incidence will increase by 45% from 2010 to 2030, with the majority of these new cancers affecting older adults [2]. The clinical, social, and health policy challenges posed by such dramatic growth in new cancer cases will be further compounded by increased interindividual variability, complexity, and vulnerability among older adults with cancer [2], which may express itself in terms of altered function involving physiological [3,4], psychological [5], and social [5] domains.

Elderly patients, including those with cancer, may present health providers with many unique challenges. Aging is inevitable and, at the level of many relevant measures, is associated with the loss of functional reserve across many organs and functional domains [6]. Nevertheless, the rate or extent of these declines, as well as the vulnerability for becoming frail, for losing one's autonomy, or for dying from a condition other than cancer varies greatly between individuals [6,7]. In the absence of a laboratory test, comprehensive geriatric assessment (Chapter 29) offers the best means of evaluating how well an individual has aged and how likely that individual is to remain healthy and independent when confronted by any number of challenges, including those associated with cancer [2]. Standardized measures of mobility performance are emerging as the most robust and reliable predictors of such vulnerability or frailty [7]. Other relevant elements of a comprehensive geriatric assessment include evaluation of cognition, affect, continence, nutrition, social isolation, multiple morbidity, polypharmacy and elder abuse. Such assessments are often neglected, not well understood or dispersed among different disciplines. As a result, multidisciplinary models of coordinated care (Chapter 31) are especially important when confronting cancer-related issues in older adults who may be frail or more vulnerable along physiological, psychological and social domains.

Cancer and Aging Handbook: Research and Practice, First Edition. Edited by Keith M. Bellizzi and Margot A. Gosney.
© 2012 Wiley-Blackwell. Published 2012 by John Wiley & Sons, Inc.

3.2 PHYSIOLOGICAL ASPECTS OF AGING

3.2.1 General Considerations

A gradual decline in physiological function represents one of the hallmarks of aging which leads to losses of homeostatic capacity, a condition which has been termed homeostenosis [6,8,9]. While these principles are becoming widely accepted, a few common misconceptions need to be dispelled:

1. Not all physiological parameters decline with aging. For example, resting heart rate and cardiac output remain unchanged with normal aging, while renal glomerular filtration rate (GFR) declines.

2. When present, such aging-related deficits tend to begin in midlife, long before the individual is typically viewed as being elderly.

3. For many systems, diminished capacity to respond to physiological challenges may become evident even without any apparent deficit under basal conditions. For example, aging is associated with a decreased capacity for the heart rate to increase in response to exercise or for normal body temperature or serum sodium concentration to be maintained during a heatwave, whereas none of these parameters are influenced by aging under basal conditions.

4. While such physiological declines have been believed to reflect normative aging, since they can be observed even in the absence of any overt disease, they tend to become even more pronounced in older individuals who are frail or disabled and/or demonstrate evidence of multiple coexisting diseases and comorbidities [3,4,6].

Viewed in this context, the body's ability to maintain homeostatic balance in the face of common extrinsic challenges is of seminal importance to frailty, which in turn reflects older adults' capacity to remain independent and avoid major disabilities. Indeed, even dating back to the nineteenth century, the term *homeostasis* has always referred to the body's attempt to maintain an internal constancy that is required for optimal function [10]. Thus, far from reflecting physiologic *stasis*, effective homeostasis actually requires that all relevant compensatory mechanisms remain suitably vibrant, responsive, and well calibrated as a means of maintaining normal function in the face of varied extrinsic challenges [6].

Several different approaches permit the clinician to identify an individual as being more frail or vulnerable. Since previous behavior may predict future responses, an individual who has already become hyperthermic and dehydrated during a previous heatwave or developed delirium following previous surgery is much more likely to develop similar problems in the future. Also, presence of underlying disability may also render individuals more vulnerable or frail. Similarly, presence of multiple coexisting deficits ranging from declines in functional performance or ADLs to the presence of specific diseases and geriatric conditions also enhances frailty. In fact, lists numbering all of the different clinical [11] or physiological [12] deficits affecting an individual, regardless of their specific nature, also increase the risk of future deficits or disabilities. Finally, evidence also exists for the presence of specific frailty phenotypes, which is especially evident in individuals who have unintentional weight loss, decreased handgrip strength, and decreased mobility and who describe a sense of exhaustion [13].

3.2.2 Blood Pressure Regulation and Cardiovascular Physiology

Basal heart rate remains unchanged, yet there is a decrease in its maximal capacity to increase in response to exercise or stress, which has been attributed to decreased responsiveness to catecholamines and a decline in the intrinsic sinus rate [14]. Similarly, at rest there is no difference in cardiac index or ejection fraction, but ability of exercise or other challenges to mediate appropriate increases in these parameters is blunted [14,15]. Aging is associated with increased ventricular stiffness, which contributes to a reduction in early diastolic filling and diastolic failure [14,16]. As a result of these changes, even older individuals with normal systolic function may develop congestive heart failure when challenged with cardiotoxic drugs such as doxorubicin [3].

The ability to maintain an adequate blood pressure in response to standing or loss of blood volume is also critical to remaining independent. Significant or symptomatic orthostatic hypotension is rare among relatively healthy community dwelling older adults [6,17]. In contrast, orthostatic hypotension becomes much more common in older individuals who are frail, suffer from relevant morbidity, take many medications, and are hospitalized or institutionalized [6,17]. Aging-related declines in vascular compliance also contribute to a higher prevalence of systolic hypertension in the elderly, which, in turn, increases the risk of hypotension by decreasing baroreceptor sensitivity and ventricular compliance beyond declines observed in normal aging [16]. Thus, elderly patients undergoing cancer therapy are at enhanced risk of developing cardiac toxicity such as congestive heart failure, arrhythmia, and hypotension [3].

3.2.3 Pulmonary System

With aging, pulmonary compliance declines, leading to decreased expiratory flow rates [18]. Respiratory drive also declines with aging, while aspiration, obstructive airway disease, decrease in mucosal clearance, and changes in immune host defense mechanisms all increase the risk pneumonia in the elderly [18,19]. These changes may render some older adults ineligible for potentially curative lung cancer surgery and may also enhance the risk of radiation-induced pulmonary toxicity [3].

3.2.4 Endocrine Physiology

Aging is associated with diminished insulin sensitivity, decreased glucose tolerance, and an increased risk of type 2 diabetes mellitus [20]. Hypothyroidism and hyperthyroidism are both common, yet serum levels of thyroid hormones and TSH are largely unaffected by aging [21]. The adrenal glands maintain their ability to secrete cortisol in response to ACTH, but the magnitude and timecourse of its diurnal secretion undergoes some change [22]. Aging is associated with gradual decreases in blood levels of growth hormone [23], as well sex hormones including testosterone, androstenedione, dehydroepiandrosterone (DHEA), and estrogen [23]. These changes contribute to an overall impaired resilience to multiple challenges, including those associated with cancer diagnosis and care diagnosis and care [4]. Age-related increases in parathyroid hormone (PTH) levels, combined with declines in gonadal hormone concentrations, contribute to the risk of osteoporosis and sarcopenia. Moreover, these physiological changes enhance the vulnerability of older individuals to the long-term risks of hormonal ablation therapies in the context of breast [24] and prostate [25] cancer.

3.2.5   Renal Physiology and Fluid Balance

Aging is associated with well-demonstrated but highly variable declines in renal function involving renal plasma flow, glomerular filtration rate (GFR), and tubular excretion [26]. Serum creatinine levels, as well as various creatinine-based equations, fail to adequately detect age-related losses in GFR since endogenous creatinine production declines in the elderly with losses in muscle mass [26]. The ability of tubules to handle water, glucose, and electrolytes is also impaired in old age. Ability of aldosterone and antidiuretic hormone (ADH) to appropriately respond to changes in fluid and salt balance is also impaired. As a result of these and other changes, older adults are less able to excrete excess fluid when fluid-overloaded [27] or to retain sodium and drink when fluid-deprived [28]. Moreover, difficulties with water disposal can predispose older individuals to develop hyponatremia, while decreased capacity to adapt to increased salt load may contribute to dependent edema, nocturia, hypertension, and congestive heart failure. As a result, older adults are at increased risk of volume depletion, prerenal azotemia, and drug-induced nephropathy [3]. Careful adjustments need to be made to doses and/or dose intervals of medications, including chemotherapy agents that are excreted through the kidneys [3]. Monitoring for nephrotoxicity is also essential, with special attention given to individuals who are on large numbers of medications, are dehydrated, or manifest evidence of underlying renal disease.

3.2.6   Gastrointestinal System

Aging results in significant declines in salivary flow rates and diminished mucosal protective mechanisms [29]. These changes enhance the risk of dry mouth, oral caries, and mucositis, especially when older adults are exposed to anticholinergic medications and chemotherapeutic agents that damage mucosal membranes [29]. Basal bloodflow to the stomach declines with aging, as does its capacity to increase in response to injury [30]. Gastric acid secretion tends to be lower in older adults, affecting their ability to liberate vitamin B_{12} from foods [31]. Decreased prostaglandin synthesis with aging also enhances the risk of gastritis when agents such as nonsteroidal antiinflammatory drugs (NSAIDs) are used [32]. Decreased gastric emptying and intestinal motility predispose older adults to reflux and constipation [30,33]. Liver bloodflow undergoes significant decline with aging, resulting in decreased hepatic drug metabolism of many drugs, particularly those metabolized by the cytochrome coenzyme system [34].

3.2.7   Blood and Immune System

Hemoglobin levels and red cell counts tend to be lower in older adults, but cannot be routinely attributed to normal aging since this may contribute to symptoms and underlying treatable causes [35]. However, erythropoiesis stimulating agents need to be used sparingly in a context other than end-stage renal failure since erythropoietin levels increase with aging and careful monitoring is required to avoid adverse effects [36]. Bone marrow cellularity and reserve also declines with aging. Aging does not impact circulating blood white cell levels, yet their ability to mobilize, to travel to the site of infection, and to destroy infectious organisms is impaired in old age [37]. Thymus involutes with aging, and T-cell precursors become defective and less responsive. Ability of precursor cells to transition to the B-cell lineage, their migration, and the nature of the humoral response are all affected by aging [38]. All of these changes increase the risk of bone marrow suppression and infection, especially in older patients receiving potent chemotherapy [4]. Finally, age-related dysregulation of cytokine production with increased levels of interleukin 6 and tumor necrosis factor alpha (TNFα) may not only contribute to the development of cancer-related symptoms such as anorexia and weight loss, but may also contribute to the development of frailty and cancer [39].

3.3 PSYCHOLOGICAL ASPECTS OF AGING

3.3.1 Mental Health and Aging

Aging does not increase the risk of developing a mental illness such as depression or anxiety. Some disorders, such as bipolar disorder or schizophrenia, typically begin in early adulthood and persist into later life. Other disorders such as major depression or phobias can begin at any point in the lifespan. The American Association of Geriatric Psychiatry [40] estimates that ~20% of the population over age 55 experience some type of mental disorder, although the prevalence of the most severe forms of these disorders, such as schizophrenia or bipolar disorder, is much smaller. However, evidence clearly shows that mental illness is not part of normal aging. Older adults with untreated mental illness have worse health status and physical functioning, reduced social connections, and more stressed caregivers. For these reasons, mental illnesses in older adults present an important public health issue [41].

Underdiagnosis and undertreatment are systemic problems for older adults [42], particularly for those with low income or from ethnic minority groups. A number of reasons appear to contribute to the under-detection and treatment of mental health problems in older adults, including stigma and related reluctance to seek help, an assumption that symptoms are part of normal aging, and presentation of purely physical symptoms [43]. Most older adults respond well to treatment when the illness or disorder is detected early.

Approximately 25% of older adults with mental health or substance abuse disorders receive mental health treatment [44]. Older adults tend to receive mental health treatment in the primary care setting rather than with mental health specialists. Although older adults report less experience using mental health services than do younger people, one study found that they are more open to referrals for mental health care from multiple sources and have more positive attitudes about mental health services than do younger adults [45,46].

In addition to biological and genetic elements that can cause mental illness, a number of other etiological factors may also relate to the onset of a mental illness. Such factors include alcohol, prescription and over-the-counter medications and herbal remedies, and nutritional deficiencies. Physical illnesses or injuries and lack of exercise can also increase the risk of experiencing a mental illness. Older adults experience losses of loved ones or of meaningful activities, as well as illnesses, more frequently than their younger peers; such stressful events increase the risk of developing certain types of mental health disorders.

Depressive disorders and symptoms of depression, followed by anxiety disorders and symptoms, occur most frequently in older adults. Substance use or abuse is another common concern. Other less common mental illnesses include bipolar disorder, schizophrenia, and personality disorders. Delirium and dementia are also commonly grouped among mental health problems in older adults.

Depression   National rates of major depressive disorder (MDD) for community dwelling adults age 18 and older are estimated at 5.3% for an episode of MDD in the prior 12 months and 12.2% for an episode at any point in the lifetime [47]. The same study reports even lower estimates for a subgroup of respondents age 65 and older: 1.6% for the previous 12 months and an 8.2% lifetime rate. These rates illustrate a likely cohort effect on mental illness prevalence rates, in that the current older cohort reports lower lifetime rates of these disorders than do their younger counterparts. The National Comorbidity Study [48] also indicates that older adults born in later cohorts demonstrate higher rates of MDD and earlier ages of onset compared to older cohorts. Middle-aged adults (50–64) report more depressive symptoms and higher lifetime rates of depression compared to adults age 65 and over [41].

For a clinical diagnosis of MDD, symptoms of depression must include depressed mood and/or lack of interest in activities in addition to four or more other symptoms not caused by a medical condition and lasting for at least 2 weeks. Additional symptoms may include feelings of worthlessness or excessive guilt, difficulty concentrating or making decisions, agitation, slowed reactions, fatigue, thoughts of death or suicide, or changes in sleep patterns or appetite [49]. Dysthymia (thyroid gland dysfunction) a mood disorder with less severe by longer lasting symptoms than MDD may occur in ≤15% of older adults and can also disrupt functioning in older adults, and therefore should also be evaluated and treated [50,51].

Depression frequently occurs simultaneously with other physical illnesses such as heart disease, cancer, and diabetes. Further, depression can slow or impede recovery from an acute illness or surgery [52]. Rates of depression for older adults in primary care, hospital, and nursing home settings significantly exceed community-based population rates, with rates of 5–10% for major depression and up to <35% for significant depressive symptoms [50].

Although community rates of major depressive disorder in older adults are relatively low overall, rates among low income minority populations are higher. One study of urban Latino and African American residents of senior housing found that 26% of respondents met criteria for major depression [53]. Younger age, more chronic conditions, and social distress related to major depressive disorder for both ethnic groups. In the general community population of older adults, psychosocial risk factors for depression include negative life events, death of a loved one, medical illness, disability and functional decline, and social isolation [54]. Older white males face a significantly higher risk of dying by suicide than other age, gender, or ethnic groups, and the risk is elevated further for white men living alone or with medical illnesses [55].

Strong evidence demonstrates that combining medication treatment with various forms of psychotherapy aids recovery and attenuates relapse, with recovery rates of ≤80% [50,56]. However, medication treatment alone is more common. Older adults with chronic comorbidities or who lack social support take longer to recover [57]. On the other hand, older adults with strong religious beliefs report lower rates of depression [58,59].

Bipolar Disorder   Bipolar disorder is characterized by cycling depression and manic phases. Fewer than 1% of the adult population have a diagnosis of bipolar disorder, which typically starts in early adulthood. Older adults with this disorder usually have had it for many years, and may continue to need treatment. Bipolar disorder can cycle through as many as four or more phases per year, or it may occur only once or twice in a lifetime. Manic symptoms include racing thoughts, excessive self-confidence, high energy and decreased need for sleep, reckless behavior or excessive spending, and delusions. Clinicians use mood stabilizers and antipsychotics to treat bipolar disorder [43].

Anxiety   National estimates for adults in the community for generalized anxiety disorder (GAD) report a 12-month prevalence of 1.6% and a lifetime prevalence of 5.1% [60], National GAD prevalence estimates for adults age 65 and older are 1.0% for a 12-month period and lifetime prevalence of 2.6% [61]. Taking all anxiety disorders together, data from the epidemiological catchment area (ECA) study suggest a rate of 5.5% among older adults [62].

Anxiety disorders include panic disorders, phobias, obsessive–compulsive disorder, and posttraumatic stress disorder. Anxiety disorders tend to begin earlier in life, with the exception of phobias, which can begin at any point [63,64]. Rates of generalized anxiety disorder among older low-income ethnic minorities are significantly higher compared with the general older population as well. Of the participants in the senior housing study described above, 12% met criteria for GAD [65].

Typical symptoms of anxiety disorders include unexplained fear, dread, or panic; edginess; agitation; difficulty sleeping; stomach, head, or chest pain; pounding heart or sweating; and preoccupation with relationships or conversations. As with depression, anxiety often accompanies medical illnesses, and symptoms of some illnesses, such as myocardial infarctions, produce symptoms similar to those in anxiety disorders [66]. Further, some medications can initiate anxiety as a side effect [67]. Anxiety often occurs simultaneously with depression as well; close to 50% of older adults with MDD also have anxiety disorders [68]. Even more than depression, anxiety is often overlooked in older adults. Successful treatments commonly include medications and/or various types of psychotherapy [50].

Substance Abuse   The term *substance abuse* refers to excessive use of alcohol, or illegal, prescription, or over-the-counter drugs; specific definitions vary somewhat by study. Lifetime rates of alcohol abuse, defined with DSM-IV criteria, are lower for older adults (6.2%) than for adults in general (13.2%) and much lower for drug abuse (0.3% vs. 7.9%) [69]. However, rates of alcohol abuse among older primary care patients range from 11% to 15% [70]. Symptoms of substance abuse include craving, impaired control, physical dependence, and tolerance. Substance abuse presents particular problems for older adults, due to interactions with changes in body composition and underlying medical conditions. Substance abuse increases the risk of both physical and mental health problems, including cognitive impairment, depression, and anxiety [42,51]. Older adults have similar or better success rates with treatment for substance abuse than do younger patients [71].

Schizophrenia   Late-life onset of schizophrenia is relatively rare. Most older adults with schizophrenia have a chronic condition that started earlier in life, typically before their mid-30s. Schizophrenia affects less than 1% of the adult population. The uncommon diagnosis of late-onset schizophrenia can be precipitated by a highly stressful life event or loss [66].

Symptoms of schizophrenia are typically categorized as positive, such as disorganized thoughts, hallucinations, and delusions, versus negative, such as flat affect or social withdrawal. Negative symptoms are more common in older people with schizophrenia [72]. Some overlap occurs between symptoms of schizophrenia and those of dementia; a differential diagnosis is critical, as successful treatments exist for schizophrenia and can enable independent function.

Personality Disorders   The term *personality disorders* refers to a group of diagnoses wherein persistent behavior patterns interfere with functioning in daily activities such as employment and relationships. This class of disorders includes obsessive–compulsive disorder, borderline personality disorder, antisocial personality disorder, and several others. Individuals with these diagnoses have chronic, inflexible beliefs or tendencies that often lead to distorted ways of viewing themselves or others [66]. Some personality disorders persist or increase in later life, while some dissipate. When new symptoms appear in later life, it is critical to distinguish them from potential symptoms of an organic disease such as dementia. Personality disorders can be triggered or worsened by life stressors. Personality disorders commonly occur together with other mental illnesses such as depression and anxiety.

3.3.2 Cognition in Later Life

Brain Structure and Function   Absent of disease-related pathology, the overall size of the brain decreases with age, accompanied by a loss of neurons. These changes develop gradually over the lifespan; in fact, the time of greatest neuronal loss occurs between 2 months of age to 18 years. Even late in life, the cerebral cortex remains somewhat adaptable, allowing for ongoing cognitive and emotional development [73]. In general, older adults experience slowing of cerebral processing and deficits in recall compared to younger adults. However, accumulated knowledge and experience may serve to counterbalance these declines [73].

Memory   Age-related declines in memory function exist in multiple types of memory, including recollection, declarative memory, episodic memory, and working memory. Other memory forms are less affected by age such as familiarity, semantic knowledge, and nondeclarative memory [74]. *Declarative*, or *explicit, memory* refers to memories of events or facts that can be consciously recalled; *nondeclarative*, or *procedural*, *memory* refers to acquired skills or other unconscious memory.

Underlying causes of age-related memory deficits include overall slowing in ability to process information, leading to difficulty in retrieving memories quickly, as well as concomitant changes in sensory perception, which can impair information processing. Various types of intervention show some success in improving memory, including cardiovascular and cognitive exercise and various memory training strategies [74]. Depression can interfere with both learning and recall, leading to notable memory deficits. Alcohol, caffeine, and sedating medications are also associated with memory problems.

Dementia   Abnormal memory impairment exists when it disrupts normal daily functioning, most commonly attributable to dementia. Dementia affects 6–8% of men and women over 65 and 50% of people 85 or older. Few types of dementia are reversible, although certain types of treatment of slow disease progression and manage some of the symptoms. The most prevalent dementia symptoms include gradual decrease in memory, attention, and judgment; disorientation; communication and word finding difficulty; inappropriate social behavior; and personality changes. Alzheimer's disease, followed by vascular dementia, are the most prevalent forms; dementia often accompanies other conditions such as Parkinson's disease, Huntington's disease, alcoholism, and AIDS. Delirium, a temporary decline in cognition and disorientation with a rapid onset secondary to various medical conditions or medications, should be distinguished from dementia.

3.4 SOCIAL ASPECTS OF AGING

This section of the chapter highlights normative age-associated social relationships encountered by older adults, and also calls attention to important variations within these normative social relationships, particularly variations according to gender, age group within later life, and racial and ethnic group membership. These normative patterns and variations are presented to help determine how they might affect the types of support and resources often needed by individuals to manage medical illnesses such as cancer. The most common social relationships experienced by individuals entering and living in later adulthood are within the family, the workplace, and in older individuals' involvement in voluntary groups and organizations. Therefore, we summarize normative patterns and variations in older adults' family structure and interactions, in work and retirement, and in volunteerism. We end with a brief overview of sources of more socially oriented community support available to all older adults in the United States through the Older Americans Act, which might prove useful to cancer-afflicted individuals and their families.

3.4.1 Family-Related Characteristics and Trends

Most older adults in the United States are either married or widowed, demonstrating the primary importance of the family as a social unit for their roles, relationships, and responsibilities. In 2008, 57% of US adults aged 65 and older were married and 30% were widowed; only 4% were never married. Owing to differential mortality rates between older women and men, 42% of older women were widowed compared to only 14% of older men, while 75% of older men and only 44% of older women were married. Gender differences in marital status become more pronounced with advanced age; in the 85+ age group, 55% of men are married compared to only 15% of women [75]. These variations suggest that older men are much more likely to maintain spousal relationships in addition to any other family roles, while older women are much more likely to engage in social interaction as single individuals with family members such as adult children and grandchildren. In the event of a chronic health condition such as cancer, these gender variations strongly suggest that older men in the United States are much more likely to turn first to their spouses for emotional and physical support, while older women are much more likely to turn to adult children or other relatives for such support.

Living arrangements reflect gender differences in marital status; in 2008, 40% of older women lived alone, compared to only 19% of older men. An additional 17%

of all older women without spouses lived with other relatives; however, this figure was much higher among African-American (32%), Asian (32%), and Hispanic (31%) older women [75]. These figures suggest that, among older women, those from racial and ethnic groups of color are more likely than non-Hispanic whites to turn to family members within their own households for emotional and physical support when living with medical illness such as cancer.

Other notable trends in family structure that will affect older adults and their family relationships are the growth of four-generation families, which adds to potential sources of family support when needed in later life, and the increasing divorce rate among middle-aged adults, which is likely to increase the proportion of people entering later adulthood as divorcé(e)s from the current figure of 9% for the 65+ population [75–77]. Increases in divorce and single-parent families in middle adulthood are known to have deleterious effects on the social and economic well-being of adults and children. Fathers in particular are affected negatively in terms of social ties and emotional bonds with children following divorce; they often remain estranged from their children into later life, which reduces their available family support in the face of illness in older age [77].

Family care givers are discussed in greater detail elsewhere in this volume (Chapter 28); however, due to gender differences in availability of spouses in older age, it is worth noting here that spouses are more likely than other family members to act as primary caregivers [78] and help with a broader range of disabilities [79] than are other family members. Given gender differences in living arrangements, it is also noteworthy that caregivers living with the family member they care for are more likely to report depressive symptoms and social isolation than caregivers living in a different household [65].

3.4.2 Work and Retirement Trends

For most people in younger and middle adulthood, the workplace is the most common nonfamily setting where social interactions are carried out. Social ties to co-workers frequently mature into friendships where health problems are shared and mutual support is provided in times of need. Therefore, trends in laborforce participation beyond middle adulthood could influence the degree to which older adults retain meaningful social relationships in the workplace. From this perspective, retirement could signal diminishing social relationships with previous coworkers, even if the major purpose of retirement is to spend time in leisure activities that could lead to development of new social ties. In fact, it has been shown that retirement decisions between spouses tend to be made jointly so that leisure activities can be synchronized to sustain and further nourish familial social relationships even as work-related social ties are diminished [80].

National data from the Current Population Survey (CPS) indicate that, in 2001, the percentage of men participating in the laborforce at age 60 was 71%, but by age 65 the corresponding figure was only 39%. For women in 2001, 53% were in the laborforce at age 60, while only 26% remained in the laborforce at age 65. The normative pattern clearly reveals that most men and women exit the workforce, and enter some type of retirement, at the "conventional" age of 65.

However, an important countervailing trend is that since 1985 the percentages of men and women remaining in the workforce at age 65 have shown clear and consistent increases after reaching historic lows that year. For men at age 65, the percentage in the laborforce increased from 32% in 1985 to 39% in 2001; for women, corresponding figures were 16% in 1985 and 26% in 2001 [81, Tables 2.2 and 2.4]. Analyses of more recent CPS figures reveal that, between 1993 and 2009, workforce participation rates for men aged 62–74 increased from 27% to 38%, and increased for women in the same age group from 17% to 28% [82]. Reasons for these changes are not well understood, but several public- and private-sector incentives to continue working were implemented during this time period [81] and, since the "great recession" beginning in 2007, older Americans may have decided to retain employment because of shrinking assets and an unexpectedly reduced standard of living [83]. Regardless of the reasons, these trends indicate that growing numbers of older adults are choosing to remain gainfully employed and that the workplace may retain or regain its function of providing a critical source of social interaction and social support well into the eighth decade of life.

Retirement itself has more recently been called an "ever-evolving institution," and the trend toward early retirement is now considered a product of history [84]. There is also no longer a linear trend whereby work life ends and retirement begins and then continues until death [81]. Many older adults retire, decide that full-time retirement is not as fulfilling as was expected, find part-time employment, and then retire again; this cycle might occur multiple times after completion of the initial working career. Most cross-sectional research finds that retirement "is rarely a crisis and typically a satisfactory experience" [84, p. 77]; this would be the normative view of retirement, based on the weight of most self-reported evidence in standardized surveys. However, when more in-depth observations are made, retirees express simultaneous positive and negative aspects of the retirement experience. For example, separation from work is viewed as an escape from anxieties related to constant deadlines and performance expectations, but also as lost opportunity for personal achievement and social connection. Unlimited time away from work allows individual control over a new organization of everyday life, but also runs the risk of increased social isolation (see Weiss [85], cited in Ekerdt [84]). The paradox of retirement could serve to help or hinder individuals' capacities to seek and find social support if and when a medical illness such as cancer becomes a part of their lives.

3.4.3 Volunteerism Trends

Although participation in volunteer activities is a lifelong endeavor for many people, volunteerism in later life, particularly after retirement, is an important source of social relationships and support for older adults. The latest figures from the CPS indicate that, in 2009, 24% of Americans age 65 and older volunteered (performed work without compensation) through or for an organization. This volunteerism rate for older Americans in 2009 was lower than for the 35–64 age group (30%), and about the same as in the 16–34 age group, and has remained unchanged since 2005 [86]. A vast range of organizations support volunteers, ranging from religious to disease-specific to environmental organizations.

A growing literature in gerontology provides substantial evidence that volunteerism is associated with a large number of positive health-related outcomes, such as improved physical function, improved self-reported health status, and reduced depressive symptomatology for older adults in both cross-sectional [87] and longitudinal [88,89] studies. Findings are inconclusive regarding whether certain subgroups of older adults benefit more than others, but gender and race appear to have no moderating effects on outcomes associated with volunteering (see Morrow-Howell et al. [87] for a review). A prevailing view contends that measurable health-related outcomes are due to socioemotional benefits derived from contributing to others in a meaningful way, which promote social integration and augment emotional support [90].

Volunteerism serves as a vehicle through which older adults could provide unpaid help to age peers with cancer, either directly through personal assistance with tasks such as transportation or grocery shopping, or indirectly by volunteering in fundraising activities at a cancer-specific community organization. Given the current higher volunteerism rates among Americans in the baby boom birth cohort (age 46–64 in 2010), it is possible that, as this cohort ages into later life, the volunteerism rates for the 65+ older age group will increase from 2009 levels and remain higher as this cohort completes its lifecycle. If so, then older individuals with medical illness such as cancer might benefit from increased voluntary support from age peers well into the future.

3.4.4 Sources of Community Support for All Older Adults

Medicare and Medicaid are well-known sources of government-financed health insurance for nearly all older adults, and for older adults with low or no income and few assets, respectively. Much less is known about government-financed sources of social, nutritional, and recreational support available to all community-dwelling older adults. The Older Americans Act (OAA) was legislated in the same year, 1965, as Medicare and Medicaid, during a period of "compassionate ageism" in the United States [91]. Under the OAA, all Americans age 60 or older, regardless of socioeconomic standing or health-related needs, have access to a wide array of services organized under the rubric of the "aging network." Congressionally appropriated funds under the OAA are disbursed by the US (federal) *administration on aging* through *state units on aging* and, within states, through *area agencies on aging*.

Core services available at all 629 area agencies on aging include information and referral assistance, home-delivered meals, congregate meals offered at senior centers, and other community locations such as churches, legal assistance, and transportation. A 2008 national survey of area agencies on aging found that more than 75% also provide case management, personal care, and homemaker services either directly or through local contracts. Additionally, more than half offer evidence-based programs to help older adults prevent or manage chronic diseases and disabilities [92]. For individuals and families living with the daily challenges of cancer, area agencies on aging can offer formal support and advice about other community resources that might address their specific health-related needs.

3.5 SUMMARY

Increasingly, cancer needs to be viewed as a disease of old age. Older patients with cancer present healthcare professionals with many complexities driven by considerations that can arise from clinical, physiological, psychological, and social perspectives. For example, in many older patients cancer does not present in isolation from other disease processes, due to the frequent presence of multiple coexisting conditions and morbidities in this age group. Furthermore, declines in physiological function also contribute to deficits in homeostatic capacity involving essentially all organ systems, potentially rendering older adults more vulnerable to a broad range of different challenges. Given the high prevalence of depression, anxiety disorders, substance abuse, and cognitive deficits in late life, clinicians must also consider psychological factors. Finally, older adults affected by cancer must not be evaluated in isolation from their families and surrounding environments. Not only does the impact of cancer extend beyond the affected individual to the entire family, but marital status, living arrangements, income, and work status all play crucial roles in determining the capacity of older adults to cope with cancer and related problems.

REFERENCES

1. Yancik R, Ries LA. Cancer in older persons: An international issue in an aging world. *Semin Oncol* 2004;**31**(2):128–136.

2. Balducci L, Colloca G, Cesari M, Gambassi G. Assessment and treatment of elderly patients with cancer. *Surg Oncol* 2010;**19**(3):117–123.

3. Sawhney R, Sehl M, Naeim A. Physiologic aspects of aging: Impact on cancer management and decision making, part I. *Cancer J* 2005;**11**(6):449–460.

4. Sehl M, Sawhney R, Naeim A. Physiologic aspects of aging: Impact on cancer management and decision making, part II. *Cancer J* 2005;**11**(6): 461–473.

5. Given B, Given CW. Cancer treatment in older adults: Implications for psychosocial research. *J Am Geriatr Soc* 2009;**57**(Suppl 2):S283–S285.

6. Kuchel GA. Aging and homeostatic regulation. In Halter JB, Hazzard WR, Ouslander JG, Tinetti ME, Wolard N, Studenski S, et al., eds. *Hazzard's Principles of Geriatric Medicine and Gerontology*, McGraw-Hill, New York, 2010, pp. 621–630.

7. Kuchel GA. Allostatic load, frailty and the future of predictive gerontology. *J Am Geriatr Soc*. 2009;**57**(9):1704–1706.

8. Lipsitz LA. Physiological complexity, aging, and the path to frailty. *Sci Aging Knowledge Environ* 2004;**16**:e16.

9. Masoro EJ, Austad SN. *Handbook of the Biology of Aging*, 6th ed., Academic Press, San Diego, 2007.

10. Cannon WB. The aging of homeostatic mechanisms. In Cannon WB, ed. *The Wisdom of the Body*, Norton, New York, 1932, pp. 202–215.

11. Song X, Mitnitski A, Rockwood K. Prevalence and 10-year outcomes of frailty in older adults in relation to deficit accumulation. *J Am Geriatr Soc* 2010;**58**(4):681–687.

12. Fried LP, Xue QL, Cappola AR, Ferrucci L, Chaves P, Varadhan R, et al. Nonlinear multisystem physiological dysregulation associated with frailty in older women: Implications for etiology and treatment. *J Gerontol A Biol Sci Med Sci* 2009;**64**(10):1049–1057.

13. Fried LP, Tangen CM, Walston J, Newman AB, Hirsch C, Gottdiener J, et al. Frailty in older adults: Evidence for a phenotype. *J Gerontol A Biol Sci Med Sci* 2001;**56**(3):M146–M156.

14. Lakatta EG. Cardiovascular system. In Masoro EJ, ed., *Aging*. Oxford Univ. Press, Oxford, UK, 1995, pp. 413–474.

15. Fleg JL, O'Connor F, Gerstenblith G, Becker LC, Clulow J, Schulman SP, et al. Impact of age on the cardiovascular response to dynamic upright exercise in healthy men and women. *J Appl Physiol* 1995;**78**:890–900.

16. O'Rourke MF, Hashimoto J. Mechanical factors in arterial aging: A clinical perspective. *J Am Coll Cardiol* 2007;**50**(1):1–13.

17. Lipsitz LA. Orthostatic hypotension in the elderly. *N Engl J Med* 1989;**321**(14):952–957.

18. Sharma G, Goodwin J. Effect of aging on respiratory system physiology and immunology. *Clin Interven Aging* 2006;**1**(3):253–260.

19. Gibson PG, McDonald VM, Marks GB. Asthma in older adults. *Lancet* 2010;**376**(9743): 803–813.

20. Meneilly GS. Diabetes in the elderly. *Med Clin North Am* 2006;**90**(5):909–923.

21. Peeters RP. Thyroid hormones and aging. *Hormones*, 2008;**7**(1):28–35.

22. Seeman TE, Robbins RJ. Aging and hypothalamic-pituitary-adrenal response to challenge in humans. *Endocr Rev* 1994;**15**(2):233–260.

23. Veldhuis JD. Aging and hormones of the hypothalamo-pituitary axis: Gonadotropic axis in men and somatotropic axes in men and women. *Ageing Res Rev* 2008;**7**(3):189–208.

24. Ghazi M, Roux C. Hormonal deprivation therapy-induced osteoporosis in postmenopausal women with breast cancer. *Best Pract Res Clin Rheumatol* 2009;**23**(6):805–811.

25. Lattouf JB, Saad F. Bone complications of androgen deprivation therapy: Screening, prevention, and treatment. *Curr Opin Urol* 2010;**20**(3):247–252.

26. Weinstein JR, Anderson S. The aging kidney: Physioical changes. *Adv Chron Kidney Dis* 2010;**17**(4):302–307.

27. Luft FC, Fineberg NS, Weinberger MH. The influence of age on renal function and renin and aldosterone responses to sodium-volume expansion and contraction in normotensive and mildly hypertensive humans. *Am J Hypertens* 1992;**5**(8):520–528.

28. Luckey AE, Parsa CJ. Fluid and electrolytes in the aged. *Arch Surg* 2003;**138**(10): 1055–1060.

29. Gonsalves WC, Wrightson AS, Henry RG. Common oral conditions in older persons. *Am Family Phys* 2008;**78**(7):845–852.

30. Morley JE. The aging gut: Physiology. *Clin Geriatr Med* 2007;**23**(4):757–767.

31. Baik HW, Russell RM. Vitamin B12 deficiency in the elderly. *Annu Rev Nutr* 1999; **19**:357–377.

32. Sostres C, Gargallo C, Lanas A. Drug-related damage of the ageing gastrointestinal tract. *Best Pract Res Clin Gastroenterol* 2009;**23**(6):849–860.

33. Bouras EP, Tangalos EG. Chronic constipation in the elderly. *Gastroenterol Clin North Am* 2009;**38**(3):463–480.

34. Cusack BJ. Pharmacokinetics in older persons. *Am J Geriatr Pharmacother* 2004;**2**(4): 274–302.

35. Balducci L. Cancer-related anemia: Special considerations in the elderly. *Oncology* 2007;**21**(1):81–86, 90.

36. Dharmarajan TS, Widjaja D. Erythropoiesis-stimulating agents in anemia: Use and misuse. *J Am Med Dir Assoc* 2009;**10**(9):607–616.

37. Wagner W, Horn P, Bork S, Ho AD. Aging of hematopoietic stem cells is regulated by the stem cell niche. *Exp Gerontol*, 2008;**43**(11):974–980.

38. Cancro MP, Hao Y, Scholz JL, Riley RL, Frasca D, Dunn-Walters DK, et al. B cells and aging: molecules and mechanisms. *Trends Immunol* 2009;**30**(7):313–318.

39. Taylor JA III, Kuchel GA. Bladder cancer in the elderly: clinical outcomes, basic mechanisms, and future research direction. *Nat Clin Pract Urol* 2009;**6**(3):135–144.

40. American Association of Geriatric Psychiatry. *Geriatrics and Mental Health—the Facts*, 2008 (retrieved 10/14/10 from http://www.aagponline.org/prof/facts_mh.asp).

41. Centers for Disease Control and Prevention, & National Association of Chronic Disease Directors. *The State of Mental Health and Aging in America Issue Brief 1: What Do the Data Tell Us?* Natl. Assoc. Chronic Disease Directors, Atlanta, GA, 2008.

42. US Dept. Health and Human Services. Older adults and mental health. In *Mental Health: A Report of the Surgeon General*, 1999, Chap. 5 (retrieved 10/14/10 from http://www.surgeongeneral.gov/library/mentalhealth/chapter5/sect1.html).

43. NAMI NH. *Mental Health, Mental Illness, Healthy Aging: A New Hampshire Guidebook for Older Adults and Caregivers*, NAMI NH. Concord, NH, 2001.

44. Mandersheid R, Agay J, Hernandez-Cartagena M, Edmond P, Male A, Parker A, et al. Highlights of organized mental health services in 1998 and major national and state trends. In Mandersheid R, Henderson M, eds. *Mental Health, United States, 2000*, Rockville, MD, US. Dept. Health and Human Services, Center for Mental Health Services, 2001.

45. Robb C, Haley WE, Becker MA, Polivka LA, Chwa HJ. Attitudes towards mental health care in younger and older adults: Similarities and differences. *Aging Mental Health* 2003;**7**:142–152.

46. Rokke PD, Scorgin F. Depression treatment preferences in younger and older adults. *J Clin Geropsychol*, 1995;**1**:243–257.

47. Hasin DS, Goodwin RD, Stinson FS, Grant BF. Epidemiology of major depressive disorder: Results from the national epidemiologic survey on alcoholism and related conditions. *Arch Gen Psychiatry* 2005;**62**(10):1097–1106.

48. Kessler RC, McGonagle KA, Zhao S, Nelson CB, Hughes M, Eshleman S, et al. Lifetime and 12-month prevalence of DSM-III-R psychiatric disorders in the United States. Results from the national comorbidity survey. *Arch Gen Psychiatry* 1994;**51**(1):8–19.

49. American Psychiatric Association. *Diagnostic and Statistical Manual of Mental Disorders*, 4th ed., APA, Washington, DC, 1994.

50. Blazer DG. Depression in late life: Review and commentary. *J Gerontol A Biol Sci Med Sci* 2003;**58**(3):249–265.

51. Knight BG, Kaskie B, Shurgot GR, Dave J. Improving the mental health of older adults. In JE, Birren, Schaie KW, eds. *Handbook of the Psychology of Aging*, 6th ed., Elsevier Academic Press, Burlington, MA, 2006, pp. 407–424.

52. Chapman DP, Perry GS, 2008. Strine TW. The vital link between chronic disease and depressive disorders. *Prevent Chron Dis* 2005;**2**(1):A14.

53. Robison J, Schensul JJ, Coman E, Diefenbach GJ, Radda KE, Gaztambide S, et al. Mental health in senior housing: Racial/ethnic patterns and correlates of major depressive disorder. *Aging Mental Health* 2009;**13**(5):659–673.

54. Bruce M. Psychosocial risk factors for depressive disorders in late life. *Biol Psychiatry* 2002;**52**(3):175–184.

55. Conwell Y. Suicide in elderly patients. In Scheider LS, Reynolds CFI, Lebowitz BD, Friedhoff AJ, eds. *Diagnosis and Treatment of Depression in Late Life*, American Psychiatric Press, Washington, DC, 1994, pp. 397–418.

56. Reynolds CF, 3rd, Frank E, Perel JM, Imber SD, Cornes C, Miller MD, et al. Nortriptyline and interpersonal psychotherapy as maintenance therapies for recurrent major depression: A randomized controlled trial in patients older than 59 years. *JAMA* 1999;**281**(1):39–45.

57. Bosworth HB, McQuoid DR, George LK, Steffens DC. Time-to-remission from geriatric depression: Psychosocial and clinical factors. *Am J Geriatr Psychiatry* 2002;**10**(5):551–559.

58. Bosworth HB, Park KS, McQuoid DR, Hays JC, Steffens DC. The impact of religious practice and religious coping on geriatric depression. *Int J Geriatr Psychiatry* 2003;**18**(10), 905–914.

59. Roff LL, Klemmack DL, Parker M, Koenig HG, Crowther M, Baker PS, et al. Depression and religiosity in African American and white community-dwelling older adults. *J Hum Behav Soc Environ* 2004;**10**(1):175–189.

60. Wittchen HU, Zhao S, Kessler RC, Eaton WW. DSM-III-R generalized anxiety disorder in the national comorbidity survey. *Arch Gen Psychiatry* 1994;**51**(5):355–364.

61. Grant BF, Hasin DS, Stinson FS, Dawson DA, June Ruan W, Goldstein RB, et al. Prevalence, correlates, co-morbidity, and comparative disability of DSM-IV generalized anxiety disorder in the USA: Results from the national epidemiologic survey on alcohol and related conditions. *Psychol Med* 2005;**35**(12):1747–1759.

62. Regier DA, Boyd JH, Burke JD, Jr, Rae DS, Myers JK, Kramer M, et al. One-month prevalence of mental disorders in the United States. based on five epidemiologic catchment area sites. *Arc Gen Psychiatry*, 1988;**45**(11):977–986.

63. Anthony JC, Aboraya A. The epidemiology of selected mental disorders in later life. In Birren JE, Sloane RB, Cohen GD, eds. *Handbook of Mental Health and Aging*, 2nd ed., Academic Press, San Diego, 1992, pp. 27–73.

64. Blazer DG, George LK, Hughes D. The epidemiology of anxiety disorder. In Salzman C, Lebowitz D, eds. *Anxiety in the Elderly: Treatment and Research*, Springer, New York, 1991, pp. 17–30.

65. Robison J, Fortinsky RH, Kleppinger A, Shugrue N, Porter M. A broader view of family caregiving: Effects of caregiving and caregiver conditions on depressive symptoms, health, work and social isolation. *J Gerontol Soc Sci* 2009;**64**B:788–798.

66. Gatz M, Kasl-Godley J, Karel MJ. Aging and mental disorders. In Birren JE, Schaie KW, eds. *Handbook of the Psychology of Aging*, 4th ed., Academic Press, San Diego, 1996, pp. 365–382.

67. Cohen G. Anxiety and general medical disorders. In Salzman C, Lebowitz BD, eds. *Anxiety in the Elderly: Treatment and Research*, Springer, New York, 1991, pp. 47–62.

68. Diefenbach, G. J., Disch, W. B., Robison, J. T., Baez, E., & Coman, E. (2009). Anxious depression among Puerto Rican and African-American older adults. *Aging Mental Health*, 2009;**13**:118–126.

69. Kessler RC, Berglund P, Demler O, Jin R, Merikangas KR, Walters EE. Lifetime prevalence and age-of-onset distributions of DSM-IV disorders in the national comorbidity survey replication. *Arch Gen Psychiatry* 2005;**62**(6):593–602.

70. Oslin DW. Late-life alcoholism: Issues relevant to the geriatric psychiatrist. *Am J Geriatr Psychiatry* 2004;**12**(6):571–583.

71. Satre DD, Mertens J, Arean PA, Weisner C. Contrasting outcomes of older versus middle-aged and younger adult chemical dependency patients in a managed care program. *J Stud Alcohol* 2003;**64**(4):520–530.

72. Meeks S, Walker JA. Blunted affect, blunted lives? Negative symptoms, ADL functioning, and mental health among older adults. *Int J Geriatr Psychiatry* 1990;**5**:233–238.

73. Scheibel AD. Structural and functional changes to the aging brain. In Birren JE, Schaie KW, eds., *Handbook of the Psychology of Aging*, 4th ed., Academic Press, San Diego, 1996, pp. 105–128.

74. Hoyer WJ, Verhaeghen P. Memory aging. In Birren JE, Schaie KW, eds., *Handbook of the Psychology of Aging*, 6th ed., Elsevier Academic Press, Burlington, MA, 2006, pp. 209–232.

75. Federal Interagency Forum on Aging-Related Statistics. *Older Americans 2010: Key Indicators of Well-being*. Federal Interagency Forum on Aging-Related Statistics, US Government Printing Office, Washington, DC, 2010.

76. Bengtson VL. Beyond the nuclear family: The increasing importance of multi-generational family relationships in American society. *J Marriage Family* 2001;(**63**):1–16.

77. Putney NM, Bengtson VL, Wakeman MA. The family and the future: Challenges, prospects, and resilience. In Pruchno RA, Smyer MA, eds. *Challenges of an Aging Society*, Johns Hopkins Univ. Press, Baltimore, 2007, pp. 117–155.

78. Lima JC, Allen SM, Goldscheider F, Intrator O. Spousal caregiving in late and midlife versus older ages: Implications for work and family obligations. *J Gerontol Soc Sci* 2008;**63**:S229–S238.

79. Stoller EP, Miklowski CS. Spouses caring for spouses: Untangling the influences of relationship and gender. In Szinovacz ME, Davey A, eds. *Caregiving Contexts: Cultural, Familial, and Societal Implications*. Springer, New York, 2008, pp. 115–131.

80. Blau DM. Labor force dynamics of older married couples. *J Labor Econ*, 1998;**16**:595–629.

81. National Research Council and the Institute of Medicine. Wegman DH, McGee JP, eds. *Health and Safety Needs of Older Workers*, Division of Behavioral and Social Sciences and Education, The National Academies Press, Washington, DC, 2004.

82. Johnson RW, Kaminski J. *Older Adults' Labor Force Participation Since 1993: A Decade and a Half of Growth*. Fact Sheet on Retirement Policy, Jan. 2010, Retirement Policy Program, Urban Institute (accessed online 10/04/10).

83. Shugrue N, Robison J. Intensifying individual, family, and caregiving stress: Health and social effects of economic crisis. *Generations* 2009;**33**:34–39.

84. Ekerdt DJ. Frontiers of research on work and retirement. *J Gerontol. Soc Sci* 2010;**65B**: 69–80.

85. Weiss RS. *The Experience of Retirement*, Cornell Univ. Press, Ithaca, NY, 2005.

86. US Dept. Labor, Bureau of Labor Statistics. *Volunteering in the United States, 2009*, Economic News Release USDL-10-0097, Jan. 26, 2010.

87. Morrow-Howell N, Hong S, Tang F. Who benefits from volunteering? Variations in perceived benefits. *Gerontologist* 2009;**49**:91–102.

88. Moen P, Dempster-McClain D, Williams R. Successful aging: A life course perspective on women's multiple roles and health. *Am J Sociol* 1992;**97**:1612–1638.

89. Pillemer K, Fuller-Rowell TF, Reid MC, Wells NM. Environmental volunteering and health outcomes over a 20-year period. *Gerontologist* 2010;**50**:594–602.

90. Tang F, Choi E, Morrow-Howell N. Organizational support and volunteering benefits for older adults. *Gerontologist* 2010;**50**:603–612.

91. Binstock RH. From compassionate ageism to intergenerational conflict ? *Gerontologist* 2010;**50**:574–585.

92. Kunkel S, Lackmeyer AE, Straker JK, Markwood S. *Area Agencies on Aging: Advancing Access for Home and Community-Based Services*, Scripps Gerontology Center, Miami Univ., Oxford, OH, 2009.

PART II

STRATEGIES FOR CANCER PREVENTION IN OLDER ADULTS

CHAPTER 4

Overview of Cancer Prevention Strategies in Older Adults

BARBARA K. DUNN and PETER GREENWALD

Division of Cancer Prevention, National Cancer Institute, Bethesda, MD

DARRELL E. ANDERSON

The Scientific Consulting Group, Gaithersburg, MD

4.1 INTRODUCTION

Cancer prevention interventions are aimed at preventing the initiation of carcinogenesis or halting the carcinogenic process before a premalignant lesion progresses to invasive cancer, with an ultimate goal of decreasing mortality due to the cancer [1]. A discussion of approaches to cancer prevention in any population, including the elderly, requires (1) a clear definition of the intended population, including the level of risk, which may be age-related/defined; (2) clarification of to what extent and in what manner cancer, the disease to be avoided, characterizes that population; and (3) what net benefit that population is anticipated to receive from active prevention measures.

4.1.1 Intended Population

In the limited clinical trials and population studies literature addressing cancer treatment and prevention in older individuals, the age range used to define this group is variously over 60, 65, or 70 years of age. These apparently arbitrarily chosen age thresholds defining what constitutes the lower limit of "elderly" have, in many cases, been used as a matter of convenience [2]. For example, until the 1950s, 60 years of age was considered elderly. This age cutoff was based in part on the life expectancy of men and women at that time and on the age at which a person was considered ready for retirement. In the early 1970s the World Health Organization (WHO) established that in developed countries 65 years constituted "elderly." The basis for this decision was the retirement age in government systems in the surveyed countries. Age 65 was chosen for men whereas age 60 was applied to women, although the actual retirement age was 65 years for both sexes. Subsequently, the Surveillance Epidemiology and End Results (SEER) database, as well as other large disease registries, incorporated the WHO age

Cancer and Aging Handbook: Research and Practice, First Edition. Edited by Keith M. Bellizzi and Margot A. Gosney.
© 2012 Wiley-Blackwell. Published 2012 by John Wiley & Sons, Inc.

groupings into their reports. Accordingly, all age groups extend from the fifth year of one decade to the fifth year of the next decade, leaving age 65 as the lower boundary of the age group 65–75. Because observational studies repeatedly reference data in SEER, age 65 emerged as a natural cutoff for the group labeled "elderly" or "older."

The lower age limit used in clinical prevention trials is generally based on the approximate age at which risk for the cancer in question begins to rise substantially. Thus, the average risk for a given cancer for a person falling into the "older" age bracket is generally higher than the average risk for the overall population; for purposes of a clinical trial, this person can be considered at "increased risk" because of his/her age alone.

Despite the historical use of a lower age limit for participation in clinical trials testing preventive efficacy for cancers associated with aging, in clinical practice the notion of being older *biologically* is more relevant to decisions regarding interventions intended to decrease mortality than is pure chronologic age [3]. This is where comorbidities and functional status feed into decisions regarding any cancer intervention, including and especially those designed for prevention [4]. In prevention, as in treatment, the ultimate goal is to prolong survival while maintaining an acceptable quality of life. Comorbidity exacerbates the already shorter length of future survival anticipated in older compared to younger persons [5,6]. Furthermore, a basic tenet of the design of trials in cancer prevention is that the tested interventions impart minimal toxicity; although important in cancer treatment as well, the emphasis on low toxicity is considerably greater in prevention, where trial participants are essentially healthy, despite being at increased risk of cancer. The balance between the benefits and adverse effects of a chemoprevention agent, for example, must be favorable enough to ensure that healthy individuals will be compliant with therapy; this concern applies especially to high-risk elderly persons [6]. Preexisting comorbid conditions and related treatments may add to or even synergize with toxicities of chemoprevention, making the bearer of such conditions, often an older individual, a poor candidate for the intervention. Therefore, careful screening for existing medical conditions should preempt mere age as an exclusion criterion for entry into trials of chemopreventive agents; a healthy older adult may be a reasonable candidate for a chemoprevention trial or preventive therapy in the general clinical setting.

Cancer Prevalence in the Target Population   The most common cancers, including those of the breast, prostate, colon, lung, and urinary bladder, are associated disproportionately with aging (Fig. 4.1a), as are other, less common types of cancer (Fig. 4.1b) [7,8]. The incidence of most of these cancers peaks in the age range of 70–80 years. The age dependence of these common epithelial cancers relates to their etiologic basis, which involves a multistep carcinogenic process taking place over many years, during which time successive oncogenic mutations and epigenetic modifications, and progressive telomere dysfunction, among other changes, accumulate in the affected tissue [9–13]. The duration of time inherent in aging provides the opportunity for the accumulation of a threshold number of oncogenic changes in DNA required for invasive cancer. In addition, normal tissues from older individuals exhibit characteristic epigenetic modifications that are similar to those typically observed in cancerous tissue [14]. Clearly, older individuals are at increased risk of these common epithelial cancers by virtue of aging, making them appropriate candidates for preventive intervention. However, the limited life expectancy of older compared to younger

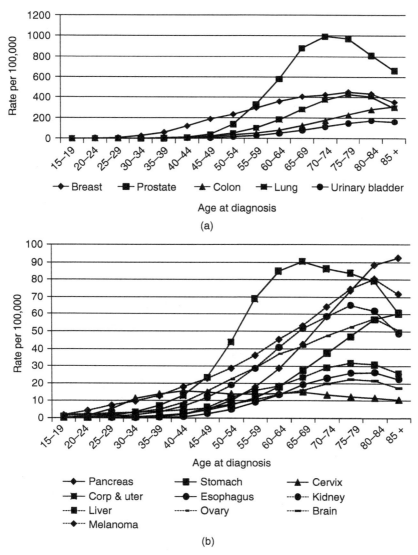

Figure 4.1   Age-specific SEER incidence rates by cancer site for (a) the most common cancers and (b) the second most common group of cancers, all ages, all races, and both sexes, 2000–2007.

individuals brings into question whether intervening with preventive agents at a later age actually will provide any benefit in terms of extending survival. This question is independent of whether comorbidities exist in a given individual.

4.1.2   Balance between Benefits and Risks of Preventive Intervention

Given the increased risk of developing the common cancers among elderly individuals, efforts at prevention in the older population would seem to be desirable. In fact, primary chemoprevention trials frequently use a minimum age requirement as an eligibility criterion in order to select for individuals at increased risk of cancer; a trial participant must be older than a given age (Table 4.1) [15–20]. For example, the National Surgical Adjuvant Breast and Bowel Project (NSABP) Prevention (P)-1: Breast Cancer Prevention Trial (BCPT) used age 60 as the lower limit of eligibility if no other risk factors were present. The P-1:BCPT investigators decided that being 60 years old, in and of itself, was associated with a sufficient increase in breast cancer risk to justify inclusion of a woman in this clinical trial, which tested the agent tamoxifen for chemopreventive efficacy. The issue here is whether candidate healthy older individuals will actually derive survival and quality-of-life benefit from preventive interventions. The few chemopreventive agents that have been validated in prospective randomized controlled clinical trials (RCTs) have been shown to impart to older participants short-term cancer incidence benefits that are comparable to those seen in younger people, where efficacy has been analyzed in relation to age (Table 4.1) [15–20]. Although pharmaceutical interventions may yield prevention benefit within the shorter anticipated future lifespan of older individuals, other lifestyle interventions might not yield their potential benefits as rapidly. Dietary modifications [21] and physical exercise [22,23] must be initiated and maintained on a long-term basis years before an individual reaches the age captured demographically as "older" or "elderly" if benefit is to be accrued. Furthermore, according to some studies, behavioral intervention must be instituted not only early but at specific stages of life [22,23], implying that a physiologic window of time exists during which susceptible tissues derive benefit in terms of cancer inhibition that will be observed much later in life. Finally, tumors in the elderly are more frequently indolent so that the limited lifespan may compete with the projected benefits of a preventive intervention. In essence, this situation is comparable to *overdiagnosis* in screening, because the intervention, even when technically effective, is superfluous since it exerts no net benefit on the clinical outcome.

In the sparse literature addressing cancer prevention in the elderly, one focus has been on *secondary prevention*, that is, prevention of second primary cancers in individuals afflicted with a localized first primary cancer treated with local and adjuvant therapy [24]. This attention to secondary prevention emerges in a context of first primaries discovered through screening, or early detection, a subject addressed in a later section of this book. It is important to remember, however, that premalignant lesions are also often detected during screening for early invasive cancer; a common example is ductal carcinoma *in situ* (DCIS) on routine mammography. In these cases, the relevant lesion may place the affected individual at increased risk of a first invasive cancer, making that person a candidate for interventions that fit into the *primary prevention*, as opposed to treatment, category. This intertwining of screening and prevention reminds us that utilization of one activity, screening, which is generally targeted to older individuals, cannot be separated from the other, primary prevention. This chapter addresses the value of approaches to primary prevention as directed to the older, or elderly, population.

Strategies for primary cancer prevention in older adults present challenges not seen, or seen to a lesser extent, in younger individuals: comorbidities, diet, mobility, lack of access to qualified geriatric specialists, and restricted living situations. In addition, adults 65 years and older are more likely to be cancer survivors and to require strategies to prevent (1) recurrence of the first primary cancer or development of second primary cancers following treatment of the first cancer and (2) development of other primary

TABLE 4.1 Phase III Prevention Trials Presenting Efficacy Results by Age

Clinical Trial [Ref(s).]	Description (Number of Participants)	Age Eligibility Requirements	Number and Age of Older Participants (% of Total Participants)	Efficacy (RR) Outcomes in Older versus Younger Participants	
P-1:BCPT [15,16]	TAM vs. placebo (13,388 women)	≥60 years or 35–59 years with additional risk factors to yield 5-year BC risk ≥1.66%	3169 (24%) women 60–69 years; 789 (6%) women ≥70 years	69 month FU [16]	7-year FU [16]
				Age (years) RR (CI)	RR (CI)
				≤49 0.56 (0.37–0.85)	0.64 (0.46–0.89)
				50–59 0.49 (0.29–0.81)	0.57 (0.38–0.84)
				≥60 0.45 (0.27–0.074)	0.49 (0.33–0.73)
STAR [17,18]	RAL vs. TAM (19,747 postmenopausal women)	≥35 years and postmenopausal with 5-year BC risk ≥1.66%	6406 (32.4%) women 60–69 years; 1706 (8.8%) women ≥70 years	3.9-year FU [17]	7-year FU [18]
				Age (years) RR (CI)	RR (CI)
				≤49 1.15 (0.37–3.74)	1.53 (0.64–3.80)
				50–59 0.93 (0.68–1.29)	1.23 (0.97–1.57)
				≥60 1.11 (0.80–1.55)	1.22 (0.95–1.58)
PCPT [19]	Finasteride vs. placebo (18,882 men)	≥55 years	7440 (39%) men ≥65 years	7-year FU [19] RR	
				Age (years)	
				<55 —	
				55–59 0.72	
				60–64 0.73	
				≥65 0.80	
REDUCE [20]	Dutasteride vs. placebo (6729 men)	50–75 years	2723 (40.5%) men ≥65 years	4-year FU [20] Relative risk reduction with Dutasteride (CI)	
				Age (years)	
				<65 24.1 (13.5–33.4)	
				≥65 22.1 (10.8–32.0)	

Notation: TAM = tamoxifen; RAL = raloxifene; FU = follow-up; RR = risk ratio; BC = breast cancer; CI = 95% confidence interval; P-1:BCPT = Prevention 1:Breast Cancer Prevention Trial; STAR = Study of Tamoxifen and Raloxifene; PCPT = Prostate Cancer Prevention Trial; REDUCE = Reduction by Dutasteride of Prostate Cancer Events study.

cancers. In sum, cancer prevention strategies for older adults may be more complicated than strategies for younger, healthy individuals. Nevertheless, data point to compelling reasons to focus on reducing risk in older adults through both lifestyle and medical strategies with the goals of increasing longevity and improving quality of life in this population.

4.2 CANCER PREVENTION STRATEGIES IN OLDER ADULTS

4.2.1 Behavioral Intervention

Eliminating Tobacco Use   At a population level, the impact of smoking reduction becomes visible approximately 20 years after the carcinogenic insult. In the United Kingdom (UK), for example, in both men and women the peaks in smoking clearly preceded the peaks in lung cancer mortality by approximately 20 years (Fig. 4.2). In women, peaks for both tobacco use and lung cancer deaths followed the equivalent peaks in men by about 20–25 years [25]. Although levels are lower and later in UK women relative to men, in women smoking prevalence peaks in 1970 (Fig. 4.2a,b) and lung cancer mortality peaks approximately in 1990 among older women (Fig. 4.2d), again pointing to a 20-year delay between tobacco exposure and mortality due to lung cancer. The optimal approach to reducing tobacco-related cancers in older people is therefore to discourage initiation of tobacco use and encourage smoking cessation while they are still young. Nevertheless, for the sizable population of older adults who still smoke tobacco (8.1% of those 65 years and older in 2009) [26], quitting smoking at any age confers some benefit for longevity and quality of life. For example, the Cancer Prevention Study II showed that the benefits of cessation extend to quitting at older ages; an otherwise healthy man at age 60–63 who smokes one pack of cigarettes or more per day reduces his risk of dying during the next 15 years by 10% if he quits smoking [27]. This reduced risk is seen for respiratory cancers, nonrespiratory cancers, and cardiovascular diseases. For overall mortality, former smokers (when compared to continuing smokers) begin to have a decline in mortality shortly after quitting, and the decline continues for at least 10–15 years, at which time the risk of all-cause mortality nearly returns to that of persons who never smoked. With the various smoking cessation strategies available today, including nicotine replacement therapies, medications such as bupropion and varenicline, and newer nicotine vaccines, clinicians have the tools needed to aggressively encourage older adults to discontinue the use of tobacco.

Physical Activity   As a lifestyle strategy for cancer prevention, increasing physical activity can have important benefits for older adults, although the greater benefit resides in starting the intervention in early adulthood. Extensive epidemiological research points, with varying levels of evidence, to beneficial effects of physical activity at specific cancer sites: convincing evidence on the risk of colon cancer; probable evidence on the risk of breast and endometrial cancers; possible evidence on cancers of the prostate, lung, and ovary; and insufficient evidence for most remaining cancer sites [28]. Clearly, physical activity (30–60 min of at least moderate activity 5 days a week) may reduce the risk of those cancers most common among older adults.

As in most cancer prevention strategies, timing of the intervention and dose (amount) are critical to reducing risk. In a review of 57 epidemiological studies on moderate recreational physical activity and breast cancer, the largest benefit (27% average risk

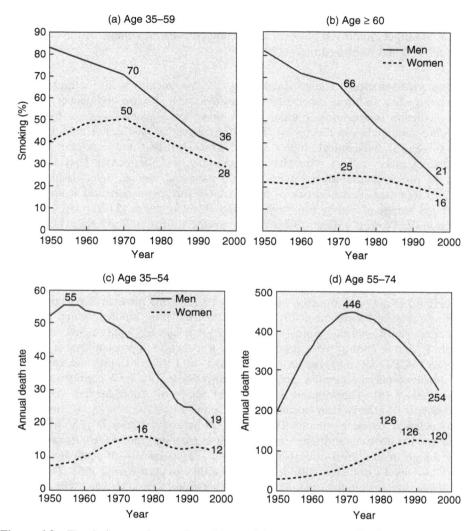

Figure 4.2 Trends in prevalence of smoking and lung cancer mortality in men and women in the United Kingdom from 1950 to 1997. (a) smoking prevalence in individuals age 35–59; (b) smoking prevalence in individuals age ≥60; (c) lung cancer mortality in individuals age 35–54; (d) lung cancer mortality in individuals age 55–74. [Figures (a)–(d) were modified from Ref. 24 and reproduced with permission from the *British Medical Journal* [25].]

reduction) was for sustained activity over the adult years, but a significant benefit (17% risk reduction) was also observed for activity in postmenopausal women over the age of 50 years [22]. The same activity level earlier in life (early adulthood or 20s) conferred only an 8% risk reduction.

Comorbidities and other factors may reduce the ability of older adults to undertake moderate exercise. This challenge, however, should not preclude designing an activity regimen that is appropriate for individuals regardless of limitations. Even among individuals with cardiovascular restrictions, diabetes, and high body mass index, studies have shown that physical exercise can have positive effects on weight loss (if needed), decreased fatigue, improved physical functioning, decreased number of falls, improved bone density, and improved mood [29].

Dietary Intervention Dietary intake can have an unequivocally favorable impact on health over a lifetime, especially on cardiovascular disease and cancer [30]. The issue of dietary intervention in older adults, however, is made less clear by the lack of intervention studies in this group. The information that has been accumulated from epidemiological and clinical studies appears to suggest that diet may play some role in reducing cancer risk at some sites. For example, the NIH-AARP Diet and Health Study (a prospective study of over 500,000 men and women age 50–71 years at baseline) found an increased risk of breast cancer for postmenopausal women with a higher percentage of energy from total fat and all fat subtypes [31,32]. An analysis of data from the Women's Health Initiative Dietary Modification Randomized Controlled Trial found a low-fat dietary pattern to be associated with a reduction in the risk of ovarian cancer in postmenopausal women [33]. An analysis of dietary data from the Prostate Cancer Prevention Trial (PCPT), conducted by the Southwest Oncology Group (SWOG) and the National Cancer Institute's Division of Cancer Prevention (NCI/DCP) (see below), found no correlation between any nutrient and prostate cancer risk. These PCPT observations were inconsistent with data from prior studies, which suggested that certain nutritional components [lycopene, longchain (ω_3) fatty acids, vitamin D, vitamin E, and selenium] were associated with a reduction in prostate cancer risk [34]. However, PCPT data suggest an increased risk of high-grade prostate cancer with high intake of polyunsaturated fats [odds ratio (OR) = 2.41, 95% confidence interval (CI) = 1.33–4.38]. The Uppsala Longitudinal Study of Adult Men, a community-based cohort of elderly men (mean age at baseline 71 years; $n = 1194$), investigated the association between vitamin D (plasma 25-hydroxyvitamin D [25(OH)D]) and cancer and cardiovascular disease mortality. More recently reported results suggest that either a high or low level of plasma vitamin D is associated with death from cancer, with a low level associated with death from cardiovascular disease [35]. The authors commented that concluding that high levels of vitamin D are associated with increased mortality may be counterintuitive, given that vitamin D has potent antiproliferative, prodifferentiative, and immunomodulatory functions in a variety of cell types. However, data from experimental studies and the National Health and Nutrition Examination Study (NHANES) III and the Framingham Heart Study also suggest that mortality increases with increasing plasma 25(OH)D levels above 40 ng/mL (100 nmol/L) [35].

One of the largest prospective studies on diet and cancer is the European Prospective Investigation into Cancer and Nutrition (EPIC), a multicenter prospective study with approximately 520,000 participants carried out in 23 centers in 10 European countries [36]. A more recent update of results supports a significant inverse association between gastric cancer risk and high levels of plasma vitamin C, some carotenoids, retinol, and α-tocopherol; high intake of cereal fiber; and high adhesion to a Mediterranean diet. Red and processed meat were associated with an increased risk of gastric cancer [36]. In addition, high intake of dietary fiber, fish, and calcium, as well as plasma vitamin D, was associated with decreased risk of colorectal cancer, whereas red and processed meat and alcohol were associated with increased risk. Interestingly, in current smokers a high intake of fruit and vegetables was associated with decreased risk of lung cancer. An increased risk of breast cancer was associated with high saturated fat intake and alcohol intake. Also, a high intake of protein and calcium from dairy products and a high serum concentration of insulin-like growth factor (IGF)1 were associated with an increased risk of prostate cancer. These results suggest that ongoing clinical research on diet can add to the scientific evidence needed to develop public health strategies. Although these data have not been presented by age group, most of the data relate to cancers with higher rates in older adults.

4.2.2 Medical and Nutritional/Bioactive Food Component (BFC) Intervention

Cancer prevention approaches that utilize pharmacologic agents (medical/chemoprevention) and individual bioactive food components (BFCs; nutritional prevention) aim to prevent, arrest, or reverse either the initiation phase of carcinogenesis or the progression of premalignant cells to invasive malignancy. Such approaches have been tested in individuals at increased risk of specific cancers, with elevated age generally contributing to the definitions of increased risk. This places the older adult clearly within the population that is eligible for investigation of these preventive interventions. Because the intended population for a chemopreventive agent or BFC is essentially healthy, although at increased cancer risk, an understanding of the risks as well as benefits of the preventive intervention must be determined. Furthermore, a natural or pharmacologic agent generally must be taken for many years in order to derive benefit, implying exposure for a prolonged period of time and necessitating careful evaluation of the cumulative, long-term risk: benefit balance. Apart from the increased likelihood of developing independent comorbidities during this extended timeframe, some of the toxicities documented for chemopreventive agents may be exacerbated in older individuals. Stark examples of such age-related toxicities are endometrial cancer and venous thromboembolic disease, which, although elevated overall in the tamoxifen arm of the BCPT, were increased primarily in ≥50-year old participants taking tamoxifen.

Well-known chemopreventive agents such as tamoxifen, raloxifene, finasteride, and dutasteride (Table 4.1) constitute only a small percentage of the chemopreventive agents that have been tested in large numbers of older adults. The importance of these trials is that they suggest the potential value of prevention in older adults for the major cancer sites. Of note, in some trials, is that the reduction in relative risk with the preventive intervention is greater in the younger participants at follow-up. For example, the PCPT results indicated a risk reduction after 7 years of follow-up of 28% in men 55–59 years of age but only 20% in those over 65 years (Table 4.1).

Large Phase III Cancer Prevention Clinical Trials with Relevance to Older Adults Large, definitive cancer prevention RCTs only have been conducted over the past two decades with most trials focusing on the major cancer sites. In the case of breast cancer, earlier adjuvant treatment trials demonstrated secondary prevention benefits from the selective estrogen receptor modulator (SERM) tamoxifen by showing a reduction in new primary cancers in the contralateral breast. These secondary outcomes led to the hypothesis that tamoxifen would prevent first primary breast cancers, leading in turn to four phase III tamoxifen prevention trials [37], The largest of these, the NSABP P-1:BCPT, was developed in conjunction with the NCI/DCP. P-1:BCPT was designed to determine whether tamoxifen would reduce the incidence of invasive breast cancer (IBC) among women with no history of breast cancer but at higher risk than the general population [15,16]. The relevance of this trial for older women is evident in its eligibility criteria, which centered around a Gail model that predicted 5-year risk of breast cancer ≥1.66%, the average risk of women 60 years of age. In P-1:BCPT, tamoxifen reduced the risk of IBC by approximately 50%, a level of efficacy that was seen in all age groups (Table 4.1). However, troublesome side effects were observed, although at very low frequency. The two major tamoxifen-associated toxicities, endometrial cancers in nonhysterectomized women and venous thromboembolic events (VTEs), were concentrated in participants >50 years, emphasizing comparable benefits but increased vulnerability to adverse effects in older women. At the same time, the SERM raloxifene, which was being tested in the Multiple Outcomes of Raloxifene Evaluation (MORE) randomized clinical trial with a primary outcome of osteoporosis, was shown to decrease the risk of IBC, a key secondary endpoint, by 76% without evident endometrial toxicity [38].

On the basis of results from P-1:BCPT and MORE, NCI/DCP and the NSABP designed the Study of Tamoxifen and Raloxifene (STAR) trial to test the promising raloxifene against tamoxifen in postmenopausal women at increased risk of breast cancer (Gail model 5-year predicted risk of breast cancer ≥1.66%) [17,18]. STAR showed that raloxifene and tamoxifen conferred equivalent reductions of IBC, but raloxifene was associated with substantially fewer adverse effects, especially uterine cancer but also a lesser increase in VTEs. Given its equivalent benefit in reducing breast cancer risk, the lower toxicity of raloxifene makes it particularly appealing for prevention in older women.

A comparable large phase III trial for prostate cancer was begun in 1993 by SWOG and the NCI/DCP. The PCPT compared finasteride to placebo in 18,882 men ≥55 years of age, again emphasizing the importance of including older individuals, the major at-risk population, in prevention trials for common cancers [19]. In 2003, the PCPT was discontinued because finasteride was definitively shown to reduce the incidence of prostate cancer (25% decrease in the finasteride group). However, a concomitant increase in high-grade prostate cancers among men who did develop prostate cancer was a finding of concern that still is being studied and discussed.

A second large phase III prostate cancer trial was the Selenium and Vitamin E Cancer Prevention Trial (SELECT), which included 37% of participants 65 years or older [39]. SELECT was based on hypotheses generated from both epidemiological data and clinical trial secondary endpoints showing that supplementation with selenium and vitamin E showed promise for the prevention of prostate cancer [40]. The Nutritional Prevention of Cancer (NPC) trial in Finland did not demonstrate a reduction in skin cancer incidence with selenium, which was its primary endpoint, but did report a lower frequency of prostate cancer in the selenium group [41]. The Alpha-Tocopherol Beta-Carotene (ATBC) trial tested vitamin E and a carotenoid for lung cancer prevention [42]. Although no beneficial effect was seen on the incidence of lung cancer with either nutrient, α-tocopherol was associated with a reduction in prostate cancer. On the basis of the promising prostate cancer findings in the two trials, SWOG and NCI/DCP recruited 35,533 men age ≥55 years (African American men ≥50 years) to the SELECT trial. Begun in 2001, SELECT was stopped in 2008 because preliminary data showed that selenium and vitamin E, taken alone or together, did not prevent prostate cancer and were unlikely ever to produce a 25% reduction, as the study was designed to show. Other causes for concern, although not statistically significant, were slight increases in prostate cancer among men taking vitamin E alone and diabetes among men taking selenium alone [39]. The implications of these results—lack of efficacy and suggestion of possible toxicity—for the older men to whom the two bioactive food components (BFCs) were targeted are still topics of much discussion.

Testing of Other Chemopreventive Agents and BFCs with Relevance to Older Adults With more than 150 chemopreventive agents having been studied since the 1980s, considerable progress has been made in potential preventive approaches for other major cancers. These investigations include smaller clinical trials. Although they have not specifically targeted older adults, the target cancers are those that disproportionately affect older populations. For example, a phase II randomized clinical trial in 375 patients with a history of resected colon polyps investigated the combination of the chemopreventive agents difluoromethylornithine (DFMO) and the nonsteroidal antiinflammatory drug (NSAID) sulindac [43,44]. Results indicated that the combination reduced polyp recurrence by 70% at 3 years, with advanced polyp recurrence reduced by 90%. This type of study exemplifies the newer approach to designing cancer chemoprevention studies that target specific genetic/molecular pathways in order to interrupt the carcinogenic process. More recent examples include the targeting of epidermal growth factor receptors for breast and other cancers; loss of heterozygosity in various genes in colon, oral, and lung cancers; and androgen receptors for prostate cancer [44].

Bioactive food components are part of a cancer prevention strategy that has been studied for more than three decades, when Doll and Peto published an inclusive analysis of quantitative estimates of the avoidable risks of cancer, estimating that approximately 35% are related to diet [45]. Subsequent studies have identified numerous BFCs that could have benefits for cancer prevention. These include vitamin D and its analogs, lycopene, soy isoflavones (genistein), indole-3-carbinol analog, and epigallocatechin-3-gallate (EGCG), which is a catechin found in abundance in green tea [46]. In the past few decades, many of the nutritional studies have focused on the major signaling pathways, which are deregulated in cancer and can be modified by one or more BFCs [47]. An example is genistein, which has been shown to induce cell cycle arrest and apoptosis in numerous cancer cell lines, including cell lines of estrogen receptor ER^+ and ER^- human breast carcinoma, prostate cancer, colon cancer, and lung cancer [48]. Although much of this research is being conducted in cancer cells and animals and in small human trials, with no concentration on older adults, the fact that these cancers affect largely older individuals suggest that their findings will likely be relevant to prevention strategies in this older population. Because diet is complex and involves a lifelong behavior, a single food component is unlikely to produce the silver bullet for cancer prevention. Yet, the accumulating knowledge of the role of diet and specific BFCs is likely to have benefits across all age groups.

4.3 OTHER ISSUES FOR CANCER PREVENTION IN OLDER ADULTS

The following issues pose barriers to implementation of cancer preventive measures in older adults.

4.3.1 Healthcare Provider Issues

Issues related to barriers to cancer prevention in older adults, as well as healthcare in general in this population, are similar across all disease categories. As one ages, especially among individuals ≥75 years, specific environmental, physical, and mental changes may occur that impede both the individual and the healthcare provider from ensuring delivery of adequate preventive care, as well as appropriate treatment when disease is diagnosed [24]. Interestingly, when preventive measures have been instituted among older individuals, they often are misdirected. For example, a recent assessment of preventive care among women age 65–80+ in an academic primary care center found that women in poor health were screened for cancer more often than healthy women [49]. Furthermore, except for women ≥80 years, healthier women received little counseling regarding exercise, depression, osteoporosis, falls, and incontinence [49]. An interesting finding was that women ≥80 years were provided with some preventive health measures from which they were unlikely to benefit [e.g., papanicolaou (Pap) smears], but did not receive others (e.g., flu vaccination) that were likely to be effective in a short time period. The issue of continued screening as a preventive measure (to identify potential cancerous lesions that have not fully developed into overt cancer) should have a higher priority in those women and men who have life expectancies greater than 5–10 years [24].

4.3.2 Access to Health-Related Information

Access to information is critical for informing older adults about healthcare facts and recommendations. The use of the Internet, either through access to websites with accurate health information, or email reminders of appointments and updates for preventive measures, is slowly being included in geriatric practice [50]. Although the Internet can be a source of factual (or misleading or unreliable) health information, it has not reached its zenith as a tool for disseminating health information to the general public. It still is a place that is generally visited by those at higher socioeconomic and education levels, and does not have widespread acceptance among many minority populations [50]. This venue affords an opportunity for prevention information to be strategically placed and advertised as more people have Internet access.

4.3.3 Barriers to Good Nutrition

Another significant barrier to implementing cancer preventive strategies related to diet and prevention with BFCs among older adults is the loss of regulators that influence hunger and sensory input related to foods. A review [51] on the "anorexia of aging" found numerous causes for changing eating habits and nutrient utilization in those 65 years and older. Sensory changes, such as a decrease in the pleasantness of a food (i.e., sensory-specific satiety) may be caused by alterations in taste bud structure in elderly individuals. Older adults also have a higher odor detection and recognition threshold, possibly due to changes in upper-airway structure and the olfactory epithelium, bulb, and nerves. In addition, older adults may take one or more of the approximately 250 medications that alter the senses of taste and smell. Gastrointestinal changes due to aging, including reduced levels of gut hormones as shown by reduced plasma levels of ghrelin, may reduce the recognition of satiety [51]. Problems with dentition, higher levels of depression and chronic disease than seen in younger adults, and social isolation also may lead to a lack of proper nutrition.

4.4 THE FUTURE OF CANCER PREVENTION IN OLDER ADULTS

The discipline of cancer prevention feeds directly into public health, addressing primarily cancers that affect large numbers of individuals. These common cancers also are the ones that disproportionately occur in older people and are therefore central to the theme of this book. The two major approaches to cancer prevention involve behavioral and medical/nutritional forms of intervention. Research into tobacco control, dietary modification, and physical exercise suggests that instituting such potentially cancer reducing behavioral modifications should ideally begin years before an individual becomes "elderly," although improvements in lifestyle are advantageous at any age in terms of benefits to general health and well-being. Definitive trials of chemopreventive agents and BFCs generally include a minimum age among the criteria for eligibility, given the increased risk of the target cancers in older people. Furthermore, the trials that have successfully demonstrated preventive activity for pharmaceutical agents show the accrued benefits to occur in participants in all age groups. Despite equivalent benefit, disproportionate toxicity in older participants needs to be carefully balanced against the preventive benefits of any agent, even in healthy older persons. Future research in cancer prevention in older people will necessarily have to address issues of comorbidity and life expectancy in addition to ongoing concerns about efficacy and adverse effects of preventive interventions.

REFERENCES

1. Dunn BK, Greenwald P. Cancer prevention I: Introduction. *Semin Oncol* 2010;**37**(3): 190–201.
2. Roebuck J. When does old age begin? The evolution of the English definition. *J Soc Hist* 1979;**12**(3):416–428.
3. Satariano WA, Ragland DR. The effect of comorbidity on 3-year survival of women with primary breast cancer. *Ann Intern Med* 1994;**120**(2):104–110.
4. Terret C, Castel-Kremer E, Albrand G, Droz JP. Effects of comorbidity on screening and early diagnosis of cancer in elderly people. *Lancet Oncol* 2009;**10**(1):80–87.
5. Extermann M, Balducci L, Lyman GH. What threshold for adjuvant therapy in older breast cancer patients? *J Clin Oncol* 2000;**18**(8):1709–1717.
6. Owusu C, Buist DS, Field TS, et al. Predictors of tamoxifen discontinuation among older women with estrogen receptor-positive breast cancer. *J Clin Oncol* 2008;**26**(4):549–555.
7. Jemal A, Siegel R, Xu J, Ward E. Cancer Statistics, 2010. *CA Cancer J Clin* 2010;**60**(5): 1–24.
8. Johnson KA. Cancer prevention in the elderly. In Hunter CP, Johnson KA, Muss HB, eds. *Cancer in the Elderly*, Marcel Dekker, New York, 2000, pp. 57–68.
9. Dunn BK, Longo DL. Molecular biology and biological markers. In Hunter CP, Johnson KA, Muss HB, eds. *Cancer in the Elderly*, Marcel Dekker, New York, 2000, pp.69–121.
10. DePinho RA. The age of cancer. *Nature* 2000;**408**(6809):248–254.

11. Blagosklonny MV, Campisi J. Cancer and aging: More puzzles, more promises? *Cell Cycle* 2008;**7**(17):2615–2618.

12. Hajjar RR. Cancer in the elderly: Is it preventable? *Clin Geriatr Med* 2004;**20**(2):293–316.

13. Dunn BK, Wagner PD, Anderson D, Greenwald P. Molecular markers for early detection. *Semin Oncol* 2010;**37**(3):224–242.

14. Bjornsson HT, Fallin MD, Feinberg AP. An integrated epigenetic and genetic approach to common human disease. *Trends Genet* 2004;**20**(8):350–358.

15. Fisher B, Costantino JP, Wickerham DL, et al. Tamoxifen for prevention of breast cancer: Report of the National Surgical Adjuvant Breast and Bowel Project P-1 Study. *J Natl Cancer Inst* 1998;**90**(18):1371–1388.

16. Fisher B, Costantino JP, Wickerham DL, et al. Tamoxifen for the prevention of breast cancer: current status of the National Surgical Adjuvant Breast and Bowel Project P-1 study. *J Natl Cancer Inst*. 2005;**97**(22):1652–1662.

17. Vogel VG, Costantino JP, Wickerham DL, et al. Effects of tamoxifen vs raloxifene on the risk of developing invasive breast cancer and other disease outcomes: The NSABP Study of Tamoxifen and Raloxifene (STAR) P-2 trial. *JAMA* 2006;**295**(23):2727–2741.

18. Vogel VG, Costantino JP, Wickerham DL, et al. Update of the National Surgical Adjuvant Breast and Bowel Project Study of Tamoxifen and Raloxifene (STAR) P-2 Trial: Preventing breast cancer. *Cancer Prev Res*. 2010;**3**(6):696–706.

19. Thompson IM, Goodman PJ, Tangen CM, et al. The influence of finasteride on the development of prostate cancer. *N Engl J Med* 2003;**349**(3):215–224.

20. Andriole GL, Bostwick DG, Brawley OW, et al. Effect of dutasteride on the risk of prostate cancer. *N Engl J Med* 2010;**362**(13):1192–1202.

21. Tyrovolas S, Panagiotakos DB. The role of Mediterranean type of diet on the development of cancer and cardiovascular disease, in the elderly: A systematic review. *Maturitas* 2010;**65**(2):122–30.

22. Friedenreich CM. The role of physical activity in breast cancer etiology. *Semin Oncol* 2010;**37**(3):297–302.

23. Friedenreich CM, Neilson HK, Lynch BM. State of the epidemiological evidence on physical activity and cancer prevention. *Eur J Cancer* 2010;**46**(14):2593–2604.

24. Balducci L. Prevention of cancer in the older person. *Cancer J* 2005;**11**(6):442–448.

25. Peto R, Darby S, Deo H, Silcocks P, Whitley E, Doll R. Smoking, smoking cessation, and lung cancer in the UK since 1950: Combination of national statistics with two case-control studies. *Br Med J* 2000 **321**(7257):323–329.

26. Centers for Disease Control and Prevention. *Behavioral Risk Factor Surveillance System*, National Center for Chronic Disease Prevention & Health Promotion. Atlanta, GA, 2009 (available at `http://apps.nccd.cdc.gov/brfss/age.asp?cat=TU&yr=2009&qkey=4396&state=US`; last accessed 10/20/10).

27. US Dept. Health and Human Services. *The Health Benefits of Smoking Cessation*, USDHHS, Public Health Service. Centers for Disease Control, Center for Chronic Disease Prevention and Health Promotion, Office on Smoking and Health. DHHS Publication (CDC) YO-K-116, 1990.

28. National Cancer Institute. *Surveillance, Epidemiology, and End Results (SEER) Program Populations (1969–2007)* NCI, DCCPS, Surveillance Research Program, Cancer Statistics Branch (available at `www.seer.cancer.gov/popdata`, released 11/09; last accessed 10/20/10).

29. Penedo FJ, Schneiderman N, Dahn JR, Gonzalez JS. Physical activity interventions in the elderly: Cancer and morbidity. *Cancer Investig* 2004;**22**(1):51–67.

30. World Cancer Research Fund/American Institute for Cancer Research. *Food, Nutrition, Physical Activity, and the Prevention of Cancer: A Global Perspective*. AICR, Washington, DC, 2007.

31. Thiebaut AC, Kipnis V, Chang SC, et al. Dietary fat and postmenopausal invasive breast cancer in the National Institutes of Health-AARP Diet and Health Study cohort. *J Natl Cancer Inst* 2007;**99**(6):451–462.

32. Gibson TM, Ferrucci LM, Tangrea JA. Epidemiological and clinical studies of nutrition. *Semin Oncol* 2010;**37**(3):282–296.

33. Prentice RL, Thomson CA, Caan B, et al. Low-fat dietary pattern and cancer incidence in the Women's Health Initiative Dietary Modification Randomized Controlled Trial. *J Natl Cancer Inst* 2007;**99**(20):1534–1543.

34. Kristal AR, Arnold KB, Neuhouser ML, et al. Diet, supplement use, and prostate cancer risk: Results from the prostate cancer prevention trial. *Am J Epidemiol* 2010;**172**:566–577.

35. Michaëlsson K, Baron JA, Snellman G, et al. Plasma vitamin D and mortality in older men: A community-based prospective cohort study. *Am J Clin Nutr* 2010;**92**(4):841–848.

36. Gonzalez CA, Riboli E. Diet and cancer prevention: Contributions from the European Prospective Investigation into Cancer and Nutrition (EPIC) study. *Eur J Cancer* 2010;**46**(14):2555–2562.

37. Arun B, Dunn BK, Ford LG, Ryan A. Breast cancer prevention trials: Large and small trials. *Semin Oncol* 2010;**37**(4):367–383.

38. Cummings SR, Eckert S, Krueger KA, et al. The effect of raloxifene on risk of breast cancer in postmenopausal women: Results from the MORE randomized trial. Multiple Outcomes of Raloxifene Evaluation. *JAMA* 1999 Jun 16;**281**(23):2189–97.

39. Lippman SM, Klein EA, Goodman PJ, et al. Effect of selenium and vitamin E on risk of prostate cancer and other cancers: The Selenium and vitamin E Cancer Prevention Trial (SELECT). *JAMA*. 2009;**301**(1):39–51.

40. Dunn BK, Richmond ES, Minasian LM, Ryan AM, Ford LG. A nutrient approach to prostate cancer prevention: The Selenium and Vitamin E Cancer Prevention Trial (SELECT). *Nutr Cancer* 2010;**62**(7):896–918.

41. Clark LC, Combs GF Jr, Turnbull BW, et al. Effects of selenium supplementation for cancer prevention in patients with carcinoma of the skin. A randomized controlled trial. Nutritional Prevention of Cancer Study Group. *JAMA* 1996;**276**(24):1957–1963.

42. Heinonen OP, Albanes D, Virtamo J, et al. Prostate cancer and supplementation with alpha-tocopherol and beta-carotene: incidence and mortality in a controlled trial. *J Natl Cancer Inst* 1998;**90**(6):440–446.

43. Meyskens FL Jr, McLaren CE, Pelot D, et al. Difluoromethylornithine plus sulindac for the prevention of sporadic colorectal adenomas: A randomized placebo-controlled, double-blind trial. *Cancer Prev Res* 2008;**1**(1):32–38.

44. Johnson KA, Brown PH. Drug development for cancer chemoprevention: Focus on molecular targets. *Semin Oncol* 2010;**37**(4):345–358.

45. Doll R, Peto R. The causes of cancer: Quantitative estimates of avoidable risks of cancer in the United States today. *J Natl Cancer Inst* 1981;**66**(6):1191–1308.

46. Greenwald P. A favorable view: Progress in cancer prevention and screening. *Recent Results Cancer Res* 2006;**174**:3–17.

47. Davis CD, Emanaker NJ, Milner JA. Cellular proliferation, apoptosis and angiogenesis: Molecular targets for nutritional preemption of cancer. *Semin Oncol* 2010;**37**(3):243–257.

48. Milner JA, McDonald SS, Anderson DE, Greenwald P. Molecular targets for nutrients involved with cancer prevention. *Nutr Cancer* 2001;**41**(1–2):1–16.

49. Schonberg MA. Preventive health care among older women in an academic primary care practice. *Womens Health Issues* 2008;**18**(4):249–256.

50. Weaver JB 3rd, Mays D, Weaver SS, Hopkins GL, Eroglu D, Bernhardt JM. Health information-seeking behaviors, health indicators, and health risks. *Am J Public Health* 2010;**100**(8):1520–1525.

51. Hays NP, Roberts SB. The anorexia of aging in humans. *Physiol Behav* 2006;**88**(3): 257–266.

CHAPTER 5

Breast Cancer Prevention

JEANNE F. NOE and HYMAN B. MUSS

University of North Carolina at Chapel Hill, Chapel Hill, NC

5.1 INTRODUCTION

Aging is the number one risk factor for breast cancer incidence and mortality [1]. In the United States and other economically advantaged populations, older adults are healthier and the average life expectancy has increased dramatically since the early 1900s. Average life expectancy for a woman born today is about 80 years. For a woman who reaches 65 years, life expectancy averages about 20 more years and for a 75-year-old, about 12 years [1,2]. As age increases, so do the biologic characteristics of breast cancers, and older patients are more likely to have tumors that are hormone-receptor-positive, lymph-node-negative, lower-grade with lower proliferation indices, and human epidermal (growth factor) receptor 2 (HER2)-negative [3,4]. Despite these generally more favorable characteristics in older compared to younger women, stage-adjusted breast cancer mortality is comparable for older and younger patients, except among the very young and very old [5,6]. Although older women are generally diagnosed with later-stage breast cancer than younger women, about 90% of older women still present in early stages (I or II) [7].

Prevention strategies for breast cancer in older women are generally similar to those recommended for younger women and include lifestyle changes and for some, pharmacotherapy. The risk of invasive breast cancer can be calculated for patients 35 years and older using validated models that include breast cancer risk factors such as age, race, age at menarche, age at birth of first child, number of first-degree relatives who have breast cancer, a history of breast biopsy and, if so, the number of biopsies, and incidence of atypical hyperplasia [8–10]. A careful family history is mandatory in older patients as some may have pedigrees suggesting a high probability of BRCA1 and BRCA2 mutations, increasing their risk. The review in this chapter focuses on breast cancer prevention strategies for older patients.

Cancer and Aging Handbook: Research and Practice, First Edition. Edited by Keith M. Bellizzi and Margot A. Gosney.
© 2012 Wiley-Blackwell. Published 2012 by John Wiley & Sons, Inc.

TABLE 5.1   Correlation between Lifestyle Risk Factors and Breast Cancer

Modifiable Lifestyle Factor	Relative Risk of Breast Cancer
Obesity at Age 50	
HRT nonusers	
BMI >31 kg/m^2 compared to ≤22.6 kg/m^2	2.07 (Morimoto [20][a])
BMI ≥40 kg/m^2 compared to 18.5–22.4 kg/m^2	2.00 (Ahn [16][a])
HRT users	
BMI>31 kg/m^2 compared to ≤22.6 kg/m^2	0.90 (Morimoto [20][a])
BMI ≥40 kg/m^2 compared to 18.5–22.4 kg/m^2	0.92 (Ahn [16][a])
Weight Gain from Age 50	
HRT nonusers	
30–39.9 kg increase compared to −1.9 to +1.9 kg	1.89 (Ahn [16][a])
Current HRT users	
30–39.9 kg increase compared to −1.9 to +1.9 kg	0.99 (Ahn [16][a])
Alcohol (10 g alcohol/drink)	
1–2 drinks/day vs. ≤ 2 drinks/week	1.13 (Allen [49], mean age 55 years)[b]
1.5–2.5 drinks/day vs. 0 drinks/day	1.13 (Collaborative group [51])[c]
>2 drinks/day vs. ≤2 drinks/week	1.29 (Allen [49], mean age 55 years)[b]
≥4 drinks/day vs. 0 drinks/day	1.46 (Collaborative [51])[c]
Postmenopausal Physical Activity	
6% decrease in breast cancer risk for each additional hour of physical activity per week (Monninkhof [28])	

[a]Adjusted for age, age at menarche, age at menopause, age at first birth, smoking, educational level, race, family history of breast cancer, fat intake, parity, alcohol consumption, physical activity (and in Ahn [16] for oophorectomy).
[b]Adjusted for age, BMI, smoking history, physical activity, HRT, ever use of oral contraceptives, socio-economic status, and region of residence.
[c]Stratified by study, age, parity, age at first birth, and smoking history.

5.2 LIFESTYLE MODIFICATION

Despite the primacy of age as a risk factor for postmenopausal breast cancer [11], women may reduce the risk of breast cancer as they age by modifying certain lifestyle behaviors, such as the amount of weight gained in adulthood, alcohol consumed weekly, and physical exercise performed regularly, even if these changes do not occur until after menopause [12]. Observational cohort and case–control studies represent the large majority of trials evaluating lifestyle risk factors (see Table 5.1) for breast cancer. This is not likely to change, given the long latency of breast cancer and the difficulties inherent in randomizing large groups of women to diet and exercise programs for prolonged periods of time [13]. However, the consistency of study results, coupled with the safety of study recommendations and their established benefit in reducing the risk of other diseases, suggests that randomized trials may not be necessary [12].

5.2.1 Increased Weight and Weight Gain

While initially perplexing, the relationship between the risk of postmenopausal breast cancer and body mass index (BMI) at menopause has now been clarified. The confusion stemmed from at least three fronts: (1) an increased BMI early in life may confer some level of protection against breast cancer throughout life [14,15]; (2) BMI at menopause represents weight gain up to that time, making it difficult to establish its independence from weight gain as a risk factor [16]; and (3) the use of hormone replacement therapy (HRT) masks the association between weight and risk of breast cancer [14,16–19].

Provided data are stratified by HRT use, studies consistently support an association between increasing BMI at menopause and an increased risk of postmenopausal breast cancer in nonusers of HRT [16,20]. The positive relationship between postmenopausal BMI and risk appears to be linear [16,21]; however, this association may eventually plateau [21]. Adult weight gain, usually defined as weight gained since the age of 18, has also been consistently associated with a higher risk of postmenopausal breast cancer in prospective cohort studies of nonusers of HRT [16,21–24]. The amount of weight gained is important; in the National Institutes of Health (NIH)-AARP observational cohort study, nonusers of HRT who gained ≥50 kg experienced a Relative Risk (RR) of 2.15 for breast cancer versus 1.18 for those who gained 2.0–9.9 kg [16]. For both weight and weight gain, the relationship to breast cancer risk remains after adjusting for known risk factors of breast cancer, including age [16,20,21–24].

Unfortunately, the relationship between weight loss and decreased risk of breast cancer is not as obvious. This may be related to the difficulty in losing and maintaining weight post-menopause, as opposed to lack of a biological effect [21]. In a 16-year follow-up report using the Nurse's Health cohort, no significant association between breast cancer and weight loss was seen, although so few women lost weight the study had limited power to examine this association [14]. In a longer-term follow-up report on the same cohort, women who never used HRT and sustained (for 4 years or longer) at least a 10kg weight loss post menopause experienced a significantly decreased breast cancer risk as compared to women who maintained weight [relative risk (RR) = 0.43] [21]. The Iowa Women's Health Study also reported RR = 0.77 in women who gained weight from age 30 to menopause but then lost weight after menopause as compared to women whose weight consistently increased [24].

5.2.2 Physical Activity

Greater than 70 distinct studies have been reported worldwide since 1985 on the association between physical activity and breast cancer risk [13,25]. These studies consistently suggest that at least some amount of physical activity is protective against breast cancer, although the amount and intensity needed to optimize this effect is unknown [26]. According to systematic reviews of the literature, the average reduction in breast cancer risk is about 25% in comparison of the most to the least physically active group, with evidence for a dose–response effect reported in the majority of studies [25]. One group has estimated a 6% decrease in breast cancer risk for each additional hour of physical activity per week, provided this level of activity is sustained [27]. Importantly, in their comprehensive review of the literature evaluating the timing of physical activity, Friedenreich and Cust reported a tendency for activity performed after the age of 50 to have a stronger effect on reducing breast cancer risk than activity performed during adolescence and early adulthood [28].

The mechanisms behind the impact of overweight, weight gain, and physical inactivity on the risk of breast cancer are interrelated, as summarized in a biological model

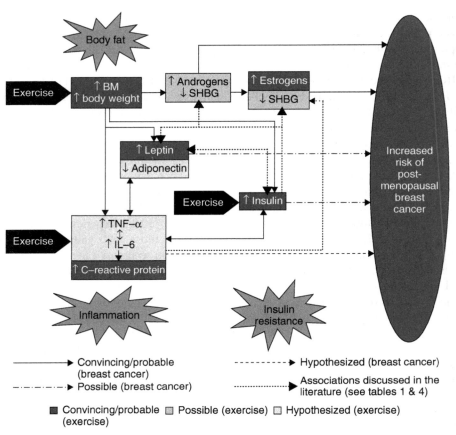

Figure 5.1 Biological model relating proposed biomarkers to long-term exercise (shading) and postmenopausal breast cancer risk (arrows). (Reprinted with permission from Neilson et al. [29], Fig. 1.)

proposed by researchers involved in physical activity and breast cancer (see Fig. 5.1) [29]. This model, based on an extensive review of the literature, correlates increased levels of several biomarkers of inflammation and body fat with an increased risk of postmenopausal breast cancer via interrelated effects on the levels of leptin, adiponectin, sex hormones, and insulin. Exercise can modulate these biomarkers by its direct effects on decreasing BMI, body weight, biomarkers of inflammation, and insulin. Insulin has been inconsistently associated with breast cancer [30–32], but strongly associated with abdominal obesity, a particular problem in postmenopausal weight gain [29,33].

The impact of exercise on blood levels of sex hormones was evaluated in three prospective controlled studies randomizing postmenopausal, overweight, sedentary women not taking HRT to 1 year of physical exercise or maintenance of normal activity [34,35]. All three studies reported a greater reduction in at least some sex hormones at 12 months and two of the studies reported increases in sex hormone binding globulin (SHBG) for the exerciser group versus the control group [35]. Results reached significance for the exerciser group as a whole in only one study for estradiol and free estradiol [35], and in the other two only when limited to those exercisers who lost ≥2% of their body fat for estrogens [35], and for androgens [34]. These data suggest that at least some of the reduction in breast cancer risk from exercise may be due to effects on serum sex hormones, although their independence from loss of body fat is not clear. Results from all three studies demonstrate the feasibility and breast cancer prevention benefit of moderately intensive, regular exercise in women up to the age of 69 [34], or 74 [35].

Investigators in one of the three trials also examined the influence of exercise on mammographic density, but failed to find any significant effect of exercise on breast density and volume of breast tissue after adjustment for standard breast cancer risk factors, including age [36].

5.2.3 Dietary Factors

Two reviews summarizing the large number of studies focusing on diet and breast cancer have been published [15,37]. A systematic review of studies published through 2005 found no association between risk of breast cancer and intake of fruits, vegetables, or vitamins A, C, and E and carotenoids. This review found either inconsistent or no association between blood levels of antioxidant vitamins and breast cancer [37]. Similarly, the World Cancer Research Fund (WCRF) drew no firm conclusions on the role of individual foods and nutrients on overall breast cancer risk after an extensive review of the literature, and indicated that the data on total fat is suggestive at best, and if present, likely modest [15,19,38].

The European Prospective Investigation into Cancer and Nutrition (EPIC) cohort investigated the relationship between consumption of meat, eggs, and dairy products, as well as dietary fat consumption with breast cancer risk in 135,529 postmenopausal women, and found only one close to significant association—a modest increase (RR = 1.13) in breast cancer risk for high processed meat consumption in the highest versus lowest quintile ($p = 0.06$ for trend) [38]. In contrast, a lower pooled risk estimate of 0.86 for postmenopausal breast cancer from a meta-analysis of 13 studies has been reported for ingestion of lignans, a major component of flaxseed and the most important class of phytoestrogens in the Western diet [39].

5.2.4 Vitamin D

Several lines of evidence have increased researchers interest in the potential role of vitamin D in preventing breast cancer, including, but not limited to the following: (1) breast cancer rates are higher in areas of the United States with lower overall ultraviolet B radiation exposure, possibly implicating lower levels of vitamin D [40]; (2) experimental studies demonstrate the role of vitamin D in regulating breast cancer cell proliferation and differentiation [41]; and (3) rodents exposed to carcinogens have fewer mammary tumors when administered vitamin D [42]. Unfortunately, more recent nested cohort studies in postmenopausal women suggest no strong association between breast cancer risk and circulating levels of vitamin D [40,43].

The International Agency for Research on Cancer (IARC) 2008 report on vitamin D and cancer concluded that studies on vitamin D intake and risk of breast cancer were generally negative for a protective role, particularly for postmenopausal women [44]. Similarly, using a cohort of postmenopausal women from the prospective prostate, lung, colorectal, and ovarian cancer screening trial, with an average age at serum collection of 62 years, no significant association between vitamin D and breast cancer for the top versus bottom quintile was discovered for either the active form of vitamin D or its precursor [43]. These results did not differ when stratified by age. A similar study using women from the prospective Cancer Prevention Study-II Nutrition Cohort reported no association between the vitamin D precursor and breast cancer for the top versus bottom quintile [40], with an average age at serum collection of 69 years. In a 2010 editorial on a series of epidemiological papers showing a lack of inverse association between vitamin D levels and six types of rarer cancer, the author emphasized that vitamin D may be teaching us the same lesson taught by vitamins A, B, C, and E; namely, that supernutritional levels of vitamins may do more harm than good [45].

While acknowledging the inconsistent results observed between vitamin D intake or blood levels and breast cancer risk, Goodwin recommends that oncologists aim for at least adequate levels of vitamin D in their breast cancer patients, with monitoring via regular measurement of blood levels [46]. This recommendation seems reasonable to apply to postmenopausal women at risk for breast cancer as well, especially given the evidence for improved bone health associated with vitamin D supplementation.

5.2.5 Alcohol

To date, the only dietary factor consistently associated with increased breast cancer risk is alcohol [47], with 13% of breast cancers attributed to alcohol, and an increase in incidence of ~11 cases per 1000 women up to age 75 years for each additional daily drink regularly consumed in the Million Women Study [48]. Pooled and meta-analyses that include scores of studies and tens of thousands of women report increases of 7–12% for each 10-g/day increment of alcohol consumed, supporting a dose–response relationship [48–50]. As noted in Table 5.1, the association between alcohol consumption and breast cancer is independent of age [48–50]. Alcohol intake has even been demonstrated to increase breast cancer risk in women positive for BRCA1 mutations [51]. Neither menopausal status, age, type of alcoholic beverage, nor HRT use modifies the impact of alcohol on breast cancer risk [48,49].

A number of mechanisms have been proposed to explain this association, including stimulation of the metabolism of carcinogens such as acetaldehyde, increases in concentrations of sex hormones [48], and interference with folate absorption and metabolism [19,33]. This latter factor increases an individual's dietary requirement for folic acid, and adequate folate intake has been shown to reduce or eliminate the excess risk due to alcohol consumption [47,52]. Several studies have reported that alcohol consumption is

TABLE 5.2 Study of Tamoxifen and Raloxifene P-2 Trial[a]

	Tamoxifen $N = 9736$ (%)	Raloxifene $N = 9754$ (%)	Relative Risk (P Value) Tamoxifen	Raloxifene
Invasive breast cancer	247 (2.5)	310 (3.2)	1.24	0.01
DCIS	111 (1.1)	137 (1.4)	1.22	0.12
Annual risk uterine cancer/1000 patients	2.25	1.23	0.55	0.003
Thromboembolism	202 (2.1)	154 (1.6)	0.55	0.007

[a] With 81-month average follow-up.

Source: Vogel et al. [59].

associated with an increased amount of mammographically dense tissue in the breast, an increasingly recognized risk factor for breast cancer [49,53]. A lack of association observed between alcohol use and the risk of ductal carcinoma *in situ* (DCIS) (whether of low or high grade) suggests that alcohol may have an effect later in the carcinogenic process [54].

5.3 PHARMACOLOGIC PREVENTION

The lifestyle modifications to prevent breast cancer apply to all women as they age. Candidates for pharmacologic prevention are limited to those at very high risk (see Table 5.3). The selective estrogen receptor modulators (SERMs) tamoxifen and raloxifene have been extensively studied in randomized clinical trials as preventive agents for early-stage breast cancer [55]. A meta-analysis of four randomized trials that included more than 12,000 patients assessed the role of tamoxifen as a preventive agent and showed a combined reduction in the risk of invasive and *in situ* cancer of 34–38%, independent of age [56]. The risk reduction was limited to patients with estrogen-receptor-positive (ER$^+$) tumors, and no risk reduction was seen for those with estrogen-receptor-negative (ER$^-$) tumors. The largest of these trials, the National Surgical Adjuvant Breast and Bowel Project (NSABP) P-1 study included 13,388 women with a five year risk of breast cancer of ≥1.66% [57]. Of note, 6% of the women in this trial were 70 years and older, and the risk reduction for invasive cancer was 55% in women 60 years and older.

Because of the major risk reductions in invasive breast cancer noted for the SERM raloxifene in osteoporosis trials, and a lower risk of endometrial cancer compared to tamoxifen, the NSABP P-2 STAR (study of tamoxifen and raloxifene) trial randomized 19,747 women to tamoxifen or raloxifene [58]. Initial results showed the treatments to be similar for breast cancer incidence. There were less cases of uterine cancer,

TABLE 5.3   Net Benefit/Risk for 10,000 Patients Using Tamoxifen for Prevention of Invasive Breast Cancer[a]

5-Year Estimated Risk of Invasive Breast Cancer (%)	Caucasian Women		Black Women	
	Age 60–69	Age 70–79	Age 60–69	Age 70–79
Intact Uterus				
2	−232	−355	−414	−513
4	−119	−242	−302	−373
6	−9	−132	−191	−262
7	47	−77	−137	−208
No Uterus				
2	−26	−132	−288	−366
4	87[b]	−19	−176	−254
6	198[c]	92*	−65	−143
7	253[c]	146*	−11	−89

[a]Negative numbers indicate that life-threatening event exceeds benefit.
[b]Weak evidence that benefit exceeds risk.
[c]Strong evidence that benefit exceeds risk.
Source: Modified from Gail et al. [60].

less thromboembolic episodes, and less cataracts in the raloxifene treated patients. The risk of strokes and fractures were similar. In a more recent update of these data [59], tamoxifen was significantly better than raloxifene in reducing the risk of invasive breast cancer but was associated with significantly more endometrial cancer and cataracts (see Table 5.2).

Despite the dramatic risk reductions for these agents, no survival advantage to date has been demonstrated. Moreover, major concerns about toxicity, especially for tamoxifen, have likely hindered the adoption of these agents into routine clinical practice. A detailed analysis by Gail and colleagues was undertaken to develop tools in which clinicians might identify women where the benefits of tamoxifen outweighed the risks [60]. The model included age, race, and specific factors related to breast cancer risk, and also included the absolute risks for tamoxifen of endometrial cancer, stroke, pulmonary embolism, deep-vein thrombosis, and fractures. Key variables in this model are race (as black women have higher risks of non–breast cancer illness than whites) and the risk of endometrial cancer. Estimated benefits and risks by age 60 years and older and hysterectomy status are presented in Table 5.3. For almost all white and black women with an intact uterus, the risks of tamoxifen exceed the projected benefits, while only white women who have had a hysterectomy derive benefit. The benefit/risk profile for raloxifene is likely to be better than for tamoxifen, but such a model is currently lacking. These data suggest that few older patients will derive major benefits from currently available SERM therapy for prevention of breast cancer; the exception is older white women at higher risk who have undergone hysterectomy. Older patients with osteoporosis might be considered for raloxifene therapy especially if their breast cancer risk over a 5-year period is high [61,62]. For most older patients, pharmacologic therapy with either tamoxifen or raloxifene is not indicated.

Aromatase inhibitors (AIs) may prove to be useful in this setting and are currently being studied as preventive agents in the IBIS II trial, a large randomized placebo-controlled study of anastrozole versus placebo [63]. At this time AIs should not be used outside of a clinical trial. Other potential agents that might reduce risk include aspirin and other nonsteroidal anti-inflammatory agents. Data are conflicting however and such drugs may have higher toxicity risks in older women [65,66]. To date, no agents have been found effective in reducing the risks of hormone receptor negative breast cancer.

5.4 SURGICAL PREVENTION

Older women with a family history of breast cancer should be considered for genetic counseling and genetic testing if appropriate. Those positive for BRCA1/2 mutations may be candidates for prophylactic mastectomy and bilateral salpingoophorectomy. Although such treatment may be considered drastic for many elders, those with expected life expectancies exceeding 5–10 years might have survival benefit from such procedures [64].

5.5 CONCLUSIONS

As women age, their physicians should stress the importance of weight control, exercise, and alcohol in moderation not just to decrease their risk of cardiovascular disease and diabetes, but breast cancer as well. Data do not support strong associations between levels of fat, fruit, or vegetable intake, or low intake and/or blood levels of vitamins, including vitamin D, and breast cancer risk. However, maintaining at least normal blood levels of vitamin D with supplementation if necessary seems reasonable, especially considering the known benefits of vitamin D for bone health. Decreasing the amount of processed meat and increasing the amount of flaxseed in the diet may help reduce risk. Pharmacologic agents such as tamoxifen and raloxifene should be considered only in older women at extremely high risk and who have a reasonable life expectancy.

Inherent in all these decisions is the effect of any of these interventions on quality of life as well as the patient's general level of health. For frail patients and those with short life expectancy most of these interventions, with the exception of exercise and preventing excessive weight gain, are unlikely to improve quality of life or life expectancy. The following recommendations apply for primary prevention of breast cancer in healthy older women:

1. Adhere to a healthy diet with generous helpings of fruits and vegetables.
2. Maintain a normal weight for age, and avoid weight gain.
3. Supplement diet with vitamin D to maintain normal range.
4. Minimize alcohol intake to several drinks weekly.
5. Exercise on a regular basis.

These recommendations promote healthy lifestyles in older patients irrespective of cancer risk. Administration of tamoxifen or raloxifene should be considered only for women at very high risk.

ACKNOWLEDGMENT

The authors wish to thank Ms. Ronda Hefner for her assistance in preparation of this manuscript.

REFERENCES

1. National Cancer Institute. *Surveillance Epidemiology and End Results Cancer Statistics Review*, NCI, Bethesda, MD, 2008 (available at http://seer.cancer.gov/csr/1975_2005/results_merged/sect_04_breast.pdf).

2. National Cancer Institute. *SEER Cancer Statistics Review, 1975-2004 NCI*, Bethesda, MD, 2007 [based on Nov. 2006 SEER data submission, posted to SEER website, 2007 (computer program); http://seer.cancer.gov.csr/1975_2004/].

3. Diab SG, Elledge RM, Clark GM. Tumor characteristics and clinical outcome of elderly women with breast cancer. *J Natl Cancer Inst* 2000;**92**(7):550–556.

4. Eppenberger-Castori S, Moore DH, Jr., Thor AD, et al. Age-associated biomarker profiles of human breast cancer. *Int J Biochem Cell Biol* 2002;**34**(11):1318–1330.

5. Tai P, Cserni G, Van De SJ, et al. Modeling the effect of age in T1-2 breast cancer using the SEER database. *BMC Cancer* 2005;**5**:130.

6. Rosenberg J, Chia YL, Plevritis S. The effect of age, race, tumor size, tumor grade, and disease stage on invasive ductal breast cancer survival in the U.S. SEER database. *Breast Cancer Res Treat* 2005;**89**(1):47–54.

7. Yancik R, Ganz PA, Varricchio CG, Conley B. Perspectives on comorbidity and cancer in older patients: Approaches to expand the knowledge base. *J Clin Oncol* 2001;**19**(4): 1147–1151.

8. *Breast Cancer Risk Assessment Tool* (available at `http://www.cancer.gov/bcrisktool/`; accessed 8/27/10).

9. Gail MH, Benichou J. Validation studies on a model for breast cancer risk. *J Natl Cancer Inst* 1994;**86**(8):573–575.

10. Gail MH, Mai PL. Comparing breast cancer risk assessment models. *J Natl Cancer Inst* 2010;**102**(10):665–668.

11. Altekruse SF, Kosary CL, Krapcho M, et al. *SEER Cancer Statistics Review, 1975–2007*, NCI, Bethesda, MD, 2010.

12. Cummings SR, Tice JA, Bauer S, et al. Prevention of breast cancer in postmenopausal women: Approaches to estimating and reducing risk. *J Natl Cancer Inst* 2009;**101**(6): 384–398.

13. Bernstein L. Exercise and breast cancer prevention. *Curr Oncol Rep.* 2009;**11**(6):490–496.

14. Huang Z, Hankinson SE, Colditz GA, et al. Dual effects of weight and weight gain on breast cancer risk. *JAMA* 1997;**278**(17):1407–1411.

15. World Cancer Research Fund, American Institute for Cancer Research *Food, Nutrition, Physical Activity, and the Prevention of Cancer: A Global Perspective*, Washington, DC, 2007.

16. Ahn J, Schatzkin A, Lacey JV, Jr., et al. Adiposity, adult weight change, and postmenopausal breast cancer risk. *Arch Intern.Med* 2007;**167**(19):2091–2102.

17. Renehan AG, Tyson M, Egger M, Heller RF, Zwahlen M. Body-mass index and incidence of cancer: A systematic review and meta-analysis of prospective observational studies. *Lancet* 2008;**371**(9612):569–578.

18. Willett WC, Talamini R, Hankinson SE, Hunter DJ, Colditz G. Nongenetic factors in the causation of breast cancer. In Harris JR, Marc EL, Monica M, Osborne CK, eds. *Diseases of the Breast*, Vol. 4, Lippincott Williams & Wilkins, Philadelphia, 2010.

19. Mahoney MC, Bevers T, Linos E, Willett WC. Opportunities and strategies for breast cancer prevention through risk reduction. *CA Cancer J Clin* 2008;**58**(6):347–371.

20. Morimoto LM, White E, Chen Z, et al. Obesity, body size, and risk of postmenopausal breast cancer: The women's health initiative (United States). *Cancer Causes Control* 2002;**13**(8):741–751.

21. Eliassen AH, Colditz GA, Rosner B, Willett WC, Hankinson SE. Adult weight change and risk of postmenopausal breast cancer. *JAMA* 2006;**296**(2):193–201.

22. Radimer KL, Ballard-Barbash R, Miller JS, et al. Weight change and the risk of late-onset breast cancer in the original Framingham cohort. *Nutr Cancer* 2004;**49**(1):7–13.

23. Feigelson HS, Jonas CR, Teras LR, Thun MJ, Calle EE. Weight gain, body mass index, hormone replacement therapy, and postmenopausal breast cancer in a large prospective study. *Cancer Epidemiol Biomark Prevent* 2004;**13**(2):220–224.

24. Harvie M, Howell A, Vierkant RA, et al. Association of gain and loss of weight before and after menopause with risk of postmenopausal breast cancer in the Iowa women's health study. *Cancer Epidemiol Biomark Prevent* 2005;**14**(3):656–661.

25. Friedenreich CM. The role of physical activity in breast cancer etiology. *Semin Oncol* 2010;**37**(3):297–302.

26. Korde LA, Micheli A, Smith AW, et al. Recruitment to a physical activity intervention study in women at increased risk of breast cancer. *BMC Med Res Methodol* 2009;**9**:27.

27. Monninkhof EM, Elias SG, Vlems FA, et al. Physical activity and breast cancer: A systematic review. *Epidemiology* 2007;**18**(1):137–157.

28. Friedenreich CM, Cust AE. Physical activity and breast cancer risk: Impact of timing, type and dose of activity and population subgroup effects. *Br J Sports Med* 2008;**42**(8):636–647.

29. Neilson HK, Friedenreich CM, Brockton NT, Millikan RC. Physical activity and postmenopausal breast cancer: Proposed biologic mechanisms and areas for future research. *Cancer Epidemiol Biomark Prevent* 2009;**18**(1):11–27.

30. Kabat GC, Kim M, Chlebowski RT, et al. A longitudinal study of the metabolic syndrome and risk of postmenopausal breast cancer. *Cancer Epidemiol Biomark Prevent* 2009;**18**(7):2046–2053.

31. Bjorge T, Lukanova A, Jonsson H, et al. Metabolic syndrome and breast cancer in the me-can (metabolic syndrome and cancer) project. *Cancer Epidemiol Biomark Prevent* 2010;**19**(7):1737–1745.

32. Agnoli C, Berrino F, Abagnato CA, et al. Metabolic syndrome and postmenopausal breast cancer in the ORDET cohort: A nested case-control study. *Nutr Metab Cardiovasc Dis* 2010;**20**(1):41–48.

33. Singletary SE. Rating the risk factors for breast cancer. *Ann Surg* 2003;**237**(4):474–482.

34. Monninkhof EM, Velthuis MJ, Peeters PH, Twisk JW, Schuit AJ. Effect of exercise on postmenopausal sex hormone levels and role of body fat: A randomized controlled trial. *J Clin Oncol* 2009;**27**(27):4492–4499.

35. Friedenreich CM, Woolcott CG, McTiernan A, et al. Alberta physical activity and breast cancer prevention trial: sex hormone changes in a year-long exercise intervention among postmenopausal women. *J Clin Oncol* 2010;**28**:1458–1466.

36. Woolcott CG, Courneya KS, Boyd NF, et al. Mammographic density change with 1 year of aerobic exercise among postmenopausal women: A randomized controlled trial. *Cancer Epidemiol Biomark Prevent* 2010;**19**(4):1112–1121.

37. Michels KB, Mohllajee AP, Roset-Bahmanyar E, Beehler GP, Moysich KB. Diet and breast cancer: A review of the prospective observational studies. *Cancer* 2007;**109**(12 Suppl):2712–2749.

38. Pala V, Krogh V, Berrino F, et al. Meat, eggs, dairy products, and risk of breast cancer in the European Prospective Investigation into Cancer and Nutrition (EPIC) cohort. *Am J Clin Nutr* 2009;**90**(3):602–612.

39. Buck K, Zaineddin AK, Vrieling A, Linseisen J, Chang-Claude J. Meta-analyses of lignans and enterolignans in relation to breast cancer risk. *Am J Clin Nutr* 2010;**92**(1):141–153.

40. McCullough ML, Stevens VL, Patel R, et al. Serum 25-hydroxyvitamin D concentrations and postmenopausal breast cancer risk: A nested case control study in the Cancer Prevention Study-II Nutrition Cohort. *Breast Cancer Res* 2009;**11**(4):R64.

41. Welsh J, Wietzke JA, Zinser GM, Byrne B, Smith K, Narvaez CJ. Vitamin D-3 receptor as a target for breast cancer prevention. *J Nutr* 2003;**133**(7 Suppl):2425S–2433S.

42. Welsh J. Vitamin D and breast cancer: Insights from animal models. *Am J Clin Nutr* 2004;**80**(6 Suppl):1721S–1724S.

43. Freedman DM, Chang SC, Falk RT, et al. Serum levels of vitamin D metabolites and breast cancer risk in the prostate, lung, colorectal, and ovarian cancer screening trial. *Cancer Epidemiol Biomark Prevent* 2008;**17**(4):889–894.

44. Working Group R. *Vitamin D and Cancer*, Vol. 5, International Agency for Research on Cancer, Lyon, France, 2008.

45. Byers T. Anticancer vitamins du jour—the ABCED's so far. *Am J Epidemiol* 2010;**172**(1):1–3.

46. Goodwin PJ. Vitamin D in cancer patients: Above all, do no harm. *J Clin Oncol* 2009;**27**(13):2117–2119.

47. Larsson SC, Giovannucci E, Wolk A. Folate and risk of breast cancer: A meta-analysis. *J Natl Cancer Inst* 2007;**99**(1):64–76.

48. Allen NE, Beral V, Casabonne D, et al. Moderate alcohol intake and cancer incidence in women. *J Natl Cancer Inst* 2009;**101**(5):296–305.

49. Key J, Hodgson S, Omar RZ, et al. Meta-analysis of studies of alcohol and breast cancer with consideration of the methodological issues. *Cancer Causes Control* 2006;**17**(6):759–770.

50. Hamajima N, Hirose K, Tajima K, et al. Alcohol, tobacco and breast cancer—collaborative reanalysis of individual data from 53 epidemiological studies, including 58,515 women with breast cancer and 95,067 women without the disease. *Br J Cancer* 2002;**87**(11):1234–1245.

51. Moorman PG, Iversen ES, Marcom PK, et al. Evaluation of established breast cancer risk factors as modifiers of BRCA1 or BRCA2: A multi-center case-only analysis. *Breast Cancer Res Treat* 2010;**124**(2):441–451.

52. Zhang SM, Willett WC, Selhub J, et al. Plasma folate, vitamin B6, vitamin B12, homocysteine, and risk of breast cancer. *J Natl Cancer Inst* 2003;**95**(5):373–380.

53. Vachon CM, Kuni CC, Anderson K, Anderson VE, Sellers TA. Association of mammographically defined percent breast density with epidemiologic risk factors for breast cancer (United States). *Cancer Causes Control* 2000;**11**(7):653–662.

54. Kabat GC, Kim M, Shikany JM, et al. Alcohol consumption and risk of ductal carcinoma *in situ* of the breast in a cohort of postmenopausal women. *Cancer Epidemiol Biomark Prevent* 2010;**19**(8):2066–2072.

55. Visvanathan K, Chlebowski RT, Hurley P, et al. American society of clinical oncology clinical practice guideline update on the use of pharmacologic interventions including tamoxifen, raloxifene, and aromatase inhibition for breast cancer risk reduction. *J Clin Oncol* 2009;**27**(19):3235–3258.

56. Cuzick J, Powles T, Veronesi U, et al. Overview of the main outcomes in breast-cancer prevention trials. *Lancet* 2003;**361**(9354):296–300.

57. Fisher B, Costantino JP, Wickerham DL, et al. Tamoxifen for prevention of breast cancer: Report of the National Surgical Adjuvant Breast and Bowel Project P-1 Study. *J Natl Cancer Inst* 1998;**90**(18):1371–1388.

58. Vogel VG, Costantino JP, Wickerham DL, et al. Effects of tamoxifen vs raloxifene on the risk of developing invasive breast cancer and other disease outcomes: The NSABP Study of Tamoxifen and Raloxifene (STAR) P-2 trial. *JAMA* 2006;**295**(23):2727–2741.

59. Vogel VG, Costantino JP, Wickerham DL, et al. Update of the National Surgical Adjuvant Breast and Bowel Project Study of Tamoxifen and Raloxifene (STAR) P-2 Trial: Preventing breast cancer. *Cancer Prevent Res* 2010;**3**(6):696–706.

60. Gail MH, Costantino JP, Bryant J, et al. Weighing the risks and benefits of tamoxifen treatment for preventing breast cancer. *J Natl Cancer Inst* 1999;**91**(21):1829–1846.

61. Cummings SR, Eckert S, Krueger KA, et al. The effect of raloxifene on risk of breast cancer in postmenopausal women: Results from the MORE randomized trial. Multiple Outcomes of Raloxifene Evaluation. *JAMA* 1999;**281**(23):2189–2197.

62. Martino S, Disch D, Dowsett SA, Keech CA, Mershon JL. Safety assessment of raloxifene over eight years in a clinical trial setting. *Curr Med Res Opin* 2005;**21**(9):1441–1452.

63. Cuzick J. IBIS II: A breast cancer prevention trial in postmenopausal women using the aromatase inhibitor anastrozole. *Expert Rev Anticancer Ther* 2008;**8**(9):1377–1385.

64. Domchek SM, Friebel TM, Singer CF, et al. Association of risk-reducing surgery in BRCA1 or BRCA2 mutation carriers with cancer risk and mortality. *JAMA* 2010;**304**(9):967–975.

65. Eliassen AH, Chen WY, Spiegelman D, Willett WC, Hunter DJ, Hankinson SE. Use of aspirin, other nonsteroidal anti-inflammatory drugs, and acetaminophen and risk of breast cancer among premenopausal women in the Nurses' Health Study II. *Arch Intern Med* 2009;**169**(2):115–121; discussion 121.

66. Zhao YS, Zhu S, Li XW, et al. Association between NSAIDs use and breast cancer risk: A systematic review and meta-analysis. *Breast Cancer Res Treat* 2009;**117**(1):141–150.

CHAPTER 6

Colorectal Cancer Prevention and Aging

ERNEST T. HAWK, SHERRI L. PATTERSON, and LOPA MISHRA

University of Texas MD Anderson Cancer Center, Houston, TX

KUSH K. PATEL

Virginia Commonwealth University, Richmond, VA

6.1   INTRODUCTION

Colorectal cancer (CRC) refers to cancers of the colon or rectum. The American Cancer Society predicted that over 140,000 new cases of CRC would be diagnosed in 2010 and over 50,000 people would die from the disease by the end of that year [1]. This makes colorectal cancer the second leading cause of death from cancer in adults. While these numbers are significant, the death rate from the disease has actually been declining since the 1980s. This is due partly to improved screening methods that lead to the detection of precancerous lesions or localized early-stage cancers that are amenable to curative excision. Despite this progress, stricter adherence to screening guidelines coupled with prevention strategies are needed to continue to drive the downward trend in incidence and death rates in CRC.

One strategy that has gained prominence for CRC prevention is cancer chemoprevention, which strives to block, reverse, or delay carcinogenesis prior to the development of invasive disease by targeting key molecular derangements with pharmacologic or nutritional agents. Chemopreventive interventions may be applied at any time during carcinogenesis, from the initial molecular defect through the accumulated molecular, cellular, and histopathologic aberrations that characterize disease progression prior to an invasive and potentially metastatic stage.

6.2   COLORECTAL CARCINOGENSIS

Colorectal tumors arise from modulation of multiple genes by mutations, epigenetic regulation, glycosylation, and microRNAs from benign to advanced cancer over a 17-year period yet generally require less than 2 years to metastasize [3]. Loss of the adenomatous polyposis coli (APC) gene (75–80%), activation of Wnt signaling, cyclin D1, c-myc, telomerase, concurrent with TGFβ type II receptor mutations in >80% of microsatellite instability positive CRCs, Smad4 mutations in (16–25% CRCs), K-RAS and TP53, and deletion on chromosome 18q, N-acetylgalactosaminyltransferase 12 (GALNT12), are required for subsequent tumor progression [2–7]. Hereditary cancer syndromes have provided powerful insights into our understanding of somatic mutations present in sporadic cancers, as well as implicated cell signaling pathways [8–11]. One example is the identification of germline, inactivating mutations in the APC gene, that encodes a 300-kD Wnt pathway adaptor protein [8,11]. Although germline mutations in APC are responsible for familial adenomatous polyposis (FAP), a rare condition affecting about 1 in 7000 individuals in the United States, somatic mutations in the APC gene are present in more than 70% of colonic adenomatous polyps and carcinoma [11]. Hereditary nonpolyposis colon cancer (HNPCC), or Lynch syndrome, involves a germline mutation in one of the DNA mismatch repair (MMR) genes, leading to defective DNA repair. Beckwith–Wiedemann syndrome (BWS) is a hereditary stem cell cancer syndrome currently linked to deregulation of an imprinted cluster on human chromosome 11p15 [6,12]. BWS is associated with an 800-fold increased risk of embryonal neoplasms of childhood and to a lesser extent, CRC. More recent studies identifying inactivation of TGFβ signaling through loss of the Smad3 adaptor β2Spectrin could potentially provide new insights into CRC development from stemlike tumor initiating cells (STICs), and targeted chemoprevention [12–14]. While over 90% of tumors are considered to be clonal and arise from a STIC, the precise identification and mechanism for STIC formation remain poorly understood [10,15–23]. Several potential markers of STIC stem cells have been proposed including CD133, CD44, musahi 1 (Msi1), DCAMLK1 (also known as DCLK1), β1 integrin subunit, EphB receptors, and most recently, Lgr5, CD44, CD34, and epithelium-specific antigen (ESA) [24–31]. Moreover, a functional role for TGFβ signaling in the intestinal stem cell niche has been demonstrated by the association of SMAD4 and BMPR1A/ALK3 mutations with human juvenile polyposis syndrome [7,12,32–36]. Studies delineating key functional pathways in colorectal STIC formation could help us effectively prevent the disease in the future. This could lead to simple strategies. For example, it is possible for vitamin D to be rendered efficacious in certain settings, such as loss of the tumor suppressor TGFβ pathway and activation of the Wnt signaling [37]. The rapid advent of relatively inexpensive whole-genome sequencing could in the future enable us to detect early colorectal cancer and treat it effectively, potentially reducing adverse events as well as the burden of cost of later disease treatment.

6.3 EVALUATION OF POTENTIAL PREVENTIVE MEASURES

6.3.1 Dietary Chemoprevention Agents

Antioxidants Antioxidants are substances or nutrients that can prevent or slow the oxidative damage to cells from free radicals. Antioxidant vitamins and minerals are commonly found in most fruits and vegetables. Some antioxidants, such as carotenoids (vitamin A precursors), retinoids (vitamin A), ascorbic acid, α-tocopherol (vitamin E), and selenium, can neutralize free radicals, thus reducing intrinsic oxidative and carcinogen-induced DNA damage. Certain studies also suggest that antioxidants may boost the immune system, resulting in the inhibition of tumorigenesis.

Although antioxidant supplementation was a compelling early hypothesis for colorectal cancer prevention, four large, well-controlled clinical trials conducted over an extended period of time failed to confirm the preventive efficacy of antioxidants against adenoma or cancer incidence [38–42]. The largest of these trials involved more than 15,000 Finnish male smokers who were administered α-tocopherol, β-carotene, or both for several years. Surprisingly, this trial reported a statistically significant 66% increase in colorectal adenomas in the α-tocopherol group compared to those who did not receive α-tocopherol [41].

The National Cancer Institute (NCI) guidelines for colorectal cancer prevention report that there is inadequate evidence to suggest that a diet high in fruits and vegetables decreases the risk of CRC, although diets rich in fruits and vegetables are recommended to promote overall health. Perhaps the most definitive analysis of their effects on CRC prevention to date is a study that examined dietary intake data based on food frequency questionnaires from 88,764 women in the Nurses' Health Study and 47,325 men in the Health Professionals Follow-up Study. The study included a total of 1,743,645 person-years of follow-up, 937 cases of colon cancer, and 244 cases of rectal cancer. On the basis of analyses adjusted for numerous covariates, the authors found no association in women or men between overall fruit and vegetable consumption and risk of colon or rectal cancer [43]. These data suggest that there is no solid relation between the use of antioxidants and CRC prevention. To what extent does the validity of the food frequency questionnaire affect the results?

The chemopreventive effect of selenium supplementation as a secondary endpoint was tested in a placebo-controlled, randomized trial of 1312 persons with a history of skin cancer. It was seen in this trial that a statistically significant 58% reduction in CRC incidence occurred among individuals randomized to selenium supplementation [44]. In 2006, a study published on selenium's effects on prevalent colorectal adenomas found significant reduced risks among the subsets of subjects with either a low baseline selenium level or among current smokers [45]. However, a placebo-controlled trial involving 35,533 men failed to identify protective effects of selenium or vitamin E supplementation on the risk of colorectal, prostate, or other cancers [46].

Folate and Methionine   Folate is a vitamin commonly found in leafy green vegetables and fresh fruits. Methionine, on the other hand, is an amino acid that can be found in red meat, chicken, and fish. Folate and methionine both supply methyl groups necessary for DNA synthesis and gene expression. Therefore, diets deficient in folate or methionine may contribute to colorectal carcinogenesis by impairing DNA synthesis, repair, or transcriptional expression [47].

Studies on folate have reported different conclusions for its efficacy in preventing cancer. One study found that higher energy-adjusted folate intake in the form of multivitamins containing folic acid was related to a lower risk for colon cancer for intake of more than 400 μg/day compared with intake of ≤200 μg/day [48]. A clinical trial conducted in 1021 men and women to assess the safety and efficacy of folic supplementation for preventing colorectal adenomas found that folic acid at 1 mg/day does not reduce colorectal adenoma risk [49]. It was even seen in this trial that there was a 67% higher risk of developing at least one advanced adenoma after two cycles of colonoscopy and a higher risk of multiple adenomas with the intake of folic acid (1 mg/day). Therefore, studies to date do not demonstrate that folate has chemopreventive potential as initially suspected, but that it might even promote colorectal neoplasia. These data highlight the importance of developing definitive data through randomized, controlled trials before making definitive inferences based on observational data alone.

Calcium Carbonate and Vitamin D   Calcium is a mineral that is required by the body for several major functions such as muscle contraction, blood vessel expansion and contraction, secretion of hormones and enzymes, and transmitting impulses throughout the nervous system. Vitamin D is a fat-soluble vitamin obtained from sun exposure, food, and dietary supplements and is important for promoting the absorption of calcium in the gut. Secondary bile acids may play an important role in colorectal carcinogenesis. Calcium binds bile and fatty acids in the form of insoluble soaps, which effectively sequester these mutagenic substances from harmful contact with epithelial cells. In addition, calcium may directly inhibit epithelial proliferation within the colorectum by modulating protein kinase C activity, stabilizing membranes, or modifying K-*ras* mutations.

Substantial data exist demonstrating that vitamin D levels are suboptimal in many Americans and that vitamin D deficiency is pervasive in the aged, with prevalence estimates ranging from 40% to 100% in this subset of the population, placing them at increased risk for falls, cardiovascular disease, immunologic impairments, and several types of cancer [50]. Although there is substantial evidence of increased CRC risk and overall mortality associated with vitamin D deficiency, there is not yet clear evidence that supplementation can reverse these risks; however, this suggestion has been made [51]. This underscores the need for randomized trials of vitamin D supplementation in aging populations.

Many different studies and trials have suggested an inverse association between calcium intake and CRC risk. A randomized placebo-controlled trial that tested the effect of calcium supplementation (3 g calcium carbonate daily) on the risk of recurrent adenoma found a modest decrease in the risk of developing at least one recurrent adenoma and in developing an average number of adenomas [52]. This study supports the suggested inverse relationship between calcium intake and CRC risk.

The chemopreventive properties of vitamin D may relate to its ability to modulate both calcium absorption and gene expression. A large epidemiological study of the American Cancer Society cohort reported a 29% reduction in CRC risk among individuals with the highest vitamin D intakes from dietary or supplemental sources [53]. A review of published observational studies found that a daily intake of 1000 IU (international units) of vitamin D and a concentration of serum 25-hydroxyvitamin D [25(OH)D] of 33 ng/mL were each associated with 50% lower risk of CRC [54]. A large, placebo-controlled trial of vitamin D and calcium in men and women between the ages of 45 and 75 years with prior adenomas is ongoing; this should provide the best evidence of the benefits and risks associated with vitamin D supplementation for CRC prevention.

Dietary Fiber   *Fiber* is crudely defined as the dietary fraction that is resistant to human digestion and absorption. Fiber may increase stool bulk and stimulate intestinal transit, thereby reducing epithelial exposure to intraluminal carcinogens. Dietary fiber also reduces procarcinogenic secondary bile acids and increases the concentration of shortchain fatty acids.

Many studies have shown dietary fiber supplementation to have an inverse relationship with colorectal cancer risk. A meta-analysis of 13 case–control studies from nine countries concluded that intake of fiber-rich foods is inversely related to cancers of both the colon and the rectum [55]. This emphasizes that a diet high in fiber leads to a lower risk of colorectal cancer. In concordance, a nested case–control study also showed that intake of dietary fiber is inversely associated with colorectal cancer risk [56]. However, two randomized, controlled trials of wheat bran fiber or a more profound dietary change involving increases in fiber, fruit, and vegetable intake as well as reduced fat failed to demonstrate reductions in recurrent adenomas over a period of several years [57,58]. Thus, to date (early 2012), the effects of fiber supplementation in reducing CRC risks have not been proved in randomized trials.

Nevertheless, the European Prospective Investigation into Cancer and nutrition (EPIC) study, which enrolled over 366,000 women and 153,000 men between the ages of 35 and 70 years, also described a significant (40%) risk reduction in CRC in those who consumed the highest versus lowest quintiles of dietary fiber, particularly for left-sided cancers, and after controlling for several potential confounders [59,60].

Polyunsaturated Fatty Acids Preclinical, clinical, and observational studies suggest that some polyunsaturated fatty acids (PUFAs), specifically ω_3, could be protective against a number of cancers, including colorectal cancer. The ω_3 fatty acids eicosapentaenoic acid (EPA) and docosahexaenoic acid (DHA) are of particular interest because they have been shown to reduce biomarkers of proliferation and inflammation in both prospective observational studies as well as short-term clinical trials [61]. By contrast, ω_6 fatty acids, found primarily in oils and animal products, are thought to be proinflammatory and therefore contribute to carcinogenesis.

Over 20,000 men between the ages of 40 and 84 years participating in the Physician's Health Study (PHS) were followed for 22 years, and their intake of fish and n-3 ω_3 fatty acid were collected via food frequency questionnaire. Results from this long-term prospective study demonstrated that ω_3 fatty acid intake may decrease the risk for colorectal cancer by as much as 40% [62]. A more recently completed randomized clinical trial comparing enteric-coated EPA versus placebo demonstrated that EPA (2 g qd × 6 months) in patients with familial adenomatous polyposis (FAP) significantly reduced rectal polyp burden (both size and number) without increasing cardiovascular risks [63].

In summary, ω_3 shows promise for both its cardiovascular and cancer prevention properties in the aging population.

6.3.2 Physical Activity

Obesity and inactivity have been associated with increased insulin resistance, which, in turn, can lead to increased serum insulin, glucose, and fatty acid levels, which can promote inflammation. Inflammation, in turn, can stimulate proliferation, inhibit apoptosis, and promote oxidative damage [64]. However, physical activity can have dramatic protective effects on the cancer. A large meta-analysis of 52 studies estimated that regular physical activity can reduce risk of colorectal cancer by 30–40%, although precisely how much, how often, and what type of exercise are required is unclear [65].

6.3.3 Pharmaceutical Agents

Nonsteroidal Antiinflammatory Drugs (NSAIDs) and COX2 Inhibitors (COXIBs) Nonsteroidal antiinflammatory drugs, or NSAIDs, are medications used primarily to treat inflammation, mild to moderate pain, and fever. Among the agents currently under investigation for the prevention of CRC, NSAIDs are the most compelling in terms of the volume, variety, and consistency of preliminary data.

Indeed, NSAIDs have been shown to exert protective effects against all clinical stages of colorectal neoplasia. The best-described activity of NSAIDs relates to the inhibition of either or both cyclooxygenase enzymes (COX1 and COX2). COX catalyzes the conversion of arachidonic acid into bioactive eicosanoids, including prostaglandins and lipoxygenases. COX2 overexpression is a common feature of colorectal preinvasive and invasive neoplasia. By inhibiting one or both COX enzymes, NSAIDs may reduce proliferation, induce apoptosis, promote immunologic surveillance, or inhibit neoangiogenesis.

There is encouraging evidence that aspirin or other NSAIDs could play a major role in CRC prevention. One randomized trial had 635 CRC survivors between the ages of 30 and 80 years assigned to 325 mg/day of aspirin versus placebo. After a median followup of 12.8 months, the study showed a significant reduction in the number of patients with incident adenomas and a significant delay in the time to a first adenoma among patients randomized to aspirin [66]. Another study randomized 1121 patients with prior colorectal adenomas to aspirin 81 or 325 mg/day versus placebo and reported 19% and 4% reductions, respectively, in the number of people with one or more adenomas [67]. The reason for the inverse dose response seen in this study is unknown.

Numerous literature reviews including one compiled by the NCI report that several epidemiological studies have identified a reduction in colon cancer incidence associated with the use of aspirin. In a report from the Health Professionals Follow-up Study of 47,000 males, regular use of aspirin (at least 2 times per week) was associated with a 30% overall reduction in CRC, including a 50% reduction in advanced cases [68].

Some trials have targeted COX enzymes. One trial that looked at the effect of aspirin on colorectal cancers overexpressing COX2 found that regular use of aspirin appears to reduce the risk of these specific cancers. It found, however, that the use of aspirin did not reduce the risk of colorectal cancers with weak or absent expression of COX2 [69]. Other trials have used COX2-selective inhibitors (COXIBs) for chemoprevention. One randomized, controlled trial in patients at very high risk due to inherited *APC* gene mutations, showed a mean 28% reduction in the number of colorectal adenomas among patients who were administered 400 mg of celecoxib twice a day over a 6-month period [70]. Two large, placebo-controlled trials of celecoxib in patients with prior sporadic adenomas also demonstrated significant reductions in recurrent adenomas, but a concomitant increase in serious cardiovascular events associated with treatment, primarily among patients at increased risk for CV disease at baseline [71–73]. The FDA has required a blackbox warning, named as such for the blackbox that appears around the text on the agent packaging, alerting consumers and healthcare professionals alike of these risks. Risk of adverse events increases in patients 65 and older, especially those taking concomitant aspirin.

More recently, investigators have pursued curcumin, a popular Indian spice, as a dietary antiinflammatory agent with chemopreventive potential owing to its ability to reduce proliferation, increase apoptosis, reduce neoangiogenesis, and blunt cell signaling through COX2 inhibition and other actions [74]. These mechanistic actions, combined with observational and preclinical data, suggest that its chemopreventive effects against colorectal neoplasia have been compelling. A few clinical studies have been done confirming curcumin's anticancer activity; however, the optimal form of the agent, dose, and administration schedule have not been decided [74,75].

Hormone Replacement Therapy Hormone replacement therapy for women who have reached menopause involves taking small doses of female hormones, such as estrogen and progesterone, in an attempt to mitigate the effects of estrogen loss (e.g., osteoporosis, hot flashes, sexual effects). Dozens of epidemiological studies have explored possible associations between exogenous estrogens (alone or in combination with progestins) and colorectal neoplasia risk. One of the more definitive trials was the NIH-sponsored Women's Health Initiative. In this trial, 16,608 postmenopausal women aged 50 79 years were randomly assigned to a combination of conjugated equine estrogens (0.625 mg/day) plus medroxyprogesterone (2.5 mg/day) or placebo. There were 43 invasive CRCs in the hormone group and 72 in the placebo group. The study concluded that short-term use of estrogen plus progestin was associated with a decreased risk of colorectal cancer [76]. Several studies have noted that protective effects against colorectal neoplasia wane after cessation of hormone replacement therapy, and this further supports a chemopreventive role for estrogen [77,78].

Statins Statins are cholesterol lowering drugs that have been proved in randomized controlled trials to prevent cardiac events. Some evidence suggests that they may significantly reduce the risk of CRC, and possibly of other cancers, as well [79]. However, a meta-analysis of studies concerning statins and cancer risk failed to identify an effect of statins on the risk of cancer and cancer mortality in randomized controlled trials [80]. A second study also shows that statin use neither increases nor decreases the incidence or mortality of CRC [81].

6.3.4 Smoking Cessation

The benefits of quitting smoking to overall health cannot be overstated. However, the exact association between smoking and colorectal cancer is still under debate. A meta-analysis of 106 observational studies was performed by a group of researchers to determine whether an association exists between smoking and colorectal cancer. The analysis found that smoking was associated with an absolute risk increase of 10.8 cases per 100,000 person-years. There was also a risk increase in patients who smoked higher numbers of packs or cigarettes a day. Overall, the study concluded that cigarette smoking is significantly associated with colorectal cancer incidence and mortality.

6.4 CONCLUSIONS

So, what can be recommended to reduce an older American's risk of colorectal cancer? The recommendations largely fall in line with what can be recommended for the general population. First, it is important to consume a diet that is varied, with an emphasis on fruits and vegetables (at least five servings per day), and limited in red and processed meats. It is also helpful to exercise regularly for at least 30 min per day, so long as the individual has no physical limitations or health concerns that would argue against it. Given the prevalence of vitamin D deficiency in the aged, it would be appropriate to have blood concentrations checked, and, if necessary, vitamin D supplementation. For women, calcium supplementation may be in order to maintain bone health, as well as for its effects in reducing colorectal neoplasia risk. Eating fish, high in ω_3 fatty acids, at least twice per week is recommended by the American Heart Association for cardioprotection and may hold the additional benefit of offering some safeguard against colorectal cancer.

Although aspirin cannot be recommended as a CRC preventive in isolation, if the individual has a 10-year CV event risk of >6–10%, aspirin is often recommended to reduce the risk of serious CV events/mortality, and if taken, can be anticipated to reduce CRC risks as well [82]. The same is true of estrogen replacement therapy—not recommended for this indication, but if an older woman is contemplating the treatment for either bone health or postmenopausal symptomatic improvement, she may have a reduced risk of colorectal cancer, as well. Finally, the benefits of quitting smoking to overall health cannot be overstated. A review of 106 observational studies revealed that cigarette smoking is associated with both colorectal cancer incidence and mortality [83].

Carcinogenesis requires replication of cellular defects and corroboration, but prevention strategies hold the potential to interrupt this process before development of physically and fiscally costly disease.

REFERENCES

1. American Cancer Society. What are the key statistics about colorectal cancer? In *Information and Resources for Cancer: Breast, Colon, Prostate, Lung and Other Forms*, ACS (available at `http://www.cancer.org/cancer/colonandrectumcancer/detailedguide/colorectal-cancer-key-statistics`; accessed 8/09/10, posted 10/27/10).

2. Markowitz SD, Bertagnolli MM. Molecular origins of cancer: Molecular basis of colorectal cancer. *N Engl J Med* 2009;**361**:2449–2460.

3. Jones S, Chen WD, Parmigiani G, Diehl F, Beerenwinkel N, Antal T, Traulsen A, Nowak MA, Siegel C, Velculescu VE, Kinzler KW, Vogelstein B, Willis J, Markowitz SD. Comparative lesion sequencing provides insights into tumor evolution. *Proc Natl Acad Sci USA* 2008;**105**:4283–4288.

4. Guda K, Moinova H, He J, Jamison O, Ravi L, Natale L, Lutterbaugh J, Lawrence E, Lewis S, Willson JK, Lowe JB, Wiesner GL, Parmigiani G, Barnholtz-Sloan J, Dawson DW, Velculescu VE, Kinzler KW, Papadopoulos N, Vogelstein B, Willis J, Gerken TA, Markowitz SD. Inactivating germ-line and somatic mutations in polypeptide N-acetylgalactosaminyltransferase 12 in human colon cancers. *Proc Natl Acad Sci USA* 2009;**106**:12921–12925.

5. Cummins JM, He Y, Leary RJ, Pagliarini R, Diaz LA Jr, Sjoblom T, Barad O, Bentwich Z, Szafranska AE, Labourier E, Raymond CK, Roberts BS, Juhl H, Kinzler KW, Vogelstein B, Velculescu VE. The colorectal microRNAome. *Proc Natl Acad Sci USA* 2006;**103**:3687–3692.

6. Feinberg AP. Phenotypic plasticity and the epigenetics of human disease. *Nature* 2007;**447**:433–440 (review).

7. Mishra L, Derynck R, Mishra B. Transforming growth factor-beta signaling in stem cells and cancer. *Science* 2005;**310**:68–71.

8. Vogelstein B, Fearon ER, Hamilton SR, Kern SE, Preisinger AC, Leppert M, Nakamura Y, White R, Smits AM, Bos JL. Genetic alterations during colorectal-tumor development. *N Engl J Med* 1988;**319**:525–532.

9. Fearon ER, Vogelstein B. A genetic model for colorectal tumorigenesis. *Cell* 1990;**61**:759–767.

10. Huang EH, Wicha MS. Colon cancer stem cells: implications for prevention and therapy. *Trends Mol Med* 2008;**14**:503–509.

11. Reya T, Clevers H. Wnt signalling in stem cells and cancer. *Nature* 2005;**434**:843–850.

12. Yao ZX, Jogunoori WS, Choufani S, Rashid A, Blake T, Yao W, Kreishman P, Amin R, Sidawy AA, Evans SR, Finegold M, Reddy EP, Mishra B, Weksberg R, Kumar R, Mishra L. Epigenetic silencing of β-spectrin a TGF-β signaling/scaffolding protein in a human cancer stem cell disorder: Beckwith-Wiedemann syndrome. *J Biol Chem* 2010;**285**:36112–36120.

13. Tang Y, Katuri V, Dillner A, Mishra B, Deng CX, Mishra L. Disruption of transforming growth factor-beta signaling in ELF beta-spectrin-deficient mice. *Science* 2003;**299**: 574–577.

14. Tang Y, Katuri V, Srinivasan R, Fogt F, Redman R, Anand G, Said A, Fishbein T, Zasloff M, Reddy EP, et al. Transforming growth factor-beta suppresses nonmetastatic colon cancer through Smad4 and adaptor protein ELF at an early stage of tumorigenesis. *Cancer Res* 2005;**65**:4228–4237.

15. Preston SL, Wong WM, Chan AO, Poulsom R, Jeffery R, Goodlad RA, Mandir N, Elia G, Novelli M, Bodmer WF, et al. Bottom-up histogenesis of colorectal adenomas: origin in the monocryptal adenoma and initial expansion by crypt fission. *Cancer Res* 2003;**63**:3819–3825.

16. Boman BM, Fields JZ, Cavanaugh KL, Guetter A, Runquist OA. How dysregulated colonic crypt dynamics cause stem cell overpopulation and initiate colon cancer. *Cancer Res* 2008;**68**:3304–3313.

17. Crosnier C, Stamataki D, Lewis J. Organizing cell renewal in the intestine: stem cells, signals and combinatorial control. *Nat Rev Genet* 2006;**7**:349–359.

18. Humphries A, Wright NA. Colonic crypt organization and tumorigenesis. *Nat Rev Cancer* 2008;**8**:415–424.

19. Dalerba P, Dylla SJ, Park IK, Liu R, Wang X, Cho RW, Hoey T, Gurney A, Huang EH, Simeone DM, et al. Phenotypic characterization of human colorectal cancer stem cells. *Proc Natl Acad Sci USA* 2007;**104**:10158–10163.

20. O'Brien CA, Pollett A, Gallinger S, Dick JE. A human colon cancer cell capable of initiating tumour growth in immunodeficient mice. *Nature* 2007;**445**:106–110.

21. Ricci-Vitiani L, Lombardi DG, Pilozzi E, Biffoni M, Todaro M, Peschle C, De Maria R. Identification and expansion of human colon-cancer-initiating cells. *Nature* 2007;**445**:111–115.

22. Ieta K, Tanaka F, Haraguchi N, Kita Y, Sakashita H, Mimori K, Matsumoto T, Inoue H, Kuwano H, Mori M. Biological and genetic characteristics of tumor-initiating cells in colon cancer. *Ann Surg Oncol* 2008;**15**:638–648.

23. Shmelkov SV, Butler JM, Hooper AT, Hormigo A, Kushner J, Milde T, St Clair R, Baljevic M, White I, Jin DK, et al. CD133 expression is not restricted to stem cells, and both CD133+ and CD133− metastatic colon cancer cells initiate tumors. *J Clin Investig* 2008;**118**:2111–2120.

24. van Es JH, van Gijn ME, Riccio O, van den Born M, Vooijs M, Begthel H, Cozijnsen M, Robine S, Winton DJ, Radtke F, et al. Notch/gamma-secretase inhibition turns proliferative cells in intestinal crypts and adenomas into goblet cells. *Nature* 2005;**435**:959–963.

25. Batlle E, Henderson JT, Beghtel H, van den Born MM, Sancho E, Huls G, Meeldijk J, Robertson J, van de Wetering M, Pawson T, et al. Beta-catenin and TCF mediate cell positioning in the intestinal epithelium by controlling the expression of EphB/ephrinB. *Cell* 2002;**111**:251–263.

26. Barker N, van Es JH, Kuipers J, Kujala P, van den Born M, Cozijnsen M, Haegebarth A, Korving J, Begthel H, Peters PJ, et al. Identification of stem cells in small intestine and colon by marker gene Lgr5. *Nature* 2007;**449**:1003–1007.

27. Holmberg J, Genander M, Halford MM, Anneren C, Sondell M, Chumley MJ, Silvany RE, Henkemeyer M, Frisen J. EphB receptors coordinate migration and proliferation in the intestinal stem cell niche. *Cell* 2006;**125**:1151–1163.

28. van de Wetering M, Sancho E, Verweij C, de Lau W, Oving I, Hurlstone A, van der Horn K, Batlle E, Coudreuse D, Haramis AP, et al. The beta-catenin/TCF-4 complex imposes a crypt progenitor phenotype on colorectal cancer cells. *Cell* 2002;**111**:241–250.

29. Kohn AD, Moon RT. Wnt and calcium signaling: Beta-catenin-independent pathways. *Cell Calcium* 2005;**38**:439–446.

30. He TC, Sparks AB, Rago C, Hermeking H, Zawel L, da Costa LT, Morin PJ, Vogelstein B, Kinzler KW. Identification of c-MYC as a target of the APC pathway. *Science* 1998;**281**: 1509–1512.

31. Todaro M, Alea MP, Di Stefano AB, Cammareri P, Vermeulen L, Iovino F, Tripodo C, Russo A, Gulotta G, Medema JP, et al. Colon cancer stem cells dictate tumor growth and resist cell death by production of interleukin-4. *Cell Stem Cell* 2007;**1**:389–402.

32. Ilyas M, Efstathiou JA, Straub J, Kim HC, Bodmer WF. Transforming growth factor beta stimulation of colorectal cancer cell lines: Type II receptor bypass and changes in adhesion molecule expression. *Proc Natl Acad Sci USA* 1999;**96**:3087–3091.

33. Xu Y, Pasche B: TGF-beta signaling alterations and susceptibility to colorectal cancer. *Hum Mol Genet* 2007;**16**(Spec 1): R14–R20.

34. Thiagalingam S, Lengauer C, Leach FS, Schutte M, Hahn SA, Overhauser J, Willson JK, Markowitz S, Hamilton SR, Kern SE, et al. Evaluation of candidate tumour suppressor genes on chromosome 18 in colorectal cancers. *Nat Genet* 1996;**13**:343–346.

35. Barnard JA, Beauchamp RD, Coffey RJ, Moses HL. Regulation of intestinal epithelial cell growth by transforming growth factor type beta. *Proc Natl Acad Sci USA* 1989;**86**: 1578–1582.

36. Takaku K, Oshima M, Miyoshi H, Matsui M, Seldin MF, Taketo MM. Intestinal tumorigenesis in compound mutant mice of both Dpc4 (Smad4) and Apc genes. *Cell* 1998;**92**:645–656.

37. Pendas-Franco N, Aguilera O, Pereira F, Gonzalez-Sancho JM, Munoz A: Vitamin D and Wnt/beta-catenin pathway in colon cancer: role and regulation of DICKKOPF genes. *Anticancer Res* 2008;**28**:2613–2623.

38. Greenberg ER, Baron JA, Tosteson TD, Freeman DH, Beck GJ, Bond JH, et al A clinical trial of antioxidant vitamins to prevent colorectal adenoma. Polyp Prevention Study Group. *N Engl J Med* 1994;**331**:141–147.

39. Bonelli L, Conio M, Picasso M, Massa P, Dodero M, Ravelli P, et al. Chemoprevention of metachronous adenomas of the large bowel (a double blind randomized trial of antioxidants (abstract), *Proc. 3rd United European Gastroenterology Week*, Oslo, abstract book, 1994, p. A61.

40. Hofstad B, Almendingen K, Vatn M, Andersen SN, Owen RW, Larsen S, et al. Growth and recurrence of colorectal polyps (a double-blind 3-year intervention with calcium and antioxidants). *Digestion* 1998;**59**:148–156.

41. Malila N, Virtamo J, Virtanen M, Albanes D, Tangrea JA, Huttunen JK. The effect of alpha-tocopherol and beta-carotene supplementation on colorectal adenomas in middle-aged male smokers. *Cancer Epidemiol Biomark Prevent* 1999;**8**:489–493.

42. Albanes D, Malila N, Taylor PR, Huttunen JK, Virtamo J, Edwards BK, et al. Effects of supplemental alpha-tocopherol and beta-carotene on colorectal cancer: Results from a controlled trial (Finland). *Cancer Causes Control* 2000;**11**:197–205.

43. Michels KB, Edward Giovannucci, Joshipura KJ, et al. Prospective study of fruit and vegetable consumption and incidence of colon and rectal cancers. *J Natl Cancer Inst* 2000;**92**:1740–1752.

44. Clark LC et al. Effects of selenium supplementation for cancer prevention in patients with carcinoma of the skin. A randomized controlled trial. Nutritional Prevention of Cancer Study Group. *JAMA* 1996;**276**:1957–1963.

45. Reid ME et al. Selenium supplementation and colorectal adenomas: An analysis of the nutritional prevention of cancer trial. *Int J Cancer* 2006;**118**:1777–1781.

46. Lippman SM, Klein EA, Goodman PJ, Lucia MS, Thompson IM, Ford LG, et al. Effect of selenium and vitamin E on risk of prostate cancer and other cancers: The Selenium and vitamin E Cancer prevention Trial (SELECT). *JAMA* 2009;**301**:39–51.

47. Choi SW, Mason JB. Folate and carcinogenesis (an integrated scheme). *J Nutr* 2000;**130**:129–132.

48. Giovannucci E, Stampfer MJ, Colditz GA, et al.: Multivitamin use, folate, and colon cancer in women in the Nurses' Health Study. *Ann Intern Med* 1998;**129**:517–524.

49. Cole BF et al. Folic acid for the prevention of colorectal adenomas: A randomized clinical trial. *JAMA* 2007;**297**:2351–2359.

50. Holick MF. Vitamin D deficiency. *N Engl J Med* 2007;**357**:266–281.

51. LaCroix AZ, Kotchen J, Anderson G, Brzyski R, Cauley JA, Cummings SR, et al. Calcium plus vitamin D supplementation and mortality in postmenopausal women: The Women's Health Initiative calcium-vitamin D randomized controlled trial. *J Gerontol A Biol Sci Med Sci* 2009;**64**:559–567.

52. Baron JA, Beach M, Mandel JS, et al.: Calcium supplements for the prevention of colorectal adenomas. Calcium Polyp Prevention Study Group. *N Engl J Med* 1999;**340**:101–107.

53. McCullough ML, Robertson AS, Rodriguez C, Jacobs EJ, Chao A, Carolyn J, et al. Calcium, vitamin D, dairy products, and risk of colorectal cancer in the cancer prevention study II nutrition cohort (United States). *Cancer Causes Control* 2003;**14**:1–12.

54. Gorham ED, Garland CF, Garland FC, et al. Vitamin D and prevention of colorectal cancer. *J Steroid Biochem Mol Biol* 2005;**97**:179–194.

55. Howe GR, Benito E, Castelleto R, et al. Dietary intake of fiber and decreased risk of cancers of the colon and rectum: Evidence from the combined analysis of 13 case-control studies. *J Natl Cancer Inst* 1992;**84**:1887–1896.

56. Dahm CC et al. Dietary fiber and colorectal cancer risk: a nested case-control study using food diaries. *J Natl Cancer Inst* 2010;**102**:614–626.

57. Schatzkin A, Lanza E, Corle D, Lance P, Iber F, Caan B, et al. Lack of effect of a low-fat, high-fiber diet on the recurrence of colorectal adenomas. Polyp Prevention Trial Study Group. *N Engl J Med* 2000;**342**:1149–1155.

58. Alberts DS, Martinez ME, Roe DJ, Guillen-Rodriguez JM, Marshall JR, van Leeuwen JB, et al. Lack of effect of a high-fiber cereal supplement on the recurrence of colorectal adenomas. Phoenix Colon Cancer Prevention Physicians' Network. *N Engl J Med* 2000;**342**:1156–1162.

59. Bingham SA, Day NE, Luben R, Ferrari P, Slimani N, Norat T, et al. Dietary fibre in food and protection against colorectal cancer in the European Prospective Investigation into Cancer and Nutrition (EPIC) (an observational study). *Lancet* 2003;**361**:1496–1501.

60. Bingham S. The fibre-folate debate in colo-rectal cancer. *Proc Nutr Sci* 2006;**65**:19–23.

61. Daniel CR, McCullough ML, Patel RC, Jacobs EJ, Flanders WD, Thun MJ, Calle EE. Dietary intake of omega-6 and omega-3 fatty acids and risk of colorectal cancer in a prospective cohort of US men and women. *Cancer Epidemiol Biomark Prevent* 2009;**18**:516–525.

62. Hall MN, Chavarro JE, Lee IM, Willett WC, Ma J. A 22-year prospective study of fish, n-3 fatty acid intake, and colorectal cancer risk in men. *Cancer Epidemiol Biomark Prevent* 2008;**17**(5):1136–1143 (erratum in ibid. 2008;**17**:2901).

63. West NJ, Clark SK, Phillips, RKS, Hutchinson JM, Leicester RJ, Belluzzi A, Hull MA. Eicosapentaenoic acid reduces rectal polyp number and size in familial adenomatous polyposis. *Gut* 2010;**59**:918–925.

64. Halle M, Schoenberg MH. Physical activity in the prevention and treatment of colorectal carcinoma. *Dtsch Arztebl Int* 2009;**106**:722–727.

65. Wolin KY, Yan Y, Colditz GA, et al. Physical activity and colon cancer prevention: A meta-analysis. *Br J Cancer* 2009;**100**:611–616.

66. Sandler RS, Halabi S, Baron JA, Budinger S, Paskett E, Keresztes R, et al. A randomized trial of aspirin to prevent colorectal adenomas in patients with previous colorectal cancer. *N Engl J Med* 2003;**348**:883–890.

67. Baron JA, Cole BF, Sandler RS, Haile RW, Ahnen D, Bresalier R, et al. A randomized trial of aspirin to prevent colorectal adenomas. *N Engl J Med* 2003;**348**:891–899.

68. Giovannucci E, Rimm EB, Stampfer MJ, et al. Aspirin use and the risk for colorectal cancer and adenoma in male health professionals. *Ann Intern Med* 1994;**121**:241–246.

69. Chan AT, Ogino S, Fuchs CS. Aspirin and the risk of colorectal cancer in relation to the expression of COX-2. *N Engl J Med* 2007;**356**:2131–2142.

70. Steinbach G, Lynch PM, Phillips RK, Wallace MH, Hawk E, Gordon GB, et al. The effect of celecoxib, a cyclooxygenase-2 inhibitor, in familial adenomatous polyposis. *N Engl J Med* 2000;**342**:1946–1952.

71. Bertagnolli MM, Eagle CJ, Zauber AG, Redston M, Solomon SD, Kim K, et al. Celecoxib for the prevention of sporadic colorectal adenomas. *N Engl J Med* 2006;**355**:873–884.

72. Arber N, Eagle CJ, Spicak J, Racz I, Dite P, Hajer J, et al. Celecoxib for the prevention of colorectal adenomatous polyps. *N Engl J Med* 2006;**355**:885–895.

73. Solomon SD, Wittes J, Finn PV, Fowler R, Viner J, Bertagnolli, MM, et al. Cardiovascular risk of celecoxib in 6 randomized placebo-controlled trials: The cross trial safety analysis. *Circulation* 2008;**117**:2104–2113.

74. Patel VB, Misra S, Patel BB, Majumdar APN. Colorectal cancer: Chemopreventive role of curcumin and resveratrol. *Nutr Cancer* 2010;**62**:958–967.

75. Cruz-Correa M, Shoskes DA, Sanchez P, Zhao R, Hylind LM, et al. Combination treatment with curcumin and quercetin of adenomas in familial adenomatous polyposis. *Clin Gastroenterol Hepatol* 2006;**4**:1035–1038.

76. Chlebowski RT et al. Estrogen plus progestin and colorectal cancer in postmenopausal women. *N Engl J Med*. 2004;**350**(10):991–1004.

77. Grodstein F, Martinez ME, Platz EA, Giovannucci E, Colditz GA, Kautzky M, et al. Postmenopausal hormone use and risk for colorectal cancer and adenoma. *Ann Intern Med* 1998;**128**:705–712.

78. Calle EE, Miracle-McMahill HL, Thun MJ, Heath CWJ. Estrogen replacement therapy and risk of fatal colon cancer in a prospective cohort of postmenopausal women. *J Natl Cancer Inst* 1995;**87**:517–523.

79. Poynter JN, Gruber SB, Higgins PD, Almog R, Bonner JD, Rennert HS, et al. Statins and the risk of colorectal cancer. *N Engl J Med* 2005;**352**:2184–2192.

80. Dale KM, Coleman CI, Henyan NN, Kluger J, White CM. Statins and cancer risk: A meta-analysis. *JAMA* 2006;**295**:74–80.

81. Jacobs EJ, Rodriguez C, Brady KA, et al.: Cholesterol-lowering drugs and colorectal cancer incidence in a large United States cohort. *J Natl Cancer Inst* 2006;**98**:69–72.

82. US Preventive Services Task Force: Aspirin for the prevention of cardiovascular disease: U.S. Preventive Services Task Force recommendation statement. *Ann Intern Med* 2009;**150**:396–404.

83. Botteri E, Iodice S, Bagnardi V, Raimondi S, Lowenfels AB, Maisonneuve P. Smoking and colorectal cancer: A meta-analysis. *JAMA* 2008;**300**:2765–2778.

CHAPTER 7

Prostate Cancer Prevention

BARBARA ERCOLE and IAN M. THOMPSON, Jr.

University of Texas, Health Science Center, San Antonio, TX

7.1 INTRODUCTION

In 2010 the National Cancer Institute estimated that approximately 217,730 new cases of prostate cancer (PCa) would be diagnosed and approximately 32,050 PCa deaths would occur by the end dur of that year [1].

7.2 RATIONALE FOR PREVENTION

American men have a 1 in 6 lifetime risk of developing PCa, making it the second most common cause of cancer death among them. More recently a concern regarding overdetection and overtreatment of the majority of prostate specific antigen (PSA) screening for detecting PCa has been raised, as these are mainly localized cancers. Since the 1990s the incidence and mortality of PCa have also been declining [2]. Although the exact cause of the decrease in mortality from PCa is unknown, it is likely multifactorial, including PSA screening, improved treatment, and chemoprevention. PSA screening has many limitations. The concept that PSA screening may have had an impact on decreased mortality rates is attractive when evaluating outcomes from radical prostatectomy series [3,4]; however, concerns about the detection of clinically insignificant/indolent disease and the economic implications of widespread screening are only some of the controversial aspects of PSA screening [5–8].

7.3 PSA SCREENING TRIALS

The impact of PSA screening on population mortality has been addressed in two large-scale studies, one in the United States and one in Europe. They have resulted in conflicting conclusions, and both studies had serious limitations. The Prostate, Lung, Colon, Ovarian, Cancer Screening Project (PLCO) trial in the United States randomized men to a fixed period of repetitive PSA screening visits versus general community

Cancer and Aging Handbook: Research and Practice, First Edition. Edited by Keith M. Bellizzi and Margot A. Gosney.
© 2012 Wiley-Blackwell. Published 2012 by John Wiley & Sons, Inc.

practice; the European Study of Screening for Prostate Cancer (ERSPC) was a similar trial that examined screening in Europe [9,10]. The US trial found no reduction in PCa mortality, while the ERSPC study found a 20% reduction with screening. Criticism of the US trial focused on significant contamination of PSA screened subjects in the control arm, relatively low rate of biopsy in those men with abnormal screening results, and short follow-up period. The ERSPC trial was criticized as well, mainly for its heterogeneity of study designs. Also, the mortality reduction was achieved as a result of an investment in a large amount of resources and time. In other words, in order to prevent one PCa death, more than 1400 men required screening and 48 men required treatment over close to a decade of follow-up.

The studies cited above have been above reanalyzed. Crawford et al. [11] reanalyzed the data for the PLCO trial by using different comorbidity strata to evaluate estimates of prostate cancer specific mortality (PCSM). In men with no or minimal comorbidity, annual screening was associated with a significant reduction in the risk of PCSM. These men were also more likely to undergo curative therapy than those with men with significant comorbidities. As the authors pointed out, these findings are hypothesis generating as the analysis was performed post randomization. The 35.7% estimate of men with no or minimal comorbidities may be an overestimate when applied to the general population. Also, the number needed to treat (NNT) was adjusted to 5; thus both overdetection and overtreatment are still a risk. Loeb et al. [12] reanalyzed the data from the ERSPC trial by analyzing the effects of varying follow-up times on number needed to screen (NNS) and NNT, as these are time-specific variables, and quoting a single timepoint may be misleading. They found that at 9 years the NNS was 1254 and NNT was 43. These variables continued to decrease with each subsequent analysis, at 10 years NNS decreased to 837 and at 12 years to 503. NNT decreased to 29 at 10 years and to 18 at 12 years. Significantly, as the number of years increases, the authors point out that the differences in the mortality between the two arms will continue to grow, and therefore the NNT estimates will continue to decrease.

Another randomized population based screening trial reported their first planned analysis on mortality outcomes in 2010 [13]. The Goteborg trial randomized 20,000 men to either screening with PSA every 2 years ($n = 10,000$) versus a control group ($n = 10,000$). The primary endpoint was PCSM and the study was analyzed according to an intention-to-screen principle. Median age of participants was 65 and prostate biopsies were performed if PSA was 3.4 ng/mL during 1995–1998 and subsequently lowered to 2.5 ng/mL after 2005. During a median follow-up of 14 years, they have thus far noted a 12.7% prostate cancer incidence in the screening group, compared to 8.2% in the control group. The cumulative relative risk reduction of death was 50% in the screening group, and they have thus far determined that NNS was 293 and NNT was 12. This report has studied only the early effects of screening, as this is a young population (median age 65) and has a comparatively short follow-up time after prostate cancer diagnosis. The relevant reduction in cancer mortality found in this study is comparable to that with breast or colorectal cancer screening. However, the authors warn that varying lead times may result in the risk of overdiagnosis.

Even though these studies are helping shed light on PSA screening, the precaution against overdetection and overtreatment is a recurring theme, and thus screening alone might not be sufficient to prevent PCa morbidity and mortality. Cost analysis for the treatment of localized PCa has been estimated at $8 billion per year in the United States [14], and some groups have argued that the treatment modalities used for cure in indolent disease is more expensive than those used in treatment of late-stage disease [7]. Strategies designed to prevent and lower the risk of PCa may prove beneficial not only in reducing the burden of disease for the individual but also in reducing the cost burden for society.

An effective prevention strategy for PCa must meet two main goals: prevent disease and modulate the risk of progression of premalignant lesions. If these goals are met, a man would not have to deal with a diagnosis of PCa. Prevention strategies should also have minimal toxicity and burden to the patient, and incur little to no cost. These concepts are not new and are present in other specialties such as in cardiology for the prevention of cardiovascular disease and in gynecology for breast cancer [15,16]. We focus our discussion around three phase III trials published to date: the Prostate Cancer Prevention Trial (PCPT), the Reduction by Dutasteride of prostate Cancer Events trial (REDUCE), and the Selenium and vitamin E Cancer prevention Trial (SELECT).

7.3.1 Chemoprevention

Five α-reductase type I and II enzymes convert testosterone into dihydrotestosterone (DHT) within prostate cells. DHT has a greater affinity for the androgen receptor in prostate tissue compared to testosterone and plays a crucial role in development of the prostate. Modulation of DHT concentration has been primarily studied via modulation of 5α-reductase type I and II enzymes. The predominant isoform in PCa tissue is type I 5α-reductase, while type II is present predominantly in normal prostatic tissue and benign prostatic hyperplasia (BPH) [17,18]. Individuals with a hereditary deficiency in the 5α-reductase enzyme type II have been noted to have abnormal development of their prostate as well as their external genitalia [19]. Preclinical data and clinical trials have demonstrated a role for 5α-reductase inhibitors in the treatment of BPH, prevention of BPH-related outcomes, and prevention of PCa [20–22]. Although not statistically significant, results from the Proscar Long-Term Efficacy and Safety Study (PLESS) helped support the notion that finasteride, a type II 5α-reductase enzyme inhibitor, may reduce the risk of PCa when compared to the placebo group ($p = 0.7$) [23]. As a result of this finding, the Prostate Cancer Prevention Trial (PCPT) was developed. PCPT was the first phase III trial conducted for the prevention of PCa.

7.3.2 Prostate Cancer Prevention Trial (PCPT)

The Southwest Oncology Group (SWOG) supported by the National Cancer Institute released the results of the PCPT in 2003 under recommendations from the Data Safety and Monitoring Committee [24]. PCPT was a randomized trial of 18,882 men randomized to either finasteride or placebo for 7 years after a 3-month placebo run-in period. Inclusion criteria included men who were ≥55 years of age, with a normal digital rectal exam (DRE) and a PSA <3.0 ng/mL. Subjects underwent a DRE and PSA test annually. Biopsies of the prostate were recommended if an abnormal DRE or PSA exceeded 4.0 ng/mL. At the end of 7 years, participants who had not already undergone a prostate biopsy were asked to undergo an end-of-study biopsy; at the time of publication 19% of study participants had not yet reached their 7-year timepoint. The primary endpoint of the study, prevalence of PCa, was met early, and thus the study results were reported. This study found a 24.8% ($p < 0.001$) relative risk reduction in the prevalence of PCa over their 7-year period in men who received finasteride.

Subgroup analysis regarding age (<55, 55–59, 60–64, and ≥65 years) demonstrated finasteride was associated with a reduction in PCa prevalence across all age strata.

Several conclusions were drawn about finasteride from the PCPT trial. Finasteride increases the ability of PSA to detect cancer and high-grade cancer. For example, if a physician uses a PSA cutoff of 4.0 ng/mL to recommend a biopsy, not only does the sensitivity of cancer detection increase from 24% to 37.8% but the sensitivity of detection of high grade disease also increases from 39.2% to 53%. Another way of looking at it is through an analysis of the area under the curve (AUC) for PSA in the finasteride group compared to the placebo group. The AUC for PSA was increased from 0.681 to 0.757 ($p < 0.001$); for Gleason 7–10 disease, it was increased from 0.781 to 0.838 ($p = 0.003$); for Gleason 8–10 disease, it was increased from 0.824 to 0.886 ($p = 0.071$). These are highly significant improvements in the performance of this biomarker for cancer detection [25]. Finasteride increases the ability of the DRE to detect cancer. The sensitivity of DRE for the detection of cancer was significantly increased among men receiving finasteride (21.3% finasteride vs. 16.7% placebo; $p = 0.013$) with no reduction in specificity. Although a similar increase was seen for high-grade disease, the difference did not attain statistical significance [26]. Finasteride improves the ability of the prostate biopsy to detect cancer and to detect high-grade cancer. This is probably best illustrated by a comparison between the placebo and finasteride groups, comparing biopsy and prostatectomy grades. In the placebo group, if high grade disease was present in the prostatectomy, only about 50% had high grade disease on biopsy. On the other hand, this rate was reduced to about 30% in the finasteride group. This 40% increase in biopsy sensitivity for high-grade cancer in the finasteride group was statistically significant ($p = 0.01$). A plausible and reasonable explanation for this outcome is the 25% reduction in gland volume in the finasteride group that leads to a more accurate sampling of the gland at time of biopsy. Redman and colleagues [27] have performed the most robust examination of the PCPT data by examining biopsies only. The bias-adjusted rates of PCa in the two groups were 21.1% (4.2% high-grade) in the placebo group versus 14.7% (4.8% high-grade) in the finasteride group. A 30% risk reduction in PCa ($p < 0.0001$) and a nonsignificant 14% increase in high-grade cancer ($p = 0.12$) with finasteride were noted when all biases were included. Thus, Redman and colleagues concluded that the overall cancer risk reduction was 30%; the reduction in risk of low-grade disease was 32%, and the impact of finasteride on high-grade disease was a risk reduction of 28%. Three independent analyses, using differing methodologies, of the PCPT data have confirmed the increase in high-grade detection of PCa in the finasteride arm to be due to detection and sampling biases as well as improvement in the performance characteristics of prostate biopsy [27–30].

7.3.3 Reduction by Dutasteride of Prostate Cancer Events Trial (REDUCE)

The effects of dutasteride on chemoprevention of PCa were tested in the REDUCE trial [31,32]. Dutasteride is a type I/II 5α-reductase inhibitor that reduces serum DHT by >90% [33,34]. Preliminary results with dutasteride and from the PCPT led to the study design of REDUCE. Andriole and colleagues demonstrated an approximate 50% reduction in PCa in the dutasteride group at 27 months (from 2.5% to 1.2%; $p = 0.002$) in a randomized trial of dutasteride for BPH ($n = 4325$) [35]. The REDUCE trial was subsequently designed and powered to further test these findings in two randomized arms: dutasteride 0.5 mg daily versus placebo [32]. Unlike PCPT, this study enrolled men who were at high risk for developing PCa based on age, PSA level, and previous suspicion of PCa that lead to a biopsy. Men in the 50–60 age range were eligible to participate if they had a PSA within 2.5–10 ng/mL, for those men in the 60–75 age range, their PSA level had to be between 3–10 ng/mL. Participants who had undergone a single biopsy within 6 months prior to enrollment and were negative were also eligible. REDUCE was a randomized, multicenter, double-blind, placebo-controlled, parallel-group study conducted for 4 years after a 4-week runin period of placebo. Biopsies were obtained at 2 and 4 years. Cancer was detected in 659 of the 3305 men in the dutasteride group compared to 858 of the 3424 men in the placebo, equating to a relative risk reduction with dutasteride of 22.8% (95% CI 15.2–29.8; $p = <0.001$) in 4 years. Subgroup analysis based on age (<65 and ≥65) demonstrated a significantly lower risk of PCa detection on biopsy with dutasteride [24.1% (95% CI 13.5–33.4) and 22.1% (95% CI 10.8–32), respectively]. There was no statistically significant increase in incidence of high-grade disease in the dutasteride arm. The overall incidence of high-grade PCa (Gleason score 7–10) was equal in both groups (6.8% vs. 6.7%) in years 3 and 4. Further breakdown of the Gleason score revealed that there were 12 Gleason score 8–10 tumors detected in the dutasteride group compared to only 1 in the placebo group ($p = 0.003$). This was an interesting find, since the incidence of Gleason score 8–10 PCa in the first 2 years, was equal between the dutasteride and the placebo groups (17 vs. 18, respectively). However, the placebo group had 141 more tumors of Gleason score 5–7 compared to the dutasteride group (558 in 3346 vs. 417 in 3239, respectively). Speculation as to why this difference occurred is due to the placebo group's higher biopsy-for-cause rates, which lead to censoring of more men from the placebo group by year 2 due to detection of PCa. A potential argument is that these same men who were censored would have been the ones to develop high-grade disease in subsequent years. Another potential explanation offered by the authors is the reduced number of high-grade PCa may have been due in part to dutasteride therapy, although this has not been confirmed. In regard to BPH endpoints, dutasteride showed a positive effect on the reduction of symptoms, mainly episodes of urinary retention. As with the initial publication of PCPT results, editorials have been published regarding REDUCE trial outcomes [36–38]. Further analysis of the large volume of data produced from the trial may lay some of the concerns to rest, mainly the effects of 5α-reductase inhibitors on high-grade PCa.

7.3.4 Selenium and Vitamin E Cancer Prevention Trial (SELECT)

The Selenium and Vitamin E Cancer Prevention Trial (SELECT), a phase III randomized, placebo-controlled trial, was designed to evaluate the efficacy of selenium and vitamin E alone and in combination in the prevention of PCa [39]. SELECT randomized 35,533 men between August 22, 2001 and June 24, 2004 to four arms: selenium (200μg/day, pure L-selenomethionine), vitamin E (400 IU/day, synthetic D,L-α-tocopherol), both, or placebo [40]. Eligibility criteria included men who were >55 years old, a PSA <4 ng/mL, and a normal DRE. Biopsies were performed if DRE was abnormal or PSA rose to >4 ng/mL, complexed PSA rose to >3.4 ng/mL, or if PSA velocity was >0.75 ng/mL per year. SELECT was planned to follow subjects for 7–12 years; however, intervention was discontinued at a median of 5.46 years because of results obtained at their second formal interim analysis. There were no statistical significant differences noted between the groups on decreasing PCa risk. Although the results did not reach statistical significance, there was an increased risk of PCa in the vitamin E group ($p = 0.06$) and of type 2 diabetes mellitus in the selenium group [RR (relative risk) = 1.07; 99% CI = 0.94–1.22; $p = 0.16$] but not in the selenium–vitamin E group. The conclusion from this study was that neither selenium nor vitamin E at the doses administered helps prevent PCa.

7.4 CONCLUSION

Completion of three phase III trials (PCPT, REDUCE, SELECT) for the study of chemoprevention of PCa is unique in the study of neoplastic disease but important because of the prevalence of PCa. However, successful completion of a prevention clinical trial does not always guarantee reaching the conclusion that the compound studied may confer a protective effect. The best example of such disappointing conclusions is illustrated by the SELECT trial, where previous randomized trials found a significant reduction in risk of PCa with selenium and vitamin E and the phase III trial found none. On the other hand, conclusions of the other two trials are promising. The conclusions from the PCPT and the REDUCE trials was that 5α-reductase inhibitors demonstrate a consistency of effect on PCa with similar magnitude of risk reduction across all risk groups. It would appear thus that 5α-reductase inhibitors should be considered an effective primary prevention strategy for men at risk of PCa including, for finasteride, a general population of men with PSAs in the lower range and, for dutasteride, men whose PSA may be higher and in whom biopsy shows no evidence of PCa at this time. These agents, employed for patients who express an interest in preventing a subsequent diagnosis of PCa and the attendant anxiety, cost, and complications of treatment or other management, could have a major impact in helping control the impact of this highly prevalent disease.

REFERENCES

1. Jemal A, Siegel R, Xu J, Ward E. Cancer statistics, 2010. *CA Cancer J Clin* 2010;**60**: 277–300.

2. Horner MJ, Ries LAG, Krapcho M, et al. *SEER Cancer Statistics Review, 1975–2006*, National Cancer Institute (`http://seer.cancer.gov/csr/1975_2006/`).

3. Jhaveri FM, Klein EA, Kupelian PA, Zippe C, Levin HS. Declining rates of extracapsular extension after radical prostatectomy: Evidence for continued stage migration. *J Clin Oncol* 1999;**17**(10):3167–3172.

4. Moul JW, Wu H, Sun L, et al. Epidemiology of radical prostatectomy for localized prostate cancer in the era of prostate-specific antigen: An overview of the Department of Defense Center for Prostate Disease Research national database. *Surgery* 2002;**132**(2):213–219.

5. Neal DE, Leung HY, Powell PH, Hamdy FC, Donovan JL. Unanswered questions in screening for prostate cancer. *Eur J Cancer* 2000;**36**(10):1316–1321.

6. McNaughton Collins M, Ransohoff DF, Barry MJ. Early detection of prostate cancer. Serendipity strikes again. *JAMA* 1997;**278**(18):1516–1519.

7. Benoit RM, Naslund MJ. The socioeconomic implications of prostate-specific antigen screening. *Urol Clin North Am* 1997;**24**(2):451–458.

8. Brawley OW, Ankerst DP, Thompson IM. Screening for prostate cancer. *CA Cancer J Clin* 2009;**59**(4):264–273.

9. Andriole GL, Crawford ED, Grubb RL 3rd, et al. Mortality results from a randomized prostate-cancer screening trial. *N Engl J Med* 2009;**360**(13):1310–1319.

10. Schroder FH, Hugosson J, Roobol MJ, et al. Screening and prostate-cancer mortality in a randomized European study. *N Engl J Med* 2009;**360**(13):1320–1328.

11. Crawford ED, Grubb R 3rd, Black A, et al. Comorbidity and mortality results from a randomized prostate cancer screening trial. *J Clin Oncol* 2011;**29**(4):355–361.

12. Loeb S, Vonesh EF, Metter EJ, Carter HB, Gann PH, Catalona WJ. What is the true number needed to screen and treat to save a life with prostate-specific antigen testing? *J Clin Oncol* 2011;**29**(4):464–467.

13. Hugosson J, Carlsson S, Aus G, et al. Mortality results from the Goteborg randomised population-based prostate-cancer screening trial. *Lancet Oncol* 2010;**11**(8):725–732.

14. National Cancer Institute. *Cancer Trends Progress Report—2007 Update*, NCI, NIH, DHHS (http://progressreport.cancer.gov).

15. Probstfield JL. How cost-effective are new preventive strategies for cardiovascular disease? *Am J Cardiol* 2003;**91**(10A):22 G-27G.

16. Kinsinger LS, Harris R, Woolf SH, Sox HC, Lohr KN. Chemoprevention of breast cancer: A summary of the evidence for the U.S. Preventive Services Task Force. *Ann Intern Med* 2002;**137**(1):59–69.

17. Bruchovsky N, Sadar MD, Akakura K, Goldenberg SL, Matsuoka K, Rennie PS. Characterization of 5alpha-reductase gene expression in stroma and epithelium of human prostate. *J Steroid Biochem Mol Biol* 1996;**59**(5–6):397–404.

18. Thomas LN, Douglas RC, Vessey JP, et al. 5alpha-reductase type 1 immunostaining is enhanced in some prostate cancers compared with benign prostatic hyperplasia epithelium. *J Urol* 2003;**170**(5):2019–2025.

19. Imperato-McGinley J, Gautier T, Zirinsky K, et al. Prostate visualization studies in males homozygous and heterozygous for 5 alpha-reductase deficiency. *J Clin Endocrinol Metab* 1992;**75**(4):1022–1026.

20. Gormley GJ, Stoner E, Rittmaster RS, et al. Effects of finasteride (MK-906), a 5 alpha-reductase inhibitor, on circulating androgens in male volunteers. *J Clin Endocrinol Metab* 1990;**70**(4):1136–1141.

21. McConnell JD, Bruskewitz R, Walsh P, et al. The effect of finasteride on the risk of acute urinary retention and the need for surgical treatment among men with benign prostatic hyperplasia. Finasteride Long-Term Efficacy and Safety Study Group. *N Engl J Med* 1998;**338**(9):557–563.

22. McConnell JD, Roehrborn CG, Bautista OM, et al. The long-term effect of doxazosin, finasteride, and combination therapy on the clinical progression of benign prostatic hyperplasia. *N Engl J Med*. 2003;**349**(25):2387–2398.

23. Andriole GL, Guess HA, Epstein JI, et al. Treatment with finasteride preserves usefulness of prostate-specific antigen in the detection of prostate cancer: results of a randomized, double-blind, placebo-controlled clinical trial. PLESS Study Group. Proscar Long-term Efficacy and Safety Study. *Urology* 1998;**52**(2):195–201; discussion 201–202.

24. Thompson IM, Goodman PJ, Tangen CM, et al. The influence of finasteride on the development of prostate cancer. *N Engl J Med* 2003;**349**(3):215–224.

25. Thompson IM, Chi C, Ankerst DP, et al. Effect of finasteride on the sensitivity of PSA for detecting prostate cancer. *J Natl Cancer Inst* 2006;**98**(16):1128–1133.

26. Thompson IM, Tangen CM, Goodman PJ, et al. Finasteride improves the sensitivity of digital rectal examination for prostate cancer detection. *J Urol*. 2007;**177**(5):1749–1752.

27. Redman MW, Tangen CM, Goodman PJ, Lucia MS, Coltman CA Jr, Thompson IM. Finasteride does not increase the risk of high-grade prostate cancer: A bias-adjusted modeling approach. *Cancer Prev Res* 2008;**1**(3):174–181.

28. Cohen Y, Liu K, Heyden N, et al. Detection bias due to the effect of finasteride on prostate volume: A modeling approach for analysis of the Prostate Cancer Prevention Trial. *J Natl Cancer Inst* 2007;**99**(18):1366–1374.

29. Pinsky P, Parnes H, Ford L. Estimating rates of true high-grade disease in the prostate cancer prevention trial. *Cancer Prev Res* 2008;**1**(3):182–186.

30. Shepherd B, Redman MW, Ankerst DP. Does finasteride affect the severity of prostate cancer? A causal sensitivity analysis. *J Am Stat Assoc* 2008;**103**(484):1392–1404.

31. Andriole G, Bostwick D, Brawley O, et al. Chemoprevention of prostate cancer in men at high risk: Rationale and design of the reduction by dutasteride of prostate cancer events (REDUCE) trial. *J Urol* 2004;**172**(4Pt 1):1314–1317.

32. Andriole GL, Bostwick DG, Brawley OW, et al. Effect of dutasteride on the risk of prostate cancer. *N Engl J Med* 2010;**362**(13):1192–1202.

33. Bramson HN, Hermann D, Batchelor KW, Lee FW, James MK, Frye SV. Unique pre-clinical characteristics of GG745, a potent dual inhibitor of 5AR. *J Pharmacol Exp Ther* 1997;**282**(3):1496–1502.

34. Clark RV, Hermann DJ, Cunningham GR, Wilson TH, Morrill BB, Hobbs S. Marked suppression of dihydrotestosterone in men with benign prostatic hyperplasia by dutasteride, a dual 5alpha-reductase inhibitor. *J Clin Endocrinol Metab* 2004;**89**(5):2179–2184.

35. Andriole GL, Roehrborn C, Schulman C, Slawin KM, Somerville M, Rittmaster RS. Effect of dutasteride on the detection of prostate cancer in men with benign prostatic hyperplasia. *Urology* 2004;**64**(3):537–541; discussion 542–533.

36. Bosland MC, Cremers RG, Kiemeney LA. Words of wisdom. Re: effect of dutasteride on the risk of prostate cancer. *Eur Urol* 2010;**58**(4):631–632.

37. Kirby RS, McNicholas TA, Fitzpatrick JM. Current prospects for the chemoprevention of prostate cancer. *Br J Urol Int* 2010;**106**(6):751–753.

38. Yu EM, El-Ayass W, Aragon-Ching JB. The use of 5-alpha reductase inhibitors for the prevention of prostate cancer. *Cancer Biol Ther* 2010;**10**(1):11–2.

39. Klein EA, Thompson IM, Lippman SM, et al. SELECT: The next prostate cancer prevention trial. Selenum and vitamin E Cancer prevention Trial. *J Urol* 2001;**166**(4):1311–1315.

40. Lippman SM, Klein EA, Goodman PJ, et al. Effect of selenium and vitamin E on risk of prostate cancer and other cancers: The Selenium and Vitamin E Cancer Prevention Trial (SELECT). *JAMA* 2009;**301**(1):39–51.

CHAPTER 8

Lung Cancer Prevention

SAMIRA SHOJAEE and KONSTANTIN H. DRAGNEV

Norris Cotton Cancer Center, Dartmouth–Hitchcock Medical Center, Lebanon, NH

8.1 INTRODUCTION

Lung cancer is the most common cause of cancer-related death worldwide [1,2]. There are approximately 1.3 million lung-cancer-related deaths worldwide. There are 220,000 new cases of lung cancer and 160,000 deaths in the United States alone every year. This mortality rate is much higher than colorectal, breast, and prostates cancer deaths combined.

8.2 LUNG CANCER EPIDEMIOLOGY

Ample evidence links lung carcinogenesis and cigarette smoking. Shopland et al. estimate that 90% of detected lung cancer cases worldwide are related to cigarette smoking [3]. More than 1 billion people smoke tobacco worldwide [4]. The risk for the development of lung cancer is directly proportional to the time period and rate of smoking and declines with smoking cessation, but remains higher than the general population [5]. Environmental tobacco exposure via passive smoking is also a risk factor for lung cancer. Its recognition led to successful introduction of smoking restrictions in the workplace, public offices, and restaurants [6,7]. Since the 1980s, due to increased public awareness of the direct relationship between cigarette smoking and lung cancer, lung cancer has begun to decline in men; however, such decreases have not been observed in women, likely due to increased prevalence of smoking in women since the 1960s [3,8,9]. Even if smoking were completely eliminated today, lung cancer would remain a major health problem for decades.

Although smoking is the most common cause of lung cancer, there are other causes, as 10% of patients with lung cancer have no history of cigarette smoking [10]. Radon found in earth's crust is a colorless, odorless gas generated by the breakdown of radioactive radium which is the result of the decayed uranium. Prolonged radon gas exposure at high levels increases risk of lung cancer by 50% [11].

Cancer and Aging Handbook: Research and Practice, First Edition. Edited by Keith M. Bellizzi and Margot A. Gosney.
© 2012 Wiley-Blackwell. Published 2012 by John Wiley & Sons, Inc.

There is a well-established association between asbestos exposure and lung cancer. This effect is synergistic when combined with the effect of tobacco smoking [12]. Other, less common causes of lung cancer in nonsmokers are occupational respiratory carcinogens such as arsenic, nickel, chromium, polyaromatic hydrocarbons (PAHs), bisether, as well as air pollution and viruses (HPV, JC virus, BK virus, CMV, simian virus 40) [13]. Reducing exposure to these agents will lead to dramatic decreases in lung cancer risk for such individuals.

Over 60% of all cases of cancer are diagnosed in men and women over 65 years of age, with 67% of cancer deaths occurring in this older group [14]. Compared to 1990, by 2020 the population is expected to increase by 12%, but the incidence of cancer will increase by 60%. Lung cancer incidence and mortality also increase with age [15]. Between 1980 and 1998, lung cancer mortality rates decreased in patients younger than 55 years of age and increased in those older than 65 [16]. With ongoing decreases in cardiovascular mortality, progress in lung cancer prevention will have a major impact on longevity of older adults, as well as the entire population.

8.3 SMOKING PREVENTION AND CESSATION

Smokers have a risk for lung cancer that is on average 10-fold higher than in lifetime never-smokers (those who smoked <100 cigarettes in their lifetime). An extensive body of evidence links cigarette smoking to lung cancer in a causative relationship. The cessation of smoking results in a slow decline in the risk of cancer development, regardless of race or ethnicity, but this risk remains elevated compared to never-smokers even more than 15 years after smoking cessation [17,18]. The relative benefit of smoking cessation appears to be greater for those persons with shorter smoking histories [5]. Stopping smoking before middle age avoids more than 90% of the risk attributable to tobacco [19]. However, if people who have been smoking for many years stop, even well into middle age, they avoid most of their subsequent risk of lung cancer (Fig. 8.1). Therefore, older adults should be strongly encouraged to quit smoking not only for the benefits in terms of cardiovascular and pulmonary disease reduction but also for improvement in their risk for lung cancer. The prevention of smoking initiation and successful smoking cessation is expected to lead to a decline in lung cancer incidence and mortality. This has been seen in states instituting more aggressive antismoking campaigns.

For individuals who want to quit, there are various cessation programs available, from behavioral modifications to pharmacologic interventions [20]. The rates of smoking cessation increase when patients are asked about smoking, and counseling is provided, as a part of primary care. Group therapy has also been found to be an effective method. While acupuncture and hypnosis may not be successful, pharmacologic interventions such as nicotine replacement therapy and administration of bupropion [21] and varenicline [22] have been shown to increase smoking cessation rates (8).

8.4 CHEMOPREVENTION

Although smoking prevention and cessation remain essential in the overall strategy for lung cancer prevention, former smokers continue to have an elevated risk for lung

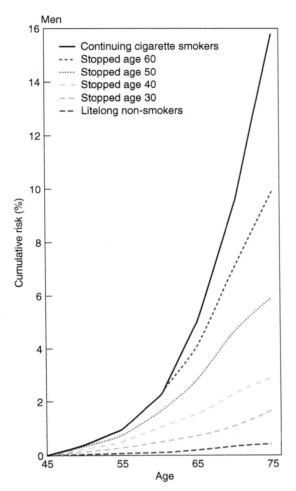

Figure 8.1 Decrease in the cumulative risk (%) of death from lung cancer up to age 75 from smoking cessation at various ages. (From Peto et al. [19].)

cancer for years after quitting [5,19,23,24]. Currently, 50% of lung cancers occur in those who have stopped smoking. Many former smokers do not develop lung cancer. Identifying individuals at higher risk for the disease will allow a more targeted approach to lung cancer prevention. Cancer incidence increases with age until the early 80s, but so do other conditions. A decision to include older adults in cancer prevention trials should be based on their functional status and physiologic rather than chronologic age. Such inclusion will allow a more precise assessment of the balance between long-term benefits and the accompanying side effects.

The cancer chemoprevention concept emphasizes intervention at early stages of carcinogenesis, even before malignancies become clinically apparent [25]. If chemoprevention is effective, this could avoid many clinical consequences of lung cancer and reduce the need for treatment of disseminated lung cancers that are often resistant to therapy. Improved understanding of the complex molecular and genetic pathways in the chronic process of lung carcinogenesis will lead to the development of diverse pharmacologic strategies for chemoprevention that target these multiple steps [26].

The selection of chemoprevention agents involves a careful process. Strong *in vitro* and animal model data should support the use of a specific approach. The choice of a given agent should not be based solely on epidemiologic data. More recent advances in tumor biology have resulted in the development of agents that target specific cellular pathways that are thought to be crucial for tumor development and progression. The chosen drug must have a favorable safety profile as it may be used for prolonged periods of time in otherwise healthy individuals who are at high -risk for developing lung cancer. The agent should be affordable and easy to administer. Alternative novel delivery approaches should also be considered [27].

8.4.1 Primary Chemoprevention

Primary chemoprevention strategies are designed to target individuals with known risk factors such as a significant smoking history, or occupational exposures to lung carcinogens. The retinoids (natural and synthetic analogs of vitamin A) are a class of agents that could exert potential clinical chemopreventive effects [28]. In 1925 Wolbach and Howe identified that vitamin A–dependent pathways are required for epithelial cell homeostasis [29]. They discovered that vitamin A deficiency in rodents caused squamous metaplasia in the trachea, as well as in other epithelial sites. This was reversed when the vitamin A deficiency was corrected. The observed changes were similar to those occurring in smokers, implicating a possible role for vitamin A in lung carcinogenesis. Epidemiological data have shown an association between vitamin A and cancer incidence as an inverse relationship was noted between vitamin A levels and incidence of cancer at specific sites [28]. These and other findings provided a basis for use of retinoids in lung cancer prevention.

The beta-Carotene and Retinol Efficacy Trial (CARET) was designed to study the effects of a combination of β-carotene and retinol on lung cancer incidence in subjects who were at high risk for the development of lung cancer [30]. The rationale was based on earlier observational epidemiologic studies. Over 18,000 subjects were enrolled in this trial, including current and former smokers, and asbestos workers. A planned interim analysis demonstrated a statistically significant increase in the relative risk for the development of lung cancer, death from any cause, and death from lung cancer [31]. These results lead to the early termination of the intervention.

The Alpha-Tocopherol Beta-Carotene (ATBC) cancer prevention study evaluated the effect of α-tocopherol (vitamin E) and β-carotene on the incidence of lung cancer in 30,000 Finnish male smokers. The selection of these agents was based almost exclusively on epidemiologic studies suggesting that a vegetable-rich diet (high in β-carotene and vitamin E) was associated with a decrease in the risk for the development of lung cancer. No effect of α-tocopherol on lung cancer incidence was observed. However, in the β-carotene arms, the relative risk of lung cancer increased. This effect was most pronounced in those subjects who smoked >20 cigarettes a day and in those who had a higher alcohol intake [32].

The Physicians' Health Study was a US randomized trial of aspirin and β-carotene in over 22,000 male physicians [33]. A minority of participants were current smokers, and just over one-third were former smokers. The primary endpoints were cardiovascular disease and cancer incidence. The study began in 1982, and the aspirin arms were closed in 1988 when a significant reduction in the incidence of myocardial infarction was noted. An analysis of the cancer incidence in the patients receiving β-carotene at the end of the study in 1995 showed no significant difference in the incidence of total cancers, lung cancer, or any other cancer. The findings from these three large studies established a negative clinical interaction between ongoing smoking and treatment with this chemopreventive agent. These adverse effects develop when carotenoids are taken in high dose by subjects who continue to smoke or who have been exposed to asbestos. This may be due to prooxidant effects of the higher concentrations of β-carotene resulting from supplementation, leading to DNA damage in individuals who continued to smoke while receiving treatment [34]. Clearly, lung cancer prevention should be combined with smoking cessation.

The Heart Outcomes Prevention Evaluation (HOPE) trial was an international study of vitamin E or placebo that enrolled nearly 10,000 subjects who were >55 years of age and had vascular disease or diabetes [35,36]. Lung cancer incidence did not differ between the vitamin E and placebo treatment arms.

8.4.2   Secondary Chemoprevention

Secondary chemoprevention approaches target individuals with identifiable preneoplastic lung lesions who are at clearly increased risk for developing lung cancer. Bronchial epithelial abnormalities can be identified in directed or blind endobronchial biopsies. There is an orderly progression of morphological changes in the bronchial epithelium from normal epithelium to metaplasia, increasing severity of dysplasia, carcinoma *in situ*, and invasive cancer [26,37] (Fig. 8.2). Theoretically, this is one of the most appropriate settings for prevention interventions to reduce risk. While this is a population at risk for invasive disease, all studies completed to date have not used cancer incidence as a primary objective. Trials of retinoids [38], nonclassical retinoids [39], folate and vitamin B_{12} [40], or antiinflammatory agents budesonide [41], and celecoxib

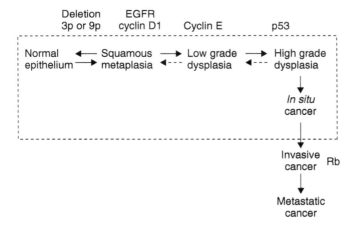

Figure 8.2   The multiple steps involved in lung carcinogenesis. This figure depicts the histological changes involved in the development of squamous cell cancers of the lung. Some preneoplastic lesions are considered reversible (solid arrow), while others may not be reversible (dotted arrow). Representative genetic alterations are also displayed. The outlined box includes potential targets for lung cancer chemoprevention. (From Dragnev et al. [26].)

[42] used either bronchial epithelial abnormalities or sputum atypia as a surrogate endpoint. There were indications that even when there was reversal posttreatment of the histological abnormalities, the improvement was limited to a short period following the intervention. Yet, the underlying genetic alterations might still have persisted [43]. It is not known whether these interventions would affect the subsequent development of invasive lung cancer.

8.4.3 Tertiary Chemoprevention

Individuals with a prior cancer of the aerodigestive tract (lung, head and neck, and esophagus) have a high rate of development of lung cancer. Patients who have undergone resection for early-stage NSCLC develop a second primary lung cancer at a rate of approximately 2% per year. Tertiary chemoprevention studies evaluate prevention strategies in patients with prior lung cancer with reduction of second primary cancers as the primary objective.

Early relatively small studies indicated benefit for retinoids (13-*cis*-retinoic acid/isotretinoin and retinyl palmitate) in reducing second primary cancer incidence [44,45]. Subsequent large trials were undertaken to confirm these results. A randomized US intergroup trial of isotretinoin in patients with resected stage I lung cancers did not show benefit. A reduction in second cancers was observed in the subset of study subjects who had never smoked [46]. A large European multicenter study also did not support a beneficial effect for retinyl palmitate and/or *N*-acetylcysteine [47]. In these trials a trend was observed for increased lung cancer incidence in patients who received the candidate preventive agent and continued to smoke, similar to the findings noted in the primary prevention studies. It is now recognized that the outcome of a chemoprevention trial may vary according to the characteristics of the subjects, such as negative in current smokers and positive in never-smokers. Such observations have a significant impact on the design of future lung chemoprevention studies.

Epidemiologic data have demonstrated lower serum levels of selenium in lung cancer patients compared with control subjects, and an association between high selenium exposure and a reduction in lung cancer risk. Selenium is an antioxidant with a mechanism of action related to oxidative stress, modulation of gene expression via DNA methylation, inhibition of COX2 expression, and other factors. A decrease in cancer incidence was observed following selenium supplementation in the Linxian Province, China [48]. A trial evaluating the role of selenium in reducing the incidence of non-melanomatous skin cancer unexpectedly showed a 26% decrease in lung cancer but did not demonstrate a decrease in the primary endpoint of skin cancer [49]. Expanding on these results, a US intergroup phase III study of selenium was conducted in patients who have had a complete resection of a stage I non–small cell lung cancer. This study was discontinued because of futility after an interim analysis showed no reduction in the incidence of second primary lung cancers [50].

8.5 LUNG CANCER CHEMOPREVENTION CHALLENGES

Clinical cancer chemoprevention trials are distinct from therapeutic trials. Chemoprevention agents are administered on a chronic basis and should have few, if any, clinical toxicities. Different populations of patients are likely to have diverse tolerability thresholds. Individuals who have already undergone a resected primary lung cancer may accept some side effects of chemoprevention agents, if this would reduce their risk of a second malignancy. Subjects at high risk for a primary lung tumor but who have not had cancer may be less amenable to a preventive drug that has side effects. Older adults face competing causes of morbidity and mortality. A relatively small risk to develop cancer in many years and a higher risk for complications from an existing nonmalignant but serious condition may render participation in a primary cancer chemoprevention trial less attractive. On the other hand, the higher risk for cancer in an older adult in generally good health but with preneoplastic lesions or prior cancer should be motivation for interventions that will reduce this risk. As life expectancy increases, effective lung cancer prevention, including smoking cessation, in older adults who have risk factors should become part of regular health maintenance. Ultimately, decisions to undergo chemopreventive interventions should be individualized and based not on age but on an estimate of the cancer risk, complication rates from the treatment, comorbidities, general functional status, and life expectancy without cancer.

Cancer chemoprevention trials require large sample sizes and long follow-up in order to achieve statistically meaningful results. Therefore, biomarkers or surrogate endpoints have been used to assess the potential for chemopreventive activity before the clinical outcomes are known [26]. These biomarkers may represent targets for lung cancer chemoprevention and may also serve as surrogate markers for response to candidate chemopreventive agents. Any individual regardless of age who is at risk for development of cancer could potentially participate in such biomarker-driven trials. Ultimately, such biomarkers will require validation in clinical trials that have cancer incidence as the primary endpoint.

The most appropriate patient population for evaluation of a particular chemoprevention strategy has not been identified. There is general agreement that former smokers should be enrolled in lung cancer prevention trials. Never-smokers are at relatively low risk for the development of lung cancer, and their inclusion will increase the size of the trial as the sample size typically is determined by the expected incidence of lung cancer in the control groups. With the potentially adverse outcomes that were reported in smokers who had received some chemopreventive agents, there is a concern about the inclusion in such trials of current smokers who are at highest risk for the development of lung cancer, unless highly successful smoking cessation is achieved.

8.6 CONCLUSIONS

Cancer chemoprevention is a rational approach to reducing the burden of lung cancer. As the molecular mechanisms of lung carcinogenesis are being unraveled, diverse strategies are introduced to reverse or arrest progression of the multistep process of lung cancer development. No effective agent for lung cancer chemoprevention has yet been identified. Selection of the individuals to be targeted for chemoprevention studies should be based on cancer risk, rather than age. Tobacco exposure is among the most preventable causes of morbidity and mortality in the United States. It is imperative not only to promote the cessation of tobacco use but also to prevent the initiation of smoking. Emphasizing that it is never too late to quit should be a constant message. Only through progress in tobacco prevention, better screening techniques, and improved molecular understanding of lung cancer, can a reduction in the incidence and mortality from lung cancer be expected to become reality.

REFERENCES

1. Jemal A, Center MM, DeSantis C, Ward EM. Global patterns of cancer incidence and mortality rates and trends. *Cancer Epidemiol Biomarkers Prevent* 2008;**19**:1893–1907.
2. Thun MJ, DeLancey JO, Center MM, Jemal A, Ward EM. The global burden of cancer: Priorities for prevention. *Carcinogenesis* 2010;**31**:100–110.
3. Shopland DR, Eyre HJ, Pechacek TF. Smoking-attributable cancer mortality in 1991: Is lung cancer now the leading cause of death among smokers in the United States? *J Natl Cancer Inst* 1991;**83**:1142–1148.
4. Jha P. Avoidable global cancer deaths and total deaths from smoking. *Nat Rev Cancer* 2009;**9**:655–664.
5. Halpern MT, Gillespie BW, Warner KE. Patterns of absolute risk of lung cancer mortality in former smokers. *J Natl Cancer Inst* 1993;**85**:457–464.
6. Fontham ET, Correa P, Reynolds P, et al. Environmental tobacco smoke and lung cancer in nonsmoking women. A multicenter study. *JAMA* 1994;**271**:1752–1759.
7. Janerich DT, Thompson WD, Varela LR, et al. Lung cancer and exposure to tobacco smoke in the household. *N Engl J Med* 1990;**323**:632–636.
8. Fiore, MC. US public health service clinical practice guideline: Treating tobacco use and dependence. *Respir Care* 2000;**45**:1200–1262.
9. Boyle P. Cancer, cigarette smoking and premature death in Europe: A review including the Recommendations of European Cancer Experts Consensus Meeting, Helsinki, October 1996. *Lung Cancer* 1997;**17**:1–60.
10. Thun MJ, Henley SJ, Burns D, et al. Lung cancer death rates in lifelong nonsmokers. *J Natl Cancer Inst* 2006;**98**:691–699.
11. Field RW, Steck DJ, Smith BJ, et al. The Iowa radon lung cancer study—phase I: Residential radon gas exposure and lung cancer. *Sci Total Environ* 2001;**272**:67–72.
12. O'Reilly KM, McLaughlin AM, Beckett WS, Sime PJ. Asbestos-related lung disease. *Am Family Phys* 2007;**75**:683–688.
13. Giuliani L, Jaxmar T, Casadio C, et al. Detection of oncogenic viruses SV40, BKV, JCV, HCMV, HPV and p53 codon 72 polymorphism in lung carcinoma. *Lung Cancer* 2007;**57**:273–281.
14. Kennedy BJ. Aging and cancer. *Oncology* 2000;**14**:1731–1733; discussion 34, 39–40.
15. Flanders WD, Lally CA, Zhu BP, Henley SJ, Thun MJ. Lung cancer mortality in relation to age, duration of smoking, and daily cigarette consumption: Results from Cancer Prevention Study II. *Cancer Res* 2003;**63**:6556–6562.
16. Wingo PA, Cardinez CJ, Landis SH, et al. Long-term trends in cancer mortality in the United States, 1930–1998. *Cancer* 2003;**97**:3133–275.
17. US Dept. Health and Human Services. *A Report of the Surgeon General: The Health Benefits of Smoking Cessation*. DHSS Publication (CDC) 1990, 90–8416.
18. Wong KY, Seow A, Koh WP, et al. Smoking cessation and lung cancer risk in an Asian population: Findings from the Singapore Chinese Health Study. *Br J Cancer* 2010;**103**:1093–1096.
19. Peto R, Darby S, Deo H, et al. Smoking, smoking cessation, and lung cancer in the UK since 1950: Combination of national statistics with two case-control studies. *Br Med J* 2000;**321**:323–329.
20. Gray J, Mao JT, Szabo E, et al. Lung cancer chemoprevention: ACCP evidence-based clinical practice guidelines (2nd edition). *Chest* 2007;**132**:56S–68S.
21. Hurt RD, Sachs DP, Glover ED, et al. A comparison of sustained-release bupropion and placebo for smoking cessation. *N Engl J Med* 1997;**337**:1195–1202.

22. Gonzales D, Rennard SI, Nides M, et al. Varenicline, an alpha4beta2 nicotinic acetylcholine receptor partial agonist, vs sustained-release bupropion and placebo for smoking cessation: A randomized controlled trial. *JAMA* 2006;**296**:47–55.

23. Ebbert JO, Yang P, Vachon CM, et al. Lung cancer risk reduction after smoking cessation: Observations from a prospective cohort of women. *J Clin Oncol* 2003;**21**:921–926.

24. Anonymous Widespread smoking cessation has halved UK lung cancer mortality. *Br Med J* 2000;**321**:0.2.

25. Sporn MB. Approaches to prevention of epithelial cancer during the preneoplastic period. *Cancer Res* 1976;**36**:2699–2702.

26. Dragnev KH, Stover D, Dmitrovsky E. Lung cancer prevention: The guidelines. *Chest* 2003;**123**:60S–71S.

27. Spinella M. J, Dmitrovsky E. Aerosolized delivery and lung cancer prevention: Pre-clinical models show promise. *Clin Cancer Res* 2000;**6**:2963–2964.

28. Hong WK, Itri LM. Retinoids and human cancer. In: Sporn MB, Roberts AB, Goodman DS eds., *The Retinoids: Biology, Chemistry, and Medicine*, 2nd ed., Raven Press, New York, 1994, pp. 597–630.

29. Wolbach SB, Howe PR. Tissue changes following deprivation of fat-soluble vitamin A. *J Exp Med* 1925;**42**:753–777.

30. Omenn GS, Goodman GE, Thornquist MD, et al. Effects of a combination of beta carotene and vitamin A on lung cancer and cardiovascular disease. *N Engl J Med* 1996;**334**: 1150–1155.

31. Omenn GS, Goodman GE, Thornquist MD, et al. Risk factors for lung cancer and for intervention effects in CARET, the Beta-Carotene and Retinol Efficacy Trial. *J Natl Cancer Inst* 1996;**88**:1550–1559.

32. The Alpha-Tocopherol, Beta-Carotene, Cancer, et al. The effect of vitamin E and beta carotene on the incidence of lung cancer and other cancers in male smokers. *N Engl J Med* 1994;**330**:1029–1035.

33. Cook NR, Le IM, Manson JE, Buring JE, Hennekens CH. Effects of beta-carotene supplementation on cancer incidence by baseline characteristics in the Physicians' Health Study (United States). *Cancer Causes Control* 2000;**11**:617–626.

34. Paiva SA, Russell RM. Beta-carotene and other carotenoids as antioxidants. *J Am Coll Nutr* 1999;**18**:426–433.

35. Lonn E, Bosch J, Yusuf S, et al. Effects of long-term vitamin E supplementation on cardiovascular events and cancer: A randomized controlled trial. *JAMA* 2005;**293**:1338–1347.

36. McQueen MJ, Lonn E, Gerstein HC, Bosch J, Yusuf S. The HOPE (Heart Outcomes Prevention Evaluation) Study and its consequences. *Scand J Clin Lab Investing Suppl* 2005;**240**:143–156.

37. Saccomanno G, Archer VE, Auerbach O, Saunders RP, Brennan LM. Development of carcinoma of the lung as reflected in exfoliated cells. *Cancer* 1974;**33**:256–270.

38. Lee JS, Lippman SM, Benner SE, et al. Randomized placebo-controlled trial of isotretinoin in chemoprevention of bronchial squamous metaplasia. *J Clin Oncol* 1994;**12**:937–945.

39. Kurie JM, Lee JS, Khuri FR, et al. N- (4-hydroxyphenyl)retinamide in the chemoprevention of squamous metaplasia and dysplasia of the bronchial epithelium. *Clin Cancer Res* 2000;**6**:2973–2979.

40. Heimburger DC, Alexander CB, Birch R, et al. Improvement in bronchial squamous metaplasia in smokers treated with folate and vitamin B12. Report of a preliminary randomized, double-blind intervention trial. *JAMA* 1988;**259**:1525–1530.

41. Lam S, leRiche JC, McWilliams A, et al. A randomized phase IIb trial of pulmicort turbuhaler (budesonide) in people with dysplasia of the bronchial epithelium. *Clin Cancer Res* 2004;**10**:6502–6511.

42. Mao JT, Fishbein MC, Adams B, et al. Celecoxib decreases Ki-67 proliferative index in active smokers. *Clin Cancer Res* 2006;**12**:314–320.

43. Mao L, El-Naggar AK, Papadimitrakopoulou V, et al. Phenotype and genotype of advanced premalignant head and neck lesions after chemopreventive therapy. *J Natl Cancer Inst* 1998;**90**:1545–1551.

44. Hong WK, Lippman SM, Itri LM, et al. Prevention of second primary tumors with isotretinoin in squamous-cell carcinoma of the head and neck. *N Engl J Med* 1990;**323**: 795–801.

45. Pastorino U, Infante M, Maioli M, et al. Adjuvant treatment of stage I lung cancer with high-dose vitamin A. *J Clin Oncol* 1993;**11**:1216–1222.

46. Lippman SM, Lee JJ, Karp DD, et al. Randomized phase III intergroup trial of isotretinoin to prevent second primary tumors in stage I non-small-cell lung cancer. *J Natl Cancer Inst* 2001;**93**:605–618.

47. van Zandwijk N, Dalesio O, Pastorino U, de Vries N, van Tinteren H. EUROSCAN, a randomized trial of vitamin A and N-acetylcysteine in patients with head and neck cancer or lung cancer. For the European Organization for Research and Treatment of Cancer Head and Neck and Lung Cancer Cooperative Groups. *J Natl Cancer Inst* 2000;**92**:977–986.

48. Blot WJ, Li JY, Taylor PR, et al. Nutrition intervention trials in Linxian, China: Supplementation with specific vitamin/mineral combinations, cancer incidence, and disease-specific mortality in the general population. *J Natl Cancer Inst* 1993;**85**:1483–1492.

49. Clark LC, Combs GF Jr, Turnbull BW, et al. Effects of selenium supplementation for cancer prevention in patients with carcinoma of the skin. A randomized controlled trial. Nutritional Prevention of Cancer Study Group. *JAMA* 1996;**276**:1957–1963.

50. Karp DD, Lee SJ, Shaw Wright GL, et al. A phase III, intergroup, randomized, double-blind, chemoprevention trial of selenium (Se) supplementation in resected stage I non-small cell lung cancer (NSCLC). *J Clin Oncol* 2010;**28**:abstr CRA7004.

PART III

CANCER SCREENING GUIDELINES FOR OLDER ADULTS

CHAPTER 9

Cancer in Older People: To Screen or Not to Screen?

CATHERINE TERRET and JEAN-PIERRE DROZ

Claude Bernard University, Lyon, France

9.1 INTRODUCTION

Aging is associated with an increasing prevalence of diseases, among which cancer holds a leading place. Approximately 43% of men and 30% of women older than 65 years will develop cancer [1]. Logically enough, the earliest detection of a tumor in the elderly population should result in the most favorable outcomes in terms of cancer mortality and patient quality of life.

Screening is defined as the early detection of cancer in asymptomatic individuals [2]. Screening is considered effective when leading to a reduction in cancer-related deaths. Large randomized trials have shown efficacy for reducing mortality from breast cancer in women aged <70 years [3] and from colorectal cancer under the age of 74 years [4].

However, little is known about true benefits and harms of cancer screening in the elderly population [5,6].

9.2 CANCER TYPES

9.2.1 Colorectal Cancer

Colorectal cancer occurs mostly in older people, with 75% of cases diagnosed after the age of 65 years. Colorectal cancers are generally adenocarcinomas, of which 60–80% derive from adenomas. Colorectal screening programs aim not only at reducing mortality of existent malignant lesions but also at preventing colorectal cancer through polypectomy.

Different screening tests have been proposed by a number of medical associations [7]. Randomized studies have shown that screening using fecal occult blood tests (FOBTs) leads to a 15–18% decrease of specific mortality in people aged 45–74 years. These results were obtained at 8–10 years from the start of screening programs [8–10].

Cancer and Aging Handbook: Research and Practice, First Edition. Edited by Keith M. Bellizzi and Margot A. Gosney.
© 2012 Wiley-Blackwell. Published 2012 by John Wiley & Sons, Inc.

Because the most appropriate interval between repeated screening tests remains unde-fined, both annual and biennial FOBT screening programs are recommended. Although the use of FOBT appears relatively easy, this test should be proposed only for older individuals who are able to comply with the instructions.

Full colonoscopy every 10 years represents the screening test of choice owing to high specificity and sensitivity [11]. A colonoscopy can detect both colon tumors and polyps. Several studies have demonstrated the effect of screening colonoscopy on colorectal cancer incidence [12]. Furthermore, more recent data have shown the procedure to be safe and effective in people aged 80 years and older [13,14]. However, conflicting results have been reported by a cross-sectional study conducted among 1244 individuals undergoing screening colonoscopy and comparing the estimated life-years saved (LYS) in very elderly ($\geq$80 years) and younger persons [15]. Although the prevalence of colon cancer increases with age, the adjusted mean extension of life expectancy and the percentage of patients who benefited from screening colonoscopy were low in the elderly group (1.7% and 16%, respectively).

9.2.2 Breast Cancer

Around 50% of breast cancer cases occur in women aged 60 years and older. Detection at an early stage has been shown to significantly improve patient prognosis [16].

There are three different breast cancer screening methods: breast self-examination (BSE), clinical breast examination (CBE), and mammograms. The effectiveness of BSE remains uncertain; existing meta-analyses and randomized trials have failed to show a significant reduction in the breast cancer mortality rate [17,18]. Moreover, to be effective, BSE requires correct training and thus cannot be safely undertaken in older women with moderate to severe cognitive impairment. Studies have shown that older women are less aware of the risk of breast cancer and have less proficiency to perform BSE [19].

Screening mammography has proved effective, since a 17% reduction in breast cancer–related death (range 15-23%) has been reported in women aged 50–69 years [20]. Little evidence exists on the benefit of screening mammography after the age of 70 years; however, trials including women aged 70–74 years have shown a trend toward a decrease in mortality (RR 0.94; 95% CI 0.60–1.64) [21]. Walter and coworkers have evaluated the potential burden of breast cancer screening in a cohort of 216 frail older women aged $\geq$55 years (mean age 81 years) [22]. Most patients had more than five comorbidities; 49% had cognitive impairment. Few women (18%) had abnormal mammography, and experienced a burden from the screening mammography (false-positive mammograms, pain or psychological distress). Four women were diagnosed with either invasive cancer [3] or ductal carcinoma *in situ* [1]. Only two of them supposedly derived benefit from cancer screening.

Clinical breast examination might represent a valuable screening tool when per-formed by trained health professionals. A Canadian randomized study comparing CBE versus mammography plus CBE has not identified any difference in mortality between the two groups [23], suggesting that CBE detects most of the breast cancers identi-fied by mammography. Conversely, mammograms fail to detect around 5-10% of the tumors uncovered at CBE. The estimated sensitivity of screening CBE is 40–69%, and its specificity is ~95% [24]. Thus, this procedure should be an integral part of any breast cancer screening program.

9.2.3   Prostate Cancer

Prostate cancer affects 679,000 men and causes 221,000 deaths worldwide each year [25]. Most men develop slow-growing tumors that are unlikely to cause serious morbidity during progression; however, patients sometimes suffer from tumors with more aggressive behaviors and would clearly benefit from early diagnosis [26].

The advantages of screening remain uncertain to date. Results of two major trials have been published in 2009. The European study ERSPC (European Randomized Study of Screening for Prostate Cancer) compared a group of more than 150,000 asymptomatic men receiving screening and follow-up to a control group [27]. Results revealed a 20% reduction in prostate cancer–related mortality and showed that 1410 and 48 asymptomatic men had to be screened and treated to prevent one death. Most positive PSA results were false-positive, leading to a considerable number of negative biopsies. The American study PLCO (Prostate, Lung, Colorectal and Ovarian Cancer Screening), which included more than 75,000 men, did not detect any significant benefit of PSA screening compared to no screening [28]. It is noteworthy that half of the men in the control group were also tested for prostate cancer using PSA, outside the protocol.

Conversely, prostate cancer screening entails substantial costs. It leads to an estimated 50% overdiagnosis [29], and to overtreatment, since the majority of prostate cancer diagnosed in patients in the screening arms had a Gleason grade of <7 and would not have required treatment [30].

9.3   BALANCE BETWEEN BENEFITS AND RISKS OF SCREENING IN ELDERLY PEOPLE

Cancer screening in elderly people involves two key issues; life expectancy and expected tumour severity. People with a life expectancy higher than 5 years are consensually considered as potential candidates for cancer screening [8,9,31]. Since most people worldwide aged ≥89 years have a life expectancy shorter than 5 years (data available on World Health Organization website, `http://apps.who.int/ghodata/?vid=720`), they cannot be considered appropriate targets for cancer screening programs.

The lack of consistent guidelines leads to a huge heterogeneity of cancer screening use in the older population. Because the estimation of individual health status or life expectancy appears to be difficult in the absence of validated methodology, we observe both overscreening and underscreening in the elderly population [32,33]. Moreover, physician recommendations have been shown to significantly influence screening behaviors [34]. These findings suggest that in order to promote adequate use of cancer screening in the elderly population, efforts should be made to enhance physicians' education on the risks and benefits of the procedure.

When studying people's attitudes toward the continuation of cancer screening in the later periods of life, Lewis and coworkers observed that most older well-educated adults were in favor of continuing screening for themselves throughout life, even against physician recommendations [35], and most believed that other elderly people living in nursing homes, or having dementia or being totally dependent should also continue to be screened. These findings suggest that there should also be efforts to improve the information given to older adults about the potential survival benefits and risks of cancer screening. In addition, the prevalence of cognitive impairment increases with age, and cancer screening poses significant ethical issues for people with cognitive decline. Studies have shown that older adults with dementia were less likely to undergo cancer screening [34,36–40]. Raik and coworkers have proposed a framework for screening mammography decision making in cognitively impaired women; this framework could be extended to other screening decisions [37]. The authors have factored in the severity of dementia, patient life expectancy, and the potential risks and benefits of cancer screening, as well as patient or surrogate preferences, when known. Their conclusion is that when screening leads to life-prolonging therapy or better quality of life, the procedure should be recommended.

The cost-effectiveness of screening requires evaluation. Extending breast cancer screening to age 79 years saved an additional 2.4 and 24.9 days of life per woman, respectively, for the entire population and among women destined to develop breast cancer, with a incremental cost >$82,000 per LYS [41]. Extending screening to lifetime would save an additional 1.1 and 12 days for the whole population and for breast cancer cases and costs >$151,000 per LYS. From a societal perspective, the cost-effectiveness of breast cancer screening is too low to warrant such screening on an annual basis beyond the age of 70 years. Similar results have been observed for prostate cancer screening, with an average 2.6-day gain in survival per person screened in the European study. One major limitation of cancer screening in the elderly population is the lack of consistent guidelines. To date only one organization recommends prostate cancer screening in male individuals [42,43]. It is important to note that there are no "negative" guidelines for breast or colorectal cancers.

9.4 PERSPECTIVES

The true benefits of cancer screening remain uncertain in the elderly population in terms of both survival improvement and cost-effectiveness. However, an individual early detection program should probably be considered for older individuals eligible for effective cancer therapy [2,44].

Breast cancer screening in elderly women should be based at least on regular CBE performed at any routine medical visit. Serial mammography may be recommended to healthy women with an estimated life expectancy higher than 3 years beyond time of visit. Women who previously participated to organised screening programs should be offered to continue regular mammography screening when the program stops, i.e. after an age varying between 69 to 74 years, with regard to their health status.

Early detection of colorectal tumors could spare individuals from undergoing emergency surgery for bowel obstruction or perforation. Furthermore, since most recurrences occur within 5 years from diagnosis, annual high–sensitivity procedures like guaiac FOBT or faecal immunochemical testing (FIT) seem appropriate for older patients able to handle them correctly, whereas full colonoscopy every 10 years may be an alternative approach for those unable to perform stool collection properly [42].

The detection of prostate cancer in older men is still questionable. Again, it should be offered to elderly individuals who have access to information about risks and benefits and to treatment options including watchful waiting. Alternatively, discontinuation of cancer screening seems reasonable for patients who have severe comorbidity, limited life expectancy, or poor health status and who are not fit for cancer treatment.

REFERENCES

1. Hayat MJ, Howlader N, Reichman ME, Edwards BK. Cancer statistics, trends, and multiple primary cancer analyses from the Surveillance, Epidemiology, and End Results (SEER) Program. *Oncologist* 2007;**12**:20–37.

2. Wilson JM. Principles of screening for disease. *Proc R Soc Med*; 1971;**64**:1255–1256.

3. Swedish Organised Service Screening Evaluation Group. Reduction in breast cancer mortality from organized service screening with mammography: 1. Further confirmation with extended data. *Cancer Epidemiol Biomark Prevent* 2006;**15**:45–51.

4. Heresbach D, Manfredi S, D'halluin PN, Bretagne JF, Branger B. Review in depth and meta-analysis of controlled trials on colorectal cancer screening by faecal occult blood test. *Eur J Gastroenterol Hepatol* 2006;**18**:427–433.

5. Terret C, Castel-Kremer E, Albrand, Droz JP. Effects of comorbidity on screening and early diagnosis of cancer in the elderly. *Lancet Oncol* 2009;**10**:80–87.

6. Quarini C, Gosney M. review of the evidence for a colorectal cancer screening programme in elderly people. *Age Ageing* 2009;**38**:503–508.

7. Levin B, Lieberman DA, McFarland B, Andrews KS, Brooks D, Bond J, et al. Screening and surveillance for the early detection of colorectal cancer and adenomatous polyps, 2008: A joint guideline from the American Cancer Society, the US Multi-Society Task Force on Colorectal Cancer, and the American College of Radiology. *CA Cancer J Clin* 2008;**58**:130–160.

8. Kronborg O, Fenger C, Olsen J, Jørgensen OD, Søndergaard O. Randomised study of screening for colorectal cancer with faecal-occult blood test. *Lancet* 1996;**348**:1467–1471.

9. Hardcastle JD, Thomas WM. Occult blood tests. *Lancet* 1989;**2**:672.

10. Faivre J, Tazi MA, El Mrini T, Lejeune C, Benhamiche AM, Dassonville F. Faecal occult blood screening and reduction of colorectal cancer mortality: A case-control study. *Br J Cancer* 1999;**79**:680–683.

11. Rex DK, Johnson DA, Anderson JC, Schoenfeld PS, Burke CA, Inadomi JM. American College of Gastroenterology guidelines for colorectal cancer screening 2008. *Am J Gastroenterol* 2009;**104**:739–750.

12. Kahi CJ, Imperiale TF, Juliar BE, Rex DK. Effects of screening colonoscopy on colorectal cancer incidence and mortality. *Clin Gastroenterol Hepatol* 2009;**7**:770–775.

13. Arora A, Singh P. Colonoscopy in patients 80 years of age and older is safe, with high success rate and diagnostic yield. *Gastrointest Endosc* 2004;**60**:408–413.

14. Karajeh MA, Sanders DS, Hurlstone DP. Colonoscopy in elderly people is a safe procedure with a high diagnostic yield: A prospective comparative study of 2000 patients. *Endoscopy* 2006;**38**:226–230.

15. Lin OS, Kozarek RA, Schembre DB, Ayub K, Gluck M, Drennan F, et al. Screening colonoscopy in very elderly patients. Prevalence of neoplasia and estimated impact on life expectancy. *JAMA* 2006;**295**:2357–2365.

16. Gamel JW, Meyer JS, Feuer E, Miller BA. The impact of stage and histology on the long-term clinical course in 163,808 patients with breast carcinoma. *Cancer* 1996;**77**:1459–1464.

17. Hackshaw AK, Paul EA. Breast self-examination and death from breast cancer: A meta-analysis. *Br J Cancer* 2003;**88**:1047–1053.

18. Kösters JP, Gøtzsche PC. Regular self-examination or clinical examination for early detection of breast cancer. *Cochrane Database Syst Rev* 2003:CD003373.

19. Hurdle DA. Breast cancer prevention with older women: A gender-focused intervention study. *Health Care Women Int* 2007;**28**:872–887.

20. Mandelblatt JS, Cronin KA, Bailey S, Berry DA, de Koning HJ, Draisma G, et al. Effects of mammography screening under different screening schedules: Model estimates of potential benefits and harms. *Ann Intern Med* 2009;**151**:738–747.

21. Nyström L, Rutqvist LE, Wall S, Lindgren A, Lindqvist M, Rydén S, et al. Breast cancer screening with mammography: Overview of Swedish randomised trials. *Lancet* 1993;**341**:973–978.

22. Walter LC, Eng C, Covinsky KE. Screening mammography for frail older women. *J Gen Intern Med* 2001;**16**:779–784.

23. Miller AB, To T, Baines CJ, Wall C. Canadian National Breast Screening Study-2: 13-year results of a randomized trial in women aged 50–59 years. *J Natl Cancer Inst* 2000;**92**:1490–1499.

24. Barton MB, Harris R, Fletcher S. Does this patient have breast cancer? The screening clinical breast examination: Should it be done? How? *JAMA* 1999;**282**:1270–1280.

25. Parkin DM, Bray F, Ferlay J, Pisani P. Global cancer statistics, 2002. *CA Cancer J Clin* 2005;**55**:74–108.

26. Johansson JE, Andren O, Andersson SO, Dickman PW, Holmberg L, Magnuson A, et al. Natural history of early, localized prostate cancer. *JAMA* 2004;**291**:2713–2719.

27. Schröder FH, Hugosson J, Roobol MJ, Tammela TLJ, Ciatto S, Nelen V, et al. Screening and prostate-cancer mortality in a randomized European study. *N Engl J Med* 2009;**360**:1320–1328.

28. Andriole GL, Grubb RL III, Buys SS, Chia D, Church TR, Fouad MN, et al. Mortality results from a randomized prostate-cancer screening trial. *N Engl J Med* 2009;**360**:1310–1319.

29. Draisma G, Etzioni R, Tsodikov A, Mariotto A, Wever E, Gulati R, et al. Lead time and overdiagnosis in prostate-specific antigen screening: Importance of methods and context. *J Natl Cancer Inst* 2009;**101**:374–383.

30. Stark JR, Mucci L, Rothman KJ, Adami HO. Prostate cancer screening: The controversy continues. *Br Med J* 2009;**339**:784–786.

31. Walter LC, Lindquist K, Covinsky KE. Relationship between health status and use of screening mammography and Papanicolaou smears among women older than 70 years of age. *Ann Intern Med* 2004;**140**:681–688.

32. Cooper GS, Fortinsky RH, Hapke R, Landefeld CS. Primary care physician recommendations for colorectal cancer screening: patient and practitioner factors. *Arch Intern Med* 1997;**157**:1946–1950.

33. Sharp PC, Michielutte R, Spangler JG, Cunningham L, Freimanis R. Primary care providers' concerns and recommendations regarding mammography screening for older women. *J Cancer Educ* 2005;**20**:34–38.

34. Blustein J, Weiss LJ. The use of mammography by women aged 75 years and older: Factors related to health, functioning, and age. *J Am Geriatr Soc* 1998;**46**:941–946.

35. Lewis CL, Kistler CE, Amick HR, Watson LC, Bynum DL, Walter LC, et al. Older adults' attitudes about continuing cancer screening later in life: A pilot study interviewing residents of two continuing care communities. *BMC Geriatr* 2006;**6**:10.

36. Heflin MT, Oddone EZ, Pieper CF, Burchett BM, Cohen HJ. The effect of comorbid illness on receipt of cancer screening by older people. *J Am Geriatr Soc* 2002;**50**:1651–1658.

37. Raik BL, Miller FG, Fins JJ. Screening and cognitive impairment: Ethics of forgoing mammography in older women. *J Am Geriatr Soc* 2004;**52**:440–444.

38. Legg JS, Clement DG, White KR. Are women with self-reported cognitive limitation at risk for underutilization of mammography? *J Health Care Poor Underserv* 2004;**15**:688–702.

39. Gorin SS, Heck JE, Albert S, Hershman D. Treatment for breast cancer in patients with Alzheimer's disease. *J Am Geriatr Soc* 2005;**53**:1897–1904.

40. Gupta SK, Lamont EB. Patterns of presentation, diagnosis, and treatment in older patients with colon cancer and comorbid dementia. *J Am Geriatr Soc* 2004;**52**:1681–1687.

41. Mandelblatt JS, Schechter CB, Yabroof KR, Lawrence W, Dignam J, Extermann M, et al. Towards optimal screening strategies for older women. *J Gen Intern Med* 2005;**20**:487–496.

42. Smith RA, Cokkinides V, Brooks D, saslow D, Brawley OW. Cancer screening in the United States, 2010. A review of current American Cancer Society guidelines and issues in cancer screening. *CA Cancer J Clin* 2012;**62**:129–142.

43. Advisory Committee on Cancer Prevention. Recommendations on cancer screening in the European Union. *Eur J Cancer* 2000;**36**:1473–1478.

44. Walter LC, Covinsky KE. Cancer screening in elderly patients. A framework for individualized decision making. *JAMA* 2001;**285**:2750–2756.

CHAPTER 10

Breast Cancer Screening

HEIDI D. NELSON

Oregon Health & Science University, Portland, OR

10.1 INTRODUCTION

Screening is a preventive service specifically intended to detect a health condition in early stages and identify individuals requiring healthcare intervention in order to improve health outcomes [1]. Individuals undergoing screening have no recognized signs or symptoms of the condition at the time of screening. An appropriate screening test must be accurate, be acceptable to users, and not cause excessive harm.

Breast cancer screening has become confusing and controversial, in part because of different understandings of what it means to screen. Women undergo mammography, other breast imaging technologies, and physical examinations for multiple reasons—diagnostic evaluations for new findings, surveillance of previous malignant and nonmalignant lesions, and monitoring of women at high risk for breast cancer, as well as for screening asymptomatic average-risk women. It is important to differentiate these purposes in order to accurately interpret evidence from studies of screening, and to understand the rationale behind clinical recommendations for screening.

10.2 RISK ASSESSMENT

Most recommendations for breast cancer screening define the screening pool as average-risk women without current abnormal physical or mammographic findings, previous breast cancer, or other important risk factors placing them at high risk for breast cancer (Fig. 10.1). The first step in screening requires determining the existence of important risk factors to correctly identify a woman's level of risk. Women with factors increasing their risk to high and moderate levels require closer monitoring than do women with minor or no risk factors. However, since the majority of women with breast cancer have no risk factors beyond age and gender, using risk factors to assure women that their risk is low could be misleading and discourage them from appropriate screening practices.

Cancer and Aging Handbook: Research and Practice, First Edition. Edited by Keith M. Bellizzi and Margot A. Gosney.
© 2012 Wiley-Blackwell. Published 2012 by John Wiley & Sons, Inc.

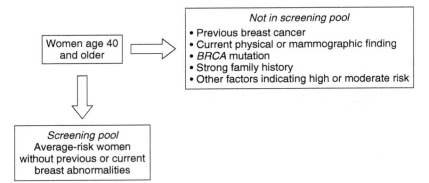

Figure 10.1   Most screening recommendations apply to average-risk women with no previous or current breast abnormalities. Women outside the screening pool fall under recommendations for monitoring high-risk women, surveillance, or diagnosis.

Although many potential risk factors have been associated with breast cancer in epidemiologic studies, few are useful for stratifying individuals into risk categories for clinical purposes [2]. Risk factors associated with high or moderate risk include known deleterious *BRCA1* or *BRCA2* gene mutations, or the presence of a mutation in a first-degree relative in the absence of testing; lifetime risk of breast cancer above 15% based on family history models; previous radiation therapy to the chest; personal history of breast cancer, ductal carcinoma *in situ* (DCIS), lobular carcinoma *in situ* (LCIS), atypical ductal hyperplasia (ADH), or atypical lobular hyperplasia (ALH); dense breasts when viewed on mammography; and the existence of Li–Fraumeni syndrome, Cowden syndrome, or hereditary diffuse gastric cancer in self or a first-degree relative (Table 10.1) [3,4].

Determining individual risk on the basis of additional risk factors is imprecise. Risk stratification models that predict an individual's risk for developing breast cancer have been evaluated for use in clinical settings, including primary care [2]. These differ from more complex models developed for genetic counseling that focus primarily on family history. The Breast Cancer Risk Assessment Tool (also referred to as the *Gail model*) was the first major breast cancer risk stratification model to be used clinically. It was derived from multivariate logistic regression analysis of identified risk factors for breast cancer using data from the Breast Cancer Detection and Demonstration Project (BCDDP) and US national data for invasive cancer from the Surveillance, Epidemiology, and End Results (SEER) program [5,6].

Subsequently developed risk stratification models use an approach similar to that for the Breast Cancer Risk Assessment Tool; however, they vary in their use of reference standards and by the variables they include. The original model included age, age at menarche, age of first birth, family history of breast cancer in first-degree relatives, number of previous breast biopsies, and history of atypical hyperplasia [5]. Subsequent models include one or more of these variables in addition to other factors, including race, body mass index (BMI) or height, estrogen and progestin use, parity, history of breastfeeding, menopause status or age, smoking, alcohol use, physical activity, breast density, and diet [2].

Risk stratification models demonstrate good calibration, with the expected number of breast cancer cases in a study population closely matching the number of breast

TABLE 10.1   Risk for Breast Cancer

High risk
  Known *BRCA1* or *BRCA2* gene mutation
  Mutation status not known, but first-degree relative (parent, brother, sister, or child) with a
    BRCA1 or *BRCA2* gene mutation
  Lifetime risk of breast cancer $\geq 20-25\%^a$.
  Radiation therapy to chest at age of 10–30 years
  Li–Fraumeni syndrome, Cowden syndrome, or hereditary diffuse gastric cancer, or having
    first-degree relatives with one of these syndromes

Moderate risk
  Lifetime risk of breast cancer $15-20\%^a$
  Personal history of breast cancer, ductal carcinoma *in situ* (DCIS), lobular carcinoma *in situ*
    (LCIS), atypical ductal hyperplasia (ADH), or atypical lobular hyperplasia (ALH)
  Extremely dense breasts or unevenly dense breasts when viewed on mammography

Minor risk
  Current use of exogenous estrogen and progestin such as menopausal hormone therapy and
    oral contraceptives
  Previous breast biopsy with benign findings
  Alcohol consumption ≥ 2 drinks per day
  Reproductive factors such as menarche after age 12, menopause after age 55, nulliparity,
    and birth of first child after age 30
  Obesity and lack of physical activity

^{a}According to risk assessment instruments used for genetic counseling that are based mainly on family history.
Sources: US National Cancer Institute [3] and American Cancer Society [4].

cancer cases observed. However, models generally have low discriminatory accuracy in predicting the probability of breast cancer in an individual. Most models perform only slightly better than age alone as a risk predictor [2], but may be useful in guiding referrals to genetic counseling services.

10.3   RECOMMENDATIONS FOR HIGH-RISK WOMEN

Strategies for high-risk women differ from those for average-risk women and may include genetic counseling and testing [7,8], earlier and more frequent mammography, and use of additional modalities such as contrast enhanced magnetic resonance imaging (MRI) and ultrasound. High-risk women may also consider the use of medications, such as tamoxifen and raloxifene [9], to reduce the risk of breast cancer.

  Women with first-degree or multiple relatives with breast or ovarian cancer are advised to seek genetic counseling in order to estimate their risks [8]. Approaches to assessing personal risk include models based on available datasets, checklists of criteria, pedigree analysis, knowledge of a deleterious mutation detected in a relative with cancer, and identification with groups known to have a higher prevalence of clinically significant *BRCA* mutations. Guidelines recommend testing for mutations only when an individual has personal or family history features suggestive of inherited cancer susceptibility, the test can be adequately interpreted, and results will aid in management [10,11]. Several characteristics are associated with an increased likelihood of deleterious *BRCA* mutations, including breast cancer diagnosed at an early age, bilateral breast cancer, history of both breast and ovarian cancer, presence of breast cancer in one or more male family members, multiple cases of breast cancer in the family, both breast and ovarian cancer in the family, one or more family members with two primary cancers, and Ashkenazi Jewish background [12–15].

The role of new technologies for monitoring high-risk women is rapidly changing. In studies of MRI and mammography in high-risk women without cancer, sensitivities of MRI ranged within 71–100% and specificities, within 81–97% [16–20]. The American Cancer Society (ACS) now recommends screening MRI along with mammography for certain high-risk groups, including women with *BRCA1* or *BRCA2* mutations, women with >20% lifetime risk of developing breast cancer as defined by risk prediction models based on family history of breast or ovarian cancer, and women who have undergone radiation therapy for Hodgkin lymphoma [21].

10.4 SCREENING APPROACHES

10.4.1 Screening Using Clinical Breast Examination

Clinical breast examination is a method of screening for breast cancer in which a clinician performs a periodic breast examination for women without known signs or symptoms of breast cancer. Women undergoing examinations to evaluate a physical or mammographic finding undergo diagnostic, not screening, breast examinations. For the screening examination, clinicians inspect the breasts for abnormalities in size or shape, and for skin changes. The examiner then thoroughly palpates the breasts and associated tissues for masses and other inconsistencies.

The clinical breast examination is relatively easy and inexpensive. Sensitivity ranges from 40% to 69%, specificity from 88% to 99%, and positive predictive value from 4% to 50%, using mammography and interval cancer as the criterion standard [22]. However, few trials evaluate the effectiveness or potential adverse effects of clinical breast examination in decreasing breast cancer mortality. In countries with widely practiced mammography screening, the utility of clinical breast examination depends on its additional contribution to mortality reduction. The Canadian National Breast Screening Study-2 (CNBSS-2) trial showed no differences between mammography with clinical breast examination versus clinical breast examination alone [23].

Trials to determine the effectiveness of clinical breast examination in reducing breast cancer mortality as the primary screening method in countries with limited healthcare resources and without mammography screening programs are inconclusive. A randomized trial comparing clinical breast examination to no screening was conducted in the Philippines; however, because of poor community acceptance, it was discontinued after one screening round [24]. Two randomized trials comparing clinical breast examination to no screening have been reported in Egypt [25] and India [26] but are inconclusive. Screening guidelines from the Canadian Task Force on Preventive Health Care [27] and US Preventive Services Task Force [28] do not promote periodic clinical breast examination for screening average-risk women for breast cancer on the basis of the lack of evidence of its effectiveness and potential adverse effects.

10.4.2 Screening Using Breast Awareness and Self-Examination

The prevention message for women has shifted from promoting monthly breast self-examinations to breast awareness [4] Awareness involves understanding how normal breasts look and feel, and reporting any new breast changes to clinicians for further evaluation. Breast awareness can be informal or through breast self-examination, and many clinicians still instruct women in its use.

Correct breast self-examination includes specific elements that improve detection of abnormalities. These include performing the examination while lying down with the arm of the examined breast placed behind the head, using the finger pads of the three middle fingers on the opposite hand to feel for lumps in the breast, applying three different levels of pressure to feel all the layers of breast tissue, and moving the fingers around the breast in an up/down pattern starting from the underarm and moving across the breast to sternum. Women are also advised to palpate their underarms, and visually examine the appearance of their breasts and skin while standing in front of a mirror with hands pressing firmly down on their hips.

While breast self-examination may provide women with a technique to improve breast awareness, its use as a screening test in itself is not supported by effectiveness trials. The sensitivity of breast self-examination ranges from 12% to 41% when compared with clinical breast examination and mammography, and is age-dependent [22]. Specificity of breast self-examination remains uncertain. A randomized trial of breast self-examination compared to none performed in St. Petersburg, Russia, a community without routine mammography screening, indicated no reduction in all-cause mortality (RR 1.07; 95% CI 0.88–1.29) [29,30]. Similar results were reported from a randomized trial conducted in Shanghai, China (RR 1.03; 95% CI 0.81–1.31) for breast cancer mortality [31]. Published meta-analyses of randomized trials [32–35] and nonrandomized studies [32–34] also indicate no significant differences in breast cancer mortality between breast self-examination and control groups. The Russian [29,30] and Shanghai [31] trials also reported that more women randomized to breast self-examination had biopsies of benign lesions than did women in control groups (Russian RR 2.05; 95% CI 1.80–2.33; Shanghai RR 1.57; 95% CI 1.48–1.68). The potential for increased unnecessary biopsies led some advisory groups to recommend not teaching breast self-examination to average-risk women for breast cancer screening purposes [27,28,36].

10.4.3 Mammography Screening for Average-Risk Women

Mammography is currently the main approach to breast cancer screening. The rationale for its use is based on the understanding that breast cancer has a known asymptomatic phase that can be identified with mammography. In addition, breast cancer can be more effectively treated in earlier stages than when clinical signs and symptoms present. Mammography screening is sensitive (77–95%), specific (94–97%), and acceptable to most women [22].

Mammography is performed using either plain film or digital technologies, although many health systems are shifting to digital. The Digital Mammographic Imaging Screening Trial (DMIST) compared the performance of film and digital mammography in a screening population of women in the United States and Canada [37]. Results indicated that the overall diagnostic accuracies of digital and film mammography were similar, although the digital method was more accurate in women under age 50 years, women with radiographically dense breasts, and premenopausal women. Contrast enhanced MRI has also been considered for screening purposes. However, there are no studies investigating MRI use in average-risk women, and use of MRI for screening women at average risk is not recommended [4].

Screening can detect a continuum of disease, ranging from noninvasive to invasive carcinoma, as well as noncancerous lesions such as benign breast cysts. Women with normal findings on mammography discontinue this round of screening at this point. If a woman has an abnormal mammographic finding, additional imaging may be recommended next to determine whether the lesion is suspicious for breast cancer and requires biopsy. Additional imaging may consist of diagnostic mammography or mammography using additional or special views (e.g., magnification, spot compression, and additional angles), a targeted breast ultrasound, or breast MRI [38,39]. If a biopsy is required, the type of biopsy performed is based on the characteristics of the lesion (e.g., palpable vs. nonpalpable; solid mass vs. microcalcifications), as well as patient and physician preferences. Current biopsy techniques include fine-needle aspiration (FNA), stereotactic core biopsy (for nonpalpable, mammographic lesions), ultrasound-guided or MRI-guided core biopsy, non-image-guided core biopsy (for palpable lesions), incisional biopsy, or excisional biopsy. These techniques vary in the level of invasiveness and amount of tissue obtained, affecting their yield and patient experience. While most women undergoing a breast biopsy initiated by mammography screening have benign pathology, the biopsy may provide a breast cancer diagnosis.

Although mammography screening has been widely practiced for many years, more recent research on its effectiveness and adverse effects has stimulated renewed debate on its relative benefits and harms. The most controversial areas concern specific ages to start and stop routine screening and the length of screening intervals. These are also issues that are not clearly resolved by existing research. A meta-analysis of breast cancer screening trials in 2009 compared women randomly selected for screening versus no screening (Table 10.2) [40]. For women age 39–49 years, eight trials provided data for the meta-analysis (Health Insurance Plan (HIP) of Greater New York [41], Canadian National Breast Screening Study-1 (CNBSS-1) [42], Stockholm [43], Malmo [43], Swedish Two-County (two trials) [43], Gothenburg trial [44], and the Age trial [45]). Trials were conducted in the UK, Sweden, Canada, and the United States using predominantly film mammography. All except the most recent trial [45] were conducted during the pretamoxifen era. Trials included multiple screening rounds that varied by trial (two to nine rounds), used various screening intervals (12–33 months), and provided 11–20 years of follow-up data. Combining results, the pooled relative risk for breast cancer mortality for women invited to mammography screening was 0.85 (95% credible interval [CrI] 0.75–0.96), indicating a 15% reduction in breast cancer mortality in favor of screening (Table 10.2).

For women age 50–59 years, six trials (CNBSS-2 [23], Stockholm [43], Malmo [43], Swedish Two-County (two trials) [43], Gothenburg [44]) provided a pooled relative risk estimate of 0.86 (95% CrI 0.75–0.99). For women age 60–69 years, two trials (Malmo [43] and Swedish Two-County (Ostergotland) [43]) provided a pooled relative risk estimate of 0.68 (95% CrI 0.54–0.87). Results for women age 70 years and older were confined to data from only one trial enrolling a small number of women age 70–74 (RR 1.12; 95% CI 0.73–1.72) [43]. A meta-analysis by the Cochrane Collaboration in 2009 included the same trials and reported similar results [46].

Additional data on mammography screening effectiveness have been reported from cohort studies of screening programs. These studies do not use randomization to determine their comparison groups subjecting them to bias. Nonetheless, their contributions are important if these limitations are considered. A study evaluating the effectiveness of mammography screening in the context of the contemporary cancer treatment era

TABLE 10.2 Breast Cancer Mortality Reduction with Mammography Screening

Age (years)	Breast Cancer Mortality RR (95% CrI)	Trials Included in Meta-Analysis
39–49	0.85 (0.75–0.96)	HIP, CNBSS-1, Stockholm, Malmo, Swedish Two-County (2 trials), Gothenburg, Age
50–59	0.86 (0.75–0.99)	CNBSS-2, Stockholm, Malmo, Swedish Two-Country (two trials), Gothenburg
60–69	0.68 (0.54–0.87)	Malmo and Swedish Two-Country (Ostergotland)
70–74	1.12 (0.73–1.72)	Swedish Two-County (Ostergotland)

Notation: CNBSS-1 = Canadian National Breast Screening Study-1; CNBSS-2 = Canadian National Breast Screening Study-2; CrI = credible interval; HIP = Health Insurance Plan of Greater New York; RR = relative risk.
Source: Based on a meta-analysis of results of randomized controlled trials of screening [40].

in Norway indicated that mammography screening reduced breast cancer mortality by 10% for women age 50–69 years [47]. In this study, mammography contributed roughly one-third of the total breast cancer mortality reduction observed over time, while improved awareness and treatment were credited with providing the most impact [47]. Other cohort studies reported results with differing degrees of effectiveness [48–53].

The beneficial impact of screening in a population depends on the estimated mortality reduction attributed to screening and the expected number of breast cancer deaths. These estimates vary by age and by other known and unknown characteristics of the population. Estimates in a US population indicate that the actual numbers of deaths prevented by screening at younger ages is only minimally influenced by the estimated mortality reduction with screening because breast cancer incidence and mortality are low. These estimates change with older age groups because breast cancer incidence is higher (Fig. 10.2).

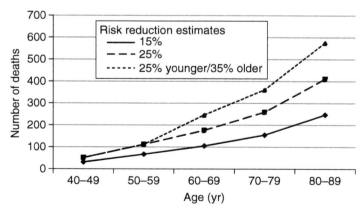

Figure 10.2 Breast cancer deaths prevented with screening. Age-specific US breast cancer mortality rates from SEER and various assumptions of screening effects provide mortality estimates for screening a hypothetical population of 100,000 women over 10 years (five rounds) at different ages.

The advantages of screening need to be considered in the context of potential disadvantages. Studies of adverse effects of mammography screening indicate that these outcomes are widespread and impose substantial burdens on individuals and health resources [40]. False-positive mammography results were common in all age groups in the Breast Cancer Surveillance Consortium (BCSC) in the United States, but rates were highest among women age 40–49 (97.8 in 1000 per screening round) [40]. Among the same women, false-negative mammography rates were lower (1.0 in 1000 per screening round), rates of additional imaging were higher (84.3 in 1000 per screening round), and rates of biopsy were lower (9.3 in 1000 per screening round) compared to older women. The BCSC results indicate that for every case of invasive breast cancer detected by a round of mammography screening in women age 40–49 years, 556 women undergo mammography; 47 women, additional imaging; and 5 women, biopsies. The yield of screening is higher for older women because fewer undergo these procedures for each breast cancer case detected. For example, for women age 60–69 years, 200 undergo mammography; 14, additional imaging; and 2, biopsies for each case detected (Fig. 10.3).

False-positive outcomes are cumulative because women undergo several rounds of screening in their lifetimes. Other sources report the cumulative risk for false-positive mammograms as 21–49% after 10 mammograms for women in general [54–56], and up to 56% for women age 40–49 years [56]. False-positive results from screening mammography had no consistent effect on most women's general anxiety and depression in a systematic review of 23 studies [57]. However, some women experienced increased breast cancer–specific distress, anxiety, and apprehension, and perceived breast cancer risk.

Overdiagnosis—the concept of diagnosing a case of breast cancer that would not become clinically evident in the absence of screening—is difficult to estimate and apply to individuals. Overdiagnosis is an important consideration in screening, however, because women experiencing overdiagnosis undergo diagnostic and treatment procedures that provide no benefit to them. Estimates of overdiagnosis range from <1% to >30% depending on the outcome measured, the woman's age, and the methods used to determine the estimates [40,58,59].

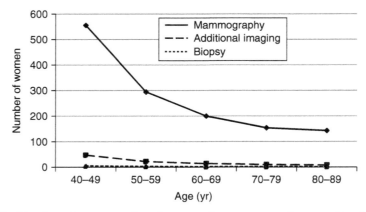

Figure 10.3 Number of women undergoing procedures per screening round to diagnose one case of invasive breast cancer. Estimates are based on data from US populations in the Breast Cancer Surveillance Consortium [40].

TABLE 10.3 Breast Cancer Screening Recommendations for Average-Risk Women

Country	Screening Mammography	
	Ages	Intervals
Australia	50–69	2 years
Austria	40 and older	2 years
Canada	50–74	2–3 years
Czech Republic	50–69	2 years
Finland	50–69	2 years
France	50–74	2 years
Netherlands	50–75	2 years
United Kingdom[a]	50–70	3 years
United States: USPSTF[b]	50–74	2 years
United States: ACS	40 and older	1 year

Abbreviations: ACS = American Cancer Society; USPSTF = U.S. Preventive Services Task Force; Program targets women age 50–69 years, but women 40–49 and 70 are also eligible.
[a] Program began an extension to women age 47–73 in 2010.
[b] Decisions about mammography screening for women age 40–49 and 75 and over should be individualized based on risk factors, other health conditions, and personal preferences.

Radiation exposure from mammography is considered a low-dose, low-energy level when using modern equipment (mean glandular dose of 7 mGy for bilateral, two-view mammography) [60]. Associations with breast cancer were inconsistent in studies of low dose exposures in a systematic review, but indicated increased risk with high dose exposure at much higher levels than routine mammography [61]. Women undergoing multiple diagnostic radiographs or therapeutic radiation for previous cancer also have increased risks for breast cancer [62].

Breast compression during mammography may cause discomfort for some women. Many women reported experiencing pain during the procedure (1–77%), but few women considered it a deterrent from future screening in a systematic review of 22 studies [61]. A review of methods to reduce pain with mammography concluded that no study has yet demonstrated an effective approach [63]. Women who received clear communication of their negative mammography results experienced minimal anxiety in a systematic review of 54 studies [64]. Some who were recalled for further testing as a result of screening demonstrated either persistent or transient anxiety.

Recommendations for mammography screening have been issued by numerous advisory groups worldwide. Recommendations vary primarily with respect to ages for beginning (40 vs. 50 years) and discontinuing (no specific age, 70 years, 75 years) routine screening, and by the length of screening intervals (1, 2, or 3 years) (Table 10.3) [4,27,28,36,65,66]. These variations reflect, in part, different interpretations of relative benefits and harms, as well as inconclusive research data about appropriate ages and optimal intervals. Recommendations from the US Preventive Services Task Force included results of statistical models designed to address these research gaps [67].

Screening practices also vary, and factors relating to screening practices likely influence the development and implementation of screening recommendations. For example, important practice differences exist between countries that have implemented national health system screening programs, such as the United Kingdom, and those that have not, such as the United States. Comparisons between clinical outcomes in the United States, using data from the Breast Cancer Surveillance Consortium (BCSC) and the National Breast and Cervical Cancer Early Detection Program, and the United Kingdom, using data from the National Health Service Breast Screening Program, highlight important discrepancies. Results indicate that recall rates and open surgical biopsy rates are twice as high in the United States than in the United Kingdom while cancer detection rates are similar [68]. These outcomes may be due to differences in healthcare delivery systems, organization of screening programs, training and practices of radiologists, quality assurance standards, malpractice climates, and patient expectations, among other factors.

10.5 CONCLUSIONS

Breast cancer screening provides an opportunity for risk stratification and early detection that can reduce mortality, but also subjects women to potential harm. After determining appropriate screening guidelines, the next essential step is implementation in public and private health systems. No screening program will be successful if the women in the screening pool do not participate. Important barriers to participation include lack of funding, limited access to facilities, cultural and language differences, and educational and literacy obstacles. Even among community breast cancer screening services that consider these barriers, strategies to engage women in screening vary in effectiveness. Five strategies for inviting women to mammography services demonstrated effectiveness compared to no interventions in a systematic review of trials [69]. These include letter of invitation, mailed educational material, letter of invitation with a phone call, phone call alone, and training activities with direct reminders for the women. While screening recommendations vary for women over age 70, many older women will continue to benefit from periodic breast cancer screening. The decision to continue screening requires consideration of each women's overall health status in order to determine the potential benefits and harms of screening on an individual basis. Continued access to screening and follow-up care is also essential to optimize screening effectiveness.

REFERENCES

1. US Preventive Services Task Force. *Guide to Clinical Prevention Services*, 2nd ed., Williams & Wilkins, Baltimore, 1996.
2. Nelson HD, Fu R, Humphrey L, Smith ME. Griffin J, Nygren P. *Comparative Effectiveness of Medications to Reduce Risk of Primary Breast Cancer in Women*, comparative effectiveness review prepared by Oregon Evidence-based Practice Center under Contract 290–2007-10057-1, Agency for Healthcare Research and Quality, Rockville, MD, April 2009 (available at www.effectivehealthcare.ahrq.gov/reports/final.cfm).
3. National Cancer Institute. *Screening Mammograms: Questions and Answers* (available at http://www.cancer.gov/cancertopics/factsheet/Detection/screening-mammograms).
4. NCI, Smith RA, Saslow D, Sawyer KA, Burke W, Costanza ME, Evans WP, et al. American Cancer Society guidelines for breast cancer screening: Update 2003. *CA Cancer J Clin* 2003;**53**(3):141–169.
5. Gail MH, Brinton LA, Byar DP, et al. Projecting individualized probabilities of developing breast cancer for white females who are being examined annually. *J Natl Cancer Inst* 1989;**81**(24):1879–1886.

6. Costantino JP, Gail MH, Pee D, et al. Validation studies for models projecting the risk of invasive and total breast cancer incidence. *J Natl Cancer Inst* 1999;**91**(18):1541–1548.

7. Nelson HD, Huffman LH, Fu R, Harris EL. Genetic risk assessment and *BRCA* mutation testing for breast and ovarian cancer susceptibility: Systematic evidence review for the U.S. Preventive Services Task Force. *Ann Intern Med* 2005;**143**(5):362–379.

8. US Preventive Services Task Force. Genetic risk assessment and *BRCA* mutation testing for breast and ovarian cancer susceptibility: Recommendation statement. *Ann Intern Med* 2005;**143**:355–361.

9. Nelson HD, Fu R, Griffin J, Nygren P, Smith MEB, Humphrey L. Systematic review: Comparative effectiveness of medications to reduce risk for primary breast cancer. *Ann Intern Med* 2009;**151**:703–715.

10. American College of Medical Genetics Professional Practice and Guidelines Committee. Genetic susceptibility to breast and ovarian cancer: Assessment, counseling, and testing guidelines executive summary, Oct. 1999 (available at `http://www.health. state.ny.us/nysdoh/cancer/obcancer/contents.htm`).

11. Statement of Clinical Oncology. Genetic testing for cancer susceptibility, adopted on February 20, 1996. *J Clin Oncol* 1996;**14**(5):1730–1736.

12. Frank TS, Deffenbaugh AM, Reid JE, et al. Clinical characteristics of individuals with germline mutations in *BRCA1* and *BRCA2*: Analysis of 10,000 individuals. *J Clin Oncol* 2002;**20**(6):1480–1490.

13. Srivastava A, McKinnon W, Wood ME. Risk of breast and ovarian cancer in women with strong family histories. *Oncology* 2001;**15**(7):889–902; discussion 902, 905–887, 911–813.

14. Shattuck-Eidens D, Oliphant A, McClure M, et al. *BRCA1* sequence analysis in women at high risk for susceptibility mutations. Risk factor analysis and implications for genetic testing. *JAMA* 1997;**278**(15):1242–1250.

15. Couch FJ, DeShano ML, Blackwood MA, et al. *BRCA1* mutations in women attending clinics that evaluate the risk of breast cancer. *N Engl J Med* 1997;**336**(20):1409–1415.

16. Kriege M, Brekelmans CTM, Boetes C, Besnard PE, Zonderland HM, Obdeijn IM, et al. Efficacy of MRI and mammography for breast-cancer screening in women with a familial or genetic predisposition. *N Engl J Med* 2004;**351**(5):427–437.

17. Kuhl CK, Schrading S, Leutner CC, Morakkabati-Spitz N, Wardelmann E, Fimmers R, et al. Mammography, breast ultrasound, and magnetic resonance imaging for surveillance of women at high familial risk for breast cancer. *J Clin Oncol*. 2005;**23**(33):8469–8476.

18. Leach MO, Boggis CRM, Dixon AK, Easton DF, Eeles RA, Evans DGR, et al. Screening with magnetic resonance imaging and mammography of a UK population at high familial risk of breast cancer: A prospective multicentre cohort study (MARIBS). *Lancet* 2005;**365**(9473):1769–1778.

19. Lehman CD, Blume JD, Weatherall P, Thickman D, Hylton N, Warner E, et al. Screening women at high risk for breast cancer with mammography and magnetic resonance imaging. *Cancer* 2005;**103**(9):1898–1905.

20. Warner E, Plewes DB, Hill KA, Causer PA, Zubovits JT, Jong RA, et al. Surveillance of BRCA1 and BRCA2 mutation carriers with magnetic resonance imaging, ultrasound, mammography, and clinical breast examination. *JAMA* 2004;**292**(11):1317–1325.

21. Saslow D, Boetes C, Burke W, et al. American Cancer Society guidelines for breast screening with MRI as an adjunct to mammography. *CA Cancer J Clin* 2007;**57**(2):75–89.

22. Humphrey LL, Helfand M, Chan BKS, Woolf SH. Breast cancer screening: A summary of the evidence for the U.S. Preventive Services Task Force. *Ann Intern Med* 2002;**137**(5):347–360.

23. Miller AB, To T, Baines CJ, Wall C. Canadian National Breast Screening Study-2: 13-year results of a randomized trial in women aged 50–59 years. *J Natl Cancer Inst* 2000;**92**(18): 1490–1499.

24. Pisani P, Parkin DM, Ngelangel C, Esteban D, Gibson L, Munson M, et al. Outcome of screening by clinical examination of the breast in a trial in the Philippines. *Int J Cancer* 2006;**118**(1):149–154.

25. Boulos S, Gadallah M, Neguib S, Essam E, Youssef A, Costa A, et al. Breast screening in the emerging world: High prevalence of breast cancer in Cairo. *Breast* 2005; **14**(5): 340–346.

26. Sankaranarayanan R, Ramadas K, Thara S, Muwong R, Prabhakar J, Augustine P, et al. Clinical breast examination: Preliminary results from a cluster randomized controlled trial in India. *J Natl Cancer Inst* 2011;**103**(19):1476–1480.

27. Canadian Task Force on Preventive Health Care. *Screening for Breast Cancer* (available at: `http://www.canadiantaskforce.ca/recommendations/2011-01-eng.html`: accessed 4/12).

28. US Preventive Services Task Force. Screening for breast cancer: U.S. Preventive Services Task Force recommendation statement. *Ann Intern Med* 2009;**151**:716–726.

29. Semiglazov VF, Moiseyenko VM, Manikhas AG, Protsenko SA, Kharikova RS, Popova RT, et al. Interim results of a prospective randomised study of self-examination for early detection of breast cancer. *Vopr Onkol* 1999;**45**:265–271.

30. Semiglazov VF, Moiseyenko VM, Bavli JL, Migmanova N, Seleznyov NK, Popova RT, et al. The role of breast self-examination in early breast cancer detection (results of the 5-years USSR/WHO randomized study in Leningrad). *Eur J Epidemiol* 1992;**8**(4):498–502.

31. Thomas DB, Gao DL, Ray RM, Wange WW, Allison CJ, Chen FL, et al. Randomized trial of breast self-examination in Shanghai: Final results. *J Natl Cancer Inst* 2002;**94**(19): 1445–1457.

32. Hackshaw AK, Paul EA. Breast examination and death from breast cancer: A meta-analysis. *Br J Cancer* 2003;**88**(7):1047–1053.

33. Baxter N; Canadian Task Force on Preventive Health Care. Preventive health care, 2001 update: Should women be routinely taught breast self-examination to screen for breast cancer? *Can Med Assoc J* 2001;**164**(13):1837–1846.

34. Tu SP, Reisch LM, Taplin SH, Kreuter W, Elmore JG. Breast self-examination: Self-reported frequency, quality, and associated outcomes. *J Cancer Educ* 2006;**21**(3):175–181.

35. Kosters JP, Gotzsche PC. Regular self-examination or clinical examination for early detection of breast cancer. *Cochrane Database Syst Rev* 2003; Issue 2. Art. CD003373 (DOI: 10.1002/14651858.CD003373).

36. Cutler D, Kulland K. *Factbox:Breast Cancer Screening Guidelines in Europe*, U.S. (available at `http://www.reuters.com/article/2010/03/27/us-cancer-breast-mammograms-factbox`: accessed 4/12).

37. Pisano ED, Gatsonis C, Hendrick E, et al. Diagnostic performance of digital versus film mammography for breast-cancer screening. *N Engl J Med*. 2005;**353**(17):1773–1783.

38. Flobbe K, Bosch AM, Kessels AG, Beets GL, Nelemans PJ, von Meyenfeldt MF, et al. The additional diagnostic value of ultrasonography in the diagnosis of breast cancer. *Arch Intern Med* 2003;**163**(10):1194–1199.

39. Bedrosian I, Mick R, Orel SG, Schnall M, Reynolds C, Spitz FR, et al. Changes in the surgical management of patients with breast carcinoma based on preoperative magnetic resonance imaging. *Cancer* 2003;**98**(3):468–473.

40. Nelson HD, Tyne K, Naik A, Bougatsos C, Chan BK, Humphrey L. Screening for breast cancer: An update for the U.S. Preventive Services Task Force. *Ann Intern Med* 2009;**151**:727–737.

41. Habbema JD, van Oortmarssen GJ, van Putten DJ, Lubbe JT, van der Maas PJ. Age-specific reduction in breast cancer mortality by screening: An analysis of the results of the Health Insurance Plan of Greater New York study. *J Natl Cancer Inst* 1986;**77**(2):317–320.

42. Miller AB, To T, Baines CJ, Wall C. The Canadian National Breast Screening Study—1: Breast cancer mortality after 11 to 16 years of follow-up. A randomized screening trial of mammography in women age 40 to 49 years. *Ann Intern Med* 2002;**137**(5P. 1):305–312.

43. Nystrom L, Andersson I, Bjurstam N, Frisell J, Nordenskjold B, Rutqvist LE. Long-term effects of mammography screening: updated overview of the Swedish randomised trials. *Lancet*. 2002;**359**(9310):909–19.

44. Bjurstam N, Bjorneld L, Warwick J, Sala E, Duffy SW, Nystrom L, et al. The Gothenburg Breast Screening Trial. *Cancer*. 2003;**97**(10):2387–96.

45. Moss SM, Cuckle H, Evans A, Johns L, Waller M, Bobrow L, et al. Effect of mammographic screening from age 40 years on breast cancer mortality at 10 years' follow-up: a randomised controlled trial. *Lancet*. 2006;**368**(9552):2053–60.

46. Gotzsche PC, Nielsen M. Screening for breast cancer with mammography. *Cochrane Database Syst Rev* 2009; Issue 4. Art. CD001877 (DOI: 10.1002/14651858.CD001877. pub3).

47. Kalager M, Zelen M, Lanmark F, Adami H. Effect of screening mammography on breast cancer mortality in Norway. *N Engl J Med* 2010;**363**:1203–1210.

48. Hellquist BN, Duffy SW, Abdsaleh S, Bjorneld L, Bordas P, Tabar L, et al. Effectiveness of population based service screening with mammography for women ages 40 to 49 years. *Cancer* 2011;**117**:714–722.

49. Hakama M, Pukkala E, Heikkila M, Kallio M. Effectiveness of the public health policy for breast cancer screening in Finland: Population based cohort study. *Br Med J* 1997;**314**:864–867.

50. Otto SJ, Fracherboud J, Looman CWN, et al. Initiation of population–based mammography screening in Dutch municipalities and effect on breast cancer mortality: A systematic review *Lancet*. 2003;**361**:1411–1417.

51. Blanks RG, Moss SM, McGahan CE, Quinn MJ, Babb PJ. Effect of NHS breast screening programme on mortality from breast cancer in England and Wales, 1990-8: Comparison of observed with predicted mortality. *Br Med J*. 2000;**321**:665–669.

52. Olsen AH, Njor SH, Bejborg I, et al. Breast cancer mortality in Copenhagen after introduction of mammography screening: Cohort study. *Br Med J* 2000;**330**:220.

53. Tabar L, Yen MF, Vitak B, Chen HHT, Smith R, Duffy SW. Mammography service screening and mortality in breast cancer patients: 20-year follow-up before and after introduction of screening. *Lancet* 2003;**361**:1405–1410.

54. Olivotto IA, Kan L, Coldman AJ. False positive rate of screening mammography. *N Engl J Med* 1998;**339**:560.

55. Hofvind S, Thoresen S, Tretli S. The cumulative risk of a false-positive recall in the Norwegian Breast Cancer Screening Program. *Cancer* 2004;**101**(7):1501–1507.

56. Elmore JG, Barton MB, Moceri VM, Polk S, Arena PJ, Fletcher SW. Ten-year risk of false positive screening mammograms and clinical breast examinations. *N Engl J Med* 1998;**338**(16):1089–1096.

57. Brewer NT, Salz T, Lillie SE. Systematic review: The long-term effects of false-positive mammograms. *Ann Intern Med* 2007;**146**(7):502–510.

58. Day NE. Overdiagnosis and breast cancer screening. *Breast Cancer Res* 2005;**7**(5):228–229.

59. Jorgensen KJ, Gotzsche PC. Overdiagnosis in publicly organised mammography screening programmes: Systematic review of incidence trends. *Br Med J* 2009;**339**:b2587.

60. Spelic DC. *Dose and Image Quality in Mammography: Trends during the First Decade of MQSA*, US Food and Drug Administration, 2003 (available at `http://www.fda.gov/CDRH/MAMMOGRAPHY/scorecard-articles.html`; accessed 6/09).

61. Armstrong K, Moye E, Williams S, Berlin JA, Reynolds EE. Screening mammography in women 40 to 49 years of age: A systematic review for the American College of Physicians. *Ann Intern Med* 2007;**146**(7):516–526.

62. John EM, Phipps AI, Knight JA, Milne RL, Dite GS, Hopper JL, et al. Medical radiation exposure and breast cancer risk: Findings from the Breast Cancer Family Registry. *Int J Cancer* 2007;**121**(2):386–394.

63. Miller D, Livingstone V, Herbison GP. Interventions for relieving the pain and discomfort of screening mammography. *Cochrane Database Syst Rev* 2008; Issue 1, Art. CD002942 (DOI: 10.1002/14651858.CD002942.pub2).

64. Brett J, Bankhead C, Henderson B, Watson E, Austoker J. The psychological impact of mammographic screening. A systematic review. *Psychooncology* 2005;**14**(11):917–938.

65. Australian Government. *BreastScreen Australia Program* (available at `http://www.cancerscreening.gov.au/internet/screening/publish.nsf/content/breastscreenabout`; accessed 4/12).

66. National Health Service Cancer Screening Programmes. *Breast Screening Programme* (available at `http://www.cancerscreening.nhs.uk/breastscreen/screening-programme.html`; accessed 4/12)

67. Mandelblatt JS, Cronin KA, Bailey S, et al. for the Breast Cancer Working Group of the Cancer Intervention and Surveillance Modeling Network (CISNET). Effects of mammography screening under different screening schedules: Model estimates of potential benefits and harms. *Ann Intern Med* 2009;**151**:738–747.

68. Smith-Bindman R, Chu PW, Miglioretti DL, Sickles EA, Blanks R, Ballard-Barbash R, et al. Comparison of screening mammography in the United States and the United Kingdom. *JAMA* 2003;**290**(16):2129–2137.

69. Bonfill Cosp X, Marzo Castillego M, Pladevall Vila M, Marti J, Emparanza JI. Strategies for increasing the participation of women in community breast cancer screening. *Cochrane Database Syst Rev* 2001; Issue 1. Art. CD002943 (DOI: 10.1002/14651858.CD002943).

CHAPTER 11

Colorectal Cancer Screening

CATHERINE QUARINI
Warneford Hospital, Oxford, UK

11.1 INTRODUCTION

Colorectal cancer is the third most common cancer in the United Kingdom (UK) [1] and the United States [2]. The lifetime risk of a person in the UK developing this disease is around 6% and worldwide it contributes to over 600,000 deaths per year.

11.1.1 Risk Factors for Development of Colorectal Cancer

Several risk factors have been identified in the development of colorectal cancer (Fig. 11.1). One of the most widely known risk factors for developing colorectal cancer is age, with over 90% of cases diagnosed in people over 50 years [2].

Previous medical history is also an important risk factor, as people who have had colorectal cancer in the past are more likely to develop it again, and people who have inflammatory bowel disease (including ulcerative colitis and Crohn's disease) are more likely to develop dysplasia and then colorectal cancer. Studies have shown that people with primary sclerosing cholangitis and ulcerative colitis have a greater risk of developing colorectal cancer than do people with ulcerative colitis alone [3].

A family history of colorectal cancer is a risk factor for an individual developing the disease; this risk is increased if the affected family member is a first-degree relative and developed the disease at a young age. About 5–10% of people who develop colorectal cancer have an inherited syndrome leading to its development; the two most common of these are familial adenomatous polyposis (FAP) and hereditary nonpolyposis colorectal cancer (HNPCC). About 1% of colorectal cancers are linked to FAP, which is caused by changes in the APC gene. People with FAP usually develop hundreds or thousands of polyps in the colon or rectum in early adult life, and by age 40 almost all people with this disorder will develop colorectal cancer if the colon is not removed. HPNCC, also known as *Lynch syndrome*, accounts for about 3–5% of all colorectal cancers, and the lifetime risk of disease in people with this condition is around 80% [2].

Cancer and Aging Handbook: Research and Practice, First Edition. Edited by Keith M. Bellizzi and Margot A. Gosney.
© 2012 Wiley-Blackwell. Published 2012 by John Wiley & Sons, Inc.

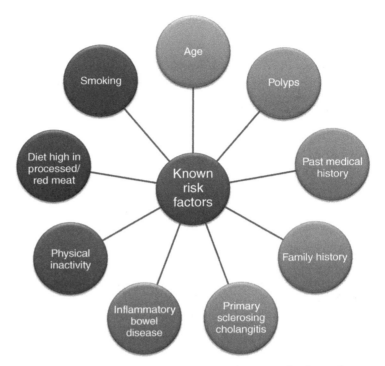

Figure 11.1 Known risk factors for the development of colorectal cancer.

Some of the known risk factors for colorectal cancer are modifiable, and these include smoking, a diet high in red and processed meats, obesity, and a sedentary lifestyle.

Findings from the 40-year follow-up in the UK Whitehall prospective cohort study [4] have shown that, compared to people who have never smoked, current smoking was associated with age-adjusted hazard ratios of 1.45 (95% CI 1.03–2.03) for colon cancer and 1.97 (95% CI 1.02 3.80) for rectal cancer. Obesity has consistently been associated with increased risk of colorectal cancer in men, but results in women have varied. The UK Million Women Study [5] found no association between BMI and the overall risk of incidence or mortality from colorectal cancer at recruitment of participants aged 50–64. However, a significant increase in risk with increasing BMI was found in premenopausal women (RR 1.61, 95% CI 1.05–2.48) but not in postmenopausal women (RR 0.99, 95% CI 0.88 1.12).

Some other possible risk factors (Fig. 11.2) in the development of colorectal cancer include high alcohol consumption, a diet low in fiber, environmental factors, exogenous hormones, low levels of selenium in the diet, and low levels of vitamin B_6. Alcohol consumption has been shown to have a weak association with the development of colorectal cancer, although more research is needed to determine whether this is a causal relationship [6]. A low-fiber diet has been suggested as a risk factor for the development of colorectal cancer, but it may be that this is actually a confounding factor, and other dietary components are more important. Ongoing research is needed regarding the role of many different environmental factors, as the incidence is far

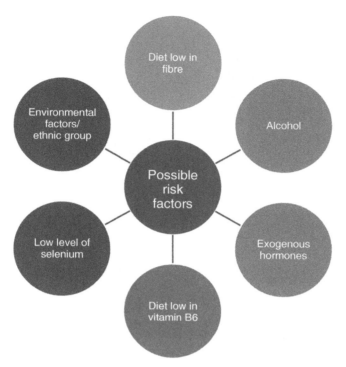

Figure 11.2   Possible risk factors for the development of colorectal cancer.

greater in industrialized countries, and it is not clear whether this can be attributed to diet, ethnicity of people in these countries, or environmental exposures that have not yet been identified. As the patterns of colorectal cancer in men and women differ, the role of oral hormone pills in women has been investigated, but no firm conclusions have been drawn on their effect on risk [7]. Animal studies have suggested that selenium from the diet may decrease the risk of colorectal cancer, but these studies have not been confirmed in humans [8]. More recent research has shown that blood levels of pyridoxal 5-phosphate, the active form of vitamin B_6, were inversely associated with risk of developing colorectal cancer [9]. This would, however, need to be followed up by large randomized controlled trials of vitamin B supplementation before any reliable conclusions about its role in cancer prevention could be drawn.

11.2   DEVELOPMENT, CHARACTERISTICS, AND TREATMENT OF COLORECTAL CANCER

11.2.1   Development

Most colorectal cancers develop from benign adenomatous polyps, with malignant transformation usually taking between one and three decades. Factors influencing malignant transformation include the type of polyp (flat polyps are at higher risk than pedunculated polyps), the histology of the polyp (those with villous architecture are

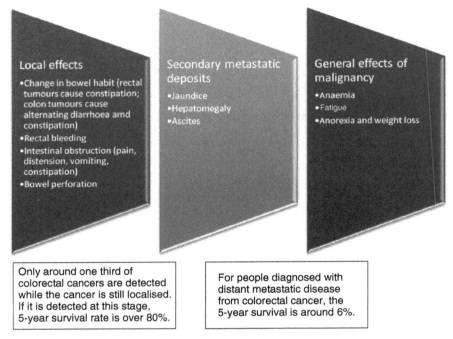

Local effects
- Change in bowel habit (rectal tumours cause constipation; colon tumours cause alternating diarrhoea amd constipation)
- Rectal bleeding
- Intestinal obstruction (pain, distension, vomiting, constipation)
- Bowel perforation

Secondary metastatic deposits
- Jaundice
- Hepatomegaly
- Ascites

General effects of malignancy
- Anaemia
- Fatigue
- Anorexia and weight loss

Only around one third of colorectal cancers are detected while the cancer is still localised. If it is detected at this stage, 5-year survival rate is over 80%.

For people diagnosed with distant metastatic disease from colorectal cancer, the 5-year survival is around 6%.

Figure 11.3   Symptoms and survival rates from colorectal cancer.

at higher risk than those with tubular architecture), and the size of the polyp (polyps >1.5 cm carry a higher risk).

11.2.2   Symptoms and Presentation

The symptoms of colorectal cancer depend on the stage of the disease. Colorectal cancer symptoms and survival rates are listed in Figure 11.3.

11.2.3   Diagnosis

Several tests may be used in the diagnosis–staging process. Colonoscopy allows biopsies to be performed at the same time for histological examination, and the diagnosis is usually confirmed after this procedure. In addition, a full blood count to detect anemia caused by bleeding from the colon, and liver function tests to assess liver involvement, should be carried out, as well as further radiological investigations including ultrasound, MRI, and CT scans to determine spread of the disease, which is important in staging.

Staging is based on the *Dukes classification* (after British pathologist Cuthbert Dukes, 1890–1977). This divides the stages of disease into four broad categories:

A—tumor confined to intestinal wall
B—tumor invasion through the intestinal wall
C—lymph nodes involved
D—distant metastases present

11.2.4 Treatment and Prognosis

Treatment and prognosis depend on the stage at which the disease is diagnosed. People with Dukes stage A disease have 5-year survival rates of over 80%, whereas those with stage D disease have 5-year survival rates of only 6%. Treatment usually consists of surgical removal of the tumor and the lymph nodes that drain it. The type of operation performed depends on the location of the tumor within the colon. Most colon cancers are found within the left colon and require a Hartmann (after French surgeon Henri A. Hartmann, 1860–1952) procedure if situated at the base of the colon, a sigmoid colectomy if situated in the lower part of the descending colon, or a left hemicolectomy if situated high in the colon. Many people with Dukes C tumors now receive postoperative chemotherapy which reduces the recurrence rate and the mortality rate.

11.3 SCREENING

11.3.1 Definition of Medical Screening

Screening is a strategy used to detect disease in people who have no symptoms of the disease being screened for, but who are at risk of developing it. The purpose of screening is to identify disease at an earlier stage than if it were left to present clinically, thus enabling treatment to be started earlier, with the intention of reducing morbidity and mortality from the disease. Screening programs may be universal, which involves offering screening to all individuals in a certain category, such as all people over a certain age, or may involve case finding, whereby a smaller group of people are screened because of the presence of risk factors, such as a family history.

The World Health Organization [10] has published a list of screening guidelines, including the following:

1. The condition should be an important health problem. This may be a condition that affects large numbers of people, or causes high morbidity or mortality.
2. There should be a treatment for the condition.
3. Facilities for diagnosis and treatment should be available.
4. There should be a latent stage of the disease. This will be the time at which the screening test ideally detects the disease.
5. There should be a test or examination for the condition.
6. The test should be acceptable to the population.
7. The natural history of the disease should be adequately understood. This is especially important in screening, as people found to have the disease will be offered treatment for a condition that has not yet caused them any symptoms. They therefore need to ensure that the natural history of the disease would lead them to develop symptoms if they do not receive treatment.
8. There should be a generally accepted policy on whom to treat.
9. The total cost of finding a case should be economically balanced in relation to medical expenditure as a whole.
10. Case-finding should be a continuous process.

11.3.2 Utility of Colorectal Cancer Screening

Screening for colorectal cancer meets many of the criteria described above. It is an important health problem, leading to a large number of deaths every year. Treatment modalities are available for the condition, and facilities are available in many parts of the world for diagnosis and treatment, but the success of treatment depends greatly on the stage at which the disease is diagnosed. The natural history of the disease, in particular its development from polyps, is understood, and there is a latent stage. Screening tests are available, and although these—in particular colonoscopy—carry some risks and side effects, they are well known so individuals can be fully informed about the tests and decide whether they find them acceptable. The total cost of finding a case and offering treatment is high, but this is comparable to many other common conditions, and cases presenting later may be more expensive to treat.

11.3.3 Methods of Screening for Colorectal Cancer

There are several methods of screening for colorectal cancer (see Table 11.1).

The *fecal occult blood test* (FOBT) detects blood in the feces. There are several types of FOBT, each testing for a different component of the blood. The most commonly used test and the one used in the UK NHS Bowel Screening Programme is the stool guaiac test, although at present there is no clear evidence determining whether guaiac or immunochemical tests perform better [11]. The stool guaiac test consists of placing a small amount of feces onto paper that has been treated with guaiac, and this step can be performed by the patient at home. The test paper is then sent to a lab where hydrogen peroxide is applied to the paper, and if blood is present, a color change to blue is seen. This occurs because the heme in hemoglobin breaks down the hydrogen peroxide. Before carrying out the stool guaiac test, people are advised to avoid iron supplements, red meat, some vegetables, and citrus fruits, which, because of their antioxidant content, can inhibit the color change reaction leading to a false-negative result.

Other types of FOBT include fecal porphyrin quantification (used mostly to detect bleeding from the upper gastrointestinal tract) and fecal immunochemical testing. Stool DNA tests are also being developed. These have high sensitivity and specificity but are not yet in widespread clinical use.

The FOBT is not very specific as it simply detects bleeding from the gastrointestinal tract; malignancy is only one of many causes, accounting for less than 10% of positive FOBT samples. Other causes include bleeding peptic ulcers, diverticular disease, benign adenomas, angiodysplasia of the colon, sickle cell anemia, and certain medications, particularly anticoagulants. A large UK study found that 35.6% of people with a positive FOBT (FOBT+) result were taking anticoagulants; 47.5% of the FOBT+ people on anticoagulants had colorectal cancer detected on colonoscopy, whereas 56.5% of FOBT+ people not on anticoagulants were found to have colorectal cancer. These findings showed that in population screening with FOBT, taking anticoagulant medication at the time of testing was associated with a significantly increased likelihood of a negative colonoscopy [12]. The FOBT is an easy and inexpensive test to administer as people can send their sample to the lab themselves. The test is noninvasive and carries no risk of physical side effects. However, because the FOBT cannot diagnose colorectal cancer, a follow-up investigation such as colonoscopy or sigmoidoscopy is needed following a positive FOBT result.

Colonoscopy can be used to screen for colorectal cancer and remove polyps, if found, for biopsy during the same procedure. It may be recommended after a positive FOBT result on initial screening, or as a first-line investigation following obvious rectal bleeding or symptoms of disease. Colonoscopy consists of endoscopic examination of the entire colon and distal small bowel by using a fiberoptic camera on a flexible tube. Patients are advised to adhere to a low-fiber diet for several days before the procedure and to take laxative medication the day before. Intravenous sedation is administered for the procedure. During the colonoscopy procedure, the entire colon can be visualized and polyps and suspicious lesions biopsied or removed. The procedure takes ~30 min and may cause some pain.

There are some risks associated with colonoscopy; the most serious is perforation (0.19% or ~1 in 500 colonoscopy cases), bleeding, and in rare cases death (0.019% or ~1 in 5000 colonoscopies) [13]. Perforation requires emergency surgery to repair the damaged bowel. Although all these occurrences are rare, if colonoscopy were widely used in screening all people over age 60, significant numbers of healthy people would be affected by these risks without deriving benefit from the test.

Virtual colonoscopy is a newer test, which is noninvasive, and involves imaging the colon using either CT or MRI scanning. CT versions carry risks associated with radiation exposure. If lesions are detected, a standard colonoscopy would then be needed to perform biopsies. Virtual colonoscopy is not yet commonly used in screening.

Sigmoidoscopy is another invasive test which is used in screening. The perforation risk is lower with sigmoidoscopy than with colonoscopy, and no sedation is required. However, sigmoidoscopy screens only up to the sigmoid colon. Tissue can be removed for biopsy during the procedure.

In some countries double-contrast barium enemas are used for screening. The colon is pumped with air and a barium enema is given, and X-rays taken after this allow the whole colon to be visualized. This is an invasive procedure, and any polyps detected then need to be biopsied or removed in a separate procedure (colonoscopy).

11.3.4   Current Colorectal Cancer Screening Practice

The UK NHS Bowel Screening Programme [14] was set up in 2006, and introduced gradually across the country until all regions were included by 2009. Screening is offered every 2 years to everyone aged 60–69. People over 70 can request a kit, but are not sent one automatically. The program does not give any guidance on an appropriate age, if any, to stop screening. An explanatory letter and FOBT test is sent by post, and people who return samples can expect results within 2 weeks. In general, for every 1000 people completing FOBT, about 20 (2%) will have a positive FOBT and be offered colonoscopy. About 80% of those advised to have a colonoscopy will do so, and around 1 in 10 people who had a positive FOBT and were offered colonoscopy will be diagnosed with colorectal cancer.

If polyps are detected on colonoscopy, the procedure for follow-up and removal of polyps depends on their number and size. It is recommended that anyone at low risk [defined as having one or two small (i.e., <1 cm) adenomas] undergo another FOBT in 2 years; those at intermediate risk (defined as having three or four small adenomas or an adenoma >1 cm) undergo colonoscopy every 3 years until two consecutive examinations are negative, and those at high risk (defined as having five or more adenomas or three or more adenomas, at least one of which is ≥1 cm) undergo

TABLE 11.1 Summary of Advantages, Disadvantages, and Uses of Colorectal Cancer Screening Tests

Test	Advantages	Disadvantages	Current Use in Screening Programs
Fecal occult blood test (FOBT)	Noninvasive and test itself does not cause physical side effects Can be carried out at home High specificity (98%) Can detect tumors throughout the large bowel Good evidence for effectiveness—evaluations of large-scale, long-term randomized controlled trials have shown that FOBT reduced mortality from colorectal cancer by about 16% Acceptable to population—several large controlled trials of FOBT in Europe and the USA demonstrated compliance rates >50%.	Low predictive value of positive test (5–10%) as FOBT simply detects bleeding and there are many other causes of bleeding Diverticular disease is the most common cause of blood in the faeces; other common causes include colonic angiodysplasia, and many anticoagulant medications Low sensitivity (50%), as not all cancers bleed, so many tumors and polyps are missed May be less effective for detection of right-sided tumors Positive FOBT alone does not diagnose colorectal cancer without follow-up tests, usually including colonoscopy, which do carry risks	UK NHS Bowel Screening Programme sends FOBT home testing kit to all people aged 60–69 every 2 years; people >70 can request a kit—people with a positive FOBT result advised to undergo colonoscopy American Cancer Society recommends people >50 at average risk carry out FOBT at home annually if no other bowel screening
Colonoscopy	Polyps seen during a screening colonoscopy can be biopsied at the same time without a further procedure Polyps can be removed before they become malignant Colonoscopy can be used to assess the entire colon	Sedation and full-bowel preparation are necessary. Risk of perforation of 1–2 per 1000 procedures; perforation can lead to hemorrhage and in some cases cause death. Expensive	UK NHS Bowel Screening Programme recommends colonoscopy after positive FOBT. American Cancer Society recommends colonoscopy after positive FOBT, sigmoidoscopy, or double-contrast barium enema

Method			
Flexible sigmoidoscopy	Biopsies can be taken at time of procedure No full-bowel preparation or sedation needed Perforation risk lower than that of colonoscopy Cheaper than colonoscopy	Risk of perforation Detects cancers only in rectosigmoid area	American Cancer Society recommends people >50 at average risk undergo annual sigmoidoscopy if no other bowel screening; follow with colonoscopy if positive
Virtual colonoscopy	Noninvasive, as involving radiological examination of colon with CT or MRI	Lesions detected require colonoscopy	New procedure; not yet sufficient evidence of effectiveness for use in screening
DNA stool examination	Sensitivity high (>90%) Specificity high (>90%)	Results currently only available from small-scale studies	New procedure; not yet sufficient evidence of effectiveness for use in screening
Double-contrast barium enema	Entire colon can be visualized by X rays taken after barium enema given and colon pumped with air	Invasive Any lesions detected then require colonoscopy so they can be biopsied	American Cancer Society recommends every 5–10 years if no other bowel screening, and follow by colonoscopy if positive

colonoscopy after 12 months, followed by colonoscopy every 3 years until they have had two negative examinations.

Screening recommendations differ between countries, but most involve a combination of FOBT as an initial screening test, followed by a more invasive but more specific test for people with a positive FOBT result. The American Cancer Society guidelines recommend that people aged >50 at average risk carry out annual FOBT tests at home, have a double-contrast barium enema every 5–10 years, or undergo sigmoidoscopy on an annual basis. If any of these procedures result in a positive test, they should be followed by colonoscopy. A screening colonoscopy alone every 10 years is another recommendation.

11.3.5 Areas of Controversy in Colorectal Cancer Screening

There are several areas of controversy in the practice of screening for colorectal cancer. Some of these are common to all screening programs, whereas others are specific to this disease.

As with any other investigation, screening tests may miss people who do in fact have the disease (false-negative result) or incorrectly test positive in people without the disease (false-positive result). False-negative tests mean that patients will be reassured that they do not have a disease when in fact they may do, and this false sense of security may lead them to ignore and not seek help for symptoms that might develop later in the course of the disease. False-positive tests create unnecessary anxiety and may prompt people to undergo unnecessary and potentially risky further tests and treatment.

Screening tests can appear to be more effective than they actually are in reducing morbidity and mortality from a condition due to lead-time bias and length-time bias. *Lead-time bias* occurs when patients are diagnosed with a disease earlier through screening than they would have been if they waited until symptoms developed, but this earlier diagnosis does not actually influence the outcome or their remaining lifespan. Because the disease is detected at an earlier point in time, the survival time from diagnosis is greater, but the patient's overall lifespan remains the same (i.e., time of death is not delayed). In this case the screening program may seem effective in increasing survival time, but in fact it has only given the person more time to worry about the diagnosis, without providing any actual benefit.

With *length-time bias*, slower-growing tumors are likely to have better prognosis than faster-growing tumors. Disease that is developing slowly is more likely to be detected at screening because more time will have lapsed before the development of symptoms in which the screening process could take place. As there is a bias for detecting disease with a better prognosis, screening tests may appear more effective than they actually are in reducing morbidity and mortality. Another problem with length-time bias is that some very slowly developing diseases may never cause the patient symptoms, so detecting it during screening and then treating it may simply cause the patient unnecessary anxiety. This is more likely to be the case in elderly people, or those with more limited life expectancy due to comorbidities.

Taking informed consent for entry into any screening program presents extra challenges because large numbers of people are usually screened so information on the test is usually sent out by post rather than given in an individual discussion. Therefore it is difficult to ensure that each person understands the risks and benefits of the screening test. Also, care must be taken to ensure that people understand that the nature of a screening test is to identify people who may be in the early stages of a disease and refer them on for diagnostic testing, rather than to definitively diagnose a disease or falsely reassure them that they do not have the disease. All screening tests carry risks, and the balance of risks and benefits from the test is likely to differ between individuals, depending on their risk factors for developing the disease. Risks such as X-ray exposure, for example, may be more justifiable for someone with a personal or family history of a condition who is more likely to develop the disease, than for someone with few risk factors.

Specific Areas of Controversy At present FOBT is offered to all people aged 60–69 in the UK, whereas those over 70 can request a test. No guidance has been given on an age at which screening should be stopped, if ever. Most screening programs worldwide do not recommend an upper age limit for screening [15]. An optimal upper age limit for screening is likely to differ between individuals, and vary according to life expectancy and comorbidities, as well as individual preferences. These can be discussed on a one-to-one basis with health professionals, but it is unlikely that a national screening program could offer advice on this issue that would be applicable to all people in this age group. However, more recent UK research into the clinical, social, and survival outcomes of people over 80 undergoing resection surgery for colorectal cancer showed that in a sample of 180 people, 30% underwent an emergency operation and most had late-stage disease. However, >80% of patients returned to the same type of accommodation as that before hospital admission and most maintained social independence, an important marker of quality of life (QOL). Researchers believe that QOL provides some rationale for presymptomatic detection of colorectal cancer in an older person, thus allowing them the opportunity of the far better clinical and survival outcomes from elective surgery for early-stage colorectal cancer rather than late emergency interventions [16]. Although the FOBT does not carry any physical health risks, colonoscopy and sigmoidoscopy both carry the risk of bowel perforation, which requires emergency abdominal surgery, and can also be fatal. Since few people undergoing screening colonoscopy will develop colorectal cancer, many people are being exposed to a potentially dangerous procedure with no health gain. Informed consent is required prior to colonoscopy, but a FOBT$^+$ individual may find it difficult and inadvisable to decide not to proceed with colonoscopy.

Informed consent is an important issue at several stages of the colorectal screening process. With FOBT it is important that people understand that it simply detects blood in the stool, which may or may not be a symptom of severe disease. It is also important that they understand that a negative FOBT result does not definitely rule out the existence of colorectal cancer. FOBT presents additional consent issues to most other screening procedures as it is carried out at home by the individuals themselves, so often the only information they are provided with for deciding whether to participate is contained in the leaflet that is supplied with the testing kit. This does not allow the information to be tailored toward the individual or take into account each individuals personal risk factors.

11.4   CONCLUSIONS

11.4.1   Research and Future Directions in Colorectal Cancer Screening

Future research in colorectal cancer screening is needed in terms of the screening tests used, and deciding who is suitable for screening.

At present the principal screening test used, the FOBT, has a low specificity, and produces large numbers of false-positive results, meaning that many people who do not actually have colorectal cancer are informed that they have a positive test result and need to undergo colonoscopy. This is because the FOBT simply tests for blood in the stools, and there are many more common reasons for blood to be present in stool samples. A screening test with a higher specificity would mean that fewer people would undergo colonoscopy and be exposed to the potential risk that it entails, and also fewer people would experience the anxiety of receiving an uncertain test result. Costs of the screening program would be reduced if fewer people were referred for colonoscopy. At present, the most promising new noninvasive screening tests appear to be DNA stool sample testing, whereby DNA from the intestinal mucosa is tested for specific mutations known to be associated with colorectal cancer. Several such point mutations have been identified in various genes, including p53, but more work is needed to build a more complete picture of gene mutations that could be tested for. DNA stool sampling is, however, very accurate, and has a high sensitivity and specificity, and so is a promising development for the future.

In the UK NHS Bowel Screening Programme everyone aged 60–69 is offered FOBT screening in the UK. This is because these people are in an age group where there is a significant risk of this disease. Offering the test to all people in a defined age group may not be the best or most efficient way of targeting resources, as different individuals within the age group are likely to be at varying degrees of risk for developing the disease, depending on other predisposing factors and comorbidities. As screening tests also carry risks, it is important to identify which individuals are likely to benefit the most from the screening test, and target these people rather than those who are unlikely to develop the disease and therefore may be exposed to the adverse effects of the test with little benefit. Future research into causes and risk factors of colorectal cancer is ongoing and is important in enabling the screening program to increasingly target those people who are most likely to benefit from it, thus reducing any unnecessary testing in others.

Current research is also needed into the issue of repeat screening tests and when to discontinue screening. At present there are no guidelines on when an individual no longer needs FOBT testing (i.e., on individual FOBT cutoff points) and whether further tests are needed. If someone who has repeatedly tested FOBT-negative in the past likely to continue to be FOBT⁻ and thus be able to reduce their screening frequency? Should a person who has many comorbidities and would be unlikely to survive a surgical operation to remove a colorectal tumor anyway, be advised to discontinue screening? Is there an age after which a majority of people could be advised to discontinue screening as the timecourse of development of the disease would significantly greater extend beyond their remaining life expectancy? Weighing up these factors means that screening decisions will increasingly be taken on a more individual, rather than population, level. This will mean that general practitioners, gastroenterologists, geriatricians, and other healthcare professionals will need to become increasingly well informed about the issues surrounding screening to enable them to help patients reach individual decisions about screening tests.

11.5 SUMMARY

To summarize, colorectal cancer is a common and serious disease, and survival rates are much higher if it is detected at an early stage.

Screening tests are available, and many countries, including the UK, have introduced screening programs. The screening tests available at the moment either have low specificity for detecting cancer or are invasive with risks of complications, so current research focuses on improving the screening processes.

REFERENCES

1. GP Notebook (www.gpnotebook.co.uk).
2. American Cancer Society (http://www.cancer.org/ColonandRectumCancer/DetailedGuide/colorectal-cancer-risk-factors).
3. Soetikno RM et al. Increased risk of colorectal neoplasia in patients with primary sclerosing cholangitis and ulcerative colitis: A meta-analysis. *Gastrointest Endosc* 2002;**56**(1):48–54.
4. Morrison DS et al. Risk factors for colonic and rectal cancer mortality: evidence from 40 years follow-up in the Whitehall 1 study. *J Epidemiol Community Health*, 2011;**65**(11):1053–8.
5. Reeves GK et al. Cancer incidence and mortality in relation to body mass index in the Million Women Study: Cohort study. *Br Med J* 2007;**335**(7630):1134.
6. Longnecker MP et al. A meta-analysis of alcoholic beverage consumption in relation to risk of colorectal cancer. *Cancer Causes Control* 1990;**1**(1):59–68.
7. Dos Santos Silver I, Swerdlow AJ. Sex differences in time trends of colorectal cancer in England and Wales: The possible effects of female hormonal factors. *Br. J. Cancer* 1996;**73**(5):692–697.
8. Finley JW et al. Selenium from high selenium broccoli protects rats from colon cancer. *J Nutr* 2000;**130**(9):2384–2389.
9. Larsson SC et al. Vitamin B6 and colorectal cancer: A meta-analysis of prospective studies. *JAMA* 2010;**303**(11):1077–1083.
10. World Health Organization. *Principles and Practice of Screening for Disease*, 1968. (available at http://whqlibdoc.who.int/php/WHO_PHP_34.pdf).
11. Burch JA et al., Centre for Reviews and Dissemination (York, UK), Diagnostic accuracy of faecal occult blood tests used in screening for colorectal cancer: A systematic review. *J. Med. Screen* 2007;**14**(3):132–137.
12. Clarke P et al. Medications with anticoagulant properties increase the likelihood of a negative colonoscopy in faecal occult blood test population screening. *Colorect Dis* 2006;**8**(5):389–392.
13. Anderson ML et al. Endoscopic perforation of the colon: Lessons from a 10-year study. *Am J Gastroenterol* 2000;**95**(12):3418–3422.
14. UK NHS Bowel Screening Programme (http://www.cancerscreening.nhs.uk/bowel).
15. Quarini C, Gosney M. Review of the evidence for a colorectal cancer screening programme in elderly people. *Age Ageing* 2009;**38**(5):503–508.
16. Clark AJ et al. Assessment of outcomes after colorectal cancer resection in the elderly as a rationale for screening and early detection. *Br J Surg* 2004;**91**(10):1345–1351.

CHAPTER 12

Prostate Cancer Screening

ANTHONY B. MILLER

University of Toronto, Toronto, Ontario, Canada

12.1 INTRODUCTION

Two tests have been advocated for screening for prostate cancer, the digital rectal examination (DRE) and the determination of the amount of prostate-specific antigen (PSA) in the blood. Although there has been a tendency to use both tests together, experience has shown the DRE is unreliable, and fails to detect many early prostate cancers detected by PSA. Further, the evidence available on the efficacy of prostate screening relates largely to PSA. Therefore, this chapter concentrates on the evidence relating to the effectiveness of screening with PSA.

Since the introduction of the PSA test, with wide adoption for screening in the United States, a number of jurisdictions in other countries with publicly funded or insurance-based health systems have agreed that PSA testing would be funded, although in Ontario and many other parts of Canada, the funding is for tests ordered for diagnosis and not screening by a physician. However, such types of funding are difficult to monitor, and it seems probable that the majority of the tests now performed in Canada and most other countries are for screening. Nevertheless, one might ask why anyone would oppose this screening test. The public and many of their physicians believe that the early detection and proper treatment of prostate cancer must be beneficial. A significant proportion of the male population, as well as many advocacy groups, it would seem, have agreed testing for elevated PSA levels is good. For example, over 25% of men over the age of 40 reported they had had a PSA screening test in a 2003 Canadian survey [1].

However, the release of mortality results on prostate cancer from two large screening trials, the prostate component of the Prostate, Lung, Colon and Ovary (PLCO) trial in the United States [2] and the European Randomized Study of Screening for Prostate Cancer (ERSPC) [3] has served to fuel the debate, exacerbated by several more recent publications from both trials. This chapter attempts to clarify the present situation and address the issue as to whether, and if so, at what ages, PSA testing should be offered.

Cancer and Aging Handbook: Research and Practice, First Edition. Edited by Keith M. Bellizzi and Margot A. Gosney.
© 2012 Wiley-Blackwell. Published 2012 by John Wiley & Sons, Inc.

12.2   PROSTATE CANCER SCREENING METHODS

12.2.1   Prostate-Specific Antigen (PSA) Screening

Potential Benefits of PSA Screening   Prostate cancer is the most common cause of death from cancer in men in most technically advanced countries [4]. It is by far the most prevalent cancer, with 30–40% of men over 60 found to have prostate cancer at autopsy [5]. The lifetime risk of a man developing microscopic prostate cancer has been estimated at 42% [6]. The sensitivity of the PSA tests depends on the cutoff level selected. If the cutoff for an abnormal PSA test is 4 ng/mL, then the sensitivity of a PSA test is about 75%, rising to over 80% if the cutoff is lowered to 3 ng/mL. However, there is a reciprocal relationship between sensitivity and specificity. If the cutoff is 3 ng/mL, the specificity is approximately 80%; thus 20% of those screened would have a false-positive result resulting in substantial numbers of men placed under supervision and many unnecessary biopsies. At a cutoff level of 4 ng/mL the specificity rises to about 90%, making it a more reasonable test as a false-positive PSA test leads only to temporary anxiety while awaiting a negative biopsy, and the unnecessary biopsies can be accepted if there is benefit from the test. Physicians console themselves that patients are always grateful for early detection of disease, especially with a favorable outcome, which is more likely to occur with early detection of most cancers. These arguments, combined with the widely held belief that early detection of any cancer must be beneficial, has made the PSA test attractive to many patents and their physicians.

Risks of PSA Screening   Although the PSA screening test can identify most men with prostate cancer with some accuracy, over 80% of them will die with the disease but from another cause, and only a small proportion of men with prostate cancer will die from the disease. The treatment of prostate cancer has modestly lowered the mortality rate, but as screening rates have increased, prostate cancer detection has increased quite dramatically, but with little improvement in mortality (Fig. 12.1 shows the situation in Canada). The more recent decline in mortality is probably attributable to prolongation of life from hormone therapy of more advanced cases, with most of them dying from other causes. Frankel et al. [6] estimated if 1 million men over 50 were screened with a PSA test cutoff at 4 ng/mL, 110,000 would have elevated PSA on the first test, 90,000 would have a biopsy, and 20,000 will be found to have cancer. Of this group 10,000 will have a prostatectomy, of whom 300 will be left with chronic incontinence, 4000 will be impotent, and 10 will die from the surgery. In the Finland component of the ESPC trial 12.5% of the screened men had at least one false-positive PSA test during the three rounds of 4-yearly screening [7]. Thus evidence of benefit is necessary to justify all this morbidity and mortality.

12.2.2   ERSPC and PLCO Randomized Screening Trials

Both trials commenced in the early 1990s. The ERSPC trial has enrolled more than 260,000 men from eight countries (Belgium, Finland, France, Italy, the Netherlands, Spain, Sweden, Switzerland) [8]. In all countries men age 55–69 were included, in Sweden men age 50–54 were also included, and in four countries men up to age 74 were included. The PLCO trial enrolled nearly 77,000 men age 55–74 from 10 centers across the United States. In both trials some men have been followed for ≥13 years, but most for 5–10 years. There have been reports on screening from both trials [8–11].

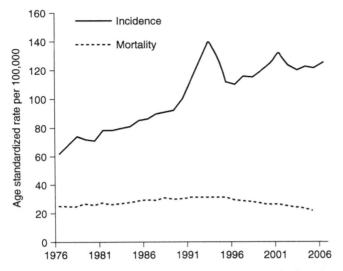

Figure 12.1 Trends in incidence and mortality from prostate cancer in Canada. [*Source:* Canadian Cancer Society Steering Committee [4].)

The first mortality results in PLCO related to all subjects randomized [2], in ERSPC to a subgroup of 182,000 men (3). The difference between this number and the total randomized as previously reported [8] is unexplained, apart from the absence of those recruited in France, where randomization did not begin until 2001.

The PLCO trial was conducted on a background of persistent, long-term advocacy of PSA screening for prostate cancer in the United States [12,13], although not all organizations share the view that screening should be offered [14]. In contrast, in the ERSPC trial, PSA screening in the population was infrequent in most countries when the trial was initiated, although it is believed that the situation changed during the course of the trial. The two trials differ in some other important respects. In PLCO, annual PSA screening to a total of six screens and four annual DRE were offered to the intervention group, in the ERSPC trial, in most countries two PSA screens at 4-year intervals was offered, although the interval was every 2 years in Sweden. The cutoff for a positive PSA was 4 ng/mL in PLCO, and in general 3 ng/mL in ERSPC, although the use of ancillary tests such as DRE and transrectal ultrasound (TRUS) varied between countries, sometimes being applied to those with a PSA <3 ng/mL. PLCO was an individually randomized trial following informed consent, as was the case in Belgium, the Netherlands, Spain, and Switzerland in ERSPC, but in the other four countries (France, Finland, Italy, Sweden) randomization on the basis of population registers was performed prior to consent, which was obtained only in those who accepted the offer of screening. In PLCO, the results of screening were reported to the participant and their physicians, and they decided on subsequent management. This resulted in placement of many people on regular PSA surveillance, rather than immediate biopsy; however, by 4 years over 80% of those with positive tests had achieved resolution (biopsy, or PSA falling to lower levels) [10]. In ERSPC immediate biopsy of those with an abnormal test result was encouraged, and treatment of those found to have cancer often was conducted under the supervision of the trial investigators. In the control groups, cancer care occurred within the community.

In both trials there was no reduction in prostate cancer mortality in the first 7 years after randomization in the screened groups compared to the control [2,3]. During years 8-10 there was a slight difference between the trials. At 10 years in PLCO, with 67% of those enrolled followed in the Andriole et al. [2] report, there was, if anything, higher mortality from prostate cancer in the intervention arm (the screened group) than in the usual care control group, although the difference was nonsignificant (RR 1.13, 95% CI 0.75–1.70). Mortality from all causes other than prostate, lung and colorectal cancer was identical in both arms. In ERSPC at 10 years, with <33.3% of those randomized followed up, the reverse occurred, with lower prostate cancer mortality observed in the screened group; however, neither the RR nor the CI at 10 years were reported. No data beyond 10 years were initially reported for PLCO. For ERSPC, all available data to the cutoff date of December 31, 2006 were reported, and included in the mortality rate ratios. There was a difference in the deaths rate from prostate cancer in the screened group compared to the control group, with a significant 20% reduction in prostate cancer mortality in the screened group compared to the control group in the core age group (men aged 55–69), and a borderline significant reduction of 15% in all subjects. Nearly all the reduction in prostate cancer deaths in the screening group were in men aged 55–59 and 65–69 at entry. There was a nonsignificant excess of prostate cancer deaths in the screened group in men aged 70–74 at entry. The decision of the ERSPC investigators to include all the available data to their cutoff date for follow-up meant that the findings in the last 2 years of follow-up came only from the two countries that enrolled subjects from 1991 (Belgium and Sweden), both enrolled far fewer subjects than the Netherlands and particularly Finland, which must have dominated the results from shorter follow-up times. In practice, the confidence intervals surrounding the point estimates of the reported mortality rate ratios in the two trials overlap, so that random chance cannot be excluded as an explanation for the apparent differences between them.

However, there are other major differences between the US and European trials that need to be considered. The first relates to the degree of background screening that occurred in the control groups. In PLCO 45% of those randomized had undergone at least one PSA test in the 3 years preceding randomization, and screening in the usual care group (opportunistic screening in the community) reached an estimated 52% by the time screening came to an end in the intervention group. Nevertheless, the level of screening in the intervention arm was substantially higher than that in the usual care arm in the early study years, and although the difference decreased later, screening levels remained distinctly higher. In ERSPC the degree of contamination was certainly less, although details are not provided in the report. The second is the different PSA cut-off level applied in the trials. This seems to have resulted in a higher detection rate of prostate cancer following screening in ERSPC than in PLCO, and substantially more overdiagnosis. It seems unlikely that this resulted in a mortality differential in ERSPC being missed in PLCO; however, as the lethality of prostate cancer increases with increasing PSA levels (as well as the converse), it has been shown in ERSPC that cancers detected by screening with a PSA of <4 ng/mL have a favorable prognosis [8]. The third possible reason for the difference in the results is differences in the application of treatment for prostate cancer. Given the way that the ERSPC trial was conducted, with treatment of screening-detected cancers directly controlled by trial investigators, but carried out in the community for those diagnosed in the control group, the potential for treatment differences existed [15]. Although the ERSPC investigators implied that this was not so [3] in Appendix 7 of their paper made available online, substantial treatment differences are seen to have occurred, with much more hormonal therapy (with or without radiotherapy) and absent information on therapy in the control arm. Unfortunately, no stage data were presented, so we do not yet know whether there were differences in treatment within the same stage. However, a publication by some of the ERSPC investigators reported that men diagnosed with prostate cancer were more likely to be treated at an academic center in the screening arm than men diagnosed in the control arm [16]. To the extent that outcomes after major surgery may be better in major referral centers than in community hospitals, this difference in treatment venue may have favored the screening arm. Further, trial arm was associated with treatment choice, especially in men at high risk for prostate cancer. Thus a high-risk control subject was more likely than a screened subject to receive radiotherapy (OR 1.43, 95% CI 1.01–2.05), expectant management (OR 2.92, 95% CI 1.33–6.42), or hormonal treatment (OR 1.77, 95% CI 1.07–2.94) than radical prostatectomy. In contrast, the policy in the PLCO trial not to mandate specific therapies after screen detection resulted in substantial similarity in treatment by stage between the two arms [2].

More recently, a report of follow-up through to 14 years of the Goteborg component of ERSPC has been published, combined with findings from some subjects who were not part of the ERSPC analysis [17]. Comparing the earlier ERSPC report [3] with this manuscript, it seems reasonable to conclude that 60% of the Goteborg cohort was included in the core age group (55–69) of ERSPC. Of the 122 deaths from prostate cancer reported in the Goteborg trial, 109 (89%) occurred in those aged 55–64 years at entry. Schröder et al. [3] did not report deaths by country, and Hugossan et al. [17] did not report how many of the Goteborg deaths were included in the core age group analysis of ERSPC, so the extent of the overlap in deaths between the two analyses is unclear. It seems reasonable, however to assume that most or all of these 109 were included in the core group analysis of Schröder et al. [3]. Indeed, the overall ERSPC result without the Goteborg (Swedish) component did not quite reach statistical significance (RR = 0.84, 95% CI 0.70–1.01) [3]. As the control group in the Goteborg trial were followed passively through national registers, and probably did not know that they were part of a trial, it seems likely that differences in treatment occurred. The Goteborg study's major finding concerning a prostate cancer mortality reduction thus seems largely derived from previously reported ERSPC data and cannot be regarded as independent validation of the findings of Schröder et al [3]. Further, in both the Goteborg and ERSPC analyses, the benefit is probably attributable to differences in treatment rather than screening.

More recently, an update on mortality in the PLCO trial has become available, with 92% of the participants followed to 10 years and 57% to 13 years [18]. At 13 years 4250 participants had been diagnosed with prostate cancer in the intervention group, and 3815 in the usual care group, for an RR of 1.12 (95% CI 1.07–1.17). At 13 years the RR (intervention/usual care group) for cumulative mortality from prostate cancer was 1.09 (95% confidence interval 0.87–1.36). These relative risk ratios are very similar to those previously reported to 10 years, providing no indication of benefit even with 3 further years of follow-up. At about the same time another analysis utilizing updated PLCO prostate mortality data through to 10 years reported a statistically significant interaction of trial arm by comorbidity status [19]. However, a similar analysis using a modified Charlson score of comorbidity through to 13 years did not confirm this [18], casting substantial doubt on the claim by Crawford et al. [19] that those with no comorbidity at baseline derive a benefit from PSA screening.

It has been concluded that wider application of improvements in prostate cancer treatment is at least in part responsible for declining prostate cancer mortality rates in most countries [20]. Even if life is only prolonged by therapy, the opportunities for competing causes of death increase, especially among older men. The WHO mortality database shows that the reductions in prostate cancer mortality have been greater in the United States than in most other countries. For the latest year for which data are available, the age-adjusted mortality rate per 100,000 for prostate cancer was 14.4 for the Netherlands (in 2008), 14.1 in Finland (in 2008), 19.5 in Sweden (in 2007), 13.6 in Switzerland (in 2007), but 10.8 in the United States (in 2005). Only for Italy (9.1 in 2007) and Spain (10.8 in 2005) are the rates comparable to the US ones (although they have been lower for some time). (The latest published rate for Belgium was 12.3 in 2004). Therefore international data suggest that either more universal screening or better treatment in the United States is responsible for the lower prostate mortality than the countries contributing the largest number of subjects to ERSPC—with the treatment explanation as the most likely.

12.3 DISCUSSION

In PLCO the screening that occurred in the usual care arm was not sufficient to eliminate the expected impacts of the annual screening in the intervention arm such as earlier diagnosis and a persistent excess of cases. Therefore what the trial was evaluating was the effect of adding an organized component of annual screening to the opportunistic screening already in place, and as far as the follow-up has continued, there is no evidence of a benefit. Indeed, there are risks, in part associated with the false-positive tests, but also with the overdiagnosis inseparable from PSA screening, especially in older men. What the trial does seem to confirm, however, would be the futility of making any attempt to set up organized screening programs in addition to what is currently ongoing in any country. There is also no evidence, from PLCO or any other screening trial, that screening by digital rectal examination (DRE) is beneficial, and therefore, DRE cannot be recommended as a substitute for PSA for screening for prostate cancer. These seem to be becoming generally accepted conclusions. Even when authors conclude that PSA screening reduces prostate cancer mortality, they also conclude that screening cannot be justified yet in the context of a public health policy [21]. Such a conclusion was also reached by the authors of a systematic review and meta-analysis of all randomized screening trials for prostate cancer [22]. Their meta-analysis failed to find a significant effect of screening on prostate cancer mortality (RR 0.88, 95% CI 0.71–1.09) and no effect on overall mortality (RR 0.99, 95% CI 0.97–1.01).

Nevertheless, the question that has to be addressed is whether the European trial results support the continuation of the opportunistic screening that is ongoing in North America and some other countries. The uncertainty that surrounds the validity of the results of ERSPC beyond 10 years makes that difficult to answer with certainty. The delay in seeing a possible benefit is certainly compatible with what is known about the long natural history of prostate cancer. If the separation between the mortality curves in ERSPC beyond 10 years is confirmed with more data, it will still be necessary to be certain that other factors, especially treatment differences between the randomized groups, are not responsible for this. However, it is important to note that both trials support the recommendation of the US Preventive Services Task Force [14] against screening men older than 69, and the European trial provides no support for screening men younger than 55.

The potential risks and disadvantages from prostate screening are considerable. In addition to the complications associated with false-positive diagnoses, and the risk of postoperative mortality in elderly men subjected to prostatectomy, there is evidence of substantial overdiagnosis, estimated in ERSPC to be 27% from a single screening test at age 55,56% for a single screening test at age 75 years. [23]. These complications have to be set against a low probability of benefit. Even if the ERSPC findings of benefit represent the truth, the investigators have estimated that 1400 men need to be screened and 45 need to undergo treatment, to save one life [3]. Thus the large majority of men who believe that their lives have been saved by PSA testing have been deceived. Raffle and Gray [24] have coined the term "the popularity paradox" for this situation: "The greater the harm from overdiagnosis and overtreatment from screening, the more people there are who believe they owe their health, or even their life, to the programme."

After the results of the UK Million Women Study [25] and the US Women's Health Initiative Study were known [26], Sackett wrote about the "arrogance of preventive medicine" [27]. He strongly attacked any intervention on healthy people that might carry more risk of harm than benefit stating "Experts refuse to learn from history until they make it themselves, and the price for their arrogance is paid by the innocent. Preventive medicine is too important to be led by them." From our present knowledge of risks and benefits attributable to prostate cancer screening and treatment, we cannot justify advocating for screening programs for prostate cancer at this time. All physicians have ethical responsibilities to inform their patients of potential risks and benefits of any procedure. However, front-line physicians cannot be expected to be constantly battling powerful public campaigns. There is a great need for alignment of all organizations with currently available evidence. Mass PSA screening cannot be justified, and most PSA screening should be discontinued to prevent more unjustified death and morbidity. So, the answer to the question men often ask their physician as to whether they should have a PSA test is "Do not screen for prostate cancer with PSA."

There are, however, a few potential conflicts of interest. Although the author declares that he has no financial relationship with any commercial organization concerned with prostate cancer screening, he has been a consultant to the Division of Cancer Prevention of the US National Cancer Institute since 1996, was chairperson of the Death Review Committee of the PLCO trial 1998–2004, has been chairperson of the Analysis Cost-effectiveness and Modelling Committee of the PLCO trial since 2004, and coauthored a number of publications on the PLCO trial [2,10,18].

ACKNOWLEDGMENTS

The initial version of the manuscript that forms the basis for this chapter was jointly written by the present author together with Emeritus Professor of Family Medicine of Queens University, Ontario, Canada, Walter Rosser. His contribution represents the sections that could provide guidance to those considering recommending PSA screening to their patients. Unfortunately, it has not been possible for Professor Rosser to have any impact on the subsequent revisions of the manuscript that has resulted in the present version.

The author would like to express his indebtedness to his colleagues in the PLCO trial, especially Barry Kramer, Paul Pinsky, and Philip Prorok, for many useful discussions on the issues considered in this chapter.

REFERENCES

1. Canadian Cancer Society/National Cancer Institute of Canada. *Canadian Cancer Statistics 2006*, Toronto, Canada, 2006.

2. Andriole GL et al., for the PLCO Project Team. Mortality results from a randomized prostate-cancer screening trial. *N Engl J Med* 2009;**360**:1310–1319.

3. Schröder FH et al., for the ERSPC Investigators. Screening and prostate-cancer mortality in a randomized European study. *N Engl J Med* 2009;**360**:1320–1328.

4. Canadian Cancer Society's Steering Committee. *Canadian Cancer Statistics 2010*, Canadian Cancer Society, Toronto, 2008.

5. Miller AB. Commentary: Implications of the frequent occurrence of occult carcinoma of the prostate. *Int J Epidemiol* 2007;**36**:282–284.

6. Frankel S et al. Screening for prostate cancer. *Lancet* 2003;**361**:1122–1128.

7. Kilpeläinen TP et al. False-positive screening results in the Finnish prostate cancer screening trial. *Br J Cancer* 2010;**102**:469–474.

8. Schröder FH. Screening for prostate cancer (PC)—an update on recent findings of the European Randomized Study of Screening for Prostate Cancer (ERSPC). *Eur Oncol* 2008;**26**:533–541.

9. Crawford ED et al. Prostate specific antigen changes as related to the initial prostate specific antigen: Data from the prostate, lung, colorectal and ovarian cancer screening trial. *J Urol* 2006;**175**:1286–1290.

10. Grubb RL et al., for the PLCO Project Team. Prostate cancer screening in the Prostate, Lung, Colorectal and Ovarian cancer screening trial: Update on findings from the initial four rounds of screening in a randomized trial. *Br J Urol Int* 2008;**102**:1524–1530.

11. Schröder FH, Roobol MJ. A comment on prostate cancer screening in the Prostate, Lung, Colorectal and Ovarian cancer screening trial: Update on findings from the initial four rounds of screening in a randomized trial. *Br J Urol Int* 2009;**103**:143–144.

12. American Urological Association (AUA). Prostate-specific antigen (PSA) best practice policy. *Oncology* 2000;**14**(2):267–272, 277–278, 280 passim.

13. American Cancer Society. *Cancer Screening Guidelines 2008* (available at http://www.cancer.org/docroot/ped/content/ped_2_3x_acs_cancer_detection_guidelines_36.asp; accessed 1/05/09).

14. US Preventive Task Force. Screening for prostate cancer: U.S. Preventive Services Task Force recommendation statement. *Ann Int Med* 2008;**149**:185–191.

15. Barry M. Screening for prostate cancer—the controversy that refuses to die. *N Engl J Med* 2009;**360**:1351–1354.

16. Wolters T et al. The effect of study arm on prostate cancer treatment in a large screening trial (ERSPC). *Int J Cancer* 2010;**126**:2387–2393.

17. Hugosson J et al. Mortality results from the Goteborg randomised population-based prostate-cancer screening trial. *Lancet Oncology* 2010;**11**:725–732.

18. Andriole GL et al. Screening for prostate cancer, a 13-year update of the results of the prostate component of the Prostate, Lung, Colon and Ovary trial. *J Natl Cancer Inst* 2012;**104**:1–8.

19. Crawford ED et al. Comorbidity and mortality results from a randomized prostate cancer screening trial. *J Clin Oncol* 2011;**29**:355–361.

20. Etzioni R, Feuer E. Studies of prostate cancer mortality: Caution advised. *Lancet Oncol* 2008;**9**:407–409.

21. van Leeuwen PJ et al. The implementation of screening for prostate cancer. *Prostate Cancer Prost Dis* 2010;**13**:218–227.

22. Djulbegovic M et al. Screening for prostate cancer: Systematic review and metaanalysis of randomised controlled trials. *Br Med J* 2010;**341**:c4543.

23. Draisma G et al. Lead times and overdetection due to prostate-specific antigen screening: Estimates from the European Randomized Study of Screening for Prostate Cancer. *J Natl Cancer Inst* 2003;**95**:868–878.

24. Raffle AE, Gray JAM. *Screening: Evidence and Practice*, Oxford Univ. Press, Oxford, UK, 2007.

25. Beral V and Million Women Study collaborators. Breast cancer and hormone-replacement therapy in the Million Women Study. *Lancet* 2003;**362**:419–427.

26. Chlebowski RT et al. Influence of estrogen plus progestin on breast cancer and mammography in healthy postmenopausal women: The Women's Health Initiative randomized trial. *JAMA* 2003;**289**:3243–3253.

27. Sackett DL. The arrogance of preventive medicine. *Can Med Assoc J* 2002;**167**:363–364.

CHAPTER 13

Other Screening Opportunities for the Future

CATHERINE QUARINI

Warneford Hospital, Oxford, UK

13.1 INTRODUCTION

This chapter begins by reviewing current cancer screening programes for elderly people, before discussing the implementation of programs to detect common cancers for which routine screening programs are not currently in place. After this, the relevance of current and future screening opportunities to elderly people is examined. Finally, the broader issues of the provision and cost of future screening opportunities, as well as the role of new technologies in realizing these opportunities, are discussed.

13.2 CURRENT CANCER SCREENING PROCEDURES FOR THE ELDERLY

Currently, screening programs are in place in the UK for breast, cervical, and colorectal cancers. There is no national screening program for prostate cancer, but men can request testing. Many of the current screening programs are relevant to elderly people, but few make specific recommendations for the elderly population or are routinely offered to elderly people.

> *Breast Screening*. Mammography is offered every 3 years to women aged 50–70 through the NHS Breast Screening Programme. The upper age limit for screening to be routinely offered will be increased to 73 by 2012 [1]. Women over 70 can request a mammogram but are not routinely invited for screening. The NHS Breast Screening Programme issues women a reminder card at the time of their last routine mammogram with details on how to request ongoing appointments. The leaflet on breast screening for women over age 70 [2] points out that the risk of breast cancer increases with age and actively encourages women to attend screening sessions, so it seems at odds with this recommendation that they are not routinely invited.

Cancer and Aging Handbook: Research and Practice, First Edition. Edited by Keith M. Bellizzi and Margot A. Gosney.
© 2012 Wiley-Blackwell. Published 2012 by John Wiley & Sons, Inc.

Cervical Screening. Women in the UK aged >65 are offered screening only if they "have not been screened since age 50 or have had recent abnormal tests" [3]. The NHS Cervical Screening Programme website explains that the natural history and progression of cervical cancer means that it is very unlikely that women over 65 who have had three consecutive negative tests would go on to develop the disease.

Colorectal Screening. The UK NHS Bowel Screening Programme [4] currently offers screening every 2 years to everyone aged 60–69. An explanatory letter and faecal occult blood test (FOBT) testing kit is sent by post. People over 70 can request a kit, but are not sent one automatically.

13.3 COMMON CANCERS FOR WHICH FUTURE SCREENING OPPORTUNITIES MAY BE AVAILABLE

Skin cancer, lung cancer, and prostate cancer are all common conditions for which methods of screening are either available or in development.

Skin   One in every three cancers diagnosed is a skin cancer [5]. Most skin cancers are either basal cell carcinomas or squamous cell carcinomas. The incidence of all types has been increasing over the past 30 years. At present there are few recommendations about screening for skin cancer by either self-examination or screening by a physician. In 2001 a review carried out for the US Preventative Services Task Force (USPSTF) found no controlled studies demonstrating that routine screening for melanoma by primary care physicians reduced morbidity or mortality from this condition [6]. More recent reviews have also concluded that at present there is not sufficient evidence to recommend appropriate screening intervals or procedures [7].

However, research has shown that there is a need for greater public education about skin cancer and the benefits of early detection. A 2009 survey of patients undergoing skin cancer screening at a US clinic revealed that most participants (80.6%) sought screening without a particular lesion that they were concerned about, but men aged >50 years, the group who are at highest risk of death from melanoma, attended screening only after being diagnosed with a skin cancer. This study considered participants' reasons for attending screening, and found that women were more likely than men to present because they were concerned about previous sun exposure (one of the main risk factors), and younger people were more likely than older people to attend because they were concerned about their family history of melanoma [8]. These findings demonstrate different reasons for attending screening and perceived risks among different population groups, which are important considerations in implementing a new screening program and targeting it at the population of interest.

At present there is no clear evidence to support the introduction of national skin cancer screening program in the UK or Europe.

Lung   Research into screening for lung cancer has been carried out in several countries, and most studies have concluded that at present screening is not recommended for asymptomatic people. However, a screening test is available, and if it is used, should be targeted only at high-risk individuals. Computerized tomography (CT) scans can be used to screen for lung cancer. At present there is little evidence to suggest that screening reduces lung cancer mortality, although a national survey of 962 primary care physicians in the United States found that many were making recommendations inconsistent with the current evidence as two-thirds thought that low-radiation-dose spiral CT screening is effective at reducing lung cancer mortality in current smokers [9].

An ongoing Dutch–Belgian randomized lung cancer screening trial (NELSON) is investigating whether screening using CT scanning will decrease lung cancer mortality compared to no screening [10]. The study participants are current smokers, and former smokers who discontinued smoking a maximum of 10 years ago and smoked heavily for >25 years.

Research in Australia has evaluated the cost-effectiveness of using low-dose spiral CT scans to screen for lung cancer and has shown that this is not cost-effective at present. This study [11] analyzed the costs and health outcomes in a hypothetical cohort of 10,000 male smokers. They compared the hypothetical outcomes from two alternatives—to screen for lung cancer every 5 years with a CT scan and then treat people who are found to have the disease, or not to screen and treat people who present symptomatically. They found that for male smokers aged 60–64 years, the increased detection rates and earlier treatment from screening would mean some increase in life expectancy, but this would come at a cost of $57,325 per life-year saved. They define a cost-effective intervention to be one in which a maximum of $50,000 is spent per life-year saved, so CT screening is not cost-effective.

Cost-effectiveness is an important consideration in developing a screening program, and is likely to be seen as more important in countries where health-care is state-funded. At present, screening all smokers over the age of 60 for lung cancer is not cost-effective. This may change if the costs of CT scanning falls, and more evidence is needed to determine whether CT screening would be cost-effective if only very high-risk individuals were targeted, such as older people who have smoked heavily for several decades.

Screening for lung cancer can be undertaken using computerized tomography. It is not currently recommended for asymptomatic people, although there is ongoing research into its use in high-risk individuals. CT scans carry health risks, and at present this screening test is unlikely to be deemed cost-effective by healthcare providers. If the cost and safety of screening methods improve, this may present a screening opportunity for the future.

Prostate Prostate cancer is the most common cancer, and the second most common cause of cancer-related deaths, in men in the UK. More than 75% of cases occur in men over 65, and most are diagnosed in those aged 70–74. The NHS screening website explains to patients that although a prostate screening trial in Europe has shown that screening reduced mortality by 20% [12], this was associated with a high level of overtreatment in people who may never have developed clinical symptoms of the disease, and at present prostate cancer does not meet the WHO criteria for screening.

Prostate-specific antigen (PSA) level is currently the best method of identifying localized disease. The UK Health Technology Assessment Programme concludes that PSA testing should be carried out only in men who have symptoms of prostate cancer and understand the uncertainties of the test, but also have a "life expectancy of at least 10 years" [13]. This criterion will exclude a proportion of elderly people.

A study of prostate cancer mortality in the UK and USA between 1975 and 2004 found that prostate cancer mortality peaked in the early 1990s in both countries, but

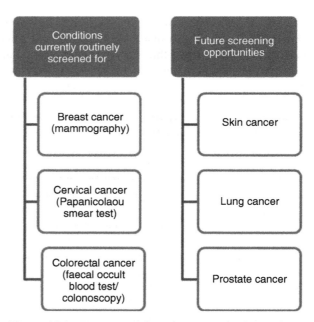

Figure 13.1   Present and future cancer screening options.

since then the mortality rate has declined 4 times faster in the United States, particularly among men over 74 years old [14]. There was a 10-fold difference in the uptake of the PSA test between the UK and the USA by 2001, and in the United States more cases of the disease are detected while still localized. However, in the United States prostate cancers tend to be treated more aggressively, with radical prostatectomy used much more commonly, even after the higher ratio of localized; nonlocalized disease was considered. Although high uptake of screening may have produced benefits for a small number of men whose aggressive prostate cancer was detected early on, and this small increase in early treatment may have affected overall mortality figures, high uptake of screening is also likely to have led to many asymptomatic men receiving unnecessary treatment. This study concluded that at present it is not possible to attribute the differences in mortality rate to screening uptake, treatment differences, or bias in practices of recording the causes of death.

Therefore the PSA test is widely available and is currently the best method of detecting localized prostate cancer. However, this test has a low specificity, and, combined with the slow development of many prostate cancers that never become symptomatic, this means that widespread use of the PSA test is currently associated with a high level of overtreatment. Screening opportunities for the future (Fig. 13.1) are likely to focus on developing more specific screening tests.

13.4   APPLICABILITY OF CURRENT CANCER SCREENING RESULTS TO ELDERLY PEOPLE

There has been little research to date on screening in elderly people, and few current guidelines recommend an upper age limit for screening. The UK Colorectal Cancer

Screening Pilot, which led to the introduction of the NHS Bowel Screening Programme, excluded people over 70 years of age because of a falloff in uptake over this age in a trial of FOBT screening. A review of this pilot scheme [15] points out that "it is worth noting that if an age cut-off of 69 years (as chosen for the England programme) rather than 74 years had been used in the Funen trial of faecal occult blood screening, 25% of detectable cancers would have been missed." A review of the guidelines for colorectal screening from many different health agencies found that none of these agencies suggest an upper age limit for screening, although most suggest beginning at 50. The exception was the Institute for Clinical Systems Improvement, which recommends FOBT screening between ages 50 and 80 [16]. With such ambiguity regarding the age at which to stop screening, it is not surprising that patients receive different advice depending on which physicians they consult. A study of 8000 US gastroenterologists revealed that 37% recommended continuing screening with the fecal occult blood test into old age or never discontinuing it [17].

Statistics from the UK NHS Breast Screening Programme report that 63,405 women aged ≥71 attended for breast screening in 2009 and the vast majority of these had requested the screening test themselves [18]. Of those screened in this age group, 1.2% were found to have invasive cancer, representing a higher percentage than for any of the age groups in which screening is routinely recommended. However, these data alone do not necessarily mean that screening should be recommended for this age group. One of the key principles of screening developed by Wilson and Junger, WHO 1968 [19], is that treatment of the condition at an early stage should be more beneficial than treatment at a later stage. Another key principle is that there should be an accepted policy on recommended treatment. These criteria may not be fulfilled for elderly people if their comorbities or life expectancy mean that they are unlikely to benefit from treatment.

In conclusion, there is little research and evidence available at present on screening specifically in elderly people. Future screening opportunities are likely to depend in part on evaluating the evidence for screening specifically in elderly people.

13.5 GUIDELINES FOR SCREENING OF THE ELDERLY

13.5.1 Need For Development of Elderly-Specific Screening Procedures

In many countries the numbers of elderly people are increasing. In the UK the percentage of the population aged ≥65 increased from 15% in 1984 to 16% in 2009, which represents an increase of 1.7 million people [20]. An even higher population increase has been in the number of those aged ≥85. In 1984 there were 660,000 people in the UK aged ≥85, whereas in 2009 there were 1.4 million people in this group, and it has been predicted that by 2034 the number of people ≥85 years will be 3.5 million, and will account for 5% of the total UK population [21]. Similar trends are being seen across Europe. Projections from the European Commission suggest that the percentage of the total population aged ≥65 will increase from 17.1% in 2008 to 30% in 2060. Likewise, the numbers of people aged ≥80 years in the European Union is expected to almost triple from 21.8 million in 2008 to 61.4 million in 2060 [22].

An increasing elderly population will mean that health services will need to focus more toward their needs. There are several questions to consider in implementing screening programmes for elderly people:

- Should there be a defined age after which screening is not recommended because the risks of intervention outweigh the benefits that may be gained after a certain age?
- Is life expectancy a more meaningful criterion for deciding whether to offer a test than simply age?
- Should the advice given to an older person who chooses to have a screening test on detection of a malignancy be different from the advice given to younger people? For example, most of the dangers of colonoscopy are from removal of polyps, and some elderly people may not have sufficient life expectancy to benefit from this. Surgery for breast or prostate cancer carries risks, and anesthetic risks increase with advancing age. The ethics of detecting a malignancy or premalignant condition and then advising the patient not to act on this knowledge are, however, complex.
- Should an individual's screening history affect the advice that person is given? If one has had negative screening tests for many years, does this mean that they are very likely to continue to have negative tests? If so, perhaps the guidelines should recommend reduced frequency of testing after a certain number of negative tests. This has already been done for cervical screening, but not for other screening programs.

In conclusion, an increasing elderly population means that policymakers and clinicians will increasingly be faced with decisions regarding screening recommendations in elderly people. Important issues to consider are life expectancy, risks and benefits from the screening test, success rates for treatment of the condition, and screening history.

13.5.2 A Proposed Model for Screening Elderly Populations

In considering future opportunities in cancer screening in elderly people, it is important to remember that life expectancy varies greatly between elderly people of the same age, depending on their comorbid conditions, and so is therefore likely to be more important in guiding screening decisions than actual age. For example, an 85-year-old woman in the upper quartile of life expectancy may have more chance of benefiting from cancer screening than a 70-year-old woman in the lower quartile.

A conceptual *screening framework* that relies partly on life expectancy estimates has already been proposed by Walker and Covinsky [23] and can be used to guide individual screening decisions, rather than using a rigid set of age-specific guidelines. The framework takes into account both quantitative estimates of the risks and benefits of tests, as well as qualitative factors, such as the patient's preferences.

The first step in the framework considers the patient's risk of dying of a screening-detectable cancer. This risk is estimated by considering the person's life expectancy and the age-specific mortality rate of the disease. The geriatrician will need to estimate whether a person's life expectancy is in the middle, upper, or lower quartiles of their age–gender cohort. This will be based on their comorbities. Next, the possible outcomes of screening tests need to be considered. For example, if this person has a positive FOBT, would further investigation with colonoscopy be appropriate? Comorbidities, life expectancy, or the person's decision that they do not want to be exposed to the risks or discomfort of the test, or the anxiety of waiting for results, may mean that it would not be appropriate. If further investigation is deemed inappropriate at the start of the process, then there is little point in carrying out FOBT, as a positive result is likely to generate anxiety without offering any later reassurance or intervention.

Finally, the risks and benefits of screening need to be weighed against the individual's situation and preferences considered. For example, a healthy 80-year-old who requests screening because of a wish to be reassured by a clear mammogram, but who has decided that if the test is positive, they would be willing to undergo further investigation and treatment, would be suitable for screening, but a 70-year-old with cardiac comorbidities and Alzheimer's disease which prevents them from being able to understand the process of screening would not be suitable, partly because, even if a malignancy is found, the person might not live for a long enough time for it to become clinically significant, and partly because the screening procedure is likely to generate anxiety but cannot provide any reassurance because of the person's cognitive decline.

Therefore, in deciding which elderly people to recommend for screening, a screening framework, which could be applied on an individual basis by geriatricians, is more appropriate than a rigid set of guidelines. Life expectancy, comorbities, and personal preference should all be considered.

13.6 FUTURE SCREENING PROSPECTS

13.6.1 Who Will Provide Screening in the Future?

As with all aspects of healthcare, there are funding considerations for screening programs. This is especially likely to be true for future opportunities for cancer screening in older people, as there are increasing opportunities to screen for diseases and an increasing elderly population. Decisions will have to be made about the priority of funding for these tests compared with other areas of healthcare. Currently in the UK the NHS provides breast, cervical, and bowel screening programs for certain population groups. This is in contrast to countries such as the United States where most screening is provided by private companies.

In the United States people have screening tests such as mammography and FOBT more frequently than the NHS provides, and screening tests at ages outside those offered in the UK. The differences between the US system and the UK NHS screening programs brings up several issues. More screening is carried out in the United States, so more asymptomatic conditions are detected at an early stage. However, all screening tests have a false-positive rate, so some people will be incorrectly informed that they have a condition and may begin treatment, whereas without the screening test they would not have been exposed to the anxiety associated with the diagnosis, and perhaps harmful effects of unnecessary treatment. Follow-up of abnormal screening results may also be different depending on the providers. A comparison of US and UK screening mammograms found that both recall rates and rates of negative open surgical biopsy rates were approximately twice as high in the United States [24], although cancer detection rates were similar between the two countries.

Many screening tests have risks associated with the procedure itself. For example, mammography involves exposing the breast tissue to a small dose of X-ray radiation, and proposed screening tests for lung cancer involve CT scans. A false-positive screening test result is likely to generate significant anxiety. The risks from the procedure needs to be balanced against the chance of obtaining benefit from the test.

There have been several recent indications that more screening in the UK may be carried out by private companies in the future. There has been an increase in private "well person" clinics offering screening tests such as cholesterol checks, which are targeted mainly at older people. Some of these providers have little infrastructure to support people who have a worrying test result, and many of these people then consult their general practitioners about the findings of a test that would not have been recommended for them. The increase in advertising for screening tests from private companies brings up the issue of the role and responsibility of these companies for offering people follow-up.

In conclusion, with an increasing elderly population and increasing screening tests available, funding decisions are likely to play a part in determining which tests can be offered to which population groups.

13.6.2   Impact of Information Technology on Future Screening Opportunities

Not only will new medical technologies change the future of screening, but new information technologies are also likely to have a large part to play in increasing screening opportunities for the future.

Currently, invitations for screening and information leaflets are sent by post, with cost limiting the amount of information that can be sent, as well as the number of reminders and appointment letters. If a person does not attend the screening session, providers have no way of knowing whether that person received the letter, or decided against the screening test. Screening providers will now be able to send people reminder emails and text messages at very low cost, and ask people to confirm their receipt of the information and to book appointments online. This will mean that more funds can be allocated for other aspects of screening programs, such as increasing the numbers of health professionals involved and targeting more resources at research.

The Internet has revolutionized public access to medical information, and people now have the opportunity to research screening methods and conditions in far greater detail than could be provided in an information leaflet. This means that they may have more knowledge and hopefully be in a better position to make an informed decision.

However, although people now have access to large volumes of information, it is not yet clear what impact this will have on the amount of time that healthcare professionals will need to spend explaining screening tests to people. Although many individuals will successfully use the Internet to research screening and therefore be less likely to need the input of healthcare staff to help them reach decisions, other people may find it more difficult to judge which sources of information are reliable. Some Internet searching may generate more questions and anxieties than it resolves, which then has an impact on the time needed for physicians to reassure and explain procedures to patients. Healthcare professionals now have a new aspect to their role in that they will need to spend time advising patients which websites are reliable sources of information and which are not.

The increasing use of information technology also raises the question of how much confidential medical information will be given via the Internet. Sending the results of screening tests to people via email means individuals have their results faster so less time is spent anxiously waiting for results, results will not be lost or delayed in the post, and the sender immediately knows if the email has not been delivered. However,

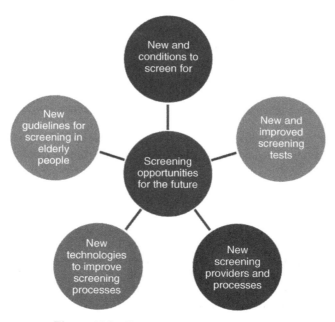

Figure 13.2   Future screening opportunities.

there are concerns over the security of online medical records. Computer security may be a particular issue for elderly people who are not computer-literate and want a family member to check their results for them—geriatricians and policy-makers will need to ensure that systems are put in place to facilitate this where appropriate.

Some elderly people also may have limited access to the Internet. Therefore paper versions of information leaflets and appointment reminders must still be available.

In conclusion, new information technology is crucial in realizing future screening opportunities (Fig. 13.2). Healthcare professionals should guide patients to reliable Internet sources of information. Care must be taken to ensure that confidentiality is maintained and that elderly people who do not use the Internet are not excluded from screening opportunities.

13.7   CONCLUSIONS

There are many challenges and opportunities for the future development of cancer screening programs in elderly people. At present, few of the screening programs already in place actively recruit elderly people, and with an increasing elderly population and increases in life expectancy, it is important that this issue be addressed. New screening tests are being developed, and these will need to be constantly reevaluated in terms of efficacy and cost before and after screening programs are implemented. In addition to advances in medicine, new technology plays a role in implementing screening programs. Future directions and opportunities in this area center around health professionals recognizing the variation in health status and preferences between different elderly people of the same age, and taking a more individualized, patient-centered approach to making screening decisions at a time of many new developments in this area.

REFERENCES

1. See `http://www.cancerscreening.nhs.uk/breastscreen/future-developments.html`.
2. See `http://www.cancerscreening.nhs.uk/breastscreen/publications/over70.pdf`.
3. See `http://www.cancerscreening.nhs.uk/cervical/about-cervical-screening.html#not-invited`.
4. NHS Bowel Cancer Screening Programme (`www.cancerscreening.nhs.uk/bowel/`).
5. World Health Organization (`http://www.who.int/uv/faq/skincancer/en/index1.html`).
6. Helfand M et al. Screening for skin cancer. *Am J Prevent Med* 2001;**20**(3 Suppl):47–58.
7. Wolff T, Tai E, Miller T. Screening for skin cancer: An update of the evidence for the U.S. Preventative Service Task Force. *Ann Intern Med* 2009;**150**(3):194–198.
8. Andrulonis R. The influence of age and sex on reasons for seeking and expected benefits of skin cancer screening. *Arch Dermatol* 2010;**146**(10):1097–1102.
9. Klabunde C et al. U.S. primary care physicians lung cancer screening beliefs and recommendations. *Am J Prevent Med* 2010;**39**(5):411–420.
10. Van Iersel CA et al. Risk based selection from the general population in a screening trial: Selection criteria, recruitment and power for the Dutch-Belgian randomised lung cancer multi-slice CT screening trial (NELSON). *Int J Cancer* 2007;**120**(4):868–874.
11. Manser R et al. Cost-effectiveness analysis of screening for lung cancer with low dose spiral CT (computed tomography) in the Australian setting. *Lung Cancer* 2005;**48**(2):171–185.
12. See `www.cancerscreening.nhs.uk/prostate`.
13. Selley S et al. *Diagnosis Management and Screening of Early Localised Prostate Cancer*. NHS Health Technology Assessment Programme, Health Technology Assessment, 1997, Vol. 1, No. 2.
14. Collin S et al. An ecological study of prostate cancer mortality in the USA and UK, 1975–2004: Are divergent trends a consequence of treatment, screening or artefact? *Lancet Oncol* 2008;**9**(5):445–452.
15. Population screening for colorectal cancer. *Drug Ther Bull* 2006;**44**(9):65–68.
16. Mahon SM. Colorectal cancer screening: A review of the evidence. *Clin J Oncol Nurs*, 2004;**8**(5):536–540.
17. Sharma V K et al. Survey of the opinions, knowledge, and practices of gastroenterologists regarding colorectal cancer screening and the use of the faecal occult blood test. *Am J Gastroenterol* 2000;**95**(12):3629–3632.
18. See `http://www.cancerscreening.nhs.uk/breastscreen/publications/nhsbsp-annualreview2009.pdf`.
19. Wilson JMG, Jungner G. *Principles and Practice of Screening for Disease*. WHO, Geneva, 1968 (available from: `http://www.who.int/bulletin/volumes/86/4/07-050112BP.pdf`)
20. See `http://www.statistics.gov.uk/cci/nugget.asp?id=949`.
21. See `http://www.statistics.gov.uk`.
22. European Commission, Eurostat. *Ageing Characterises the Demographic Perspectives of the European Societies* (available at `http://epp.eurostat.ec.europa.eu`).
23. Walter L, Covinsky C. Cancer screening in elderly patients: A framework for individualized decision making. *JAMA* 2001;**285**(21):2750–2756.
24. Smith-Bindman et al. Comparison of screening mammography in the United States and the United Kingdom. *JAMA* 2003;**290**(16):2129–2137.

PART IV

CANCER TREATMENT

CHAPTER 14

General Principles in Older Adults with Cancer

MARTINE EXTERMANN

Senior Adult Oncology Program, H. Lee Moffitt Cancer Center & Research Institute, Tampa, FL

14.1 INTRODUCTION

In this chapter, we will address a cluster of general issues pertaining to the treatment of older cancer patients. We will focus on aspects that have a broad validity across several types of cancer and treatments. The specific aspects will be addressed in the respective chapters.

14.2 GENERAL GUIDELINES

The following general guidelines are recommended for tailoring cancer treatment methods to the needs of the elderly population:

1. *Recognize that the older cancer population is diverse.* The first general principle is an intellectual step, involving integration, in the treatment plan, of the fact that there is diversity in the elderly population. Whereas young adults can be expected as a rule to be in good general condition apart from their cancer, this is not true of older patients. This does not mean, however, that all older patients are frail [1]. One can be 77 and in solid physical condition, like space-shuttling Senator John Glenn, or one can be 77, and going to the bathroom may feel akin to a space expedition. Although the prevalence of frailty increases with age, still only a third or less of the nonagenarians are frail [1]. In determining the risk of individual severe side effects from chemotherapy, the older patients' variability in health status weighs 2–3 times as much as the variability in the toxicity of the chemotherapy regimens [2].

2. *Do not think age, think life expectancy.* As a consequence of variable health and functional condition, older patients of a same age can have very variable life expectancies. An 85-year-old man in the top quartile of life expectancy in the United States has a life expectancy of 7.9 years, which is more than triple the life expectancy

Cancer and Aging Handbook: Research and Practice, First Edition. Edited by Keith M. Bellizzi and Margot A. Gosney.
© 2012 Wiley-Blackwell. Published 2012 by John Wiley & Sons, Inc.

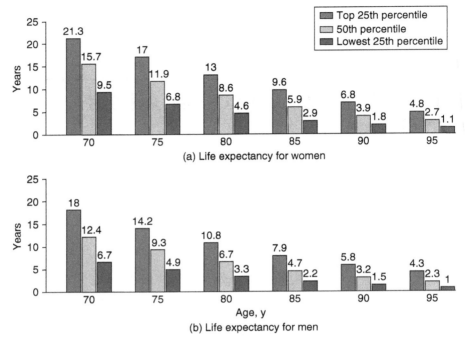

Figure 14.1 Life expectancies for women (a) and men (b) in the United States. (Adapted from Walter and Covinsky [3], with permission.)

of a man of similar age in the bottom quartile (2.2 years), and also more than a 70-year-old man in the bottom quartile (6.7 years) [3] (Fig. 14.1). This is a major argument for the proper integration of a thorough assessment of comorbidity, functionality, and general functional reserve with a comprehensive geriatric assessment (CGA) as part of optimal care of the older patient. Life expectancy considerations are especially critical in the adjuvant setting for early-stage cancers. Figure 14.2 shows examples of 5-year survival of various diseases compared to cancer.

3. *Quantify and time the treatment benefits and risks.* Proper quantification of the benefits is crucial in older patients. In younger patients, benefits usually can be directly transferred from clinical trials to the patient. In older patients, such endeavors can be more difficult. Older patients are underrepresented in clinical trials [4]. The median age of the patients enrolled in large studies is often several years below the median age at which the cancer occurs in the general population. Physicians often assume some generally discounted benefit in older patients. However, the data are much more heterogeneous. Sometimes the side effects of the treatment and the related early mortality and dose reductions cancel the benefit observed in younger patients. Such is the case, for example, for high-dose AraC consolidation in AML, or possibly adding bevacizumab to carboplatin and paclitaxel in older patients with non–small cell lung cancer [5,6]. In other cases, the effectiveness and side effects are stable as age advances, for example, for adjuvant 5-Fluorouracil (5FU)-based chemotherapy in stage III colon cancer (at least until the age of 80) [7]. In other cases, the treatment might offer greater proportional benefit in older patients than in younger ones. Adding rituximab to CHOP chemotherapy led to a greater improvement in the survival of diffuse large B cell

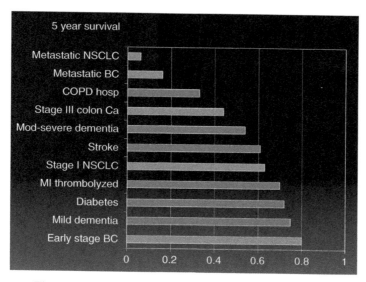

Figure 14.2   Rates of 5-year survival for various diseases.

lymphoma patients in older patients than younger ones [8]. Finally, there may be a divergence of benefits in older patients. For example, for older women with hormone-receptor-positive breast cancer, the impact of adjuvant chemotherapy and hormonal therapy on disease-free survival is weakly affected by age and comorbidity, whereas the survival benefit becomes seriously curtailed by competing mortality [9]. The latter observation leads us to an important point that is rarely emphasized in younger patients: the timing of maximum expected benefit. In patients with metastatic disease, the question is usually straightforward; the expected benefits are immediate (e.g., symptom control, tumor shrinkage), and so are the side effects of treatment. In the adjuvant setting, the question is more prominent, as the goal of an immediate treatment is to prevent an eventual relapse years later. An example is the use of adjuvant chemotherapy in early-stage breast cancer. As noted above, the incremental benefit on survival diverges from that on disease-free survival as life expectancy decreases for women with hormone-receptor-positive breast cancer. This is due to the fact that the relapse rate is relatively constant over time, and that several lines of hormone therapy and chemotherapies are available even after relapse, allowing for years of survival with the disease. In contrast, for hormone-receptor-negative breast cancer, the maximum mortality risk is in the first 3–4 years after the initial diagnosis and the risk tapers afterward [10] (Fig. 14.3). Therefore, for a similar incremental benefit to studies of young patients, an older woman with a limited life expectancy will be more likely to experience a survival benefit of adjuvant chemotherapy if she has a hormone-receptor-negative than a positive breast cancer. Similarly, as most colon cancers relapse within the first 5 years after surgery, the benefit of chemotherapy can be expected to be preserved for most patients with a (remaining) life expectancy of >5 years. On the other hand, in a slowly evolving disease such as a low-risk chronic lymphocytic leukemia, it is highly unlikely that an aggressive chemotherapy such as FCR will produce any survival benefit over a less intensive one, but a resultant secondary thrombocytopenia might affect the patient for years.

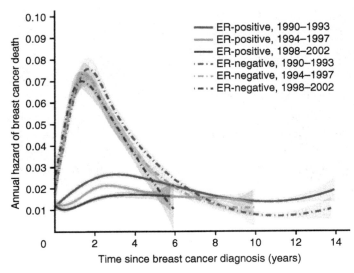

Figure 14.3 Annual death rate from breast cancer by receptor status. (Reproduced from Jatoi et al. [10], with permission.)

4. *Prevent the need for emergency interventions.* One key characteristic of aging is a decrease in functional reserve, and this decrease varies from organ to organ (for a review, see Ref. 11). Interestingly, the baseline organ function is usually very well maintained. As a result, elective surgical procedures, for example, carry little more risk of complications and mortality than younger patients with similar conditions. Conversely, emergency surgery is associated with much more morbidity and mortality in elderly people [12,13]. This topic is addressed in more detail in Chapter 15. Therefore, when building a treatment plan, two things should be considered. In an elective setting, one should ask: If I do not treat now, what are the chances that an emergency need for intervention might arise in the future? (This question might arise in a decision about resecting a colon cancer in a patient with comorbidities.) In an emergency setting, the question becomes: Can I control the situation and improve the patient status before performing a specific oncology intervention? For example, one might choose to stent an obstructing sigmoid lesion, or delay chemotherapy for a high-grade lymphoma until a pneumonia is resolved. In contrast, an AML patient might need to start chemotherapy immediately despite having pneumonia. Every effort should be made to prevent the need for emergency action in older cancer patients. This includes a proactive supportive care approach during treatment as detailed below.

5. *Use models to be objective.* The prediction of treatment outcome in a situation where multidimensional variables occur as with the older patient is difficult. Trained oncologists have difficulty integrating in their treatment plan more than three variables at one time [14]. Our interpretation of the patient's desires might be biased by cultural expectations [15,16], and our reading of the literature is selective because of time constraints. Therefore, good quality decision models based on systematic reviews of available data are very precious. Such models exist, for example, for the adjuvant treatment of breast, colon, and lung cancer (see www.adjuvantonline.com) or for initial treatment of prostate cancer [17]. These strategies allow an objective quantification of

benefits that can be weighed against potential risks in the individual discussion with the patient. As there will never be therapeutic studies focusing only on—say—older women with lung cancer, diabetes, and coronary artery disease, there is a clear need for more such models in geriatric oncology.

6. *Always calculate creatinine clearance*. As a result of progressive nephron loss, the creatinine clearance rate decreases with age. As older patients also have a large variation in body size and composition, a serum creatinine within the normal range established for young patients offers a decreasing reflection of actual kidney function. In fact, most 85-year-old patients with a normal serum creatinine have a stage III or higher renal insufficiency [18]. Therefore, it is very important to calculate the creatinine clearance of older patients. Several formulas are available. There is some divergence in the reporting of their accuracy. In general, the Cockroft–Gault formula tends to underestimate a little the clearance, whereas the modification of diet in renal disease (MDRD) formula tends to overestimate it [19]. Adjusting for body surface area does not significantly modify the performance of these indices. It should be noted that the Cockroft–Gault formula is the only one that has been validated for adjustment of chemotherapy dosages.

7. *Beware of drug interactions*. Older patients take multiple medications [18]. The number is steadily rising from an average of four in the mid-1990s, to six a decade later [20,21]. This presents significant risks for interaction of existing drugs with chemotherapy. Chemotherapy drugs can alter the effect of noncancer drugs; the best known effect is probably the interaction between 5FU and oxaliplatin with anticoagulation. However, the reverse is also true. Patients experiencing drug interactions level 1 according to Drug Interaction Facts software were twice as likely to have severe toxicities from their chemotherapy, and 3 times more likely if the interaction directly involved one of the chemotherapy agents [22]. Therefore a careful review of the list of a patient's medications, including over-the-counter ones, CAM, and nutriceuticals, is necessary prior to initiating oncologic treatment. Every effort should be made to pare down the list, or choose alternate medications with less interactions. If a drug needs to be maintained, adequate mitigating procedures should be taken (e.g., weekly testing of INR for patient on FOLFOX and warfarin). The need for medications should be regularly reassessed during chemotherapy. Modification of antihypertensive or antidiabetic treatments are frequently needed, due to weight loss, lack of appetite, steroid use, and other factors.

14.3   THE TWO-STEP APPROACH

As a general approach to the treatment of older cancer patients, we suggest a two-step process in daily oncology practice, illustrated in Figure 14.4.

Several short screening instruments are available with some validation in geriatric oncology, such as the Senior Adult Oncology Program 2 (SAOP2) questionnaire, the VES13, the Triage Risk Screening Tool, the G8, and the Groningen Frailty Index. Their sensitivity varies, so their use should be associated with further testing [23]. In our 7 years of clinical experience with the SAOP2 screening questionnaire, about half of our new patients will screen negative, and half will require a team assessment [24]. In practice, the diagnostic, staging, and treatment planning procedures often take a couple of weeks to assess. This provides ample time to refer the patient for a geriatric

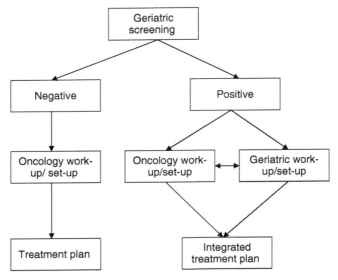

Figure 14.4   General approach to treatment planning in an older cancer patient.

consultation, or for a multidisciplinary team evaluation. Then with both evaluations, an integrated treatment plan can be developed.

14.4   PROACTIVE SUPPORTIVE CARE

In the experience of the author, this is the most critical key to treatment success in older patients. The key role of baseline assessment is to prevent complications and their associated risk of deconditioning. Careful follow-up should aim at detecting problems early and correcting them aggressively. In a pilot series of older breast cancer patients, the mean number of unaddressed/underaddressed problems was six, with three more developing over 6 months. Complications such as postoperative delirium are associated with an increased risk of institutionalization, functional dependence, and mortality after hospital discharge [25,26]. Level I evidence interventions are available to reduce the risk of delirium in hospitalized elderly people [27,28]. The use of predictive models for toxicity from chemotherapy and prophylactic growth factors and other supportive measures upfront can noticeably reduce the risk of severe complications. One should be aware that half of the serious toxicities from chemotherapy occur in the first cycle of treatment [2,29].

14.5   CONCLUSIONS

The use of the basic principles outlined in Section 14.2 and the approaches discussed in Sections 14.3 and 14.4 should go a long way in providing the general oncologist with better tools to handle the treatment of older cancer patients, which represents a rapidly growing proportion of everybody's practice. More specialized aspects can be found in the following disease-specific chapters.

REFERENCES

1. Fried LP, Tangen CM, Walston J, et al. Frailty in older adults: Evidence for a phenotype. *J Gerontol A Biol Sci Med Sci* 2001;**56**:M146–M156.

2. Extermann M, Boler I, Reich R, Lyman GH, Brown RH, DeFelice J, Levine RM, Lubiner ET, Reyes P, Schreiber FJ, Balducci L. Predicting the risk of administering chemotherapy in older patients. The CRASH score (Chemotherapy Risk Assessment Scale for High-age patients): *Cancer* 2011. [Epub ahead of print]

3. Walter LC, Covinsky KE. Cancer screening in elderly patients: A framework for individualized decision making. *JAMA* 2001;**285**:2750–2756.

4. Hutchins LF, Unger JM, Crowley JJ, et al. Underrepresentation of patients 65 years of age or older in cancer-treatment trials. *N Engl J Med* 1999;**341**:2061–2067.

5. Mayer RJ, Davis RB, Schiffer CA, et al. Intensive postremission chemotherapy in adults with acute myeloid leukemia. Cancer and Leukemia Group B. *N Engl J Med* 1994; **331**:896–903.

6. Ramalingam SS, Dahlberg SE, Langer CJ, et al. Outcomes for elderly, advanced- stage non small-cell lung cancer patients treated with bevacizumab in combination with carboplatin and paclitaxel: Analysis of Eastern Cooperative Oncology Group Trial 4599. *J Clin Oncol* 2008;**26**:60–65.

7. Sargent DJ, Goldberg RM, Jacobson SD, et al. A pooled analysis of adjuvant chemotherapy for resected colon cancer in elderly patients. *N Engl J Med* 2001;**345**:1091–1097.

8. Sehn LH, Donaldson J, Chhanabhai M, et al. Introduction of combined CHOP plus rituximab therapy dramatically improved outcome of diffuse large B-cell lymphoma in British Columbia. *J Clin Oncol* 2005;**23**:5027–5033.

9. Extermann M, Balducci L, Lyman GH. What threshold for adjuvant therapy in older breast cancer patients? *J Clin Oncol* 2000;**18**:1709–1717.

10. Jatoi I, Chen BE, Anderson WF, et al. Breast cancer mortality trends in the United States according to estrogen receptor status and age at diagnosis. *J Clin Oncol* 2007;**25**: 1683–1690.

11. Kevorkian R. Physiology of aging. In Pathy M, Sinclair, AJ, Morley JE, eds. *Principles and Practice of Geriatric Medicine*, 4th ed., Wiley, Hoboken, NJ, 2006, pp. 37–46.

12. Keller SM, Markovitz LJ, Wilder JR, et al. Emergency and elective surgery in patients over age 70. *Am Surg* 1987;**53**:636–640.

13. Faiz O, Haji A, Bottle A, et al. Elective colonic surgery for cancer in the elderly: An investigation into postoperative mortality in English NHS hospitals between 1996 and 2007. *Colorect Dis* 2011;**13**(7):779–785.

14. Loprinzi CL, Ravdin PM, de Laurentiis M, et al. Do American oncologists know how to use prognostic variables for patients with newly diagnosed primary breast cancer? *J Clin Oncol* 1994;**12**:1422–1426.

15. Slevin ML, Stubbs L, Plant HJ, et al. Attitudes to chemotherapy: Comparing views of patients with cancer with those of doctors, nurses, and general public. *Br Med J* 1990;**300**: 1458–1460.

16. Extermann M, Albrand G, Chen H, et al. Are older French patients as willing as older American patients to undertake chemotherapy? *J Clin Oncol* 2003;**21**:3214–3219.

17. Alibhai SM, Naglie G, Nam R, et al. Do older men benefit from curative therapy of localized prostate cancer? *J Clin Oncol* 2003;**21**:3318–3327.

18. Giannelli SV, Patel KV, Windham BG, et al. Magnitude of underascertainment of impaired kidney function in older adults with normal serum creatinine. *J Am Geriatr Soc* 2007;**55**:816–823.

19. Lamb EJ, Webb MC, Simpson DE, et al. Estimation of glomerular filtration rate in older patients with chronic renal insufficiency: Is the modification of diet in renal disease formula an improvement? *J Am Geriatr Soc* 2003;**51**:1012–1017.

20. Corcoran ME: Polypharmacy in the older patient with cancer. *Cancer Control* 1997;**4**: 419–428.

21. Popa M, Wallace, K, Brunello, A, Extermann, M. The impact of polypharmacy on toxicity from chemotherapy in elderly patients: Focus on cytochrome P-450 inhibition and protein binding effects. *Proc Am Soc Clin Oncol* 2008;**26**:503s.

22. Extermann M, Druta M, Wallace K, Brunello A, Balducci L. *Drug Interactions Assessed with Drug Interaction Facts™ Are Associated with Increased Risk of Chemotoxicity in Older Cancer Patients Receiving Chemotherapy*, American Association of Cancer Research, Denver, CO, 2009, Abstract 5450.

23. Extermann M. Evaluation of the senior cancer patient: Comprehensive geriatric assessment and screening tools for the elderly. In Schrijvers D, Aapro M, Zakotnik B, Audisio R, van Halteren H, Hurria A, eds. *Handbook of Cancer in the Senior Patient*, Informa Healthcare, New York/London, 2010, pp. 13–21.

24. Johnson D, Blair, J, Balducci, L, Extermann, M, Crocker, T, McGinnis M, Vranas P. The assessment of clinical resources in a senior adult oncology program, *Proc. Eur. Oncology Nursing Soc. Meeting*, Innsbruck, Austria, 2006.

25. McCusker J, Cole M, Abrahamowicz M, et al. Delirium predicts 12-month mortality. *Arch Intern Med* 2002;**162**:457–463.

26. McCusker J, Cole M, Dendukuri N, et al. Delirium in older medical inpatients and subsequent cognitive and functional status: A prospective study. *Can Med Assoc J* 2001;**165**: 575–583.

27. Inouye SK, Bogardus ST Jr., Charpentier PA, et al. A multicomponent intervention to prevent delirium in hospitalized older patients. *N Engl J Med* 1999;**340**:669–670.

28. Vidan MT, Sanchez E, Alonso M, et al. An intervention integrated into daily clinical practice reduces the incidence of delirium during hospitalization in elderly patients. *J Am Geriatr Soc* 2009;**57**:2029–2036.

29. Crawford J, Dale DC, Kuderer NM, et al. Risk and timing of neutropenic events in adult cancer patients receiving chemotherapy: The results of a prospective nationwide study of oncology practice. *J Natl Comprehen Cancer Netw* 2008;**6**:109–118.

CHAPTER 15

Surgery for Older Adults with Cancer

LYNDA WYLD and MALCOLM WALTER RONALD REED

Department of Oncology, The University of Sheffield, Royal Hallamshire Hospital, Glossop, UK

THOMPSON GORDON ROBINSON

University Hospitals of Leicester NHS Trust, Leicester, UK

15.1 INTRODUCTION

Surgery is the mainstay of treatment for the majority of human solid tumors, including breast, colorectal, gastric, oesophageal, prostate, gynecological, and lung cancers. The majority of cancers develop in the older population, with 64% of cancers being diagnosed in those >65 (CRUK website), where the incidence of cancers is 11-fold greater than in younger patients [1]. For example, one-third of all breast cancers occur in those >70, 70% of colorectal cancers occur in people >65 [2] and 60% of lung cancers in those age >70. Therefore the majority of cancer surgery is performed on older individuals. While surgery for many of these cancers is well tolerated, the risks of morbidity and mortality are higher in almost every cancer site, and accordingly there is widespread evidence that practice varies with age. Evidence of omission of surgery altogether in older people with these cancers is widespread in the literature [3–5], although the more recent trend has been for this effect to decrease [6].

Surgeons are increasingly willing to offer surgery to older and more frail individuals optimizing pre-, peri-, and postoperative surgical care to improve outcomes [4]. The underlying cause of this is multifactorial and includes improved preoperative preparation, improved anesthesia, improved surgery (including minimally invasive surgery), and better aftercare. In addition, the life expectancy of the UK population has increased dramatically from 60 years in the 1960s to the mid-80s at the present time, and it is predicted that it will continue to rise in the next 30 years [7,8]. This has been associated with improved performance status in older patients at a given age, so what may have been viewed as high risk in the 1970s in a 75-year-old may now be seen as routine practice, for example, liver resection for secondary colorectal carcinoma.

It is becoming accepted that older age is not a barrier to effective treatment but rather a challenge to be met. This has still not translated into high-quality research evidence in many disease sites [9], so there is still much progress to be made.

Cancer and Aging Handbook: Research and Practice, First Edition. Edited by Keith M. Bellizzi and Margot A. Gosney.
© 2012 Wiley-Blackwell. Published 2012 by John Wiley & Sons, Inc.

This chapter reviews the variance of surgical practice and outcomes in older cancer patients with common cancers (colorectal, gastric, lung, breast, and prostate) and then discusses some of the factors that have supported progress in these fields.

15.2   DISEASE-SITE-SPECIFIC VARIANCE IN SURGICAL PRACTICE WITH OLDER AGE

Colorectal Cancer   Colorectal cancer is very much a disease of older people with 70% of cases occurring in individuals age >65 [2] and 30–40% in those >75 [2]. Surgery is the only means of curative treatment, and because of the nature of colorectal surgery, which breaches a major body cavity and often necessitates prolonged general anesthesia, surgery is associated with significant morbidity and mortality. The rates of both death and serious morbidity are increased in older individuals. The 30-day mortality rate is 6 times greater in >85 compared to the 75–84-year age group and almost 3 times higher in the >75 versus the <75 groups [10]. The more complex rectal procedures, such as low anterior resection and abdominoperineal resection, both requiring careful dissection of the mesorectum from the pelvis and increasingly undertaken after radiotherapy, have a higher morbidity in the older age group [10]. Not surprisingly, therefore, a 2007 UK audit of colorectal cancer patients showed significantly increased rates of Hartmann's procedure, colonic stenting, and formation of dysfunctioning and permanent stomas, all of which are quicker, simpler, and less morbid procedures in patients >75 years [10]. Unfortunately, although patients are more likely to survive these interventions, they may have sub-optimal long-term outcomes. Overall, while curative resection is performed in 75% of patients between ages 65 and 74, only 67% of patients over age 85 [11] undergo curative resection, and the rate of nonsurgical treatment in this age group is 3.5 times greater. One reason for this is that older patients are more likely to present as an emergency [11], although more advanced disease (nodal or liver metastases and high-grade disease) is more common in younger patients [12].

However, mortality rates in older patients undergoing elective colorectal resection have fallen from over 8% to 5% between 2000 and 2005 [10], due, in part, to better preoperative preparation and patient selection. In addition, screening in a younger age group has been introduced, and this may impact positively on the percentage of cases presenting with obstruction or perforation, both of which have higher morbidity and mortality rates. Laparoscopic colorectal surgery is also becoming increasingly practiced and may also impact on morbidity and mortality rates (see text below). Outcomes may therefore continue to improve.

Gastric Cancer   Gastric cancer is a disease that predominantly affects the older population, with 66% occurring in the >70 and 32% in the >80 groups [13]. As with colorectal cancer, definitive treatment is surgery in the form of partial or total gastrectomy or esophagogastrectomy for lesions at the gastroesophageal junction. This type of surgery involves breaching one or sometimes two body cavities, a lengthy general anesthetic and an upper abdominal or abdominothoracic incision, which are painful and can compromise mobility and lung function postoperatively. Preoperative nutritional status is often compromised, and this may contribute to morbidity. Consequently, this type of surgery in older patients may be associated with significant mortality and morbidity and may be less well tolerated. There is a fourfold increase in 30-day mortality between the >70 (8.6%) and the <50 groups, (2.1%) [14], although other series have shown lesser degrees of difference, for example, a 30-day mortality of 3% in patients both <75 and >75 in a series from Italy, although 7% of frailer older subjects were excluded from surgery altogether [15]. Mortality rates have reduced dramatically in all age groups, but especially the elderly. A large French study showed mortality rates of 8 versus 26% in the <70 versus the >70 groups during 1976–1983, falling to 3.5 and 10% during 1984–1995 [16], with further improvements since then [17]. Morbidity rates are also affected by age, increasing in older subjects (23 vs. 29%, in <75 or >75 groups [15] and 19.2 vs. 23.8, in <70 or >70 groups [18], although this may reflect increasing levels of comorbid disease rather than age per se [15,18].

Review of data from over 30 years ago (as of early 2012) shows that in the UK only 20% of patients over 80 years received any form of surgery and most received no treatment at all [19]. In contrast, more recent audits now show 57% of the >80 group undergoing potentially curative resection compared with 71% of those <80. Although advanced disease stage was the most common reason for excluding patients from surgery, 30 patients were excluded for reasons of age in the </>80 age groups [20]. There is no doubt that this percentage has dropped significantly since the 1960s [6,17] with the average age of surgically treated patients rising and patients with advanced age being offered surgery. This may reflect increasing confidence in outcomes as mortality rates in this series dropped from 6% to <0.7% despite the increased age of the patients [6].

Non–Small Cell Lung Cancer   Lung cancer is also a disease predominantly affecting older people with 60% occurring in the >70 and 25% in the >80 groups [21]. Once again, for the majority of cases, surgery is the only chance of cure for those who present with operable disease. This inevitably involves breaching the thoracic cavity, which is associated with a significant risk of morbidity and mortality. This is due to damage to the respiratory musculature, reduction of remaining lung capacity, postoperative pain, and a range of other surgical and anesthetic complications [22]. Added to this, elderly people have reduced lung capacity [FEV_1 (forced expiratory volume) falls year on year after 35 years of age], and because the majority of lung cancers are caused by cigarette smoking, there is a high prevalence of chronic obstructive pulmonary disease in these patients, which compromises their tolerance to surgery and increases the risks of postoperative complications. Older patients with lung cancer are more likely to have chronic obstructive pulmonary disease (COPD) than younger lung cancer patients (19% of <65 vs. 30% of >65 groups [23]), further increasing the risks. Consequently, the risk of 30-day mortality for open or thoracoscopic surgery is strongly influenced by age (3.5% at <65 years, 7.3% at >70 and 8.1% at >80 [24] and 4 vs. 1% mortality for </>75 [25]). However, in the 1990s, video-assisted thoracosopic surgery (VATS) was introduced, enabling lobectomy and wedge resection with several 2-cm incisions compared to the typical single 20–25-cm incision. This type of surgery is thought to be oncologically safe and is associated with reduced postoperative pain, earlier discharge, and reduced morbidity rates [25]. It is safe and gives good results in older patients [26–27]. Indeed, there is evidence that it may be associated with lower morbidity and mortality in older patients. Berry and colleagues found 30-day morbidity and mortality reduced in thoracoscopic rather than open lobectomy patients over the age of 75 years (8% vs. 4.3% mortality and 68% vs. 52% morbidity) [25].

As with many other cancer sites, there has been a trend for increasing rates of surgery in older patients. The same is true for lung cancer patients with a rising percentage of those >70 undergoing surgery [28].

Breast Cancer Breast cancer is again a disease with a high incidence in older women, with a third of all cases occurring in women over 70 [29]. The mainstay of curative therapy is surgery, in the form of either mastectomy or lumpectomy. Some form of axillary surgery is also performed, either a staging procedure such as sentinel lymph node biopsy (SLNB) to sample a percentage of lymph nodes with removal of all axillary nodes performed if there are proven metastases. Despite the psychological impact of mastectomy, it is body surface surgery, breaching no major body cavity, and is therefore generally well tolerated. In some cases it may be performed under local or regional anesthesia. The mortality is therefore very low, and it is impossible to determine whether current mortality rates following breast cancer surgery are higher in older women, as most recent audits show overall mortality rates of 0–0.2% and are therefore too low to derive meaningful statistical analyses of the impact of age [30–32]. The morbidity associated with breast cancer surgery includes not only the physical adverse event (hematoma, wound infection, flap necrosis, and lymphedema), which are variably affected by age, being generally increased [32–34], but also the psychological effects of loss of a breast.

In contrast to many of the other common cancers, there is an alternative to surgery for frail older women. The majority of breast cancers in older women are sensitive to estrogen [35] and may be controlled, at least in the short to medium term, by antiestrogens such as tamoxifen. This is referred to as *primary endocrine therapy* and gives equivalent survival but reduced rates of local disease control when compared to surgery and adjuvant endocrine therapy [36] and is used in ≤40% of women over age 70 in the UK [3,4,37,38], representing a much higher proportion than in other European countries. As disease control may be lost after a few years, patients treated with Primary endocrine therapy (PET) should have a predicted life expectancy of <5 years. As a consequence of the option of PET, despite the low risks of breast cancer surgery, rates of nonsurgical treatment remain high in the UK [39]. The rate of nonsurgical treatment is variable between clinicians and UK health regions, however, which raises concerns that some women may be selected inappropriately, and thus possibly under- or overtreated. This may be a factor contributing to inferior disease outcomes in the UK compared to European averages [40].

Prostate Cancer Prostate cancer is again more common with increasing age, with 56% occurring in men >70 years and 19% in those over 80 [41]. The incidence has risen substantially since the 1970s with the increasing use and availability of prostate-specific antigen (PSA) screening. The mortality has fallen over the same period, although some of this fall may reflects the fact that some of the PSA-detected cancers might never have become symptomatic during the patient's lifetime. Unlike most of the cancers discussed so far, there are a range of options available to treat prostate cancer with good effect. The simplest, for low-risk cancer in older subjects, is surveillance only plus or minus endocrine manipulation. This tends to be reserved for subjects with a predicted life expectancy of <10 years (usually taken as age 80), although some would suggest that outcomes may be better in selected older men with more definitive therapy [42] and others, that selection is not stringent enough [43].

For example, in a series of 13,154 cases of radical prostatectomy at the Mayo clinic (USA), only 19 were over age 80 (0.14%) [44]. For higher-risk disease, radical prostatectomy and/or radiotherapy (external beam with or without brachytherapy) may be used. In terms of cancer outcomes, there is little to choose between these two options (although there have been few good-quality RCTs, and cohort studies rarely control adequately for selection bias), but the long-term side effects may be slightly worse with radiotherapy; the short-term, worse with surgery [45]. These effective nonsurgical options mean that frailer older subjects may be spared the significant risks of radical prostatectomy. Further discussion will focus on surgery and how this is influenced by age.

Radical retropubic prostatectomy, for the reasons outlined above, is not routinely performed on the oldest elderly (85+) and very infrequently in those over 80. Most studies therefore report outcomes based on comparison between males <70 and *largely healthy* males over age 70. Mortality rates in reported series are therefore low, as unfit or frail older males are not routinely offered surgery. The 30-day mortality is low, usually <1% in modern series [45–47], but is affected by age (0.18% in 50–59-year-olds vs. 0.59% in 70–79-year-olds) [47]. Similarly, morbidity is linked to age, being highest in older males [46].

In terms of trends, rates of surgery have varied with time: highest in the early 1990s but falling steadily in older males as radiotherapy techniques were found to be efficacious. A significant contribution to the fall in mortality in this period is thought to be due to the use of radiotherapy in subjects with significant comorbidity [48]. The International Society for Geriatric Oncology (SIOG) has published guidelines to aid clinicians in deciding how to select men for each of these treatment modalities on the basis of age and fitness.

Since 2000, laparoscopic and robotic prostatectomy have been the focus of much interest and do seem to offer improvements in volume of blood loss, duration of inpatient stay, and morbidity [49]. Use in men over 70 is feasible [50], but there is little published evidence on whether it is beneficial in older males compared to nonsurgical therapies or open surgery.

15.3 ADVANCES IN SURGICAL PRACTICE

As can be seen for most of the surgical cancer sites listed above (and many others), there are strong trends for increasing use of potentially curative surgery and significant improvements in outcomes among older patients [6,15,18]. This reflects improvements in a wide range of surgical and related areas:

1. Surgical techniques
    a. Minimally invasive techniques
    b. Centralization of surgery in specialized units
    c. Reduced intraoperative blood loss
    d. Alternative procedures (SLNB and wide local excision in breast cancer, colonic and esophageal stents, radiotherapy in prostate cancer).
2. Improvements in pre- and postoperative support
    a. Pre- and postoperative nutritional support and optimization
    b. Chronic disease optimization

3. Improved anesthetic techniques
   a. Routine use of epidurals and spinal anesthesia
   b. Increased understanding of the pharmacology of drugs in the elderly population
   c. New anesthetic drugs and techniques
4. Improved aftercare and rehabilitation
5. Improvements (age for age) in the general level of fitness of the older population compared to the 1970s
6. Availability of effective, nonsurgical therapies, (radiotherapy and hormonal therapy for prostate cancer and hormonal therapy for breast cancer) for higher-risk surgical patients

These issues are discussed in detail below.

15.3.1   Improvements in Surgical Techniques

Minimally Invasive Surgery   In the late 1980s and early 1990s, surgical practice was first introduced to the concept of minimally invasive surgery by means of laparoscopy. Over the ensuing 20 years the range of procedures that can now be accomplished laparoscopically has expanded significantly and includes many cancer operations. These include VATS, wedge excision lobectomy, pneumonectomy, laparoscopically assisted colonic and rectal resections, gastric [51] and esophageal surgery, and radical prostatectomy (among others). It is now well established that the morbidity–mortality of laparoscopic procedures is lower than the corresponding open procedure in most cases, due to reduced postoperative pain [55], lower rates of pulmonary [56] and thrombotic complications, and reduced surgical metabolic stress. Time to discharge is also reduced [55–57] and quality of life enhanced [58]. While there remain concerns about the increased time to undertake these procedures and increased operative costs [57], increased surgical skill, training, and equipment now mean that in many cases surgeries take less time. Elderly people may benefit from these techniques, and much research has focused on this aspect more recently. A study series in Japan found no significant difference in outcome between patients <70 or >70 undergoing laparoscopically assisted gastrectomy [59]. The MRC CLASICC trial of open versus laparoscopic colorectal cancer surgery found no difference in outcome between patients over and under age 70 [60].

Centralization of Surgery in Specialized Units   Because of the complex and demanding nature of many cancer operations, outcomes may be improved by undertaking such surgery in specialist units with high surgeon case numbers [52]. This has been found to be the case with a range of cancer procedures (gastrectomy [14], hepatectomy, pancreatectomy [61], and pneumonectomy [62] as well as many others). Accordingly, in the UK, United States, and Europe there has been a move to centralize the care of such cancers in high-volume units.

Reduced Intraoperative Blood Loss   Prior to the 1980s most surgical procedures were undertaken with sharp, or scalpel-based, dissections. Over the years, intraoperative bleeding rates and consequently transfusion rates have been reduced by a number of technical improvements in surgery, including the use of diathermy dissection, use of argon beam and harmonic scalpels, diathermy scissors, and laparoscopic instruments that coagulate vessels as they cut them. In addition there is improved understanding of coagulopathy and enhanced availability of specialist blood products to reverse bleeding disorders. Finally, there are now a range of products that promote coagulation in operative sites. As a result, the use of blood products and intraoperative and postoperative blood loss rates have steadily fallen, reducing morbidity and mortality rates globally. This enhanced control of intra/postoperative bleeding is beneficial to older subjects who have reduced cardiac reserve, which may compromise their tolerance of hypovolemia and anemia.

Alternative Procedures   In several types of cancer, surgical morbidity has been reduced by changes in practice as it has been realized that less morbid procedures may give equivalent oncological outcomes to more traditional techniques. Examples include the increasing use of wide local excision (plus radiotherapy) in breast cancer and the realization that axillary lymph node clearance is not necessary for disease control in all women with breast cancer but can be safely substituted by SLNB or limited sampling in those with uninvolved axillas. This is associated with lower morbidity rates (particularly lymphedema) in breast cancer patients [63]. In lung cancer there is a trend toward wedge resection for small lesions, which is associated with a reduced morbidity when compared to lobectomy. In prostate cancer, the option of surveillance or radiotherapy is available instead of radical prostatectomy and in limb sarcomas, it is no longer felt necessary to amputate, as limb sparing surgery (plus or minus radiotherapy) is now known to be associated with equivalent disease control. The use of stents in colonic, esophageal, gastric, and pancreatic cancers may avoid the need for surgery altogether or permit disease and patient optimization (relief of obstruction, improved nutrition, enhanced operability with neoadjuvant chemotherapy) prior to subsequent surgical treatment.

15.3.2   Improvements in Preoperative Preparation

Pre- and Postoperative Nutritional Support and Optimization   Malnutrition is a common occurrence in patients with many forms of cancer; it is particularly prevalent in cancers of the gastrointestinal tract. Malnutrition is also more common in the older population and is a well recognized indicator of frailty. The causes in older patients are multifactorial and include depression, social isolation, immobility, anorexia, and chronic illness [64]: Older age is a risk factor for malnutrition in cancer patients, and $\leq 47\%$ of older patients with gastrointestinal cancers will manifest evidence of malnutrition [65,66].

The presence of preoperative malnutrition is a negative risk factor for both morbidity and mortality following surgery [67]. This fact is being increasingly recognized and addressed. Perioperative nutritional support has been shown to reduce both morbidity and mortality rates [68,69]. Awareness of the link between older age and nutrition is vital to ensure that this risk factor is adequately addressed.

Chronic Disease Optimization [53]   As previously discussed, the proportion of the United Kingdom's population over the age of 65 years continues to increase, with an estimated total remaining life expectancy of 11.6 and 17.2 years for males and females currently aged 65 years, respectively [70]. With increasing age comes an increased risk of comorbidity, and associated disability and functional dependency, such that disability-free remaining life expectancy is currently only 11.6 years for a male aged 65 years and 13.9 years for a female [70]. It is therefore important in the oncological management of an older patient that there be an assessment of the biological, not chronological, age. A geriatrician has expertise in the comprehensive assessment of the older person, including the diagnosis of specific morbidity associated with aging (the "geriatric giants"), which may have implications for the diagnosis and management of cancer [71]. For example, one in three individuals aged >70 years will fall each year, with 10% of falls resulting in injury and skeletal metastases increasing the risk of a pathological fracture with falling. A geriatric multidisciplinary team has expertise in identifying reversible causes and interventions to reduce falls and associated fractures. Furthermore, age-related impairment in vision and hearing may impact adversely on discussions to inform cancer treatment and compliance, as well as increasing the risk of postoperative delirium, which will be discussed later. However, common causes are often easily reversible: cataract extraction under local anesthetic and wax removal to treat the commonest cause of conductive hearing loss.

However, it is important that a comprehensive assessment does not focus solely on comorbidity, but also on function in personal and extended activities of daily living, cognition, depression, and nutrition. All these factors are more likely to influence outcomes, including mortality, length of hospital stay, institutionalization, and hospital readmission, than age per se in a hospital-based general medical population aged ≥60 years [72]. There are specific examples of interventions based on comprehensive geriatric assessment that produced positive benefits on cancer outcome. Extermann and colleagues assessed the prevalence of geriatric problems amenable to intervention in a small study of older breast cancer patients, reporting a significant number of multidisciplinary team interventions, with positive influence on treatment outcome and: compliance with treatment and qualification for inclusion in randomized controlled trials [73]. In a consecutive series of 250 older breast cancer patients, Stotter and colleagues reported that the use of a comprehensive geriatric assessment to identify and treat reversible causes of comorbidity, functional dependence, and cognitive impairment could be used to predict life expectancy and tailor best treatment; patients who are fit for the best surgical treatment are more likely to survive for 2 years [74].

Assessment of Fitness for Surgery   While rates of surgery for most cancer types have increased, there are still variable proportions of patients who are offered nonsurgical therapy because of concerns about their level of fitness to withstand surgery; this is an area of surgical practice where research is needed to provide guidance. It is no longer appropriate to simply use arbitrary age cutoffs because, as the life expectancy and level of fitness of older people increases, the age cutoff will continually move upward. Assessment needs to be based on evidence-based indicators of frailty and poor-health. A number of generic and disease-specific tools have been developed to help with such decisions, but few have been rigorously tested in trials [75]. These are reviewed in Table 15.1.

15.3.3 Improved Anesthetic Techniques

Routine Use of Epidurals and Regional and Local Blocks   Regional blocks may be used in place of, or as a supplement to, general anesthesia and may improve surgical outcome. For example, use of peri- and intraoperative epidural anesthetic infusions as

TABLE 15.1   Summary of Comorbidity Indices for Outcome Prediction

Index	Factors Assessed	Evaluation	Reference
Charlson index	Weighted index of number and severity of defined comorbid diseases	Predicts 1-year mortality in women with breast cancer with moderate accuracy; disease spectrum assessed is limited, and disease interactions cannot be accounted for	26
Satariano–Ragland	Weighted index of 7 comorbid diseases, (myocardial infarction, heart disease, other cancer, respiratory, gallbladder, and liver problems)	Validated predictor of 3-year survival for women with breast cancer aged 40–84 years; limited by small number of conditions assessed but is simple and easy to administer	20
Comprehensive prognostic index	Assesses age, stage of cancer, and comorbid disease	Broader range of comorbidities, enabling interactions between diseases to be taken into account; can be used to predict 1-year mortality	27
Comprehensive geriatric assessment (CGA)	Detailed assessment of comorbidity, functional status, cognitive function, and depression scores	Complex and time-consuming to administer, but may be at least as effective as the Karnofski performance status at outcome prediction, although further work is being done to establish its efficacy	28,29
Karnofski performance status	Widely used but crude scoring system of functional status in oncology patients of any age	Does correlate with mortality posttreatment for a variety of cancers and is easy to use; may be insensitive in the elderly where multiple comorbidities may be present and interact	29
ASA	Widely used but crude scoring system of comorbidity for patients of any age	Multiple comorbidities in the elderly diminish its sensitivity in groups 2 and 3; probably most widely used scoring system for preoperative risk assessment; not a cancer-specific tool.	
Functional status	Assessment of ADL and IADL	These measures of functional ability have been used to predict non-cancer-specific mortality with some success	30

well as providing significantly improved postoperative pain control and reduced overall mortality (reduced by one-third [76]) is associated with an approximate halving of the rates of postoperative myocardial infarction [77], postoperative pulmonary atelectasis and chest infections, and deep-vein thrombosis/pulmonary embolism (DVT/PE) [76]. Their use in older patients needs to be exercised with caution because of reduced cardiac reserve and increased incidence of atherosclerosis, which may reduce patients' tolerance of hypotension. Older patients may also have raised sensitivity to agents used, and doses may need to be reduced or shortacting agents used [78]. In some forms of cancer surgery, use of such regional blocks may obviate the need for general anesthesia altogether, which, for patients with significant pulmonary disease, may increase the feasibility of surgery. Good examples of this are in breast surgery, where mastectomy may be performed under local infiltration anesthesia [79], intercostal nerve block [80], paravertebral block [81], or a high thoracic epidural [82].

Increased Understanding of Pharmacology and Pharmacokinetics of Drugs in Elderly Individuals Older individuals not only have higher rates of comorbid disease that will interact with anesthesia and surgery but also undergo physiological senescence in most of their body systems. Consequently, their sensitivity to and ability to clear many drugs are altered significantly.

Furthermore, several significant co-morbidities are elevated, with angina rates increasing from 0.68% in 45–54-year-olds to almost 5% in those over 75 [83], with dementia increasing from <1% in 65–69-year-olds to 40% in those over 90 [84] and rates of arrhythmia quadrupling between ages 45 and 75 [85]. Physiological senescence causes reductions in cardiac, respiratory, and renal reserves [33] and reduced cognitive and motor function [84]. In addition, many older patients are already on regular medication, which may interact with anesthetic drugs.

As a consequence, dose reductions for certain anesthetic agents may be needed; for example, elderly people are much more sensitive to the effects of opiates than are younger patients, which increases the risk of short-term effects such as acute confusional (delirium) states and respiratory depression. It is well recognized that older people may suffer from delirium in the postoperative period. In some cases this is the result of acute hypoxia secondary to basal pulmonary collapse, chest infection, and the use of opiates suppressing respiration. Other common causes include wound, urinary tract, or pulmonary infections, or deranged fluid and acid–base balance. In older individuals, especially those with a basal degree of cognitive decline, removing them from their familiar home environment, with its social and functional clues, has a destabilizing effect that may be sufficient to cause what was thought to be someone with good cognitive function to become acutely confused.

For reasons that are not entirely clear, older people may also suffer prolonged postoperative cognitive dysfunction, which is linked with both age and duration of anesthesia and may affect >14% of those >70 years undergoing general anesthesia [86]. The precise etiology of this phenomenon is not clear but may relate to neurotoxic effects of certain anesthetic agents or their interaction with the CNS cholinergic system, which is linked to cognition [87].

New Anesthetic Drugs and Techniques Anesthesia is traditionally regarded as a low-risk process, with one death per 100,000 anesthetics [88]. However, this may be misleading, as most perioperative deaths occur sometime after surgery and mortality is diluted by the large number of simple operations on relatively fit people. There are patients with comorbidities requiring major surgery who have a very high risk of morbidity and mortality. Comorbidity and frailty tend to increase with age; therefore older patients need special individualized consideration. Aging impairs handling of drugs even in older people with few or no obvious comorbidities [89], and to complicate matters further, the drugs that they receive have often been tested on a population younger and with fewer comorbidities than the population who actually receive the drug in practice [90]. Although the inclusion of elderly subjects in clinical trials is becoming more widely accepted, the problem still exists in currently registered trials [91].

It does not suffice to just think about the intraoperative process. It is necessary to consider the whole perioperative package of preoperative care, preparation, intraoperative care, and postoperative care. Failure in any of these areas will adversely affect outcome, especially in the more frail patients undergoing the more invasive surgery. However, even in high-risk patients undergoing major surgery there are techniques that will reduce morbidity and mortality. These can include perioperative goal-directed therapy [92]. Unfortunately, preoperative optimization is sometimes misinterpreted as a reason for a prolonged delay before emergency surgery rather than the use of appropriate resuscitation, promptly followed by surgery to allow source control of sepsis, bleeding, or other acute problems to take place. Elective surgery should be thoroughly planned with a full discussion of the options available and with abnormalities corrected where possible well before surgery. This is especially relevant for older individuals, where the majority of cases will manifest an abnormality that should be investigated and optimized. Similarly, during the preoperative assessment the state of cognition should be assessed and other important factors, such as the presence of living wills, should be established. In cases of hip fracture, pre- or postoperative intervention recommended by dedicated geriatricians can reduce the incidence of postoperative delirium, clearly indicating the need for more organized perioperative ward care [93]. This is very important, because delirium not only complicates the delivery of many types of care but also may well indicate the presence of sepsis or other medical abnormalities.

Even in routine surgery, management of existing drug therapy has the potential to impact on the patient. Older patients often suffer the effects of halting their routine medication in the perioperative period, due to deliberate and sometimes inappropriate or unnecessarily early withdrawal (such as misinterpretation of preoperative starvation leading to a failure to take drugs on the day of surgery). For many drugs, this may be relatively unimportant because of their long half-lives or because of the nature of the treatment. However, this early withdrawal often equally applies to antiarrhythmic drugs or other key medication. After surgery postoperative ileus may be a problem, and in some cases an alternative is not readily available, but should be discussed with the pharmacist. Diabetes is increasingly common in the older patient, and adequate control of blood sugar is important in the perioperative period to reduce cardiac and infective complications. The need for conversion to sliding-scale insulin should always be anticipated, with the patient stabilized on this regime for several hours before proceeding to elective surgery.

Both surgery and anesthesia can produce major physiological changes for a patient. General anesthesia (GA) usually involves anesthetic agents that also produce vasodilatation and a fall in blood pressure, which is complicated further by the effects of positive pressure ventilation, which, by decreasing venous return, will further drop cardiac output and organ perfusion. This may in particular produce effects on renal and cerebral perfusion. In peripheral surgery this can be avoided by using regional or local anesthesia. The recent widespread adoption of ultrasound-guided nerve blockade has greatly increased the accurate placement of local anesthetics for limb surgery, so removing the need for general anesthesia in some cases and even reducing the need for epidural or spinal placement. This is especially valuable where cardiac valvular lesions such as aortic stenosis preclude the use of spinal anesthesia.

Nonetheless, the commonest forms of regional anesthesia are spinal and epidural techniques, both of which can be prolonged by the use of catheters. However, the former is largely for intraoperative use, because of the risks of infection entering the subarachnoid space, rather than a technique that can readily be extended into the postoperative period. There is conflicting evidence regarding survival benefit beyond the first month for spinal and epidural anesthesia over and above GA [88]. However, Rasmussen et al. did show a survival benefit for regional blockade at 3 months and a significant difference in postoperative cognitive dysfunction at 1 week, although this was no longer a feature at 3 months [94,95].

Postoperative cognitive dysfunction (POCD) is present in 26% of older patients at 1 week after major surgery and can be detected at 24 h in 47% of elderly patients after sevoflurane anesthesia or propofol anesthesia for minor surgery [96]. Unfortunately, there is a paucity of studies including the >85 age group. However, there is evidence for a lower degree of postoperative delirium in patients receiving lower amounts of sedation during regional anesthesia [97]. Sleep disturbances are common after anesthesia and critical illness, and although the etiology is multifactorial, drug factors are of major importance. Sedative and analgesic drugs, especially those used to facilitate mechanical ventilation, can be extremely disruptive. Even the withdrawal of opioid analgesic drugs during the recovery phase can lead to disruption of sleep with a return to high levels of rapid eye movement (REM) sleep and disturbed respiratory patterns. Delirium is often worse at night and adds to the difficulty of maintaining adequate oxygenation, fluid intake, drug compliance, and general care.

There is growing concern regarding the potential link between anesthesia and the onset or progression of neurodegenerative disorders. The Consensus Statement of the First International Workshop on Anaesthetics and Alzheimer's Disease makes a number of key points, including the presentation of evidence from animal models of an increase in brain tissue caspase activation, B-amyloid peptide, B acting cleavage enzyme, and phosphorylated τ, all of which can contribute to Alzheimer progression [98]. The evidence on examining brain slices that have been exposed to isoflurane is conflicting, with both protective and stressing effects occurring. However, there is evidence of postoperative cognitive decline in clinical studies of unclear etiology. Hypothermia causes τ hyperphosphorylation and so should be avoided in the perioperative period. There is a clear need for further work in this area, and if the evidence becomes convincing, then eventually a ranking of the potential of anesthetic drugs for influencing this effect would occur. Older rats appear to have increased difficulty with spatial learning and with memory after anesthesia. In a 7-year study of modifiable risk factors for dementia in a population with a mean baseline age of 73, anesthesia was found to significantly increase the chances of dementia, producing a Cox model hazard ratio of 1.28 [99].

Increasing age is associated with slow metabolism of drugs, which may lead to a further degree of cerebral impairment in the postoperative period. Aging impairs handling of drugs even in older people with few or no obvious comorbidities [100].

There is therefore potential benefit in using drugs that are easily metabolized or are inhaled volatile agents that can largely be exhaled. Unfortunately, the situation is not as clearcut as it appears at first sight. Remifentanil is a rapid-offset drug that is metabolized by plasma cholinesterase, and so its removal is little affected by impaired renal or hepatic function. For many anesthetists, it has largely replaced nitrous oxide, which has complicated effects on the bone marrow and is toxic to the gut. Unfortunately, its rapid metabolism means that very soon after the patient emerges from anesthesia, all its analgesic effects disappear, and other longeracting agents or regional blockade are needed to provide pain relief. In terms of postoperative analgesia, elderly patients may be more sensitive to opiates than younger patients. Unfortunately, alternatives such as nonsteroidal antiinflammatory drugs (NSAIDs) exert major hepatic and renal effects (although perhaps surprisingly there is some evidence that long-term administration may reduce the incidence of dementia) and a risk of producing gastric bleeding [101]. The concerns over renal function are especially the case in hypovolemic conditions, and so the acute administration of NSAIDS in the postoperative period is an area of great concern in older people.

Renal failure is a common cause of death in elderly individuals after surgery, but because cardiac failure is also common in this age group, the need for precise titration of fluid to the patients' requirements becomes even more important. This will mean a low threshold for the use of urinary catheter placement (despite the risks of urosepsis), arterial line, CVP measurement, and the use of more sophisticated techniques such as transesophageal Doppler measurement or the use of another tool for assessing cardiac output and related parameters.

Can the problems related to anesthesia in older people be reduced with newer drugs? Some are designed to be cleaner in their effects, such as oxycodone, which has fewer adverse effects than morphine. Some are reformulations of older drugs, such as intravenous paracetamol, which has an important opiate sparing effect and is valuable as long as dosage is correct. Volatile agents have different characteristics, and as a result there is increasing interest in the neuroprotective effects of xenon. However, at present studies are small, but although anesthesia emergence is accelerated by xenon, disappointingly, it has not so far been shown to reduce delirium in the small studies that have been conducted.

In summary, the older patient needs appropriate selection and preparation for surgery, together with care throughout the perioperative period. Organ dysfunction and delirium pose a real risk, so maintaining suitable cardiovascular performance is vital if this is not going to become even more of a problem. There is increasing interest in reducing the problems for older people associated with anesthesia and surgery. So far most of the impact has been to reduce the duration of short-term complications, which is important to reduce the costs and difficulties encountered in early postoperative care, but longer-term improvements are vital, as the size of the older population increases.

15.3.4 Improved Aftercare and Rehabilitation

Since 2000 interest has focused on improved outcome after major surgery using enhanced recovery programs (so-called fast-track surgery [102]). These programs have related mainly to colorectal surgery but have also been applied in other surgical fields [54,103]. These are based around protocol-driven pathways for adequate analgesia (thoracic epidural), early mobilization, and early feeding. They are associated with reduced length of hospital stay, improved morbidity rates, earlier return of bowel function, and enhanced oral nutritional intake [102]. Several studies have looked at their applicability to older patients and found that the protocols are effective in the majority, but not all older subjects [104].

Irrespective of diagnosis, the admission of an elderly person to hospital may be associated with progressive functional decline and an increased risk of mortality at 1 year following discharge; multivariate predictors include increased mortality, including male gender, past history of congestive cardiac failure or cancer, activities of daily living status at discharge, and biochemical markers of renal impairment and malnutrition [105]. Once again, functional status is highlighted as an important predictor, and is modifiable by a proactive rehabilitation intervention from day 1, rather than referral as a last resort [106]. Rehabilitation is an individualized problem solving and educational process aimed at reducing disability and handicap experienced by an individual as a consequence of disease, requiring multidisciplinary leadership. In addition, it is important to reiterate the impact of delirium; an acute, transient, global disorder of fluctuating cognition and attention with a noticeable decline in the sleep–wake cycle. Common in the elderly hospitalized population, it is associated with an increased risk of morbidity and mortality, delayed and reduced functional recovery, and increased lengths of hospital stay. Many risk factors can be identified preoperatively: polypharmacy, drug interactions, sedative withdrawal, impaired vision and hearing, anxiety and depression, and cognitive impairment; thus a proactive multicomponent intervention utilizing the skills of a geriatrician and the wider multidisciplinary team is often beneficial [107,108].

15.3.5 Improvements (Age for Age) in General Level of Fitness of Older Population

In the near future, the proportion of older people is expected to continue to increase; the fastest-growing cohort are the oldest elderly $\geq$90 years. Already, 50% of cancer diagnoses are in patients aged >70 years, and this proportion will inevitably increase as older people survive other disorders. While the elderly population may have multiple problems that interfere with cancer treatment, including comorbidity, functional dependence, cognitive decline, and depression, a significant and increasing number will be healthy and independent. The Medical Research Council Cognitive Function and Ageing Study collected data on prevalent and incident disability from a number of UK sites, and estimated that only ~16% of individuals age $\geq$65 years had a disability. Of these, approximately 20% were either independent or did not need help on a daily basis [109]. Even in the oldest elderly ($\geq$90 years), although there is an increased risk of frailty, comorbidity, and cognitive impairment compared to the younger elderly (65-84 years), a reported 25% of males and 11% of females will have no disability in personal or extended activities of daily living [110].

15.4 SUMMARY

The practice of surgery and anesthesia has changed significantly since the 1970s, and rates of successful surgical treatment for older individuals have increased significantly. There are still problems to be addressed. As the boundaries of practice have been extended, it is no longer possible to put simple age limits on who is or isn't fit for surgery, and more complex algorithms are needed that factor in frailty, comorbidity, age, and disease characteristics. Tools are available (Charlson Index, ASA score, POS-SUM, IADL, CGA) to assist in the assessment of surgical and anesthetic risk, but these have rarely been tested in the context of clinical trials. Advances in surgical and anesthetic techniques with time also mean that these data will need to be reacquired every decade to reflect improvements in practice.

This is an area of research where more work is urgently required. In the meantime, each patient needs to be carefully assessed to determine whether surgery is the safest and best option for them, with active patient involvement in the decision making process. In some cases, this may involve multidisciplinary assessment with the input of surgeons, geriatricians, anesthetists, and therapist (physio-, occupational, and nutritional therapists).

ACKNOWLEDGMENT

The authors would like to thank Dr. G. Mills (Sheffield Teaching Hospitals NHS Trust) for his contribution to this chapter.

REFERENCES

1. Yancik R. Cancer burden in the aged: An epidemiologic and demographic overview. *Cancer* 1997;**80**(7):1273–1283.
2. Faivre J, Lemmens VE, Quipourt V, Bouvier AM. Management and survival of colorectal cancer in the elderly in population-based studies. *Eur J Cancer*. 2007;**43**(15):2279–2284.
3. Wyld L, Garg DK, Kumar ID, Brown H, Reed MW. Stage and treatment variation with age in postmenopausal women with breast cancer: Compliance with guidelines. *Br J Cancer* 2004;**90**(8):1486–1491.
4. Lavelle K, Todd C, Moran A, Howell A, Bundred N, Campbell M. Non-standard management of breast cancer increases with age in the UK: A population based cohort of women > or = 65 years. *Br J Cancer*. 2007;**96**(8):1197–1203.
5. Wishart GC, Greenberg DC, Chou P, Brown CH, Duffy S, Purushotham AD. Treatment and survival in breast cancer in the eastern region of England. *Ann Oncol* 2010;**21**(2):291–296.
6. Hyung WJ, Kim SS, Choi WH, Cheong JH, Choi SH, Kim CB, et al. Changes in treatment outcomes of gastric cancer surgery over 45 years at a single institution. *Yonsei Med J* 2008;**49**(3):409–415.
7. Tuljapurkar S, Li N, Boe C. A universal pattern of mortality decline in the G7 countries. *Nature* 2000;**405**(6788):789–792.
8. Christensen K, Doblhammer G, Rau R, Vaupel JW. Ageing populations: The challenges ahead. *Lancet* 2009;**374**(9696):1196–1208.
9. Bayer A, Tadd W. Unjustified exclusion of elderly people from studies submitted to research ethics committee for approval: Descriptive study. *Br Med J* 2000;**321**(7267): 992–993.
10. Tan E, Tilney H, Thompson M, Smith J, Tekkis PP. The United Kingdom National Bowel Cancer Project—epidemiology and surgical risk in the elderly. *Eur J Cancer* 2007;**43**(15): 2285–2294.

11. Colorectal Cancer Collaborative Group. Surgery for colorectal cancer in elderly patients: A systematic review. Lancet 2000;**356**(9234):968–974.

12. O'Connell JB, Maggard MA, Liu JH, Etzioni DA, Ko CY. Are survival rates different for young and older patients with rectal cancer? *Dis Colon Rectum* 2004;**47**(12):2064–2069.

13. CRUK (Cancer Research UK). *Stomach Cancer: Key Facts*, 2010 (available at, http://infocancerresearchukorg/cancerstats/types/stomach/).

14. Smith JK, McPhee JT, Hill JS, Whalen GF, Sullivan ME, Litwin DE, et al. National outcomes after gastric resection for neoplasm. *Arch Surg* 2007;**142**(4):387–393.

15. Orsenigo E, Tomajer V, Palo SD, Carlucci M, Vignali A, Tamburini A, et al. Impact of age on postoperative outcomes in 1118 gastric cancer patients undergoing surgical treatment. *Gastric Cancer* 2007;**10**(1):39–44.

16. Msika S, Benhamiche AM, Tazi MA, Rat P, Faivre J. Improvement of operative mortality after curative resection for gastric cancer: Population-based study. *World J Surg* 2000;**24**(9):1137–1142.

17. Saif MW, Makrilia N, Zalonis A, Merikas M, Syrigos K. Gastric cancer in the elderly: An overview. *Eur J Surg Oncol* 2010;**36**(8):709–17.

18. Jeong O, Park YK, Ryu SY, Kim YJ. Effect of age on surgical outcomes of extended gastrectomy with D2 lymph node dissection in gastric carcinoma: Prospective cohort study. *Ann Surg Oncol* 2010;**17**(6):1589–1596.

19. Winslet MC, Mohsen YM, Powell J, Allum WH, Fielding JW. The influence of age on the surgical management of carcinoma of the stomach. *Eur J Surg Oncol* 1996;**22**(3):220–224.

20. Coniglio A, Tiberio GA, Busti M, Gaverini G, Baiocchi L, Piardi T, et al. Surgical treatment for gastric carcinoma in the elderly. *J Surg Oncol* 2004;**88**(4):201–205.

21. CRUK. *Lung Cancer: Key Facts*, 2010 (available at http://infocancerresearchukorg/cancerstats/keyfacts/indexhtm).

22. Jaklitsch MT, Pappas-Estocin A, Bueno R. Thoracoscopic surgery in elderly lung cancer patients. *Crit Rev Oncol Hematol* 2004;**49**(2):165–171.

23. van de Schans SA, Janssen-Heijnen ML, Biesma B, Smeenk FW, van de Poll-Franse LV, Seynaeve C, et al. COPD in cancer patients: Higher prevalence in the elderly, a different treatment strategy in case of primary tumours above the diaphragm, and a worse overall survival in the elderly patient. *Eur J Cancer* 2007;**43**(15):2194–2202.

24. Ginsberg RJ, Rubinstein LV. Randomized trial of lobectomy versus limited resection for T1N0 non-small cell lung cancer. Lung Cancer Study Group. *Ann Thorac Surg* 1995;**60**(3):615–622; discussion 22–23.

25. Berry MF, Hanna J, Tong BC, Burfeind WR Jr, Harpole DH, D'Amico TA, et al. Risk factors for morbidity after lobectomy for lung cancer in elderly patients. *Ann Thorac Surg* 2009;**88**(4):1093–1099.

26. Heerdt PM, Park BJ. The emerging role of minimally invasive surgical techniques for the treatment of lung malignancy in the elderly. *Anesthesiol Clin.* 2008;**26**(2):315–324, vi–vii.

27. Shaw JP, Dembitzer FR, Wisnivesky JP, Litle VR, Weiser TS, Yun J, et al. Video-assisted thoracoscopic lobectomy: State of the art and future directions. *Ann Thorac Surg.* 2008;**85**(2):S705–S709.

28. Koike T, Yamato Y, Asamura H, Tsuchiya R, Sohara Y, Eguchi K, et al. Improvements in surgical results for lung cancer from 1989 to 1999 in Japan. *J Thorac Oncol.* 2009;**4**(11):1364–1369.

29. CRUK. *Breast Cancer: Key Facts*, 2010 (available at http://infocancerresearch ukorg/cancerstats/types/breast/).

30. National Mastectomy and Breast Reconstruction Audit, 2011. The NHS Information Centre. (www.ic.nhs.uk).

31. El-Tamer MB, Ward BM, Schifftner T, Neumayer L, Khuri S, Henderson W. Morbidity and mortality following breast cancer surgery in women: National benchmarks for standards of care. *Ann Surg* 2007;**245**(5):665–671.

32. Hynes DM, Weaver F, Morrow M, Folk F, Winchester DJ, Mallard M, et al. Breast cancer surgery trends and outcomes: Results from a National Department of Veterans Affairs study. *J Am Coll Surg*, 2004;**198**(5):707–716.

33. Wyld L, Reed M. The role of surgery in the management of older women with breast cancer. *Eur J Cancer* 2007;**43**(15):2253–2263.

34. Houterman S, Janssen-Heijnen ML, Verheij CD, Louwman WJ, Vreugdenhil G, van der Sangen MJ, et al. Comorbidity has negligible impact on treatment and complications but influences survival in breast cancer patients. *Br J Cancer* 2004;**90**(12):2332–2337.

35. Diab SG, Elledge RM, Clark GM. Tumor characteristics and clinical outcome of elderly women with breast cancer. *J Natl Cancer Inst* 2000;**92**(7):550–556.

36. Hind D, Wyld L, Reed MW. Surgery, with or without tamoxifen, vs tamoxifen alone for older women with operable breast cancer: Cochrane review. *Br J Cancer* 2007;**96**(7): 1025–1029.

37. Lavelle K, Moran A, Howell A, Bundred N, Campbell M, Todd C. Older women with operable breast cancer are less likely to have surgery. *Br J Surg*. 2007;**94**(10):1209–1215.

38. Golledge J, Wiggins JE, Callam MJ. Age-related variation in the treatment and outcomes of patients with breast carcinoma. *Cancer* 2000;**88**(2):369–374.

39. Cheung SGN, Lagord C, Williams L, Kearins O, Lawrence G. All Breast Cancer Report. *A UK Analysis of All Symptomatic and Screen-Detected Breast Cancers Diagnosed in 2006*, West Midlands Cancer Intelligence Unit, 2009.

40. Thomson CS, Forman D. Cancer survival in England and the influence of early diagnosis: What can we learn from recent EUROCARE results? *Br J Cancer* 2009;**101**(Suppl 2): S102–S109.

41. CRUK. *Key Fact: Prostate Cancer*, 2010 (available at http://infocancerresearch ukorg/cancerstats/types/prostate/indexhtm).

42. Wong YN, Mitra N, Hudes G, Localio R, Schwartz JS, Wan F, et al. Survival associated with treatment vs observation of localized prostate cancer in elderly men. *JAMA* 2006;**296**(22):2683–2693.

43. Jeldres C, Suardi N, Walz J, Saad F, Hutterer GC, Bhojani N, et al. Poor overall survival in septa- and octogenarian patients after radical prostatectomy and radiotherapy for prostate cancer: A population-based study of 6183 men. *Eur Urol* 2008;**54**(1):107–116.

44. Thompson RH, Slezak JM, Webster WS, Lieber MM. Radical prostatectomy for octogenarians: how old is too old? *Urology* 2006;**68**(5):1042–1045.

45. Alibhai SM, Leach M, Warde P. Major 30-day complications after radical radiotherapy: A population-based analysis and comparison with surgery. *Cancer* 2009;**115**(2):293–302.

46. Alibhai SM, Leach M, Tomlinson G, Krahn MD, Fleshner N, Holowaty E, et al. 30-day mortality and major complications after radical prostatectomy: Influence of age and comorbidity. *J Natl Cancer Inst* 2005;**97**(20):1525–1532.

47. Alibhai SM, Leach M, Tomlinson G, Krahn MD, Fleshner N, Naglie G. Rethinking 30-day mortality risk after radical prostatectomy. *Urology* 2006;**68**(5):1057–1060.

48. Bubolz T, Wasson JH, Lu-Yao G, Barry MJ. Treatments for prostate cancer in older men: 1984–1997. *Urology*. 2001;**58**(6):977–982.

49. Ficarra V, Novara G, Artibani W, Cestari A, Galfano A, Graefen M, et al. Retropubic, laparoscopic, and robot-assisted radical prostatectomy: A systematic review and cumulative analysis of comparative studies. *Eur Urol*. 2009;**55**(5):1037–1063.

50. Poulakis V, Witzsch U, de Vries R, Dillenburg W, Becht E. Laparoscopic radical prosta-tectomy in men older than 70 years of age with localized prostate cancer: Comparison of morbidity, reconvalescence, and short-term clinical outcomes between younger and older men. *Eur Urol* 2007;**51**(5):1341–1348; discussion 9.

51. Yamada H, Kojima K, Inokuchi M, Kawano T, Sugihara K. Laparoscopy-assisted gastrec-tomy in patients older than 80. *J Surg Res* 2010;**161**(2):259–263.

52. Gruen RL, Pitt V, Green S, Parkhill A, Campbell D, Jolley D. The effect of provider case volume on cancer mortality: Systematic review and meta-analysis. *CA Cancer J Clin* 2009;**59**(3):192–211.

53. Rossi M, Iemma D. Patients with comorbidities: what shall we do to improve the outcome. *Minerva Anestesiol* 2009;**75**(5):325–327.

54. Wang D, Kong Y, Zhong B, Zhou X, Zhou Y. Fast-track surgery improves postopera-tive recovery in patients with gastric cancer: a randomized comparison with conventional postoperative care. *J Gastrointest Surg* 2010;**14**(4):620–627.

55. Lee WJ, Wang W, Chen TC, Chen JC, Ser KH. Totally laparoscopic radical BII gastrectomy for the treatment of gastric cancer: A comparison with open surgery. *Surg Laparosc Endosc Percutaneous Tech* 2008;**18**(4):369–374.

56. Francescutti V, Choy I, Biertho L, Goldsmith CH, Anvari M. Gastrectomy and esopha-gogastrectomy for proximal and distal gastric lesions: A comparison of open and laparo-scopic procedures. *Surg Innov* 2009;**16**(2):134–139.

57. Murray A, Lourenco T, de Verteuil R, Hernandez R, Fraser C, McKinley A, et al. Clinical effectiveness and cost-effectiveness of laparoscopic surgery for colorectal cancer: system-atic reviews and economic evaluation. *Health Technol Assess* 2006;**10**(45):1–141,iii–iv.

58. Kim YW, Baik YH, Yun YH, Nam BH, Kim DH, Choi IJ, et al. Improved quality of life outcomes after laparoscopy-assisted distal gastrectomy for early gastric cancer: Results of a prospective randomized clinical trial. *Ann Surg* 2008;**248**(5):721–727.

59. Tokunaga M, Hiki N, Fukunaga T, Miki A, Ohyama S, Seto Y, et al. Does age matter in the indication for laparoscopy-assisted gastrectomy? *J Gastrointest Surg* 2008;**12**(9):1502–1507.

60. Jayne DG, Thorpe HC, Copeland J, Quirke P, Brown JM, Guillou PJ. Five-year follow-up of the Medical Research Council CLASICC trial of laparoscopically assisted versus open surgery for colorectal cancer. *Br J Surg* 2010;**97**(11):1638–1645.

61. Skipworth RJ, Parks RW, Stephens NA, Graham C, Brewster DH, Garden OJ, et al. The relationship between hospital volume and post-operative mortality rates for upper gastroin-testinal cancer resections: Scotland 1982–2003. *Eur J Surg Oncol* 2010;**36**(2):141–147.

62. Begg CB, Cramer LD, Hoskins WJ, Brennan MF. Impact of hospital volume on operative mortality for major cancer surgery. *JAMA* 1998;**280**(20):1747–1751.

63. Fleissig A, Fallowfield LJ, Langridge CI, Johnson L, Newcombe RG, Dixon JM, et al. Post-operative arm morbidity and quality of life. Results of the ALMANAC randomised trial comparing sentinel node biopsy with standard axillary treatment in the management of patients with early breast cancer. *Breast Cancer Res Treat* 2006;**95**(3):279–293.

64. Morley JE. Anorexia in older persons: epidemiology and optimal treatment. *Drugs Aging* 1996;**8**(2):134–155.

65. Correia MI, Caiaffa WT, da Silva AL, Waitzberg DL. Risk factors for malnutrition in patients undergoing gastroenterological and hernia surgery: an analysis of 374 patients. *Nutr Hosp*. 2001 Mar-Apr;**16**(2):59–64.

66. Beguiristain Gomez A, Medrano Gomez MA, Uriarte Zaldua C, Alvarez Caperochipi J. Preoperative nutritional status in geriatric patients with digestive neoplasm. *Nutr Hosp* 1991;**6**(6):364–374.

67. Sorensen J, Kondrup J, Prokopowicz J, Schiesser M, Krahenbuhl L, Meier R, et al. EuroOOPS: An international, multicentre study to implement nutritional risk screening and evaluate clinical outcome. *Clin Nutr* 2008;**27**(3):340–349.

68. Minig L, Biffi R, Zanagnolo V, Attanasio A, Beltrami C, Bocciolone L, et al. Reduction of postoperative complication rate with the use of early oral feeding in gynecologic oncologic patients undergoing a major surgery: A randomized controlled trial. *Ann Surg Oncol* 2009;**16**(11):3101–3110.

69. Wu MH, Lin MT, Chen WJ. Effect of perioperative parenteral nutritional support for gastric cancer patients undergoing gastrectomy. *Hepatogastroenterology* 2008;**55**(82–83): 799–802.

70. Jagger C, Matthews R, Matthews F, Robinson T, Robine J-M, Brayne C, and the MRC-CFAS Investigators. The burden of diseases on disability-free life expectancy in later life. *J Gerontol Med Sci* 2007;**62A**:408–414.

71. Gosney M. Contribution of the geriatrician to the management of cancer in older patients. *Eur J Cancer* 2007;**43**:2153–2160.

72. Campbell SE, Seymour DG, Primrose WR, for the ACMEplus project. A systematic literature review of factors affecting outcome in older medical patients admitted to hospital. *Age Ageing* 2004;**33**:110–115.

73. Extermann M, Meyer J, McGinnis M, Crocker TT, Corcoran M-B, Yoder J, Haley WE, Chen H, Boulware D, Balducci L. A comprehensive geriatric intervention detects multiple problems in older breast cancer patients. *Crit Rev Oncol Hematol* 2004;**49**:69–75.

74. Stotter A, Tahir M, Pretorius R, Robinson T. Experiences of a multidisciplinary elderly breast cancer clinic: Using the right specialists, in the same place, with time. In Reed MW, Audisio RA: eds. *Management of Breast Cancer in Older Women*, Springer, 2010.

75. Gosney M. Clinical assessment of elderly people with cancer. *Lancet Oncol* 2005;**6**: 790–797.

76. Rodgers A, Walker N, Schug S, McKee A, Kehlet H, van Zundert A, et al. Reduction of postoperative mortality and morbidity with epidural or spinal anaesthesia: Results from overview of randomised trials. *Br Med J* 2000;**321**(7275):1493.

77. Beattie WS, Badner NH, Choi P. Epidural analgesia reduces postoperative myocardial infarction: A meta-analysis. *Anesth Analg* 2001;**93**(4):853–858.

78. Tsui BC, Wagner A, Finucane B. Regional anaesthesia in the elderly: A clinical guide. *Drugs Aging* 2004;**21**(14):895–910.

79. Oakley N, Dennison AR, Shorthouse AJ. A prospective audit of simple mastectomy under local anaesthesia. *Eur J Surg Oncol* 1996;**22**(2):134–136.

80. Atanassoff PG, Alon E, Weiss BM. Intercostal nerve block for lumpectomy: Superior postoperative pain relief with bupivacaine. *J Clin Anesth* 1994;**6**(1):47–51.

81. Greengrass R, O'Brien F, Lyerly K, Hardman D, Gleason D, D'Ercole F, et al. Paravertebral block for breast cancer surgery. *Can J Anaesth* 1996;**43**(8):858–861.

82. Lynch EP, Welch KJ, Carabuena JM, Eberlein TJ. Thoracic epidural anesthesia improves outcome after breast surgery. *Ann Surg* 1995;**222**(5):663–669.

83. Zaher C, Goldberg GA, Kadlubek P. Estimating angina prevalence in a managed care population. *Am J Managed Care* 2004;**10**(11 Suppl):S339–S346.

84. Brayne C, Matthews FE, McGee MA, Jagger C. Health and ill-health in the older population in England and Wales. The Medical Research Council Cognitive Function and Ageing Study (MRC CFAS). *Age Ageing* Jan;**30**(1):53–62.

85. De Bacquer D, De Backer G, Kornitzer M. Prevalences of ECG findings in large population based samples of men and women. *Heart* 2000;**84**(6):625–633.

86. Moller JT, Cluitmans P, Rasmussen LS, Houx P, Rasmussen H, Canet J, et al. Long-term postoperative cognitive dysfunction in the elderly ISPOCD1 study. ISPOCD investigators. International Study of Post-Operative Cognitive Dysfunction. *Lancet* 1998;21:**351**(9106):857–861.

87. Severn A. Anaesthesia and the preparation and management of elderly patients undergoing surgery. *Eur J Cancer* 2007;**43**(15):2231–2234.

88. Jenkins K, Baker AB. Consent and anaesthetic risk. *Anaesthesia* 2003;**58**:962–984.

89. Avorn J. Including elderly people in clinical trials. *Br Med J* 1997;315(7115):1033–1034.

90. Martin K, Bégaud B, Latry P, Miremart–Salame G, Fourrier A and Moore N. Differences between clinical trials and postmarketing use. *Br J Clin Pharmacol* 2004; **57**: 86–92.

91. Cherubini A, Oristrell J, Pla X, Ruggiero C, Ferretti R, Diestre G, Clarfield AM, Crome P, Hertogh C, Lesauskaite V, Prada GI; Szczerbinska K, Topinkova E, Sinclair Cohen J, Edbrooke D, Mills GH. The persistent exclusion of older subjects from ongoing trials on heart failure. *Arch Intern Med* 2011;**171**(6):550–6.

92. Pearse R, Dawson D, Fawcett J, Rhodes A, Grounds RM, Bennett ED. Early goal-directed therapy after major surgery reduces complications and duration of hospital stay. A randomised, controlled trial [ISRCTN38797445]. *Crit Care* 2005;**9**:R687–R693.

93. Marcantonio ER, Flacker JM, Wright RJ, Resnick. Reducing delirium after hip fracture: A randomized trial. *J Am Geriatr Soc* 2001;**49**(5):516–522.

94. Williams-Russo P, Sharrock NE, Mattis S, Szatrowski TP, Charlson ME. Cognitive effects after epidural vs general anesthesia in older adults. A randomized trial. *JAMA.* 1995;**274**(1):44–50.

95. Rasmussen LS, Johnson T, Kuipers HM, Kristensen D, Siersma VD, Vila P, Jolles J, Papaioannou A, Abildstrom H, Silverstein JH, Bonal JA, Raeder J, Nielsen IK, Korttila K, Munoz L, Dodds C, Hanning CD, Moller JT. Does anaesthesia cause postoperative cognitive dysfunction? A randomised study of regional versus general anaesthesia in 438 elderly patients. ISPOCD2 (International Study of Postoperative Cognitive Dysfunction) Investigators. *Acta Anaesthesiol Scand* 2003;**47**(3):260–266.

96. Rohan D, Buggy DJ, Crowley S, Ling FKH, Gallagher H, Regan C, Moriarty DC. Increased incidence of postoperative cognitive dysfunction 24 hr after minor surgery in the elderly. *Can J Anesth* 2005;**52**(2):137–142.

97. Sieber FE, Zakriya KJ, Gottschalk A, Blute MR, Lee HB, Rosenberg PB, Mears SC. Sedation depth during spinal anesthesia and the development of postoperative delirium in elderly patients undergoing hip fracture repair. *Mayo Clin Proc* 2010;**85**(1):18–26.

98. Baranov D, Bickler PE, Crosby EJ, Culley DJ, Eckenhoff MF, Eckenhoff RE, Hogan K, Gevtovic–Todorovic V, Palotas A, Peronansky M, Planel E, Silverstein JH, Wei Whittington RA, Xie Z, Zou Z. et al. Consensus statement: First International Workshop on Anesthetics and Alzheimer's Disease. *Anesth Analg* 2009;**108**:1627–1630.

99. Ritchie K, Carrière I, Ritchie CW, Berr C, Artero S, Ancelin M-L. Designing prevention programmes to reduce incidence of dementia: Prospective cohort study of modifiable risk factors. *Br Med J* 2010;**341**:c3885.

100. Avorn J. Including elderly people in clinical trial. *Br Med J* 1997;**315**(7115):1033–1034.

101. Szekely CA, Thorne JE, Zandi PP, Ek M, Messias E, Breitner JC, Goodman SN. Non-steroidal anti-inflammatory drugs for the prevention of Alzheimer's disease: A systematic review. *Neuroepidemiology* 2004;23(4):159–169.

102. Gouvas N, Tan E, Windsor A, Xynos E, Tekkis PP. Fast-track vs standard care in colorectal surgery: A meta-analysis update. *Int J Colorect Dis* 2009;24(10):1119–1131.

103. van Dam RM, Hendry PO, Coolsen MM, Bemelmans MH, Lassen K, Revhaug A, et al. Initial experience with a multimodal enhanced recovery programme in patients undergoing liver resection. *Br J Surg* 2008;**95**(8):969–975.

104. Scharfenberg M, Raue W, Junghans T, Schwenk W. "Fast-track" rehabilitation after colonic surgery in elderly patients—is it feasible? *Int J Colorect Dis* 2007;**22**(12):1469–1474.

105. Walter LC, Brand RJ, Counsell SR, Palmer RM, Landefeld CS, Fortinsky RH, Covinsky KE. Development and validation of a prognostic index for 1-year mortality in older adults after hospitalization. *JAMA* 2001;**285**:2987–2994.

106. Gosney M. Geriatric oncology. *Age Ageing* 2009;**38**:644–645.

107. Jin F, Chung F. Minimizing perioperative adverse events in the elderly. *Br J Anaesth* 2001;**87**:608–624.

108. Gosney M. Acute confusional states and dementia's: Peri-operative considerations. *Current Anaesth Crit Care* 2005;**16**:34–39.

109. Melzer D, McWilliams B, Brayne C, Johnson T, Bond J. Profile of disability in elderly people: Estimates from a longitudinal population study. *Br Med J* 1999;**318**:1108–1111.

110. Xie J, Matthews F, Jagger C, Bond J, Brayne C. The oldest old in England and Wales: A descriptive analysis based on the MRC Cognitive Function and Ageing Study. *Age Ageing* 2008;**37**:396–402.

CHAPTER 16

Chemotherapy in Older Adults with Cancer

MATTI S. AAPRO

Clinique de Genolier, Genolier, Switzerland

HANS WILDIERS

University Hospitals Leuven, Leuven, Belgium

16.1 INTRODUCTION

Physiology and body functions are known to alter with increasing age. These changes can have a considerable impact on the pharmacokinetic (PK) processes of absorption, distribution, metabolism, and excretion of administered drugs.

For many drugs, these changes are not clinically relevant, but for drugs with low therapeutic index, such as those used in chemotherapy, this can have dramatic consequences. Increased drug levels can lead to increased side effects in elderly people who already have diminished reserve capacities to deal with these toxicities.

This chapter discusses two important issues related to specific chemotherapeutic agents in older patients: (1) specific aspects of the pharmacology of different chemotherapeutic drugs in older adults, focusing on clinical implications and (2) general and specific side effects of practical recommendations and future perspectives.

16.2 GENERAL PHARMACOLOGICAL ISSUES RELATED TO CHEMOTHERAPY IN ELDERLY CANCER PATIENTS

Age can have an effect on most pharmacokinetic parameters, including absorption, volume of distribution, hepatic drug metabolism, and excretion [1].

Diminished absorption can occur because of atrophic gastritis, decreased gastric motility and secretions, or decreased intraluminal surface area, possibly resulting in reduced effectiveness. However, it is still controversial whether decreased absorption actually occurs with age [2].

Polypharmacy with multiple concomitant medications can alter absorption by binding drugs in the gastrointestinal tract, by changing absorption or pH, and by competition for carrier sites [3].

The volume of distribution (V_d) is a function of body composition, serum protein profile, and blood cells. A progressive increase in body fat and a decline in body

Cancer and Aging Handbook: Research and Practice, First Edition. Edited by Keith M. Bellizzi and Margot A. Gosney.
© 2012 Wiley-Blackwell. Published 2012 by John Wiley & Sons, Inc.

water content generally occur with increasing age. These changes tend to reduce the V_d of water-soluble drugs, such as anthracyclines, and increase those of fat-soluble compounds, such as carmustine. Plasma albumin levels can decrease because of the aging process and/or because of concomitant pathophysiological processes that will clearly influence the concentration of the unbound or free fraction of drug in the plasma, especially those that are highly protein-bound [4,5,6].

Hepatic function is also modified by aging; decreases in liver size (by 18–44%), bloodflow, albumin production, and cytochrome P450 function have all been reported. Also, drug interactions at the level of hepatic metabolization (or to a lesser extent at other levels such as drug binding or renal elimination) are an important issue in elderly individuals because drug prescription increases with increasing age [4,7].

The decreasing renal excretion of drugs is the most predictable and easily measurable pharmacokinetic change, as the glomerular filtration rate (GFR) declines on average with age by ~1 mL/min per year from the age of 40 years [8]. For drugs that are predominantly renally excreted, the dose usually needs to be reduced when the creatinine clearance (CrCl) is below 60 mL/min.

Despite previous knowledge, great uncertainty exists regarding the optimal dose of chemotherapy for older patients. This is not dissimilar from the case for younger patients in whom identical drugs can also have dramatic differences in pharmacology with subsequent over- or underdosing in some patients. It is hoped that pharmacogenomics in the near future will allow for better titration of the chemotherapy doses in different individuals. Because interindividual heterogeneity, related to differences in aging processes and development of comorbid diseases, increases with age, dose individualization is of utmost importance in older patients. At present, we can use available data on pharmacology to titrate the doses, and this can already eliminate partial differences in drug exposure. Dose adaptation in elderly patients is a double-edged sword. On one hand, overdosing can lead to important toxicity. Elderly individuals also have much less capability to deal with toxicity related to diminished functional reserve capacities. Dehydration can lead more quickly to renal insufficiency, and neutropenia can lead to more dramatic infections and treatment-related/induced death [9]. On the other hand, great care is warranted when making dose reductions because the antitumor effect may also decrease. For instance, a 50% initial dose reduction of cyclophosphamide, doxorubicin, vincristine, and prednisone (CHOP) in patients age 65 years and older is inferior to the full dose in patients with non-Hodgkin's lymphomas (NHL) [10]. Also, less intensive chemotherapy, such as etoposide, mitoxantrone, and prednimustine (VMP), is less effective than standard CHOP chemotherapy in NHL in those >69 years of age [11]. However, the VMP schedule is still effective with an objective response rate of 50%, less toxicity, and fewer toxic deaths.

Hematological growth factors could help in maintaining dose intensity while decreasing hematological toxicity but do not alleviate nonhematological toxicities. A lot depends on the clinical situation and goals of therapy. In a curative setting, such as lymphomas, dose intensity is critical and should be maintained if possible to optimize chances of cure. In an adjuvant setting, several studies suggest that low-dose or soft chemotherapy is associated with decreased efficacy. In breast cancer, cyclophophamide, methotrexate, and fluorouracil (CMF) chemotherapy is not as effective if a dose intensity of 85% cannot be reached [12].

A more recent study showed that classical chemotherapy with doxorubicin and cyclophosphamide (AC) or CMF is superior to capecitabine; the latter is an oral drug incorrectly thought to be more easily manageable in elderly patients. In a metastatic setting, there is no hard proof that dose intensity is crucial. The main goals of treatment are palliative, which is controlling disease as long as possible while causing as little toxicity as possible.

16.3 PHARMACOLOGY AND SIDE EFFECTS OF SPECIFIC ANTICANCER DRUGS IN ELDERLY INDIVIDUALS

Data on drugs commonly used can be found in several reviews [13–15].

16.3.1 Alkylating Agents

Cyclophosphamide (CPA) can be given orally and is very well absorbed, with a true bioavailability close to 100%. CPA by itself is inactive and is transformed in the liver into active metabolites, which are ultimately eliminated by hepatic metabolism and in 20–25% by renal excretion. One study of 44 women with breast cancer, aged 35–79 years and treated with CPA and doxorubicin, showed no age-related differences in the clearance of CPA [16]. An accumulation of toxic alkylating metabolites is expected in renal insufficiency, justifying a dose reduction of 20–30%, depending on the degree of renal insufficiency [17]. At the pharmacodynamic level, it has been shown that circulating monocytes in older people (>72 years vs. <25 years of age) are less able to recuperate from CPA-induced DNA damage [18], which can explain the increased risk of myelosuppression, the predominant toxicity of CPA in elderly patients.

16.3.2 Platinum Compounds

Cisplatin is an important drug in several tumor types, but the metabolism of cisplatin is not fully understood. It is partly excreted renally (20–70%), and dose adjustment recommendations have been made: 75% of the regular dose for CrCl $\leq$60 mL/min and 50% for CrCl $\leq$45 mL/min; no data are available for CrCl $\leq$30 mL/min [19]. However, the irreversible plasma protein binding of cisplatin also should be considered as an important elimination process as only the unbound plasma cisplatin concentrations represent the active fraction. Plasma protein binding of cisplatin is greater than the plasma protein binding of other platinum compounds (e.g., carboplatin). In addition to renal function, age is an independent and significant predictor of the area under the curve (AUC) of the free ultrafilterable platinum fraction (U-Pt) and total plasma platinum, with a higher AUC with increasing age [20]. The maximum concentration (C_{max}) of U-Pt has been shown to correlate significantly with nephrotoxicity [21], and it may be appropriate to reduce the rate of infusion in older patients [22]. Renal function should be considered as a major pharmacodynamic parameter for cisplatin as renal insufficiency represents the major toxicity, together with magnesium wasting, nausea and vomiting, peripheral neuropathy, auditory impairment (which can be problematic since age-related hearing loss is already frequent), and myelosuppression. Severe nausea and vomiting have been markedly reduced by the use of adequate antiemetic treatment regimens. Intravenous hydration has reduced acute nephrotoxicity to <5%.

In conclusion, increased AUC and toxicity in elderly patients prohibit the use of high-dose cisplatin. Cisplatin could be used at the lower range of dosage (e.g., 60 mg/m^2) and at a reduced infusion rate (e.g., >24 h).

Carboplatin, in contrast to cisplatin, has very limited protein binding. It is completely eliminated through the kidneys and has a unique method of dosing based on the GFR and the targeted AUC that has permitted individualization of the carboplatin dose for maximum effect with tolerable side effects. The Calvert formula [where AUC = AUC of carboplatin (mg mL^{-1} min^{-1})] provides an accurate and safe dose [23]:

$$\text{Dose (mg)} = \text{target AUC (GFR} + 25)$$

There is some controversy over the optimal way of determining GFR [24]. Several methods are available; the most popular is determination of creatinine clearance, which involves 24-h urine collections, or from the Cockcroft–Gault equation using serum creatinine. Because of the low incidence of nonhematologic toxicity and the quite similar efficacy, carboplatin can replace cisplatin in the palliative setting or when adverse effects of cisplatin are problematic.

Oxaliplatin, like cisplatin, is strongly protein-bound. The kidneys eliminate approximately 30–50% of the drug, and the AUC of the free fraction correlates with CrCl. However, in patients with normal or moderately impaired renal function (CrCl range 27–57 mL/min), no increased toxicity was observed, suggesting that it can be safely administered without dose adjustment or hydration in moderate renal dysfunction [25]. Patients with a severe decrease in GFR should have a dose reduction. In the meta-analysis from Goldberg and colleagues that involved patients receiving FOLFOX 4 for colorectal cancer [26], there was no difference in toxicity or efficacy between younger and (selected) older patients. Also, the combination of oxaliplatin and capecitabine was feasible and effective in older patients, and there was no relationship between response and patient age, Eastern Cooperative Oncology Group performance status, or the ability to perform activities of daily living (ADLs) or instrumental ADLs [27,28]. The rate of neurotoxicity secondary to oxaliplatin-based chemotherapy has not been shown to be any greater in older than in young patients. There is no data to support dose reduction based on age alone.

16.3.3   Taxanes

Paclitaxel and docetaxel are extensively metabolized in the liver. The majority of paclitaxel and docetaxel is protein-bound (97% and 94%, respectively). Only a small amount is excreted renally, and in principle, these drugs can be employed at full doses even if renal function is impaired. Both drugs are extensively metabolized in the liver by the cytochrome P450 system and are excreted in bile, resulting in increased toxicity when administered to patients with impaired liver function [29]. Neuropathy can be troublesome and debilitating, especially for elderly patients with unsteady balance. An extensive review on the use of taxanes in elderly breast cancer patients provides more details [30].

Paclitaxel was developed as a three weekly schedule but is currently often used as a weekly regimen because toxicity is diminished while efficacy is at least as good and in breast cancer is even better as in 3-weekly (i.e., once every 3 weeks) regimens [31]. A Cancer and Leukemia Group B trial showed a modest but significant decrease in clearance of total paclitaxel with increasing age and also an increase in white blood cell nadir, although this did not result in increased fever and neutropenia [32]. This decreased clearance seems partly induced by decreased clearance of the formulation vehicle Cremophor EL. Moreover, unbound paclitaxel might be a better predictor of clinically relevant exposure than total paclitaxel [33]. There is still controversy on the effect of age on paclitaxel pharmacology. However, several trials indicate the feasibility of both 3-weekly and weekly paclitaxel in elderly patients. There is no basis for a dose reduction based on age alone.

Docetaxel undergoes extensive metabolization by cytochrome CYP3A4, which is by far the strongest predictor of docetaxel clearance and, together with albumin/1-acid glycoprotein (AAG), accounts for 72% of the interpatient variation in clearance [34]. Attempts have been made to predict docetaxel PK by measurement of CYP3A4 activity by the erythromycin breath test or by plasma AAG concentration or urinary cortisol ratio, but this is difficult to implement in routine clinical care. Population PK studies suggest that docetaxel clearance decreases with age and hypoalbuminemia, but by only 7% and 8%, respectively [35]. Small, specific phase I trials in elderly cancer patients treated with docetaxel every 3 weeks have been performed with contradictory results [36,37]. As with paclitaxel, weekly dose docetaxel regimens have been investigated, and they seem to decrease toxicity without loss of efficacy [38], except perhaps in prostate cancer, where a 3-weekly regimen was slightly more effective than weekly docetaxel [39]. Neutropenia was limited with weekly regimens, but fatigue and lacrimation were often incapacitating. Various dosages (e.g., 20–35 mg/m^2 weekly or 60–100 mg/m^2 every 3 weeks) and regimens (rest weeks at various timepoints) have been used. There is no significant data to support dose modification of docetaxel based on age alone. Docetaxel pharmacokinetics are at most only minimally influenced by age. Any age-related changes are minimal compared with interpatient variability in metabolism. Elderly patients are more vulnerable to adverse effects; however, interpatient variability is greater than age-related variability. In principle, standard regimens of docetaxel can be used (e.g., 30–36 mg/m^2 weekly with a rest week at regular timepoints or 75 mg/m^2 every 3-weekly regimen). The choice between weekly and 3-weekly regimens can depend on the setting (e.g., in prostate cancer, 75 mg/m^2 every 3 weeks is the standard) and on potential adverse effects (if neutropenia should be avoided, weekly regimens are preferred). Nanoparticle-bound paclitaxel is a promising taxane formulation with low risk of allergy not requiring corticosteroids, but no studies have yet been undertaken specifically in older patients.

16.3.4 Topoisomerase Interactive Agents

The pharmacokinetics of etoposide are quite unpredictable and vary considerably between individuals; even more variability is to be expected in the elderly patient. The oral formulation poses even more problems than the intravenous formulation because intestinal absorption can also vary significantly [40]. Impaired renal function leads to a decrease in drug clearance rates, and dose modification has been proposed [14]. Increased age was a significant predictor of decreased etoposide clearance, increased AUC, and increased hematological toxicity, and in elderly patients with normal organ function, a small dose reduction and/or careful monitoring is advised [41,42].

Irinotecan (CPT11) is converted by decarboxylation in the liver into the active metabolite SN38, which is 1000 times more cytotoxic than the parent compound. Only a small amount is excreted in the urine, indicating that dose adjustment is not needed in patients with renal dysfunction. It can be given as a weekly or 3-weekly dose. The weekly and 3-weekly regimens showed similar efficacy and quality of life but differences in toxicity [43]. Therapy with CPT11 is feasible in older patients, but some studies indicate somewhat higher toxicity, mainly delayed diarrhea [44,45], which can be problematic in older individuals who are less able to deal with dehydration. A pharmacokinetic study demonstrated clearly that age is a significant independent predictor of the AUC of CPT11 [46]. It has been suggested that patients >70 years, patients with prior pelvic irradiation, or patients with poor performance status should start at reduced doses. However, there are no good data to support a specific dose modification. A more recent retrospective but large study [47] demonstrated no difference in toxicity and efficacy in older patients and recommended standard dosing. Further studies are necessary to demonstrate whether a reduced initial dose is preferable in elderly cancer patients.

Topotecan is ~40% renally excreted, but there is also a substantial concentration in bile [48]. Dose adjustments are required in extensively pretreated patients and in those with moderate (but not mild) renal impairment because of the risk of increased toxicity. A specific dose modification has been proposed, based on CrCl, for the standard daily intravenous dose of 1.5 mg/m^2 for 5 days every 3 weeks [49]. Weekly regimens seem to be effective with a decreased risk of hematological toxicity [50].

16.3.5 Antimetabolites

Methotrexate (MTX) is excreted mainly by the renal route and is inhibited by nonsteroidal anti inflammatory drugs, cephalosporins, and several other drugs. The dose of MTX should be adjusted according to renal function, and recommendations have been proposed [51]. Increased toxicity has been observed in elderly patients receiving low-dose, long-term methotrexate. The methotrexate half-life and clearance have been shown to be significantly prolonged in older patients [52]; therefore, the dose should be adjusted in the elderly population, based on renal function.

5-Fluorouracil (5FU) pharmacokinetics are only marginally influenced by age [53,54]. At most, 15–20% of the drug is excreted renally; some authors suggest a dose reduction to 80% in severe renal failure, but this is not really evidence-based [55].

Some studies have suggested increased toxicity in elderly individuals [56,57], while a pooled analysis of adjuvant chemotherapy for resected colon cancer in 3351 elderly patients [58] showed no significant interactions between age, efficacy, and toxicity (except for leukopenia in one of the seven trials studied). It seems that otherwise healthy older patients with colorectal cancer obtain benefits from adjuvant chemotherapy that do not differ much from those experienced by younger patients, while the benefits might be much lower in elderly patients with comorbidities and impaired functional status [59]. The data suggest no reason to reduce the dose for intravenous fluoropyrimidines, unless there is severe renal dysfunction or comorbidity. There are some data to suggest that women may be at higher risk of toxicity than men because of a decrease in the enzyme used to metabolize 5FU in women compared to men [54].

Capecitabine is an oral prodrug of 5FU that is extensively metabolized in the liver to 5FU, and >70% of the dose is recovered in the urine. This necessitates dose reduction in patients with renal dysfunction [60]. The pharmacokinetics of capecitabine are not affected by age in patients with normal renal function [61]. Studies in elderly breast cancer patients showed that the dose of capecitabine might be reduced from 1250 to 1000 mg/m^2 with equal efficacy but reduced toxicity [62].

Gemcitabine seems to require dose adaptation in patients with hepatic and renal dysfunction on the basis of clinical pharmacokinetic data [63]. However, there is a lack of correlation between pharmacokinetic parameters and toxicity that has made it impossible to provide any specific dose recommendations. Nevertheless, caution is required in patients with renal or hepatic impairment. The total clearance and half-life of gemcitabine are influenced by age and gender, with a longer half-life with increasing age and in men [64]. However, gemcitabine as a single agent causes minimal toxicity in elderly patients, and the side effect profile does not seem to be affected by patient age, leading to dose recommendations in elderly people that are no different from those for the general population [65–67].

16.3.6 Antitumor Antibiotics

Doxorubicin is probably the most commonly used anthracycline drug. It is metabolized and excreted primarily through the hepatobiliary route, while renal excretion is very low, not necessitating dose adjustment in case of renal failure. Increased peak plasma levels have been observed in older patients [13,68]. Some studies suggest that the drug's peak concentration correlates with efficacy, whereas toxicity is most likely a function of both peak and exposure [69]. Anthracyclines can cause cardiac dysfunction, and older patients are at higher risk. This increased incidence of anthracycline-related cardiomyopathy over the age of 70 years is most likely due to a combination of factors, including a higher prevalence of preexisting conditions restricting the functional reserve of the myocardium. In a situation such as adjuvant therapy for early breast cancer, where a large proportion of patients are cured, treatment-induced cardiac toxicity can be troublesome. A large study used the Surveillance, Epidemiology, and End Results Medicare database and included women aged 66–80 years, with no history of chronic heart failure (CHF) and who were diagnosed with stage I–III breast cancer from 1992 to 2002 [70]. A total of 43,338 women were included. Anthracycline-treated women were younger, with fewer comorbidities and more advanced disease than women who received nonanthracycline or no chemotherapy ($p = 0.001$ for each). The adjusted hazard ratio for CHF was 1.26 (95% confidence interval 1.12–1.42) for women aged 66–70 years treated with anthracycline compared with other chemotherapy. It was concluded that women aged 66–70 years who received adjuvant anthracyclines had significantly higher rates of CHF. The difference in rates of CHF continued to increase through more than 10 years of follow-up. The benefit of adjuvant chemotherapy in breast cancer can be rather small and might be counterbalanced by treatment-induced toxicity. The expected advantages and disadvantages should always be balanced when taking treatment decisions. Also, in NHL, doxorubicin in elderly patients has been extensively studied. Large prospective studies of elderly patients (aged >60 years) with NHL receiving doxorubicin (50 mg/m^2) in the CHOP regimen have shown that this regimen can be used in older patients but is associated with a higher degree of toxicity and a death rate of 7.6–15%, due to toxicity [71,72].

Several attempts have been made to deal with increased toxicity in older people, including dose reduction, alternative administration regimens, removal of doxorubicin from the multidrug regimen, and the use of hematological growth factors. Great care is warranted when doxorubicin is combined with new therapies such as trastuzumab, a recombinant monoclonal antibody against HER2, where a clear additive cardiotoxic effect occurs [73]. When doxorubicin is administered by continuous infusion or in small daily doses, the incidence of drug-related cardiotoxicity seems to be reduced significantly [69]. Weekly low-dose doxorubicin has also been studied in elderly patients with the potential benefit of inducing less neutropenia and lower peak plasma levels, which may both be related to cardiac toxicity. Desrazoxane can also reduce cardiac toxicity, but this needs to be confirmed and investigated specifically in the elderly population [74]. In addition, it is unclear whether the addition of desrazoxane may impact anti-tumor efficacy. Liposomal formulations of doxorubicin have been shown to prevent cardiotoxicity while providing comparable antitumor activity [75]. They may be very beneficial in elderly patients with anthracycline-sensitive disease, but the experience in this group is limited.

There are no strict guidelines for the dose adjustment of doxorubicin on the basis of age, but great care is recommended in an older person given the observed increased toxicity, and doses higher than $50-60$ mg/m^2 should be avoided. It has been suggested that in patients over the age of 70 years, regardless of coexisting heart disease, a cumulative doxorubicin dose of 450 mg/m^2 should not be exceeded, whereas in younger patients, a 550-mg/m^2 threshold is used [76]. Several other strategies (slower infusion rate, low-dose weekly regimens, liposomal forms, etc.) have been proposed in an effort to reduce the toxicity.

16.4 GENERAL SIDE EFFECTS OF CHEMOTHERAPY IN OLDER ADULTS WITH CANCER

Several drug-specific side effects that increase in older patients have been mentioned in the previous section. Elderly patients have a decreased tolerability to chemotherapy in general, with increased incidence of various toxicities. Myelosuppression and mucositis are less drug-specific and will be discussed briefly. The greater incidence and severity of toxicity in this age group mean that they require more supportive care. The aggressive and effective management of toxicity associated with chemotherapy is, therefore, crucial in this population.

16.4.1 Myelosuppression

Myelosuppresion is the major dose-limiting toxicity of many modern chemotherapeutic drugs. Retrospective analyses of data from clinical trials in patients with solid tumors show no correlation between age and myelosuppression [77–80]. These retrospective studies show that age itself should not be a contraindication for cancer therapy. Severe selection bias was, however, present in these studies, thus limiting the generalizability of these conclusions to the general older population. Elderly individuals are underrepresented in clinical studies, particularly patients above the age of 80 years. Moreover, conventional enrollment criteria ensure that older patients have disproportionately few comorbidities and a good performance status.

In contrast, age was found to be a definite independent risk factor for neutropenia in patients older than 60 years with lymphoma in a number of prospective clinical trials of CHOP or regimens with equivalent toxicity [81–87]. The conclusion is that age is clearly associated with a greater risk of grade 4 neutropenia, neutropenia-related infection, and mortality. Not only the incidence but also the severity of myelosuppression increase in older patients receiving chemotherapy, resulting in longer hospital stays and higher inpatient mortality [88].

The risk of neutropenia and its complications, including death, is highest in the early cycles of chemotherapy [81,89,90]. Because of this risk and the potential for better outcomes, prophylaxis with a colony stimulating factor beginning in the first cycle should be considered in elderly patients [91]. Age-related data on anemia and thrombocytopenia are less available but are probably also relevant.

16.4.2 Mucositis

Chemotherapeutic drugs such as irinotecan and fluorouracil are well known to induce intestinal mucositis, and liposomal anthracyclines cause more oral mucositis than do classic anthracyclines; however, many other chemotherapeutic drugs also can induce mucositis to varying degrees. Older people seem to be more susceptible to mucosal toxicities, such as cystitis, gastritis, stomatitis, and intestinal mucositis, which can lead to diarrhea [92–94]. In studies of 5FU-containing regimens for colorectal cancer or CMF for breast cancer, advanced age predicted more frequent and more severe diarrhea and stomatitis [93–95]. Mucositis can lead to dehydration and can become life threatening, and elderly individuals are more prone to this [93,94].

16.5 PRACTICAL RECOMMENDATIONS

Specific recommendations can be made when chemotherapy is considered in elderly cancer patients [15]:

1. Tailor treatment to each individual patient. Treatment individualization is important in oncology but is even more important in the elderly patient because interindividual heterogeneity dramatically increases with increasing age.
2. Perform some form of geriatric assessment at ≥70 years of age [96].
3. Consider administering supportive or protective agents, such as hematological growth factors or antiemetics, which can play a key role in diminishing toxicity in the elderly patient [97].
4. Beware of the risk of drug interactions. Because many elderly patients are on multiple medications, drug interactions can adversely influence the pharmacokinetics of anticancer drugs [98].
5. Monitor patient compliance. For intravenous drugs, this is not an issue, but for oral drugs such as capecitabine or temozolomide, or for supportive drugs such as antiemetics and growth factors, this is important.
6. Consider the possibility of less toxic therapy. Older cancer patients (>70 years) undergoing classical chemotherapy have a higher risk of experiencing toxicity. Several studies show that chemotherapy is generally well tolerated with a limited impact on independence, comorbidity, and quality of life, but selection bias might be present. Targeted therapies do not induce classic side effects of chemotherapy in general (hair loss, neutropenia, nausea, and vomiting) and are certainly promising for elderly individuals, but care is warranted because specific side effects might also occur. Angiogenesis inhibitors, for instance, can cause thrombosis and hypertension, and age is an important risk factor.
7. Maintain adequate hydration. Elderly patients have a tendency to drink less, especially when feeling ill, and are more intolerant of dehydration. Poor hydration can lead to decreased clearance and increased toxicity, especially for drugs subject to renal excretion.

8. Define the aim of chemotherapy.

9. Check renal function in elderly cancer patients. The International Society of Geriatric Oncology has made specific guidelines on the determination of renal function [24] as well as on dose adaptation of specific chemotherapeutic agents in renal dysfunction [99]. Prior to drug therapy in elderly patients with cancer, assessment and optimization of hydration status and evaluation of renal function to establish any need for dose adjustment are required. Serum creatinine alone is insufficient as a means of evaluating renal function. More accurate tools, including creatinine clearance methods, such as the Cockcroft–Gaultmethod (CG) procedure, are available and are generally good indices of renal function status of the patient. However, in elderly patients, CG and other similar formulas are not as accurate as in the younger population. More recently developed tools, such as the modification of diet in renal disease (MDRD) equation, may be the estimation of choice in elderly patients, whereas the CG estimate can be used in subjects younger than 65 years. However, the MDRD has generally not been validated for dose calculation of chemotherapy, and the CG may be more practical. Moreover, in extremes of obesity and cachexia and at very high and low creatinine values, no single tool is really accurate. The best estimate of GFR is provided by direct methods such as 51Cr-EDTA or inulin measurement. Within each drug class, preference may be given to agents less likely to be influenced by renal clearance. Within each drug class, preference may be given to agents less likely to be toxic to the kidneys or for which appropriate methods of prevention for renal toxicity exist. Coadministration of known nephrotoxic drugs, such as nonsteroidal antiinflammatory drugs (NSAIDs), should be avoided or minimized.

10. Be aware of clinical data for specific chemotherapy drugs [13,14]. As mentioned, many clinical and pharmacological data on pharmacokinetics of chemotherapy are available. However, it should be stated that dose adaptation based on age-related pharmacological changes is an invalidated approach because clinical trials prospectively testing the efficacy and toxicity of age-related dose adaptation versus standard dosing are lacking [99,100].

16.6 CONCLUSIONS AND FUTURE PERSPECTIVES

Management of the elderly patient with cancer represents an increasingly common challenge. Physicians and oncologists should be familiar with the age-related changes in physiology that affect the disposition and response to drugs in older patients. The impact of these changes on the availability, efficacy, and toxicity of most classical anticancer drugs is not always well documented. In general, and for most drugs, age itself is not a contraindication to full-dose chemotherapy. Cancer chemotherapy in the elderly population may best be considered as an example of the need for dose optimization in individual patients. By considering the basic principles of the pharmacokinetics and pharmacodynamics of these agents, therapy can be optimized. For most agents, it is not possible to provide clear level I guidelines for dose modification on the basis of age. However, one should consider the statement that "if it was not due to the extreme variability, medicine would be a science and not an art." The geriatric population is predominantly a heterogeneous population at all levels, and therefore it will be very difficult to provide simple guidelines. Despite these difficulties, if the important physiological changes in elderly patients are kept in mind, severe toxicity or toxic deaths can be avoided. The fine balance between increased efficacy plus higher toxicity and potentially lesser efficacy, but better tolerability, can frequently swing to the latter because it is just this severe toxicity that is often unacceptable to elderly patients. The decision to modify the dose of an anticancer agent still lies with the bedside clinician, who must integrate knowledge of pharmacology with the type of cancer and condition of the elderly patient, as well as the intention of therapy. It is evident that more pharmacological studies of anticancer agents in this population are required. It is reassuring that there is more interest and focus on the elderly population such as the increasing development of clinical trials specifically directed at this group.

ACKNOWLEDGMENT

This work has drawn on material from Hans Wildler and Matti Aapro, Pharmacology and unique side-effects of chemotherapy in older adults, in Arti Hurria and Harvey Jay Cohen (eds.), *Practical Geriatric Oncology* (2010), © Cambridge Univeristy Press. Reproduced with permission.

REFERENCES

1. Vestal RE. Aging and pharmacology. *Cancer* 1997;**80**:1302–1310.
2. Johnson SL, Mayersohn M, Conrad KA. Gastrointestinal absorption as a function of age: xylose absorption in healthy adults. *Clin Pharmacol Ther* 1985;**38**:331–335.
3. Skirvin JA, Lichtman SM. Pharmacokinetic considerations of oral chemotherapy in elderly patients with cancer. *Drugs Aging* 2002;**19**:25–42.
4. Wallace SM, Verbeeck RK. Plasmaprotein binding of drugs in the elderly. *Clin Pharmacokinet* 1987;**12**:41–72.
5. Yuen GJ. Altered pharmacokinetics in the elderly. *Clin Geriatr Med* 1990;**6**:257–267.
6. Egorin MJ. Cancer pharmacology in the elderly. *Semin Oncol* 1993;**20**:43–49.
7. Balis FM. Pharmacokinetic drug interactions of commonly used anticancer drugs. *Clin Pharmacokinet* 1986;**11**:223–235.
8. Brenner BM, Meyer TW, Hostetter TH. Dietary protein intake and the progressive nature of kidney disease: The role of hemodynamically mediated glomerular injury in the pathogenesis of progressive glomerular sclerosis in aging, renal ablation,and intrinsic renal disease. *N Engl J Med* 1982;**307**:652–659.
9. Muss HB, Woolf S, Berry D, et al. Adjuvant chemotherapy in older and younger women with lymph node-positive breast cancer. *JAMA* 2005;**293**:1073–1081.
10. Dixon DO, Neilan B, Jones SE, et al. Effect of age on therapeutic outcome in advanced diffuse histiocytic lymphoma: the Southwest Oncology Group experience. *J Clin Oncol* 1986;**4**:295–305.
11. Tirelli U, Errante D, Van Glabbeke M, et al. CHOP is the standard regimen in patients ≥70 years of age with intermediate-grade and high-grade non-Hodgkin's lymphoma: Results of a randomized study of the European Organization for Research and Treatment of Cancer Lymphoma Cooperative Study Group. *J Clin Oncol* 1998;**16**:27–34.
12. Bonadonna G, Valagussa P. Dose-response effect of adjuvant chemotherapy in breast cancer. *N Engl J Med* 1981;**304**:10–15.

13. Wildiers H, Highley MS, de Bruijn EA, et al. Pharmacology of anticancer drugs in the elderly population. *Clin Pharmacokinet* 2003;**42**:1213–1242.

14. Lichtman SM, Wildiers H, Chatelut E, et al. International Society of Geriatric Oncology chemotherapy taskforce: evaluation of chemotherapy in older patients—ananalysis of the medical literature. *J Clin Oncol* 2007;**25**:1832–1843.

15. Wildiers H. Mastering chemotherapy dose reduction in elderly cancer patients. *Eur J Cancer* 2007;**43**:2235–2241.

16. Dees EC, O'Reilly S, Goodman SN, et al. A prospective pharmacologic evaluation of age-related toxicity of adjuvant chemotherapy in women with breast cancer. *Cancer Investig* 2000;**18**:521–529.

17. Moore MJ. Clinical pharmacokinetics of cyclophosphamide. *Clin Pharmacokinet* 1991;**20**:194–208.

18. Rudd GN, Hartley JA, Souhami RL. Persistence of cisplatin-induced DNA interstrand crosslinking in peripheral blood mononuclear cells from elderly and young individuals. *Cancer Chemother Pharmacol* 1995;**35**:323–326.

19. Kintzel PE, Dorr RT. Anticancer drug renal toxicity and elimination: Dosing guidelines for altered renal function. *Cancer Treat Rev* 1995;**21**:33–64.

20. Yamamoto N, Tamura T, Maeda M, et al. The influence of ageing on cisplatin pharmacokinetics in lung cancer patients with normal organ function. *Cancer Chemother Pharmacol* 1995;**36**:102–106.

21. Reece PA, Stafford I, Russell J, et al. Creatinine clearance as a predictor of ultrafilterable platinum disposition in cancer patients treated with cisplatin: Relationship between peak ultrafilterable platinum plasma levels and nephrotoxicity. *J Clin Oncol* 1987;**5**:304–309.

22. Baker SD, Grochow LB. Pharmacology of cancer chemotherapy in the older person. *Clin Geriatr Med* 1997;**13**:169–183.

23. Calvert AH, Newell DR, Gumbrell LA, et al. Carboplatin dosage: Prospective evaluation of a simple formula based on renal function. *J Clin Oncol* 1989;**7**:1748–1756.

24. Launay-Vacher V, Chatelut E, Lichtman SM, et al. Renal insufficiency in elderly cancer patients: International Society of Geriatric Oncology clinical practice recommendations. *Ann Oncol* 2007;**18**:1314–1321.

25. Massari C, Brienza S, Rotarski M, et al. Pharmacokinetics of oxaliplatin in patients with normal versus impaired renal function. *Cancer Chemother Pharmacol* 2000;**45**:157–164.

26. Goldberg RM, Tabah-Fisch I, Bleiberg H, et al. Pooled analysis of safety and efficacy of oxaliplatin plus fluorouracil/leucovorin administered bimonthly in elderly patients with colorectal cancer. *J Clin Oncol* 2006;**24**:4085–4091.

27. Feliu J, Salud A, Escudero P, et al. XELOX (capecitabine plus oxaliplatin) as first-line treatment for elderly patients over 70 years of age with advanced colorectal cancer. *Br J Cancer* 2006;**94**:969–975.

28. Comella P, Natale D, Farris A, et al. Capecitabine plus oxaliplatin for the first-line treatment of elderly patients with metastatic colorectal carcinoma: Final results of the Southern Italy Cooperative Oncology Group Trial 0108. *Cancer* 2005;**104**:282–289.

29. Venook AP, Egorin MJ, Rosner GL, et al. Phase I and pharmacokinetic trial of paclitaxel in patients with hepatic dysfunction: Cancer and Leukemia Group B9264. *J Clin Oncol* 1998;**16**:1811–1819.

30. Wildiers H, Paridaens R. Taxanes in elderly breast cancer patients. *Cancer Treat Rev* 2004;**30**:333–342.

31. Seidman AD, Berry D, Cirrincione C, et al. Randomized phase III trial of weekly compared with every-3-weeks paclitaxel for metastatic breast cancer, with trastuzumab for all HER-2 overexpressors and random assignment to trastuzumab or not in HER-2 nonoverexpressors: Final results of Cancer and Leukemia Group B protocol 9840. *J Clin Oncol* 2008;**26**:1642–1649.

32. Lichtman SM, Hollis D, Miller AA, et al. Prospective evaluation of the relationship of patient age and paclitaxel clinical pharmacology: Cancer and Leukemia Group B (CALGB 9762). *J Clin Oncol* 2006;**24**:1846–1851.

33. Smorenburg CH, ten Tije AJ, Verweij J, et al. Altered clearance of unbound paclitaxel in elderly patients with metastatic breast cancer. *Eur J Cancer* 2003;**39**:196–202.

34. Hirth J, Watkins PB, Strawderman M, et al. The effect of an individual's cytochrome CYP3A4 activity on docetaxel clearance. *Clin Cancer Res* 2000;**6**:1255–1258.

35. Bruno R, Vivier N, Veyrat-Follet C, et al. Population pharmacokinetics and pharmacokinetic-pharmacodynamic relationships for docetaxel. *Investig New Drugs* 2001;**19**:163–169.

36. Girre V, Beuzeboc P, Livartowski A, et al. Docetaxel in elderly patients: phase I and pharmacokinetic study [abstract number 2113]. *J Clin Oncol* 2005;**16**:162.

37. Zanetta S, Albrand G, Bachelot T, et al. A phase I trial of docetaxel every 21 days in elderly patients with metastatic breast cancer [abstract]. *Ann Oncol* 2000;**11**(Suppl 4):73.

38. Hainsworth JD, Burris HA 3rd, Litchy S, et al. Weekly docetaxel in the treatment of elderly patients with advanced non-small cell lung carcinoma: A Minnie Pearl Cancer Research Network phase II trial. *Cancer* 2000;**89**:328–333.

39. Tannock IF, de Wit R, Berry WR, et al. Docetaxel plus prednisone or mitoxantrone plus prednisone for advanced prostate cancer. *N Engl J Med* 2004;**351**:1502–1512.

40. Souhami RL, Spiro SG, Rudd RM, et al. Five-day oral etoposide treatment for advanced small-cell lung cancer: Randomized comparison with intravenous chemotherapy. *J Natl Cancer Inst* 1997;**89**:577–580.

41. Joel SP, Shah R, Slevin ML. Etoposide dosage and pharmacodynamics. *Cancer Chemother Pharmacol* 1994;**34**(Suppl):69–75.

42. Miller AA, Rosner GL, Ratain MJ, et al. Pharmacology of 21-day oral etoposide given in combination with I.V. cisplatin in patients with extensive-stage small cell lung cancer: A Cancer and Leukemia Group B study (CALGB9062). *Clin Cancer Res* 1997;**3**:719–725.

43. Fuchs CS, Moore MR, Harker G, et al. Phase III comparison of two irinotecan dosing regimens in second-line therapy of metastatic colorectal cancer. *J Clin Oncol* 2003;**21**:807–814.

44. Aparicio T, Desrame J, Lecomte T, et al. Oxaliplatin- or irinotecan-based chemotherapy for metastatic colorectal cancer in the elderly. *Br J Cancer* 2003;**89**:1439–1444.

45. Sastre J, Marcuello E, Masutti B, et al. Irinotecan in combination with fluorouracil in a 48-hour continuous infusion as first-line chemotherapy for elderly patients with metastatic colorectal cancer: A Spanish cooperative group for the treatment of digestive tumors study. *J Clin Oncol* 2005;**23**:3545–3551.

46. Miya T, Goya T, Fujii H, et al. Factors affecting the pharmacokinetics of CPT-11: The body mass index, age and sex are independent predictors of pharmacokinetic parameters of CPT-11. *Investig New Drugs* 2001;**19**:61–67.

47. Chau I, Norman AR, Cunningham D, et al. Elderly patients with fluoropyrimidine and thymidylate synthase inhibitor-resistant advanced colorectal cancer derive similar benefit without excessive toxicity when treated with irinotecan monotherapy. *Br J Cancer* 2004;**91**:1453–1458.

48. Herben VM, ten Bokkel Huinink WW, Beijnen JH. Clinical pharmacokinetics of topotecan. *Clin Pharmacokinet* 1996;**31**:85–102.

49. O'Reilly S, Armstrong DK, Grochow LB. Life-threatening myelosuppression in patients with occult renal impairment receiving topotecan. *Gynecol Oncol* 1997;**67**:329–330.

50. Armstrong DK. Topotecan dosing guidelines in ovarian cancer: Reduction and management of hematologic toxicity. *Oncologist* 2004;**9**:33–42.

51. Gelman RS, Taylor SG. Cyclophosphamide, methotrexate, and 5 fluorouracil chemotherapy in women more than 65 years old with advanced breast cancer: The elimination of age trends in toxicity by using doses based on creatinine clearance. *J Clin Oncol* 1984;**2**:1404–1413.

52. Kristensen LO, Weismann K, Hutters L. Renal function and the rate of disappearance of methotrexate from serum. *Eur J Clin Pharmacol* 1975;**8**:439–444.

53. Port RE, Daniel B, Ding RW, et al. Relative importance of dose, body surface area, sex, and age for 5-fluorouracil clearance. *Oncology* 1991;**48**:277–281.

54. Milano G, Etienne MC, Cassuto-Viguier E, et al. Influence of sex and age on fluorouracil clearance. *J Clin Oncol* 1992;**10**:1171–1175.

55. Young AM, Daryanani S, Kerr DJ. Can pharmacokinetic monitoring improve clinical use of fluorouracil? *Clin Pharmacokinet* 1999;**36**:391–398.

56. Stein BN, Petrelli NJ, Douglass HO, et al. Age and sex are independent predictors of 5-fluorouracil toxicity—analysis of a large-scale phase-III trial. *Cancer* 1995;**75**:11–17.

57. Weinerman B, Rayner H, Venne A, et al. Increased incidence and severity of stomatitis in women treated with 5-fluorouracil and leucovorin [Abstract 1176]. *Proc Am Soc Clin Oncol* 1998.

58. Sargent DJ, Goldberg RM, Jacobson SD, et al. A pooled analysis of adjuvant chemotherapy for resected colon cancer in elderly patients. *N Engl J Med* 2001;**345**:1091–1097.

59. Balducci L. The geriatric cancer patient: equal benefit from equal treatment. *Cancer Control* 2001;**8**:1–25.

60. Poole C, Gardiner J, Twelves C, et al. Effect of renal impairment on the pharmacokinetics and tolerability of capecitabine (Xeloda) in cancer patients. *Cancer Chemother Pharmacol* 2002;**49**:225–234.

61. Cassidy J, Twelves C, Cameron D, et al. Bioequivalence of two tablet formulations of capecitabine and exploration of age, gender, body surface area, and creatinine clearance as factors influencing systemic exposure in cancer patients. *Cancer Chemother Pharmacol* 1999;**44**:453–460.

62. Bajetta E, Procopio G, Celio L, et al. Safety and efficacy of two different doses of capecitabine in the treatment of advanced breast cancer in older women. *J Clin Oncol* 2005;**23**:2155–2161.

63. Venook AP, Egorin MJ, Rosner GL, et al. Phase I and pharmacokinetic trial of gemcitabine in patients with hepatic or renal dysfunction: Cancer and Leukemia Group B 9565. *J Clin Oncol* 2000;**18**:2780–2787.

64. Lichtman SM, Skirvin JA. Pharmacology of antineoplastic agents in older cancer patients. *Oncology* 2000;**14**:1743–1755.

65. Shepherd FA, Abratt RP, Anderson H, et al. Gemcitabine in the treatment of elderly patients with advanced non-small cell lung cancer. *Semin Oncol* 1997;**24**:S7-50–S7-55.

66. Martin C, Ardizzoni A, Rosso R. Gemcitabine: safety profile and efficacy in non-small cell lung cancer unaffected by age. *Aging* 1997;**9**:297–303.

67. Martoni A, Di Fabio F, Guaraldi M, et al. Prospective phase II study of single-agent gemcitabine in untreated elderly patients with stage IIIB/IV non-small-cell lung cancer. *Am J Clin Oncol* 2001;**24**:614–617.

68. Robert J, Hoerni B. Age dependence of the early-phase pharmacokinetics of doxorubicin. *Cancer Res* 1983;**43**:4467–4469.

69. Legha SS, Benjamin RS, Mackay B, et al. Reduction of doxorubicin cardiotoxicity by prolonged continuous intravenous infusion. *Ann Intern Med* 1982;**96**:133–139.

70. Pinder MC, Duan Z, Goodwin JS, et al. Congestive heart failure in older women treated with adjuvant anthracycline chemotherapy for breast cancer. *J Clin Oncol* 2007;**25**:3808–3815.

71. Sonneveld P, Deridder M, Vanderlelie H, et al. Comparison of doxorubicin and mitoxantrone in the treatment of elderly patients with advanced diffuse non-Hodgkins-lymphoma using CHOP versus CNOP chemotherapy. *J Clin Oncol* 1995;**13**:2530–2539.

72. Coiffier B, Lepage E, Briere J, et al. CHOP chemotherapy plus rituximab compared with CHOP alone in elderly patients with diffuse large-B-cell lymphoma. *N Engl J Med* 2002;**346**:235–242.

73. Slamon DJ, Leyland-Jones B, Shak S, et al. Use of chemotherapy plus a monoclonal antibody against HER2 for metastatic breast cancer that overexpresses HER2. *N Engl J Med* 2001;**344**:783–792.

74. Swain SM, Whaley FS, Gerber MC, et al. Cardioprotection with dexrazoxane for doxorubicin-containing therapy in advanced breast cancer. *J Clin Oncol* 1997;**15**: 1318–1332.

75. Harris L, Batist G, Belt R, et al. Liposome-encapsulated doxorubicin compared with conventional doxorubicin in a randomized multicenter trial as first-line therapy of metastatic breast carcinoma. *Cancer* 2002;**94**:25–36.

76. Buzdar AU, Marcus C, Smith TL, et al. Early and delayed clinical cardiotoxicity of doxorubicin. *Cancer* 1985;**55**:2761–2765.

77. Gelman RS, Taylor SG. Cyclophosphamide, methotrexate, and 5-fluorouracil chemotherapy in women more than 65 years old with advanced breast cancer: The elimination of age trends in toxicity by using doses based on creatinine clearance. *J Clin Oncol* 1984;**2**:1404–1413.

78. Ibrahim NK, Frye DK, Buzdar AU, et al. Doxorubicin-based chemotherapy in elderly patients with metastatic breast cancer: tolerance and outcome. *Arch Intern Med* 1996;**156**: 882–888.

79. Begg CB, Carbone PP. Clinical trials and drug toxicity in the elderly: the experience of the Eastern Cooperative Oncology Group. *Cancer* 1983;**52**:1986–1992.

80. Giovanazzi-Bannon S, Rademaker A, Lai G, et al. Treatment tolerance of elderly cancer patients entered on to phase II clinical trials: An Illinois Cancer Center study. *J Clin Oncol* 1994;**12**:2447–2452.

81. Bastion Y, Blay JY, Divine M, et al. Elderly patients with aggressive non-Hodgkin's lymphoma: disease presentation, response to treatment, and survival—a Groupe d'Etude des Lymphomes de l'Adulte study on 453 patients older than 69 years. *J Clin Oncol* 1997;**15**:2945–2953.

82. Bertini M, Freilone R, Vitolo U, et al. P-VEBEC: A new 8-weekly schedule with or without rG-CSF for elderly patients with aggressive non-Hodgkin's lymphoma(NHL). *Ann Oncol* 1994;**5**:895–900.

83. Gomez H, Mas L, Casanova L, et al. Elderly patients with aggressive non-Hodgkin's lymphoma treated with CHOP chemotherapy plus granulocyte-macrophage colony-stimulating factor: Identification of two age subgroups with differing hematologic toxicity. *J Clin Oncol* 1998;**16**:2352–2358.

84. O'Reilly SE, Connors JM, Howdle S, et al. In search of an optimal regimen for elderly patients with advanced-stage diffuse large-cell lymphoma: results of a phase II study of P/DOCE chemotherapy. *J Clin Oncol* 1993;**11**:2250–2257.

85. Sonneveld P, Deridder M, Vanderlelie H, et al. Comparison of doxorubicin and mitoxantrone in the treatment of elderly patients with advanced diffuse non-Hodgkins-lymphoma using CHOP versus CNOP chemotherapy. *J Clin Oncol* 1995;**13**:2530–2539.

86. Tirelli U, Zagonel V, Serraino D, et al. Non-Hodgkins lymphomas in 137 patients aged 70 years or older—a retrospective European Organization for Research and Treatment of Cancer lymphoma group—study. *J Clin Oncol* 1988;**6**:1708–1713.

87. Zinzani PL, Storti S, Zaccaria A, et al. Elderly aggressive-histology non-Hodgkin's lymphoma: First-line VNCOP-B regimen experience on 350 patients. *Blood* 1999;**94**:33–38.

88. Morrison VA, Picozzi V, Scott S, et al. The impact of age on delivered dose intensity and hospitalizations for febrile neutropenia in patients with intermediate-grade non-Hodgkin's lymphoma receiving initial CHOP chemotherapy: a risk factor analysis. *Clin Lymphoma* 2001;**2**:47–56.

89. Gomez H, Hidalgo M, Casanova L, et al. Risk factors for treatment-related death in elderly patients with aggressive non-Hodgkin's lymphoma: Results of a multivariate analysis. *J Clin Oncol* 1998;**16**:2065–2069.

90. Zinzani PL, Pavone E, Storti S, et al. Randomized trial with or without granulocyte colony stimulating factor as adjunct to induction VNCOP-B treatment of elderly high-grade non-Hodgkin's lymphoma. *Blood* 1997;**89**:3974–3979.

91. Balducci L, Repetto L. Increased risk of myelotoxicity in elderly patients with non-Hodgkin lymphoma—the case for routine prophylaxis with colony-stimulating factor beginning in the first cycle of chemotherapy. *Cancer* 2004;**100**:6–11.

92. Balducci L, Corcoran MB. Antineoplastic chemotherapy of the older cancer patient. *Hematol Oncol Clin N Am* 2000;**14**:193–212.

93. Crivellari D, Bonetti M, Castiglione-Gertsch M, et al. Burdens and benefits of adjuvant cyclophosphamide, methotrexate, and fluorouracil and tamoxifen for elderly patients with breast cancer: The International Breast Cancer Study Group trial VII. *J Clin Oncol* 2000;**18**:1412–1422.

94. Stein BN, Petrelli NJ, Douglass HO, et al. Age and sex are independent predictors of 5-fluorouracil toxicity—analysis of a large-scale phase-III trial. *Cancer* 1995;**75**:11–17.

95. Popescu RA, Norman A, Ross PJ, et al. Adjuvant or palliative chemotherapy for colorectal cancer in patients 70 years or older. *J Clin Oncol* 1999;**17**:2412–2418.

96. Extermann M, Aapro M, Bernabei RB, et al. Use of comprehensive geriatric assessment in older cancer patients: Recommendations from the taskforce on CGA of the International Society of Geriatric Oncology (SIOG). *Crit Rev Oncol Hematol* 2005;**55**:241–252.

97. Aapro MS, Cameron DA, Pettengell R, et al. EORTC guidelines for the use of granulocyte-colony stimulating factor to reduce the incidence of chemotherapy-induced febrile neutropenia in adult patients with lymphomas and solid tumours. *Eur J Cancer* 2006;**42**:2433–2453.

98. Loadman PM, Bibby MC. Pharmacokinetic drug interactions with anticancer drugs. *Clin Pharmacokinet* 1994;500.

99. Lichtman SM, Wildiers H, Launay-Vacher V, et al. International Society of Geriatric Oncology (SIOG) recommendations for the adjustment of dosing in elderly cancer patients with renal insufficiency. *Eur J Cancer* 2007;**43**:14–34.

100. Wildiers H, Highley MS, de Bruijn EA, et al. Pharmacology of anticancer drugs in the elderly population. *Clin Pharmacokinet* 2003;**42**:1213–1242.

CHAPTER 17

Radiotherapy in Older Adults with Cancer

IAN KUNKLER

University of Edinburgh, Western General Hospital, Edinburgh, UK

17.1 INTRODUCTION

Cancer in elderly individuals, particularly over the age of 70, represents a growing healthcare challenge [1]. Cancer is predominantly a disease of the second half of life and with increasing life expectancy, and the proportion of individuals over the age of 75 is predicted to triple and over 85 years to double by 2030 [2]. The burden in this age group will rise inexorably. It is of note that the global increase in cancer in this age group is predominantly in the developing world. This is of relevance to radiation oncology because access to modern radiotherapy equipment is often limited in developing regions. Substantial and sustained investment in radiation oncology equipment and staffing will be needed to meet this challenge. The evidence base for radiation oncology, often included as part of multimodality therapy with surgery and systemic therapy, is well established for a wide range of solid tumors. This includes tumors of the CNS, head and neck, lung, breast, esophagus, bladder, prostate, testis, rectum, cervix, endometrium, and skin as well as the sarcomas.

The definition of what constitutes the threshold for defining patients as elderly is not agreed on. Previously the borderline between middle and old age was 65 years. The National Institute of Aging defined "elderly" as those in the age group of 65 years and older [3]. They provided three subgroups of the elderly: the young elderly (65–74 years), the older elderly (75–85 years), and the oldest elderly, over the age of 85 years. Life expectancy also needs to be taken into consideration. For a 70-year-old man, remaining life expectancy in the general population is about 14.2 years and for an 85-year-old man, 5.2 years [4].

This chapter focuses on the technical and clinical issues relevant to the management of older adults with solid tumors managed by the radiation oncologist. It does not deal with breast radiation in older patients, which is covered in Chapter 3.

Cancer and Aging Handbook: Research and Practice, First Edition. Edited by Keith M. Bellizzi and Margot A. Gosney.
© 2012 Wiley-Blackwell. Published 2012 by John Wiley & Sons, Inc.

17.2   CLINICAL ASSESSMENT OF OLDER PATIENTS IN RADIATION ONCOLOGY

Selection for radiation therapy with curative or palliative intent will take account of the stage of disease, general medical condition, any physical and psychological factors and risks of toxicity that may influence the safe delivery of radiotherapy. Robust methodologies are needed to differentiate patients suitable for radical radiotherapy and those for whom palliative radiotherapy [5] or supportive care alone may be more appropriate. Comorbidities rise with age and need to be carefully documented in the assessment process, as well as weight loss and performance status [6]. Those particularly relevant to radiation oncology are grouped in two categories [6]. In the first group comorbidity prevents radiotherapy being delivered. This includes dementia and Parkinson's disease for which the immobility required for treatment is impossible to achieve. Cognitive deficits may be sufficient to preclude patients being treated with external beam irradiation if they are not able to lie on the treatment couch without moving during treatment setup and beam ON time when the patient is alone in the treatment room. However, most patients without major cognitive deficits with the aid of immobilization devices (head or body shell) can be treated conventionally with external beam irradiation. Patients with rheumatological conditions of the cervical spine may not be able to achieve the hyperextension of the neck needed for some head and neck treatments. The second group includes underlying pathologies that are exacerbated by radiotherapy such as chronic cardiopulmonary disease. Respiratory function may be too poor to consider radical radiotherapy to the lung or oesophagus. In general a forced expiratory volume (FEV_1) of less than one liter (<1 L) is a contraindication to radical radiotherapy for these sites. Beams arrangements may have to be modified to avoid cardiac pacemakers. Occasionally they may have to be resited if their avoidance from the beam would compromise adequate irradiation of the clinical target volume.

In addition, there are logistical barriers that limit access to radiation therapy for older patients. These include difficulties with transport and social support. Attending for several weeks of treatment 5 days a week is burdensome. Patients may be dependent on family members to provide transport, which may be difficult for working relatives or older spouses or partners to provide. Hospitalizing the older patient may induce social isolation, anxiety, and depression [7], particularly when patients are separated from their normal family/social support structures. There is evidence that bias of the physician, patient, or patient's family or misunderstanding about the benefits and risks of treatment may compromise access to curative or palliative radiotherapy [8,9]. As with surgery and systemic therapy, older patients are less likely to receive standard radiation therapy [10]. The lower levels of radiotherapy (RT) in older patients may relate to beliefs that RT is less well tolerated in this age group [11]. However, there is no evidence of any systematic compromise of radiation planning and delivery in older patients [12]. As Pignon and Scalliet [11] point out, most patients treated with radiotherapy are old and tolerate the treatment well. However, historically most patients at least over the age of 70 were excluded from clinical trials. There is, therefore, little level I evidence to underpin best radiotherapy practice in older patients. We are largely dependent on retrospective series of older patients irradiated for cancers at different sites, with different age thresholds, reporting of morbidity, dose fractionation schedules, and variable periods of follow-up. As with all retrospective series, selection bias may be operating and firm conclusions on safety and efficacy may be difficult to draw.

In addition, there may be some publication bias against inconclusive studies that have attempted to relate age to different late radiation-induced toxicities [13]. There is a pressing need to establish clinical trials in older patients to strengthen the evidence base for best practice. In addition, there is a dearth of clinical guidelines for radiation therapy in older patients, which might contribute to standardizing practice in this age group.

17.3   TECHNOLOGICAL ADVANCES IN RADIATION ONCOLOGY

Avoidance of acute and late radiation-induced toxicity remains as important in older individuals as it does in their younger counterparts. There have been important advances in radiation oncology that have reduced the risks of radiation-induced toxicity. In modern radiotherapy practice the introduction of conformal CT-based radiotherapy planning with the beam collimated to minimize irradiation of surrounding normal tissue has reduced toxicity. This is well illustrated in a randomized trial of prostate cancer where limiting the dose to the rectum using conformal radiotherapy reduced the risks of acute and late rectal damage compared to standard pelvic irradiation [14]. Injection of contrast is often needed for CT planning, and care needs to be taken to ensure that renal function measured by creatinine clearance is adequate in older patients [6], particularly those who have diabetes or hypertension.

Similarly, the ability to modulate dynamically the fluence of the X-ray beam using intensity-modulated radiotherapy (IMRT) can diminish unwanted dose to critical structures such as radiosensitive structures (e.g., the parotid glands in head and neck cancer) and reduce disabling radiation induced xerostomia [15]. Techniques of extracranial stereotactic body irradiation have been introduced more recently [16]. These allow very focal irradiation of the clinical target volume to be achieved, while minimizing irradiation of adjacent normal structures (e.g., in the irradiation of small-volume non–small cell lung cancer in patients unfit for surgery). A number of linear accelerators with fully adapted stereotactic radiotherapy delivery systems are available (e.g., Novalis TX, Brain LAB, Elekta Axesse, Tomotherapy, and CyberKnife). Comorbidities often limit access to radiotherapy in older patients. The CyberKnife system, for example, is an image-guided robotic system in which a compact linear accelerator is mounted on a six-joint robotic arm (see Fig. 17.1). This allows flexibility in the generation of beam patterns and produces very conformal, nonisocentric plans with very sharp falloff in dose outside the planning target volume (Fig. 17.2). In a study of 345 cases of elderly patients treated with the CyberKnife from a single center predominantly for primary and metastatic liver tumors, head and neck cancer in previously irradiated sites, bone metastases, and primary non–small cell lung cancer, treatment was as well tolerated as in young patients [17]. The authors argue that the CyberKnife should be the preferred form of treatment in frail elderly patients, particularly because of the smaller number of treatment sessions.

17.4   MODIFICATION OF STANDARD RADIOTHERAPY
IN OLDER PATIENTS

Three key questions must to be addressed in considering any modification of radiation therapy in older patients [6]:

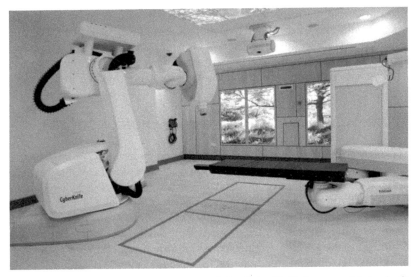

Figure 17.1   The major hardware components of the CyberKnife image-guided robotic stereotactic ablative radiotherapy system. (Reproduced by permission of Accuray Inc.)

Should the total dose be reduced?

Should the volume irradiated be reduced?

Should a hypofractionated (fewer doses of higher dose per fraction) regime be used?

Careful consideration should be given before reducing the conventional radical dose since for many tumors there is a dose–response relationship that may compromise local control [18,19]. There is little published information on the impact of reducing the irradiated volume in older patients. The risk of doing so may be a "geographic" miss and local failure, particularly at sites such as the prostate and lung, which are affected by physiological motion. There is some evidence that confining the irradiated volume to the gross tumor volume rather than allowing a margin for microscopic spread to generate a clinical target volume (CTV) improves tolerance in a small series of 57 nonagenarians treated by radical radiotherapy to a variety of primary sites [20].

Traditionally radical radiotherapy is conducted over 3–7 weeks for most solid tumors. However, efforts to shorten the duration of treatment by delivering fewer higher-dose treatments may actually result in lower local control rates due to inferior biological effects and greater late radiation induced toxicity or both [21]. With greater life expectancy, patients are increasingly likely to survive long enough to experience late treatment toxicity, which compromises quality of life. Few of these hypofractionated dose fractionation schedules have been submitted to clinical trial but have mainly been tested empirically and adopted. A difficult balance has to be struck between local control, survival, and treatment tolerance. Some hypofractionated regimes appear in nonrandomized studies to be comparable to standard longer conventionally fractionated radiotherapy. For example, patients treated by radiotherapy in two fractions of 7 Gy each with concomitant carboplatin for locally advanced non–small cell cancer who were over the age of 70 seemed to have outcomes similar to classical fractionation in younger patients [22].

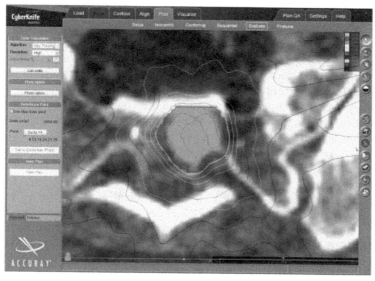

Figure 17.2 Axial slice from the CyberKnife plan of a sacral metastasis. The planning target volume is shown in red overlay. The treatment is prescribed to the 80% isodose (green line). The other isodose lines shown are 95% (red), 90% (orange), 70% (white), 60% (yellow), 50% (pink), 40% purple, 30% (light blue), 20% (blue), and 10% (dark blue). (Reproduced with permission from Martin A, Gaya A. Stereotactic body radiotherapy: A review. *Clin Oncol* 2010;**22**:157–172.)

17.4.1 Head and Neck Cancer

Head and neck cancer is a heterogeneous disease and commonest in the fifth and sixth decades of life. The highest incidence of many head and neck cancers is over the age of 70 years. For example, in a retrospective study undertaken by the Italian Geriatric Oncology Group, 12% (1112 in 9422) of head and neck cancers were in patients over the age of 70 years [23]. A higher estimate of 24% for head and neck cancer over the age of 70 is given by Muir et al. [24]. The three commonest primary sites in elderly patients are the larynx, oropharynx, and oral cavity [25]. Older patients are more likely to have locally advanced (T4) disease but fewer neck metastases [26] and to have second primary tumors (4% in a series of 331 patients from Institut Gustave Roussy, Paris over the age of 70 [25]. As with other cancer sites, the threshold age for the definition of "elderly" varies, and there is no consensus [27]. There are no head and radiotherapy trials specifically confined to the elderly population, so we have to extrapolate from trials that include but are not confined to an elderly group. Older patients tend to be less well represented in trials than in patients treated outside trials. Only 12% of the EORTC head and neck trials were over the age of 70 [28]. However, since the EORTC removed an age limit from radiotherapy protocols, in excess of half of radiotherapy trial protocols develop since 1995 have followed this recommendation [29].

Since the 1990s the intensity of treatment for head and neck cancer has increased with more extensive surgical resections, high-dose radiotherapy, and the addition of adjuvant chemotherapy, each with its own toxicities. This increase in intensity of treatment is a particular issue for older patients in whom the number of comorbidities (particularly hypertension and coronary insufficiency) rises with age. This presents the clinician with a dilemma as to whether treatment should be curative or palliative in intent and how issues of cure, toxicity, quality of life, and health economics should be balanced. The key question is whether treatment is radical or palliative in intent. Assessment of whether older patients are likely to be able to tolerate combined therapy requires a careful assessment of patient fitness. A number of studies have shown that radical surgery and radiotherapy can be safely carried out in older patients with significant morbidities without increasing the risk of complications [25] and that the response in older patients treated aggressively matches that in younger patients. However matters are complicated by the fact that in 4–10% of older patients treated with curative interest, the extent of disease is underestimated and patients die of an undetected second primary tumor [30].

Radiotherapy remains, with surgery, a key treatment modality for head and neck cancer either alone or in combination with surgery and chemotherapy. As a treatment that allows organ conservation and retention of normal physiological function (e.g., of swallowing), it is of particular benefit to older patients where comorbidities preclude surgery. Radical radiotherapy alone is curative for early-stage tumors of the larynx, tonsil, and base of tongue. The development of combination radiotherapy and chemotherapy to improve locoregional control and survival presents major issues of toxicity in older patients. Very careful pre-assessment is needed to ensure that patients are fit for treatment and that their general medical conditions and nutrition are addressed before, during, and after radiotherapy. Within the EORTC radiotherapy trials, albeit a highly selected population of fitter patients, there was no difference in tumor response to radiotherapy and in survival between older and younger patients [28].

17.4.2   Dose and Fractionation

In general, irradiation of the primary tumor and clinical lymphadenopathy requires a dose of ≥70 Gy to achieve tumor control. The conventional dose per fraction is 1.8 Gy. For subclinical microscopic disease in the neck in patients who have not undergone surgery, doses of ≥50 Gy were needed at doses of 2 Gy per fraction. For patients who have undergone surgery, normal vascularity of the tissues is reduced and higher doses of the order of 60–65 Gy are needed to achieve regional control. For patients treated with palliative intent, doses of the order of 30 Gy in 10–15 daily fractions are commonly used.

17.4.3   Altered Fractionation

Accelerated fractionation schedules have been designed to counter tumor proliferation during treatment. Two large European radiotherapy trials (EORTC 22851 [31], 22791) and a US trial (RTOG 90-03) [32] have evaluated hyperfractionation in head and neck cancer. In the EORTC trial 22851 [31] patients were included up to the age of 75 years with performance status ≤2. In the EORTC 22791 trial there was no stratification by age. Details of the age distribution of the trial were not included in the results of either trial. In the RTOG trial, half of the patients were over the age of 60 years. The locoregional control rate was improved in the accelerated and hyperfractionated schedules compared to conventional fractionated radiotherapy. However, it was at the expense of increase acute and late toxicity [32].

17.4.4 Side Effects of Radiotherapy

Studies of radiation-induced toxicity in older patients do not show any consistent pattern. In a series of patients from Institut Gustave Roussy, no differences were found in mucosal tolerance in older patients. The incidence of severe mucositis was 17% (57 of 331 cases). Of these cases, 54% (31 in 57) required nasogastric feeding [26].

17.4.5 Impact of Comorbidities on Local Control

Substantial comorbidity is associated with a higher incidence of complications after radical radiotherapy and impaired quality of life [33]. This may adversely affect local control. For example, the 5-year survival in patients with laryngeal cancer is reported to decline from 74% to 15% when major comorbidities are present [33].

17.4.6 Urological Cancer

Prostate Cancer Prostate cancer is the commonest cancer in older men [2] and, in the United States, has a median age at diagnosis of 68 years with its peak incidence in men 75 years or older [34]. In Germany radical prostatectomy is less likely to be offered to men over the age of 75 years, and radical radiotherapy is the only curative therapy [35]. In addition, radiation therapy is also used to palliate symptoms of advanced disease.

While there is no level I evidence underpinning the use of radical radiotherapy for prostate cancer in older patients, the risk of dying from prostate cancer for men aged 75–84 was minimally improved with radical prostatectomy or radical radiotherapy [36]. Patients treated by radical radiotherapy or radical prostatectomy between the ages of 65 and 80 in the Surveillance, Epidemiology, and End Results (SEER) database with low- or intermediate-risk prostate cancer had superior 5- and 10-year survival rates compared to a policy of "watchful waiting" [37]. Biochemical recurrence-free survival and toxicity from radical radiotherapy were similar for older and young patients. Indeed, patients ≥75 years had superior biochemical recurrence-free survival, despite controlling for tumor grade, stage, radiation dose, and pretreatment PSA [35]. If androgen deprivation is added to radical radiotherapy for high-risk prostate cancer, there is a higher risk of toxicity. Particular care should be taken before advocating this approach in older patients. Toxicity levels of this combined therapy vary between studies. However, where there are comorbidities, in particular a previous myocardial infarction, complications are more frequent [38].

Brachytherapy has theoretical advantages over external beam therapy in prostate cancer because of the brevity of treatment and potentially lower risk of complications. In addition, recuperation after brachytherapy may be faster than after surgery [39]. However, a much higher rate of urinary complication and requirements for invasive procedures was found in older patients in the SEER study of patients undergoing interstitial therapy during at least 2 years of follow-up [40].

Bladder Cancer Bladder cancer has a relatively poor prognosis reflecting aggressive biology, frequently advanced disease at presentation, old age, and associated comorbidities. The median age of onset is 70 years [41]. The peak incidence of urothelial cancer of the bladder is 85 years in California [42]. In the series of studies by Duncan and Quilty [43] of 900 patients from Edinburgh treated by radical radiotherapy, the mean age was 66 years.

Opinion is divided on the role of radical radiotherapy for invasive bladder cancer. For the large part this reflects the lack of randomized trials comparing outcomes of muscle invasive bladder cancer for cystectomy and for radical radiotherapy. For patients with bladder cancer invading muscle, radical radiotherapy offers equivalent long-term survival to cystectomy [44]. There is no established role for radiotherapy for noninvasive bladder cancer [45]. Radical cystectomy remains the curative treatment of choice for muscle invasive or refractory non-muscle-invasive bladder cancer in North America [46]. The advantage for the older patient with radiotherapy is that organ preservation is possible in 75% of long-term survivors [47]. Nonetheless, elderly patients with invasive bladder cancer fare poorly with only 11.6% achieving 5-year survival among 44 patients over the age of 79 treated by radical radiotherapy in a nonrandomized series [43]. In selected older patients where fitness to tolerate radical radiotherapy is uncertain, split-course therapy can be adopted. This allows all patients to receive a palliative dose of radiotherapy in the first phase of treatment. Only those patients tolerating the first phase proceed after a planned rest to a second phase so that the total dose is radical. This has the advantage of avoiding exposure to a radical dose for those patients experiencing significant toxicity from a palliative dose. In a series of 76 patients treated between 1987 and 1992, 25% of all patients, 36% of those completing treatment, and 51% who underwent follow-up cystoscopy had a complete response [48]. However, in other series the results of split-course radiotherapy have been inferior to conventional continuous radical radiotherapy [49,50].

17.4.7 Improvements in Delivery of Radiotherapy for Prostate and Bladder Cancer

Modern developments in radiotherapy have the potential for improving outcomes for radical radiotherapy for both bladder and prostate cancer. In the UK the gross tumor volume is normally the whole of the bladder plus a margin for subclinical disease. Partial bladder irradiation can allow some dose escalation with only 7% of patients experiencing relapse in the bladder [51]. However, the bladder is often difficult to identify accurately on cross-sectional imaging and may change shape during radiotherapy. Bladder filling may alter its shape, as may rectal filling [52]. A margin of 15–20 mm is normally added to create the clinical target volume to account for microscopic spread. However, inter- and intrafractional changes in the bladder are a persistent challenge for tumor localization. Predictive organ localization (A-POLO) is one approach being explored. The daily target volume and plan is chosen on an individual basis, based on the pattern of the patient's bladder filling [52], which tends to be consistent over time. These adaptive radiotherapy solutions need to be prospectively evaluated to assess their impact on local control and toxicity.

Organ motion is a problem for local radiotherapy of prostate cancer. The greatest movement is in the anteroposterior direction. Daily online imaging of the prostate during radiotherapy is desirable to account for differences in inter/intrafraction position of the prostate. Image-guided radiotherapy (IGRT) has the potential for improving the accuracy of radiotherapy delivery and local control. However, image acquisition, analysis, and repositioning is time-consuming. The CyberKnife is one form of IGRT that has software that allows the X-ray beam to track the target organ as it moves. Implanted fiducials in the prostate can be tracked using a stereoscopic X-ray system, with the beam adjusted by moving the head of the linear accelerator robotically. Hypofractionated schedules with the CyberKnife are possible with total doses of the order of 37–37.5 Gy at 7–7.5 Gy per fraction. Prospective studies are in progress to assess the role of the CyberKnife in this setting [53].

17.4.8 Pelvic Malignancy

Cervical Cancer While cancer of the cervix is predominantly a disease of young women, there is a late peak in women over the age of 70 years [54]. Localized cancers of the cervix are usually treated by a combination of intracavitary therapy and external beam irradiation. For more advanced disease, combined chemoradiotherapy has become standard. There is limited information on differences in local control and toxicity in older patients. In an analysis of the radiotherapy arm of 1619 patients with pelvic malignancy (uterine, anal, rectum, prostate, and bladder) included in nine EORTC trials, survival was comparable for cancer of the uterus in women in ages 55–70 and >70 years [55]. There was a trend toward older patients experiencing more diarrhea. When adjustment had been made for radiotherapy dose, acute urinary complications were observed equally in each age range. Complaints about sexual function before and after radiotherapy were marked in older patients. However, older patients did have partial recovery of sexual function. In a study of 398 patients with stage I–III cervical cancer treated with radical radiotherapy, local control equivalent to that in younger patients was achieved when comparable treatment was given [56]. Older age was not associated with an increase in acute and late complications.

However, in a study of younger patients with cervical cancer [≤64 years, young elderly (65–74 years) and older elderly patients (≥75 years)], no difference in disease specific survival or toxicity from radical radiotherapy was found in older patients [57].

Rectal Cancer About 80% of rectal cancers occur in the elderly population, with 50% over the age of 70 and 20% over the age of 80 years [58]. The treatment of stage III and IV rectal cancer involves surgical resection and preoperative or postoperative radiotherapy. In Europe strategies can be divided into preoperative radiotherapy alone (short course) or a combination of chemotherapy and radiotherapy (long course) [59]. The wide adoption of total mesorectal excision has substantially reduced rates of pelvic recurrence.

Only ~25% of older patients have been recruited into clinical trials of adjuvant therapy [60]. Meta-analyses have shown that preoperative radiotherapy has a significant, if modest, impact on survival, but no survival benefit has been demonstrated for postoperative radiotherapy [61,62]. Both preoperative and postoperative radiotherapy reduce the risk of local recurrence of rectal cancer. Martijn and Vulto [58] studied four trials of adjuvant peri-operative radiotherapy in which there was no age limit in the eligibility criteria. Two studies from Scandinavia compared surgery and surgery plus short-course preoperative radiotherapy (25 Gy in five daily fractions over 1 week). These demonstrated a reduction in local recurrence from preoperative radiotherapy. In the Stockholm I trial there was an increase in the postoperative mortality in patients ≥75 years [63,64], reflecting the large irradiated volume and the parallel opposed treatment technique. The causes of death were mainly cardiovascular and infective. In the Stockholm II trial [65] a smaller pelvic volume was irradiated using a multifield technique, and mortality was reduced to 20% compared to 8% in the Stockholm I trial. Martijn and Vulto [58] identified 10 population studies of the management of rectal cancer in relation to age. A number of these studies showed that older patients were less likely to receive radiotherapy. Paszat et al. [66] showed that patients over the age of 80 were less likely to receive radiotherapy after resection. In another study analyzing the use of radiotherapy with/without chemotherapy, patients ≥65 years were less likely to receive radiotherapy postoperatively or radiotherapy combined with chemotherapy if they were >69 years [67]. In an audit of the treatment of rectal cancer during 1995–2004 in Sweden [68], patients ≥75 years were less likely to receive preoperative radiotherapy (34.3% vs. 67.2%, $p = <0.001$).

While concerns among clinicians about radiotherapy-induced toxicity may explain lower rates of uptake of perioperative radiotherapy, age was not found to be a factor in increasing radiation-induced toxicity in the study by Pignon et al. [55]. Similar conclusions were drawn in an Italian retrospective study of adjuvant radiotherapy in patients ≥75 years [69]. It may be that comorbidities such as diabetes, hypertension, and vascular disease increase the risks of significant radiation-induced small bowel injury in older patients, but this remains uncertain.

In older, frail patients for whom chemotherapy is planned, preoperative radiotherapy (25 Gy in five fractions) with a delay of 6–8 weeks before surgery, significant tumor cytoreduction and a high proportion of RO resections were achieved with patients with T4 rectal cancer [70].

For older patients too frail for radical radiotherapy, short-course palliative radiotherapy (20–30 Gy in 5–10 daily fractions) may provide useful control of pain, rectal discharge, and bleeding.

17.4.9 Thoracic Malignancy

Lung Cancer Lung cancer is the principal cause of cancer mortality in Western countries. The median age at the time of diagnosis in the United States is 71 years, with 69% of patients ≥65 years and 36% ≥75 years [71]. Lung cancer has become more of an issue in the elderly population as, since the 1990s, mortality has fallen in patients under the age of 50 and risen in those 70 years and older [71]. However, older patients are less likely to receive standard care probably as a result of concerns about comorbidities and efficacy and toxicity of treatment. Comorbidities occur in nearly 70% of older patients compared to 50% in younger patients [72]. Radiotherapy has both a curative and palliative role for non-small cell lung cancer in this age group. The topic has been reviewed by Batymen et al and Redmond et al [73,74]. It is the most commonly applied treatment in the older age group [75], although most of the evidence for efficacy is drawn from retrospective series [73]. Level I evidence on the role of radiotherapy in older patients is extremely sparse. Only one randomized trial posing a radical radiotherapy question in this age group has been conducted [76]. The latter closed prematurely because of toxicity.

Non–Small Cell Lung Cancer (NSCLC) Radical radiotherapy alone in older patients can achieve a median survival of ≤37 months for stage I/II disease [77–80]. Much more limited survival (8 months) is achieved for stage III disease. Age per se is not an adverse prognostic factor for NSCLC treated by radical radiotherapy [81,82]. Combined analysis of a number of EORTC trials showed no difference in overall survival whether patients were under or ≥ 70 years [83]. Data are even more sparse on radical radiotherapy in octogenarians. One small study of 21 patients showed a response rate of 77% and an interruption free completion rate of 95% [84].

Doses of ≤ 66 Gy are well tolerated by older patients with grade 3/4 oesophagitis occurring in <4% [84–86]. No difference in acute or late radiation-induced toxicity was found in six EORTC radiotherapy trials in patients ≤ 70 years or >70 years [83].

For inoperable stage I non–small cell lung cancer, stereotactic body radiotherapy (SBRT) delivering a limited number of hypofractionated doses to a well-defined target with limited margins is an attractive new development on theoretical and practical grounds in older patients. The limited overall duration of therapy and low toxicity are benefits. A number of early-phase trials have been conducted without excluding older patients. Dose fractionation regimes have varied from 24 to 60 Gy in two to eight fractions with local control rates of 83–96% at 2–3 years [73]. Tolerance of SBRT among older patients seems to be good.

For locally advanced non–small cell lung cancer, concurrent chemoradiation is standard practice. However, no completed phase III trials have compared radiation alone versus chemoradiation. A Japanese clinical trial with this design (with daily carboplatin administration in the combined modality) was discontinued early because of four treatment-related deaths [76]. Retrospective series of combined modality therapy in general do not show any adverse effect of age on survival.

Small Cell Lung Cancer   The standard of care for limited-stage small cell lung cancer has been chemoradiation with four cycles of cisplatin and etoposide and thoracic irradiation to 45 Gy. In a subset analysis of the Intergroup 0096 trial on which this standard was based, there was a significant increase in grade 4 or 5 toxicity (61% vs. 84%, $p < 0.01$) and treatment-induced mortality (1% vs. 10%, $p = 0.01$) in patients over the age of 70 compared to those 70 years and younger [87]. To reduce toxicity, less intensive regimes of two cycles of carboplatin and etoposide with accelerated hyperfractionated radiotherapy (45 Gy in 1.5-Gy fractions twice daily) have been evaluated in phase II studies in older patients. A complete response rate of 57% and 2- and 5-year overall survival rates of 32% and 13%, respectively, have been reported with the chemoradiation schedule [88].

Whether older patients should be candidates for prophylactic whole-brain irradiation (PCI) after a complete response to chemoradiation is uncertain [74]. Patients treated with PCI are more likely to develop permanent neurocognitive deficits [89].

Palliative Radiotherapy for Lung Cancer   For both non–small cell and small cell lung cancer, palliative radiotherapy plays a valuable role in the relief of dyspnea, hemoptysis, and cough. Randomized trials examining different dose and fractionation regimes have produced conflicting results [90]. A meta-analysis [90] showed equivalent palliation of specific symptoms by high- and low-dose irradiation. However symptom scores after high-dose palliative radiotherapy were lower. While the 1 year overall survival improved by 4.8% by dose fractionation schedules of 35 Gy biological equivalent dose, levels of radiation induced oesophagitis were also higher.

17.4.10   Esophageal Cancer

Esophageal cancer is the sixth leading cause of cancer mortality worldwide, with a particularly high incidence in Japan. In Europe, North America, and Japan, the peak age is in the elderly population (70–79 years). Combined modality therapy with surgery, chemotherapy, and radiotherapy has been widely adopted. With the higher risks of complications from this combined approach, there is an understandable caution in applying the approach to older as well as younger patients. For example, in a small nonrandomized study of 34 patients aged ≥75 years [91] treated by full-dose chemoradiation for esophageal cancer during 2002–2008, acute grade ≥4 toxicity occurred in 38.2% of the patients, and 70.6% of the patients had to be hospitalized [91]. There were four treatment-related deaths. With a median follow-up of 14.5 months, median survival was only 12 months.

Despite recognition of the importance of including older patients in clinical trials, clinicians tend to be conservative, preferring less intensive treatment for older patients [92].

In a prospective nonrandomized trial from Japan [93], 51 patients ≥80 years [18 TI (35%) and 33 T2 (65%)] were treated by primary radiotherapy alone (66 Gy over 6.5 weeks). The planning target volume (PTV) was defined as the clinical target volume (CTV) plus a sufficient margin for organ motion and setup error. Prophylactic nodal irradiation was not permitted. Overall survival at 3 years was 39% with a median survival of 30 months. Actual grade ≥3 toxicity was 26%. These results are comparable to outcomes in younger patients. They reflect what is achievable in octogenarians when close attention is given to radiotherapy planning and delivery in this age group.

17.4.11 Brain Tumors

The incidence of brain tumors has been rising in older patients [94] and is highest among the 75–84-year age group [95]. Frailty, multiple comorbidities, and higher risk of radiation-induced neurotoxicity present major challenges. In addition, advanced age has been demonstrated to be an adverse prognostic factor in primary brain tumors in several trials of anaplastic astrocytomas and glioblastoma multiforme [96,97]. The poorer prognosis may be related to aggressive tumor biology or to characteristics of an older population [98]. However, older patients with favorable prognostic factors and good performance status should not be excluded from standard therapy on the basis of age alone. Surgery followed by postoperative radiotherapy provides the best treatment outcomes for malignant gliomas [99]. This was based on randomized trials of the Brain Tumor Study Group, which showed a survival advantage from radiotherapy compared to supportive care alone (median survival 36 vs. 14 weeks) [100]. However, while older patients were included in these trials, the specific benefit to older patients was uncertain [98]. A more recent retrospective analysis of 2836 patients over the age of 70 with glioblastoma from the SEER registry showed that radiotherapy significantly improved cancer-specific survival (HR 0.43,95% CI 0.38–0.49) after adjusting for surgery, tumor size, age at diagnosis, and ethnicity [101]. In a prospective randomized trial of GBM in patients >70 years, there was a limited survival benefit from radiotherapy compared to supportive care (29.1 weeks vs. 16.9 weeks) [102]. The dose chosen (50 Gy) was lower than the conventional dose (60 Gy), and it is unclear whether the lower dose would confer benefit similar to that in younger patients.

17.4.12 Hypofractionation

Hypofractionation, providing fewer doses at higher doses per fraction, has been explored. The total dose is reduced to combat the increased risk of neurotoxicity.

A randomized comparison of a shorter hypofractionated fractionation regime (40 Gy in 15 fractions) in patients with glioblastoma in patients over the age of 60 years compared to 60 Gy in 6 weeks showed no difference in median survival (5.1 vs. 5.6 months) [103]. The advantage to the shorter fractionation regime was that it was better tolerated and more patients completed treatment than with the longer regime. Quality of life measurements using the functional assessment of cancer therapy (FACT) scale were collected on 45% of the study population, which was insufficient to draw any meaningful conclusions. Short-course radiotherapy may therefore be appropriate for some older patients, particularly those with impaired performance status. For those with good performance status, 60 Gy over 6 weeks is a reasonable choice.

17.4.13 Lymphomas

Hodgkin's Disease Improvements in outcomes for Hodgkin's disease have come from combination chemotherapy and better radiotherapy techniques. However, improvements in survival have not extended to elderly patients. Advanced age at presentation is an independent poor prognostic factor in Hodgkin's disease. A number of reasons have been hypothesized for the adverse effect of age on outcome. These include more aggressive biology, increased comorbidity and intolerance of standard therapy, more severe toxicity, and treatment related mortality [104]. In a retrospective series of 4251 patients with Hodgkin's disease, older patients were more likely to have mixed cellularity disease, B symptoms, raised ESR, and poor performance status [105]. For early stage unfavourable Hodgkin's disease involved field (IF-RT) has been shown to be as effective as extended field radiotherapy (EF-RT) [106]. In a retrospective study of 1204 patients with HD randomized to four cycles of chemotherapy followed by radiotherapy (30 Gy extended field plus 10 Gy boost to bulky disease, or 30 Gy IF-RT plus 10 Gy) to bulk disease, freedom from treatment failure (64% vs. 87%), overall survival (70% vs. 94%) at 5 years was lower in older patients. Acute toxicity was higher with EF radiotherapy [107]. EF-RT should therefore be avoided in older patients.

Non-Hodgkin's Lymphoma In Europe and North America more than 50% of non-Hodgkin's lymphomas (NHL) occur in patients over the age of 65 years. NHL is a very heterogeneous disease. Old age has been identified as a poor prognostic factor with shorter overall and disease-free survival compared to younger patients matched for clinical and histological features [108,109]. The principles of the use of radiotherapy to sites of bulky disease after initial doxorubicin-based chemotherapy is underpinned by a phase III trial in intermediate/high-grade non-Hodgkin's lymphoma comparing eight cycles of cyclophosphamide, adriamycin, vincristine, and prednisolone (CHOP) or three cycles of CHOP followed by involved field radiotherapy (40–55 Gy) showing both treatment regimes are effective [110]. Nearly half the patients were over the age of 60. In a retrospective nonrandomized single institutional series of 205 NHL over the age of 80, their characteristics and prognostic factors were similar to those of younger patients. However, the median survival was only 2.2 years. The principal cause of death was disease progression, implying that this group of patients had been undertreated. The principles of combined modality therapy should therefore be applied equally to both older and younger patients.

17.5 SUMMARY AND CONCLUSIONS

The elderly population potentially benefiting from radical and palliative radiotherapy is growing rapidly. However, there are few randomized trials specifically addressing the benefits in terms of locoregional control and survival of radical (curative) radiotherapy in older cancer patients. There are important advances in radiation technology (such as intensive modulated radiotherapy and stereotactic body irradiation) that may reduce radiation-induced toxicity and/or shorten the duration of treatment. Prospective clinical trials are needed to evaluate the impact of these new technologies in the older population on loco-regional control, survival, and quality of life. The evidence base for radiotherapy in older patients was reviewed for a wide range of solid tumors in this chapter.

REFERENCES

1. Lamont DW, Gillis CR, Caird FI. Epidemiology of cancer. In Caird FI, Brewin TB, eds. *Cancer in the Elderly*, London, 1990, p. 915.
2. Jemal A, Siegel R, Ward E et al. Cancer statistics. *CA Cancer J Clin* 2007;**57**:43–66.
3. Parker SL, Tong T, Bolden S, et al. Cancer statistics. *CA Cancer J Clin* 1997;**47**:5–27.
4. Yancik R, Ries LA, Cancer in older persons, magnitude of the problem—how we apply what we know? *Cancer* 1994;**74**:1995–2003.
5. Havlik RJ, Yancik R, Long S, et al. The National Institute on Aging and the National Cancer Institute SEER collaborative study on comorbidity and early diagnosis of cancer in the elderly. *Cancer* 1994;**74**:2101–2106.
6. Durdux C, Boisserie T, Gisselbrecht M. Radiation therapy in elderly subjects. *Cancer Radiother* 2009;**13**:609–614.
7. Peters L, Sellick K. Quality of life of cancer patients receiving inpatient and home-based palliative care. *J Adv Nurs* 2006;**53**:524–533.
8. Berkman B, Rohan B, Sampson S. Myths and biases related to cancer in the elderly. *Cancer* 1994;**74**:2004–2008.
9. Newcomb PA, Carbone PP. Cancer treatment and age: Patient perspectives. *J Natl Cancer Inst* 1993;**85**:1580–1584.
10. Mor V, Masterson-Allen S, Goldberg RJ, et al. Relationship between age at diagnosis and treatment received by cancer patients. *J Am Geriatr Soc* 1985;**33**:585–589.
11. Pignon T, Scalliet P. Radiotherapy in the elderly. *Crit Rev Oncol Hematol* 1998;**27**: 129–130.
12. Steinfield AD, Diamond JJ, Hanks GE et al. Patient age as a factor in radiotherapy. Data from the patterns of care study. *J Am Geriatr Soc* 1989;**17**:335–338.
13. Scalliet P. Radiotherapy in the elderly. *Eur J Cancer* 1991;**27**:3–5.
14. Dearnaley DP, Khoo VS, Norman AR. Comparison of side effects of conformal and conventional radiotherapy in prostate cancer: A randomised trial. *Lancet* 1999;**353**:267–272.
15. Eisbruch A. Radiotherapy: IMRT reduces xerostomia and improves quality of life. *Nat Rev Clin Oncol* 2009;**6**:567–568.
16. Martin A, Gaya A. Stereotactic body radiotherapy: A review. *Clin Oncol* 2010;**22**: 157–172.
17. Dewas S, Dewas-Vautravers C, Servent V et al. Results and special considerations when treating elderly patients with Cyberknife: A review of 345 patients. *Crit Rev Oncol Haematol* 2011;**79**:308–314.

18. Giraud P, Helfre S, Lavole A et al. Non-small cell bronchial cancers Improvement in chance of survival with conformational radiotherapy. *Cancer Radiother* 2002;**7**:125s–34s.

19. Zelefsky MJ, Leibel SA, Gaudin PB et al. Dose escalation with three-dimensional conformal radiation therapy affects the outcome in prostate cancer. *Int J Radiat Oncol Biol Phys* 1998;**41**:491–500.

20. Ikeda H, Ishikura S, Oguchi M, et al. Analysis of 57 nonagenarians cancer patients treated by radical radiotherapy: A survey of eight institutions. *Jpn J Clin Oncol* 1999;**29**:378–381.

21. Scalliet P, Pignon T. Radiotherapy in the elderly. In Balducci L, Lyman G, Erschler W, eds. *Comprehensive Geriatric Oncology*. Harwood Academic, London, 1996.

22. Donato V, Zurio A, Bonfilli P. Hypofractionated radiation therapy for advanced non-small cell lung cancer. *Tumori* 1999;**85**:174–176.

23. Olmi P, Ausili-Cefaro G, Loreggian L. Radiotherapy in the elderly with head and neck cancer. *Rays* 1997;**22**:77–81.

24. Muir CS, Fraumeni JF Jr, Doll R. The interpretation of time trends. *Cancer Surv*. 1994;**19–20**:5–21.

25. Metges JP, Eschwege F, de Crevoisier R, et al. Radiotherapy in head and neck cancer in the elderly: A challenge. *Crit Rev Oncol Hematol* 2000;**34**:195–203.

26. Lusinchi A, Bourhis J, Wibault P, et al. Radiation therapy for head and neck cancers in the elderly. *Int J Radiat Oncol Biol Phys* 1990;**18**:819–823.

27. Syrigos KN, Karachalios D, Karapanagiotou EM, et al. Head and neck cancer in the elderly: An overview on the treatment modalities. *Cancer Treat Rev* 2009;**35**:237–245.

28. Pignon T, Horiot JC, Van den Bogaert W, et al. No age limit for radical radiotherapy in head and neck tumours. *Eur J Cancer* 1996;**32A**:2075–2081.

29. Horiot JC. Radiation therapy and geriatric oncology patient. *J Clin Oncol* 2007;**25**: 1930–1935.

30. Lippmann SM, Hong WK. Second malignant tumors in head and neck squamous cell carcinoma: The overshadowing threat for patients with early stage disease. *Int J Radiat Oncol Biol Phys* 1989;**17**:691–694.

31. Horiot JC, Bontemps P, van den Bogaert W, et al. Accelerated fractionation (AF) compared to conventional fractionation (CF) improves loco-regional control in the radiotherapy of advanced head and neck cancers: results of the EORTC 22851 randomized trial. *Radiother Oncol* 1997;**44**:111–1121.

32. Fu KK, Pajak RF, Trotti A, et al. Radiotherapy Therapy Oncology Group (RTOG) phase III randomised study to compare hyperfractionation and two variants of accelerated fractionation to standard fractionation radiotherapy for head and neck squamous cell carcinoma: first report of RTOG 9003. *Int J Radiat Oncol Biol Phys* 2000;**48**:7–16.

33. Grenman R, Chevalier D, Gregoire V, et al. Treatment of head and neck cancer in the elderly. European Consensus (panel 6) of the EUFOS Congress in Vienna 2007. *Eur Arch Otorhinolaryngol* 2010;**267**:1619–1621.

34. Horner MJ, Ries LAG, Krapcho M, Neyman N, Aminou R, Howlader N, Altekruse SF, Feuer EJ, Huang L, Mariotto A, Miller BA, Lewis DR, Eisner MP, Stinchcomb DG, Edwards BK, eds. *SEER Cancer Statistics Review 1975–2006*, National Cancer Institute, Bethesda, MD, 2000 (http://seer.cancer.gov/csr/1975_2006/, based on 11/08 SEER data submission, posted to SEER website in 2009).

35. Geinitz H, Zimmermann FB, Thamm R, et al. 3D conformal radiation therapy for prostate cancer in elderly patients. *Radiother Oncol* 2005;**76**:27–34.

36. Hoffman R, Barry M. Health outcomes in older men localised prostate cancer: Results from prostate cancer outcomes study. *Am J Med* 2006;**119**(5):418–425.

37. Wong Y, Mitra N, Hudes G. Survival associated with treatment vs observation of localized prostate cancer. *JAMA* 2006;**296**:2683–2693.

38. D'Amico A, Chen M, Renshaw A, et al. Comorbidities affect benefit of combined radiation, androgen suppression. *Proc 2008 Genitourinary Cancer Symp.*, San Francisco, Feb. 2008 (Abstract 11).

39. Sandhu A, Mundt AJ. Radiation therapy for urologic malignancies in the elderly. *Urol Oncol: Semin Orig Investig* 2009;**27**:643–652.

40. Chen A, D'Amico A, Neville B, et al. Patient and treatment factors associated with complications after brachytherapy. *J Clin Oncol* 2006;**24**:5298–5304.

41. Messing EM. Urothelial tumors of the bladder. In Wein AJ, Kavoussi LR, Novick AC, Partin AW, Peters CA, eds. *Campbell Walsh Urology*, 9th ed., Saunders-Elsevier, Philadelphia. 2008, Chap. 75, pp. 2407–2446.

42. Schultzel M, Saltzstein SL, Downs TM, et al. Late age (85 or older) peak incidence of bladder cancer. *J Urol* 2008;**79**:1302–1305.

43. Duncan W, Quilty PM. The results of a series of 963 patients with transitional cell carcinoma of the urinary bladder primarily treated by radical megavoltage X-ray therapy. *Radiother Oncol* 1986;**7**:299–300.

44. Kotwal S, Choudhury A, Johnston C, et al. Similar treatment outcomes for radical cystectomy and radical radiotherapy in invasive bladder cancer treated at a United Kingdom specialist treatment centre. *Int J Radiat Oncol Biol Phys* 2008;**70**:456–463.

45. Harland SJ, Kynaston H, Grigor K, et al. A randomised trial of radical radiotherapy for management of pTI3 NX M0 transitional cell carcinoma of the bladder. *J Urol* 2007;**178**:807–813.

46. Shariat F, Shariat MD, Milowsky M, et al. Bladder cancer in the elderly. *Urol Oncol* 2009;**27**:653–667.

47. Shipley WU, Kaufman DS, Tester WJ, et al. Overview of bladder cancer trials in the Radiation Oncology Group. *Cancer* 2003;**97**(Suppl 8):2115–2119.

48. Phillips HA, Howard GCW. Split course radical radiotherapy for bladder cancer in the elderly. Nonsense or commonsense? A report of 76 patients. *Clin Oncol* 1996;**8**:35–38.

49. Salminem E. Split-course radiotherapy for urinary bladder cancer. *Radiother Oncol* 1989;**15**:327–331.

50. Davidson SE, Symonds RP, Snee MP, et al. Assessment of factors influencing the outcome of radiotherapy for bladder cancer. *Br J Urol* 1990;**66**:288–293.

51. Cowan RA, McBain CA, Ryder WD, et al. Radiotherapy for muscle invasive cancer of the bladder: results of a randomised trial comparing conventional whole bladder with dose-escalated partial bladder radiotherapy. *Int J Radiat Oncol Biol Phys* 2004;**59**:197–207.

52. Button MR, Staffurth JN. Clinical application of image-guided radiotherapy in bladder and prostate cancer. *Clin Oncol* 2010;**22**:698–706.

53. Townsend N, Huth B, Ding W, et al. Acute toxicity after Cyberknife-delivered hypofractionated radiotherapy for prostate cancer. *Am J Clin Oncol* 2011;**34**:6–10

54. See www.cancerresearchuk.org/cancerstats/types/cervix/incidence.

55. Pignon T, Horiot JC, Bolla M, et al. Age is not a limiting factor for radical radiotherapy in pelvic malignancies. *Radiother Oncol* 1997;**42**:107–120.

56. Mitchell PA, Waggoner S, Rotmensch J, et al. Cervical cancer in the elderly treated with radiation therapy. *Gynecol Oncol* 1998;**71**:291–298.

57. Ikushima H, Takegawa Y, Osaki K, et al. Radiation therapy for cervical cancer in the elderly. *Gynaecol Oncol* 2007;**7**:339–343.

58. Martijn H, Vulto JCM. Should radiotherapy be avoided or delivered differently in elderly patient with rectal cancer? *Eur J Cancer* 2007;**43**:2301–2306.

59. Papmichael D, Audisio R, Horiot JC, et al. Treatment of the elderly colorectal cancer patient: SIOG expert recommendations. *Ann Oncol* 2009;**20**:5–16.

60. Talarico L, Chen G, Pazdur R. Enrollment of elderly patients in clinical trials for cancer drug registration: A 7-year experience by the US Food and Drug Administration. *J Clin Oncol* 2004;**22**:4626–4631.

61. Camma C, Giunta M, Fiorica F, et al. Preoperative radiotherapy for resectable rectal cancer: a metanalysis. *JAMA* 2000;**284**:1008–1015.

62. Colorectal Cancer Collaborative Group. Adjuvant radiotherapy for rectal cancer: A systematic overview of 8507 patients from 22 randomised trials. *Lancet* 2001;**358**:1291–304.

63. Cedermark B, Johansson H, Rutqvist LE, et al. The Stockholm I trial of preoperative short term radiotherapy in operable rectal carcinoma. A prospective randomised trial. Stockholm Colorectal Cancer Study Group. *Cancer* 1995;**75**:2269–2275.

64. Marjnen CA, Kapitejn D, van de Velde CH, et al. Acute side effects and complications after short-term preoperative radiotherapy combined with total mesorectal excision in primary rectal cancer: Report of a multicentre randomized trial. *J Clin Oncol* 2002;**20**:817–825.

65. Folkesson J, Birgisson H, Pahlman L, et al. Swedish Rectal Cancer Trial: longlasting benefits from radiotherapy on survival and local recurrence rate. *J Clin Oncol* 2005;**23**: 5644–5650.

66. Paszat LF, Brundage MD, Groome PA et al (1999). A population-based study of rectal cancer: permanent colostomy as an outcome. *Int J Radiat Oncol Biol Phys* 1999;**45**: 1185–1191.

67. Schrag D, Gelfand SE, Bach PB, et al. Who gets adjuvant treatment for stage II and III rectal cancer? Insight from surveillance, epidemiology and end results—Medicare. *J Clin Oncol* 2001;**19**:3712–3718.

68. Jung B, Pahlman L, Johansson R, et al. Rectal cancer treatment and outcome in the elderly: An audit based on the Swedish rectal cancer registry 1995–2004. *BMC Cancer* 2009;**9**:68.

69. Fiorica F, Cartei F, Carau B, et al. Adjuvant radiotherapy on older and oldest elderly rectal cancer patients. *Arch Gerontol Geriatr* 2009;**49**:54–59.

70. Radu C, Berglund K, Pahlman L et al. Short course preoperative radiotherapy with delayed surgery in rectal cancer: a retrospective study. *Radiother Oncol* 2008;**87**:343–349.

71. Owonikoko TK, Ragin CC, Belani CP et al. Lung cancer in elderly patients: An analysis of the surveillance, epidemiology and end results database. *J Clin Oncol* 2007;**25**:5570–5577.

72. Janssen-Heijnen ML, Schipper RM, et al. Prevalence of co-morbidity in lung cancer patients and its relation with treatment: A population-based study. *Lung Cancer* 1998;**21**: 105–113.

73. Bayman N, Alam N, Faivre-Finn C. Radiotherapy for lung cancer in the elderly. *Lung Cancer* 2010;**68**:129–136.

74. Redmond KJ, Song DY. Thoracic irradiation in the elderly. *Thor Surg Clin* 2009;**19**:391–400.

75. Smith TJ, Penberthy L, Desch CE, et al. Differences in initial treatment patterns and outcomes of lung cancer in the elderly. *Lung Cancer* 1995;**13**:235–252.

76. Atagi S, Kawahara M, Tamura T, et al. Standard thoracic radiotherapy with or without concurrent daily low-dose carboplatin in elderly patients with locally advanced non-small cell lung cancer: A phase III trial of the Japan Clinical Oncology Group (JCO9812). *Jpn J Clin Oncol* 2005;**35**:195–201.

77. Lonardi F, Coeli M, Pavanato G, et al. Radiotherapy for non-small cell lung cancer in patients aged 75 and over: safety, effectiveness and possible impact on survival. *Lung Cancer* 2000;**28**:43–50.

78. San Jose S, Arnaiz MD, Lucas A, et al (2006). Radiation therapy alone in elderly with early stage non-small cell lung cancer. *Lung Cancer* 2006;**52**:149–154.

79. Tombolini V, Bonanni A, Donato V, et al. Radiotherapy alone in elderly patients with medically inoperable stage IIIa and IIIb non-small cell lung cancer. *Cancer Res* 2000;**20**: 4929–4933.

80. Furuta M, Hayakawa K, Katano S, et al. Radiation therapy for stage I-II non-small cell lung cancer in patients aged 75 years and older. *Jpn J Clin Oncol* 1996;**26**:97–98.

81. Aristibal SA, Meyerson M, Caldwell WI, et al. Age as a prognostic indicator in carcinoma of the lung. *Radiology* 1976;**121**:721–723.

82. Palma DA, Tyldesley S, Sheehan F, et al. Stage I non-small cell lung cancer (NSCLC) in patients aged 75 years or older. Does age determine survival after radical treatment? *J Thor Oncol* 2010;**5**:818–824.

83. Pignon T, Gregor A, Schaake Koning C, et al. Age has no impact on acute and late toxicity of curative thoracic radiotherapy. *Radiother Oncol* 1998;**46**:2399–2448.

84. Zachariah B, Balducci L, Venkattaramanabalaji GV, et al. Radiotherapy for cancer patients age 80 or older: A study of effectiveness and side effects. *Int J Radiat Oncol Biol Phys* 1997;**39**:1125–1129.

85. Pergolizzi S. Santacaterina A, Renzis CD, et al. Older people with non-small cell lung cancer in clinical stage IIIA and co-morbid conditions. Is curative radiation feasible? Final results of a prospective study. *Lung Cancer* 2002;**37**:201–206.

86. Yu HM, Liu YF, Yu JM, et al. Involved field radiotherapy is effective for patients 70 years or older with early stage non-small cell lung cancer. *Radiother Oncol* 2008;**87**:29–34.

87. Yuen AR, Zou G, Turrisi GT, et al. Similar outcome of elderly patients in Intergroup trial 0096: Cisplatin, etoposide, and thoracic radiotherapy administered once or twice daily in limited stage small cell lung carcinoma. *Cancer* 2000;**89**:1953–1960.

88. Jeremic B, Shibamoto Y, Acimovic L, et al. Carboplatin, etoposide and accelerated hyper-fractionated radiotherapy for elderly patients with limited small cell lung carcinoma: A phase II study. *Cancer* 1998;**82**:836–841.

89. Crossen JR, Garwood D, Glatstein E, et al. Neurobehavioral sequelae of cranial irradiation in adults: A review of radiation induced encephalopathy. *J Clin Oncol* 1994;**12**:627–642.

90. Fairchild A, Harris K, Barnes E, et al. Palliative thoracic radiotherapy for lung cancer: A systematic review. *J Clin Oncol* 2008;**26**:4001–4011.

91. Mak RH, Mamon HJ, Miyamoto DT, et al. Toxicity and outcomes after chemoradiation for esophageal cancer in patients aged 75 or older. *Dis Esophagus* 2010;**23**:316–323.

92. Kawashima M, Ikeda H, Yorozu A, et al. Multi-institutional survey of radiotherapy for octogenarian squamous cell carcinoma of the thoracic esophagus: Comparison with the results of surgery reported from Japan. *Nippon Igaka Houshasen Gakkai Zasshi* 1999;**50**:72–78.

93. Kawashima M, Kagami Y, Toita T, et al. Prospective trial of radiotherapy for patients 80 years of age or older with squamous cell carcinoma of the thoracic esophagus. *Int J Radiat Oncol Biol Phys* 2006;**64**:1112–1121.

94. Greg NH, Ries LG, Yancik R, et al. Increasing annual incidence of primary malignant brain tumours in the elderly. *J Natl Cancer Inst* 1998;**82**:1621–1624.

95. Central Brain Tumor Registry of the United States. *2009 CBTRUS Statistical Report: Primary Brain and Central Nervous System Tumors Diagnosed in the United States in 2004-5* (available at http//www.cbtrus.org/reports/2009-NPCR-04-05/ CBTRUS-NPCR2004-2005-Report-pdf).

96. Chang CH, Horton J, Schoenfeld D, et al. Comparison of postoperative radiotherapy and combined postoperative radiotherapy and chemotherapy in the multidisciplinary management of malignant gliomas. A joint Radiation Therapy Oncology Group and Eastern Cooperative Oncology Group study. *Cancer* 1983;**52**:997–1007.

97. Shapiro WR, Geen SB, Burger PC, et al. Randomised trials of three chemotherapy regimens and two radiotherapy regimens in postoperative treatment of malignant glioma. *J Neurosurg* 1998;**71**:1–9.

98. Nayak L, Iwamoto FM. Primary brain tumors in the elderly. *Curr Neurol Neurosci Rep* 2010;**10**:252–258.

99. Hochberg FH, Pruitt A. Assumptions in the radiotherapy of glioblastoma. Assumptions in the radiotherapy of glioblastoma. *Neurology* 1980;**30**:907–911.

100. Walker MD, Alexander E Jr, Hunt WE, et al. Evaluation of BCNU and/or radiotherapy in the treatment of anaplastic gliomas. A cooperative clinical trial. *J Neurosurg* 1978;**49**:333–343.

101. Scott J, Tsai Y-Y, Chinnaiyan P, et al. Effectiveness of radiotherapy for elderly patients with glioblastoma. *Int J Radiat Oncol Biol Phys* 2011;**81**:206–210

102. Keime-Guibert F, Chinot GO, Taillandier L, et al. Radiotherapy for glioblastoma in the elderly. *N Engl J Med* 2007;**356**:1527–1535.

103. Roa W, Brasher PM, Bauman G, et al. Abbreviated course of radiation therapy in older patients with glioblastoma multiforme: A prospective randomized clinical trial. *J Clin Oncol* 2004;**22**:1583–1588.

104. Wedein C, Bjorkholm M, Biberfeld P, et al. Prognostic factors in Hodgkin's disease with special reference to age. *Cancer* 1984;**52**:1202–1208.

105. Engert A, Ballova V, Haverkamp H, et al. Hodgkin's lymphoma in elderly patients: A comprehensive retrospective analysis from the German Hodgkin's study group. *J Clin Oncol* 2005;**23**:5052–5060.

106. Engert A, Schiller P, Josting A, et al. Involved field radiotherapy is equally effective and less toxic compared with extended-field radiotherapy after 4 cycles of chemotherapy in patients with early-stage unfavourable Hodgkin's lymphoma: Results of the HD8 trial of the German Hodgkin's Lymphoma Study Group. *J Clin Oncol* 2003;**21**:3601–3608.

107. Klimm B, Eich HT, Haverkamp H, et al. Poorer outcome of elderly patients treated with extended-field radiotherapy compared with involved-field radiotherapy after chemotherapy for Hodgkin's lymphoma: An analysis from the German Hodgkin Study Group. *Ann Oncol* 2007;**18**:357–363.

108. Dixon DO, Neilan B, Jones SE, et al. Effect of age on therapeutic outcome in advanced diffuse histiocytic lymphoma: The South West Oncology Group experience. *J Clin Oncol* 1986;**4**:295–305.

109. d'Amore F, Brincker H, Christiansen BE, et al. Non-Hodgkin's lymphoma in the elderly. A study of 602 patients aged 70 or older from a Danish population based registry. The Danish LYEO-Study Group. *Ann Oncol* 1992;**3**:379–386.

110. Miller TP, Dahlberg S, Cassady R, et al. Chemotherapy alone compared with chemotherapy plus radiotherapy for localised intermediate and high grade non-Hodgkin's lymphoma. *N Eng J Med* 1998;**339**:21–26.

PART V

COMMON CANCERS IN THE ELDERLY

CHAPTER 18

Breast Cancer

LAURA BIGANZOLI and CATHERINE OAKMAN
Hospital of Prato, Prato, Italy

RICCARDO A. AUDISIO
St. Helens Teaching Hospital, Merseyside, UK

IAN KUNKLER
University of Edinburgh, Western General Hospital, Edinburgh, UK

18.1 INTRODUCTION

Worldwide, nearly a third of breast cancer cases occur in patients over the age of 65 years [1]. In more developed countries this proportion rises to more than 40% [1]. The population is aging because of improvements in healthcare and nutrition. Given the relationship between breast cancer incidence and age, breast cancer will be an increasingly common diagnosis as the absolute number of women over age 65, and even over 85 years, grows.

Awareness of the need for recommendations to ensure optimal, individualized treatment of older women with breast cancer is increasing. Attempts have been made by several organizations, including the International Society of Geriatric Oncology (SIOG) [2] and the National Comprehensive Cancer Network (NCCN) [3], to create recommendations. However, several obstacles have been identified. Few women older than 65 years are included in randomized clinical trials; thus reliable data of treatment efficacy and toxicity in this population are lacking. Functional status, social support, the presence of comorbidities, and estimations of life expectancy must be considered to maximize benefit and minimize risk for these patients. Exploration of patient expectations is a key component in management.

18.2 GENERAL ASPECTS OF BREAST CANCER

18.2.1 Tumor Biology

Older women have characteristic differences in the biology of breast cancer compared with younger women. Advanced age at diagnosis of breast cancer is associated

Cancer and Aging Handbook: Research and Practice, First Edition. Edited by Keith M. Bellizzi and Margot A. Gosney.
© 2012 Wiley-Blackwell. Published 2012 by John Wiley & Sons, Inc.

with more favorable tumor biology, evidenced by increased hormone sensitivity, lower expression of the human epidermal growth factor receptor 2 (HER2), and lower grades and proliferative indices [4]. Nevertheless, breast cancer in most elderly patients is diagnosed at a more advanced clinical stage with a higher rate of large primary tumors, locally advanced disease, and metastatic disease [5].

Prognostic factors retain the same significant value in older and younger postmenopausal patients. Tumor size, lymph node status, histological grade, presence or absence of vascular invasion, estrogen receptor (ER) and progesterone receptor (PgR) status, HER2 status, and the tumor proliferative rate are all important parameters to be considered when estimating the risk of relapse. Of note, 20–30% of older patients have an aggressive biological phenotype, characterized by lack of ER and PgR expression. There are indications that in contrast with younger patients in whom HER2-positive tumors are associated with ER-negative status, HER2-positive tumors in elderly woman are paradoxically ER-positive [6].

Some studies suggest that breast cancers are not less aggressive in older versus younger women. A single institution analysis by Singh et al. of 2136 postmastectomy patients who did not undergo systemic adjuvant therapy showed that the likelihood of developing distant metastases was significantly higher among elderly women compared with younger women, even for similar tumor biology [7]. Additional studies are required to evaluate the biological properties of breast tumors in older and younger women, and to investigate the influence of host-related characteristics, such as age and the presence of comorbidities, on tumor growth.

18.2.2   Patient Life Expectancy

Life expectancy is better predicted by health status than age alone; therefore, function and comorbidities should be taken into account. Different instruments have been developed to estimate life expectancy. Lee et al. developed and validated a potentially useful prognostic tool for clinicians to estimate 4-year mortality risk in which each patient is stratified into high, intermediate, or low risk of mortality, based on age, gender, self-reported comorbid conditions, and functional measures [8]. Ravdin et al. developed a computer program (www.adjuvantonline.com) to estimate prognosis and the benefits of chemotherapy and/or endocrine therapy [9]. In this program, relapse-free and overall survival are estimated on the basis of age, the effects of comorbidity, and standard biological features. This is the only tool that can estimate both breast cancer–specific mortality and death from other causes for individual patients. However, it is critical to note that the prognostic and predictive estimates are derived from data for younger women, aged 36–69 years, from the Surveillance, Epidemiology and End Results (SEER) database and Early Breast Cancer Trialists' Collaborative Group 2000 Overview, respectively.

18.2.3   Breast Cancer Mortality and Competing Causes of Death

The mortality burden of breast cancer increases with increasing age. The percentage of women in the United States 50 and 70 years old who will die of breast cancer within 10 years is 0.4% and 0.9%, respectively [10].

Competing causes of death assume a large role in determining survival in older breast patients. An analysis of data from the SEER database for approximately 400,000 patients with breast cancer diagnosed between 1973 and 2000 found that as the age of diagnosis increased, the risk for death from breast cancer decreased relative to the risk for death from other causes. However, among patients aged 70 years or older, death from breast cancer still accounted for a significant percentage of mortality, especially in patients with high-risk disease [11].

Satariano and Ragland performed a population-based study of 3-year mortality rates of approximately 1000 women with breast cancer and identified comorbidity as a strong predictor of survival independent of age, disease stage, tumor size, treatment, race, and social/behavioral factors [12]. Women with three or more particular comorbid medical diagnoses had a 20-fold increase in non-breast-cancer-related death and a fourfold increase in all-cause mortality compared with breast cancer patients with no comorbid conditions. The issue of comorbidities is often coupled with the challenge of polypharmacy and important potential drug interactions.

18.2.4 Patient Assessment

It is of key importance to quantify the risk that individual patients have of dying from breast cancer, or developing symptoms due to local or systemic relapse or progression, or treatment side effects, within their estimated lifetime. The risk of morbidity from cancer, related to disease relapse or progression, is generally defined by tumor stage and biology at diagnosis.

The main challenge remains identification of older patients who on limited assessment appear to be healthy, but who are at higher risk of functional decline or even death. According to SIOG, collaboration with geriatricians and comprehensive geriatric assessment (CGA) are of paramount importance in detecting unaddressed problems, improving functional status and possibly improving survival in elderly patients with cancer [2]. CGA provides a thorough review of the overall health of older patients, allowing tailoring of treatment based on assessment of each patient deemed to be fit, vulnerable, or frail. Beyond its clinical importance, CGA is a valuable research tool as it provides better categorization of patients for enrolment in clinical trials and enables comparison of homogenous cohorts of elderly patients. Therefore CGA should always be considered when evaluating elderly cancer patients. It is time-consuming; however, abbreviated screening tools are being implemented to overcome this issue.

Metabolomics is a science that studies metabolites and small molecules. It allows the simultaneous identification and quantification of thousands of metabolites, with creation of a metabolomic profile. Metabolomic assessment of systemic biofluids may provide a portrait of physiological and pathological metabolic status for an individual [13]. Lawton et al. assessed plasma metabolites from healthy adults and found that the relative concentrations of nearly 100 compounds were statistically altered with age [14]. In many cases these changes are consistent with theories of aging (e.g., increased oxidative stress markers consistent with the free-radical theory of aging). In other cases the biological significance of these variations remains speculative. According to the authors, evaluation of the plasma metabolome provides a rapid and powerful method for examining physiological perturbations in aging and other biological processes. A prospective evaluation of the metabolomic profile of elderly women with breast cancer is ongoing, aiming to identify a metabolomic spectrum that correlates with the overall health of the patient.

18.2.5 Patient Expectation

Expectations of elderly breast cancer patients and the impact of these expectations on treatment decisions have been evaluated. It has been consistently shown that the level of acceptance of treatment does not differ among younger and older patients. However, the priority of older women is to ensure that their quality of life and independence remain unaffected [15,16]. Another feature is that elderly women rely heavily on "expert" advice in making their treatment choices [16–19]. Therefore, physicians should provide clear information on disease prognosis, treatment options, and possible related side effects when counseling elderly women with breast cancer. Patients should also be informed about the negative impact of undertreatment on disease outcome [20].

18.3 SURGERY

18.3.1 Surgery for Breast Cancer in Older Women

Many older women are fit for standard surgical therapy, but increasing age, frailty, and comorbidity may raise concerns about their fitness for certain treatment modalities. It has been reported that older women do not receive the same surgical treatment as younger women [21]. Surgery may be omitted or minimized, and axillary staging is less likely to be performed. The impact of these changes on local and systemic disease control has been explored in observational studies. Few randomized clinical trials have been performed. Rates of local control are inferior when surgery is omitted, and there is some suggestion that systemic disease control rates are impaired in elderly groups [20]. Survival in this age group is heavily influenced by competing causes of death and general medical conditions.

Surgery is usually well tolerated, and operative mortality is exceptionally rare, owing to modern anesthetic techniques (general, regional, and local) [2] and accurate patient selection. However, surgery is perceived as hazardous in the case of extreme age, severe comorbidity, and frailty. For this reason it is crucial to define frailty when dealing with oncogeriatric series undergoing surgery. The routine use of assessment tools is highly recommended.

Finally, it must be noted that the evidence base for modified surgical management strategies in elderly patients is poor, due to a lack of good quality primary research in this age group and the inherent difficulties in studying disease processes, patient-related variance, and treatment variance in such a heterogeneous patient group.

18.3.2 General History of and Indications for Breast Cancer Surgery

Surgery is the mainstay of treatment for younger women and, until the 1980s, was also the mainstay of treatment for all except the frailest older person [22,23]. At that time the concept of primary endocrine therapy (PET) was first suggested by researchers in Scotland [24]. This idea gained in popularity when trials demonstrated that there was no survival disadvantage to omission of surgery in women over the age of 70 years. Despite inferior local control rates, long-term follow-up showed little detriment in overall survival, with only one of the trials showing a slight but significant improvement in survival with surgery. It is worth remembering that the cause of death can be difficult to establish in patients with numerous associated medical conditions. Breast cancer–specific mortality in this age group is difficult to determine from the literature. This is due to the fact that outcomes are rarely adjusted to reflect patient comorbidity, there is widespread disease understaging in older women as many either have no surgery or limited surgery (often excluding axillary staging), and finally, overall treatment is often substandard when compared to younger patients. These factors result in inaccurate comparisons with younger women's outcomes. Progress in this area can be achieved through randomized trials or detailed observational studies that accurately stratify patient outcome according to age, disease stage and health status.

In favor of the surgical approach is the fact that operative mortality associated with surgery for breast cancer is negligible (0–0.3%) in most historic series. Most of the surgical procedures are of fairly short duration and patients are ambulatory immediately afterward. In many cases, the surgery can also be performed under local or regional anesthesia, further reducing the risks. Morbidity is also generally low, although lymphedema, wound infection, delayed healing requiring numerous clinical visits, and the psychological morbidity associated with the loss of a breast may cause some older women considerable distress and should not be underestimated. Very little evidence has been collected to document the quality of life achieved after surgical management, but anecdotal experience confirms that most patients agree that they would consider surgery again and would recommend a surgical approach to their friends, despite the original anxiety regarding surgery.

18.3.3 Surgery of the Primary Breast Cancer

There are two main surgical approaches to the treatment of primary breast cancer: mastectomy or wide local excision plus radiotherapy, as clearly demonstrated in the 1980s with two large trials [25,26]. Regrettably, both of these trials excluded patients over 70 years. Thus, strictly speaking, there is no evidence to support this approach in older women. Overall survival for these two approaches is equivalent, while there is a slightly higher rate of long-term local control for women who undergo a mastectomy.

The importance of local control on long term overall survival outcomes has been highlighted in the overview analysis of the Early Breast Cancer Trialists' Collaborative Group [27] demonstrating the importance of adequate local treatment in the management of operable breast cancers. Adequate local control of disease is important, irrespective of the patient's age, and this may have a significant impact on survival in women with a (remaining) life expectancy of 10–15 years. Therefore, a fit 70-year-old woman with a predicted life expectancy of 15 years should receive treatment as per standard guidelines based on evidence from trials recruiting younger women. However, in women of advanced age or with associated comorbidity (with a life expectancy restricted to ≤5 years) it is not unreasonable to consider alternative approaches.

For a woman of any age, the "absolute" indication for mastectomy is multifocal disease within more than one quadrant of the breast. In the absence of neoadjuvant therapy, mastectomy may be mandated by a large primary tumor in patients with a relatively small breast. Mastectomy may be warranted if the cosmetic result of conservative surgery would be unfavorable. In addition, mastectomy may be mandated in patients with an extensive in situ component to their invasive cancer. A further important indication for mastectomy is patient preference. A recent UK audit demonstrated that a significant proportion of patients with small tumors suitable for breast conservation surgery prefer mastectomy if given a choice [28]. Finally, access to adjuvant radiotherapeutic facilities should also be taken into account; quality of life should be considered at all times, and the stress of long-term, long-distance travel to receive radiotherapy must be remembered when tailoring treatment plans.

Older women may be less concerned about the impact of mastectomy on their body image and perhaps more anxious about the time and inconvenience that radiotherapy may entail. Nonetheless, the loss of the breast is still a major cause of psychological distress for many older women. This observation is further supported by the common observation of how an increasing number of older women are asking for breast preservation as well as breast reconstruction.

The decision of whether to operate only rarely revolves around the issue of fitness to undergo general anesthesia. Wide local excision is almost always possible under local anesthetic. Furthermore, a series of mastectomies performed under local anesthetic has proved feasible and rarely necessitated the use of harmful levels of local anesthetics [29].

18.3.4 Surgery to the Axilla

Two reasons support adequate axillary staging:

1. In patients in whom there is clear clinical or biopsy-proven nodal disease, axillary clearance is indicated to prevent local progression. Increasingly, preoperative axillary ultrasound and biopsy of suspicious nodes is gaining acceptance, and reducing the need for a two-stage surgical procedure to the axilla (i.e., sentinel lymph node biopsy followed by delayed clearance, where the sentinel node cannot be assessed intraoperatively). Routine axillary clearance has been superseded by a much less invasive approach, namely, sentinel lymph node biopsy (SLNB) [30–32]. SLNB involves the injection of a radioisotope-labeled and/or blue dye into the breast prior to surgery to localize the first lymph node in the breast drainage nodal chain. The radioactive and/or blue-colored sentinel nodes are identified and removed at surgery. The degree of axillary dissection is greatly reduced, and the procedure is associated with a lower morbidity than standard axillary management [30]. A number of studies in younger patients have demonstrated the accuracy of SLNB, improved quality of life, and reduced morbidity associated with this technique [30–32]. In many ways the SLNB approach is ideally suited to older patients where the potential morbidity associated with more radical axillary surgery may have a greater impact on arm function.

2. The extent of axillary nodal disease must be determined to estimate prognosis and select appropriate adjuvant therapies. As older women are much less likely to be offered adjuvant chemotherapy, axillary staging may be considered less important. However, axillary positivity will also determine whether a woman is advised to have adjuvant chest wall or supraclavicular fossa radiotherapy. Therefore, unless a woman is judged too frail to undergo these treatments, axillary staging should be considered.

Potential morbidity of axillary dissection has prompted research into whether axillary dissection may be avoided in some older patients. Median 15-year follow-up of a nonrandomized, retrospective study of older patients with T1N0 disease treated by surgery and adjuvant tamoxifen with or without axillary dissection revealed no survival difference and a cumulative incidence of axillary disease in the group without axillary dissection of 5.8% [33]. Two randomized studies have shown that avoiding axillary clearance in older patients with clinically node-negative, operable disease did not significantly effect breast cancer mortality and overall survival [34,35]. The incidence of subsequent axillary events was very low (2%). In both trials, all women were treated with adjuvant tamoxifen—the majority of women as expected in this age group had hormone-receptor-positive disease. With the current approach of sentinel node sampling, there are no data on whether axillary dissection can be avoided in the presence of positive sentinel nodes.

18.4 ALTERNATIVE APPROACHES IN PATIENTS WITH RESTRICTED LIFE EXPECTANCY

A small number elderly women with breast cancer will present with extreme frailty due to very advanced age or associated conditions and for whom remaining life expectancy will be predicted to be very short. A number of minimally invasive procedures have been proposed, including percutaneous tumor excision, radiofrequency ablation, focused ultrasound ablation, interstitial laser ablation, and cryotherapy. These techniques may be associated with improved cosmetic results, reduced psychological morbidity, and short hospital stay. They require close collaboration with the radiology department. While these techniques might be suitable for frail individuals, they should still be regarded as investigational until more data are made available [36–39].

18.4.1 Radiotherapy

Local control in breast cancer is as important for older patients as it is for their younger counterparts, whether after mastectomy or after breast conserving surgery [40–42]. Radiotherapy, in conjunction with surgery, continues to play a key role in achieving this. The Oxford overview of randomized trials of adjuvant radiotherapy demonstrates that good local control contributes to reducing breast cancer mortality [27]. There is little level I evidence for the role of adjuvant radiotherapy in breast cancer, largely due to historical exclusion of patients over the age of 70 from clinical trials. Extrapolation of the results of trials of adjuvant radiotherapy in younger patients to older patients may not be appropriate, given the different biology of breast cancer in older patients and the competing risks of non–breast cancer mortality in this age group. In general, older patients tend to have more favorable biological prognostic factors than younger patients, with a higher proportion of hormone-receptor-positive tumors. For example, in a retrospective study of 1755 patients with operable breast cancer from Institute Curie, 81% had hormone-receptor-positive tumors [43]. This advantage is counterbalanced by exclusion of older patients from national breast screening programs. As a result, presentation with locally advanced disease with associated poor prognosis is still seen.

As detailed below, for older patients with breast cancer, postoperative whole-breast irradiation after breast conserving surgery remains the standard of care. Postmastectomy radiotherapy is advised for high-risk patients. In intermediate-risk breast cancer, its role is controversial. Tolerance of radiotherapy in general is good in older patients and does not impair quality of life. Multimodality therapy should not be withheld from older patients.

Advances in Radiotherapy Older radiotherapy techniques that led to excess radiation-induced cardiac toxicity and mortality have been replaced by three-dimensional (3D) planning [44] and breath holding techniques [45] to minimize cardiac irradiation in left-sided tumors. In successive cohorts of patients treated in the United States, radiation-induced cardiac mortality has fallen [46]. This almost certainly reflects the introduction of 3D planning for breast cancer. Ischemic heart disease is more common in older patients. While the cardiac sequelae of adjuvant breast irradiation may take 10 years to manifest themselves, this latency may be within the life expectancy of older patients with early breast cancer. At least the same priority should be given to minimizing cardiac irradiation in older as in younger patients.

Postoperative Radiotherapy Following Breast Conserving Surgery It remains controversial as to whether there is any subgroup of patients from whom postoperative radiotherapy can be omitted. The current consensus is that no such group has been identified. Whole-breast radiotherapy reduces the risk of ipsilateral breast tumor recurrence (IBTR) in all subgroups, although the absolute benefit in low-risk, small (<2 cm), well-differentiated, hormone-receptor-positive, node-negative tumors is small. The only randomized trial to address the issue of the omission of postoperative radiotherapy in low-risk women after breast conserving surgery is the US Cancer and Leukemia Group B (CALGB) trial [47,48]. In this trial, 636 women, 70 years or older with T1N0M0 breast tumors, were randomized after breast conserving surgery and tamoxifen to whole-breast irradiation or no further treatment. The difference in local recurrence was 3% at 5 years (4% vs. 1%) in favor of adjuvant irradiation (Table 18.1) [47]. Breast edema, skin fibrosis, and pain were more frequent in the irradiated group. In an accompanying editorial [49] the value of radiotherapy was questioned, given the small difference in local recurrence. No axillary surgical staging procedure was required, so it is possible that the some higher-risk, node-positive patients were included. In addition, as the authors acknowledge, the trial was underpowered. It is well recognized that there is a persistent pattern of local recurrence of 1% per year at least up to 10 years [50]. This concern is validated by the update of the CALGB trial (Table 18.1) showing that at a median follow-up of 10.5 years, the difference in local recurrence has increased to 7% (9% vs. 2%). Of the 43% of patients who had died, only 7% of the deaths were due to breast cancer, reflecting the competing risks of death from non–breast cancer causes, predominantly vascular.

The Oxford overview of randomized trials of postoperative radiotherapy after breast conservation showed that a 16% reduction in 5-year ipsilateral breast tumor recurrence is associated with a 5% reduction in 15-year breast cancer mortality [27]. This led

TABLE 18.1 Local Control and Survival in CALGB Trial of Lumpectomy, Tamoxifen (Tam) with or without Postoperative Irradiation in Women Age >70 Years

| Number of Patients | Local Recurrence | | Overall Survival | | | |
	RT (%)	No RT (%)	Tam RT (%)	Tam RT (%)	Med FU (years)	Reference
636	2	9	61	63	5	48
636	1	4	87	86	10.5	47

to the conclusion that for every four local recurrences, one breast cancer death was avoided. There were very few patients (<700) over the age of 70 in the overview, so it is unclear whether this reduction in mortality applies equally to older as well as to young patients. However with increasing life expectancy and more effective systemic therapy with aromatase inhibitors, it is possible that local control may reduce breast cancer mortality in older patients, albeit probably to a lesser extent. Two additional trials shed light on this issue. The Italian 55–75 trial [51] randomized 749 women with T (<2.5-cm) N0/1,M0 breast cancer to whole-breast irradiation (50 Gy in 2-Gy fractions) after quadrantectomy and systemic therapy. For N0 patients, SLNB was undertaken. SLNB-positive patients were additionally treated by axillary clearance. This trial is not directly comparable to the CALGB trial since it was not exclusive to older patients and higher-risk patients with one to three involved nodes were included as well as hormone-receptor-positive and -negative tumors. At a median follow-up of 53 months, the cumulative incidence of IBTR was 2.5% in the surgery alone arm and 0.7% in the surgery-plus-radiotherapy arm. The smaller difference in IBTR (1.8%) in the Italian 55–75 trial compared to the CALGB trial largely reflects the greater volume of breast tissue resected by quadrantectomy compared to lumpectomy. The PRIME II trial [52] is still in the follow-up phase and has yet to report. It randomized over 1300 patients with T < 3 cm pathologically axillary-node-negative breast cancer after breast conserving surgery (minimum 1 mm clear margin) and adjuvant endocrine therapy to whole-breast irradiation (40–50 Gy) or no whole-breast radiotherapy. Accrual was completed in 2009. Other randomized trials of breast conserving surgery with/without postoperative radiotherapy that included but was not limited to older patients do not provide an answer to the question of the omission of postoperative radiotherapy after breast conserving surgery in elderly women. In a Canadian trial [53], age was an independent risk factor with a higher locoregional recurrence rate (LRR) in women over the age of 50. However, a low-risk group with a LRR <10% could not be identified. In the Milan III trial, women over the age of 55 years had a lower risk of recurrence (3.8%) versus 8.8% for the whole population. In the Scottish conservation trial [54], there was a trend to a lower recurrence rate with age, particularly between 60 and 70 years. No difference in local recurrence was observed in the NSABP B06 trial for women older or younger than 50 years [55]. The upper age of the trial, however, is not stated. At present international consensus is that postoperative radiotherapy after breast conserving surgery should be the standard of care for all fit patients irrespective of age [2]. It should be noted however that 5-year local recurrence rates in more recently published studies of breast conservation are falling to ~3% [56]. In part this is due to better systemic therapy, particularly the introduction of aromatase inhibitors. So the absolute benefits in local control from whole-breast irradiation for older patients are likely to diminish.

Breast Boost after Breast Conserving Surgery   There is level I evidence that a boost of irradiation to the site of excision after breast conserving surgery improves local control in older as well as young patients. The EORTC boost trial randomized over 5000 T1/2N0/1M0 patients after breast conserving surgery with clear margins and whole-breast irradiation (50 Gy) to a boost of 16 Gy in eight fractions or no boost. The original analysis [57] at 5 years of follow-up showed that the benefit in local control was only statistically significant in women under the age of 50. However, at 10 years of follow-up [58], all age groups were shown to benefit, although the reduction in local recurrence (7.3% vs. 3.8%) was only 3.5% in the >60-year age group. On this basis all patients including patients over the age of 60 should be considered for a boost.

Impact of Adjuvant Whole-Breast Radiotherapy on Quality of Life It might be assumed that the quality of life of older patients treated with postoperative radiotherapy would be worse than for patients treated by breast conserving surgery and adjuvant endocrine therapy alone, due to the burden of attending for several weeks of radiotherapy. However, there is good evidence that adjuvant radiotherapy is well tolerated by the majority of older patients [59,60]. The only trial to address this issue is the PRIME I trial. It randomized 255 T1/2N0M0 patients treated by breast conserving surgery and endocrine therapy to whole-breast radiotherapy (40–50 Gy) or no further therapy. There was no overall difference in global quality of life measured by the EORTC breast modules [61] at a follow-up of 15 months. This implies that, while quality of life is in general a relevant issue in selecting patients for treatment, it should not be a major factor in determining whether older patients are recommended to receive postoperative radiotherapy.

Postmastectomy Irradiation While the overall benefits of postmastectomy radiotherapy (PMRT) in high-risk postmenopausal patients are supported by level I evidence [62], the specific benefit in an elderly population is difficult to establish since they constitute a small subgroup among the patients of widely differing ages studied [63]. PMRT has been established as the standard of care for all fit postmenopausal patients with high-risk breast cancer (four or more involved axillary nodes) based on the Danish Breast Cancer Cooperative 82 c trial [62]. In this trial, a 9% survival advantage was observed from the addition of locoregional radiotherapy after mastectomy in patients <70 years old who received 2 years of tamoxifen. The risk of locoregional recurrence (LLR) in this trial was independent of age. The duration of adjuvant tamoxifen was shorter than the current standard of 5 years, so the absolute benefit of PMRT may have been overestimated. In addition there was criticism of the quality of axillary surgery where the average number of nodes was less than the current standard of at least 10 nodes in a level III clearance. It is also of interest that the survival advantage in postmenopausal patients emerged only after 5 years. This suggests that older patients with a life expectancy of <5 years are unlikely to derive a survival benefit and there is a less pressing case for PMRT. For patients over the age of 70 there are no level I data but there are nonrandomized data to suggest that the survival advantage of PMRT may extend to women over the age of 70 [64]. A retrospective survey comparing women aged 50–69 to those ≥ 70 treated by mastectomy without PMRT showed in the group with four or more involved axillary nodes that the LRR were respectively 16.8% and 30.8% at a median follow-up of 8.3 years [65]. This implies that high-risk older women may be at higher risk of LRR than younger and that chronological age should not be a barrier to the application of PMRT. For patients at intermediate risk of recurrence with one to three involved axillary nodes, the role of PMRT is controversial and is currently being studied in the MRC SUPREMO trial [66], which has no upper age limit of eligibility. There is limited information on what impact the Danish trial [62] had on the adoption of PMRT in older patients. Using data from the SEER cohort, the use of PMRT increased markedly in 1997. However, from 1998 to 2002, nearly 50% of eligible patients were still not receiving PMRT [67]. PMRT was particularly likely to be omitted in women of $\geq$ 85 years old, or those with moderate to severe comorbidities. There was also marked variation in the usage of PMRT between regions. These observations imply that there is little consensus on how PMRT should be applied to older patients.

Hypofractionated Dose Fractionation Regimes   Shorter radiation regimes than the internationally recognized standard of whole-breast irradiation of 50 Gy in 25 fractions over 5 weeks would be particularly attractive to older patients to reduce the burden of lengthy periods of outpatient attendance and associated fatigue. While there is no randomized trial testing hypofractionation in older patients, the results of two UK trials [68,69] and a one Canadian trial [70] are likely to be practice changing for older as well as younger patients. Both trials show that breast cancer is sensitive to the fraction size and that fewer larger fractions provide equivalent local control with similar or reduced breast toxicity. In the UK START A trial, two postoperative hypofractionated dose fractionation regimes, 39 Gy in 13 fractions of 3.2 Gy and 41.6 Gy in 13 fractions of 3 Gy, were compared with 50 Gy in 25 fractions in 2236 women treated by mastectomy or breast conserving surgery [68]. All regimes were given over 5 weeks. The 5-year LRR were 3.6%, 3.5%, and 5.2% for 50, 41.6, and 39 Gy, respectively [68]. In the START B trial, 40 Gy in 15 fractions over 3 weeks was compared to 50 Gy in 25 fractions over 5 weeks in 2215 women after primary surgery. The 5-year LRRs were 2.2% and 3.3% for 40 Gy and 50 Gy regimes, respectively. Breast cosmesis was superior in the 40-Gy arm. In both trials the shorter regimes provided similar locoregional control to the standard 50 Gy. The National Institute for Clinical Excellence (NICE) has adopted 40 Gy in its 15-fraction dose fractionation regime as the new UK standard for adjuvant postoperative radiotherapy [70]. In the Canadian trial [71], 1234 patients with T1/2 axillary-node-negative breast cancer were randomized after breast conserving surgery with clear margins to a hypofractionated regime (42.5 Gy in 16 fractions over 3.5 weeks) of whole-breast irradiation or to 50 Gy in 25 fractions over 5 weeks. No boost was given to the site of excision. At 10 years the local recurrence rate was 6.7% in the standard arm and 6.2% in the test arm. Breast cosmesis was similar in both arms of the trial. There has been little consensus on the generalizability of the findings of the START and Canadian hypofractionation trials. The more recent ASTRO consensus statement recommends that hypofractionated whole-breast irradiation (HF-WBI) is confined to women 50 years or older with T1/2N0 disease not receiving chemotherapy or nodal irradiation [72]. There is uncertainty about the long-term effects of hypofractionated radiotherapy on the heart. The ASTRO consensus statement therefore advises that hypofractionated whole-breast irradiation (HF-WBI) is used only where the heart is excluded from the radiation fields. The results of other hypofractionated dose fractionation regimes have been reported in nonrandomized studies. Kirova et al. in a series of 317 patients aged $\geq$ 70 years treated with 32.5 Gy in five fractions once weekly of 6.5 Gy found similar cause-free, local recurrence-free and metastasis-free survival to conventionally fractionated radiotherapy of 50 Gy in 25 daily fractions over 5 weeks [73]. Acute skin toxicity with the HF-WBI regime was acceptable and no different from the conventionally fractionated patients of similar age. Cosmesis was also similar. However, late complications measured on the LENT-SOMA (late effects normal tissue-subjective, objective management, analytic) showed a higher incidence of grade 1/2 fibrosis (33%) with HF-WBI compared with conventionally fractionated therapy (15%). Similar rates of late effects were seen using the same hypofractionated regime by Ortholan et al. [74].

Partial Breast Irradiation   Partial breast irradiation (PBI) in which adjuvant irradiation is delivered exclusively or in higher dosage to the primary site than the rest of the breast is being investigated in a number of randomized trials. The rationale for this approach is that local recurrences predominantly occur at or close to the site of excision [25,55]. A number of techniques are being studied in clinical trials including external beam import low [75], intraoperative kilovoltage (TARGIT [76] (Fig. 18.1)/electron therapy (ELIOT, Fig. 18.2) [77] and intraoperative or postoperative brachytherapy [78]. The rationale and indications for these techniques have been reviewed [79]. Of particular interest to older patients are single-fraction intraoperative techniques that avoid the inconvenience of attendance for several weeks of daily outpatient radiotherapy.

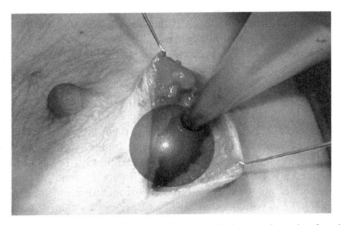

Figure 18.1   Targeted intraoperative radiotherapy technique using the intrabeam system: (a) placement of applicator in tumor bed; (b) delivery of X-ray source to tumor bed using a surgical support stand. During X-ray delivery, the sterile applicator is connected to a sterile drape to cover the stand. (Reproduced with kind permission from *Lancet* [80].)

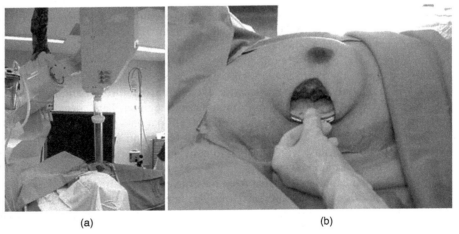

(a)	(b)

Figure 18.2   The linear accelerator used for ELIOT and thoracic wall protection. (Reproduced with kind permission from *Breast Cancer Research Treatment* 2010;**124**(1):141–151.)

The only published randomized trial of PBI is the TARGIT A trial [80] in predominantly low-risk postmenopausal patients randomized to intraoperative radiotherapy (IORT) with the Intrabeam device (Fig. 18.1) using 50-kV X rays (20 Gy to the surface of the applicator) or to whole-breast irradiation. The local recurrence rate was very low in both arms of the trial, but the follow-up was relatively short (4 years). The Kaplan–Meier estimate of ipsilateral breast tumour recurrence at 4 years was 1.20% (95% CI 0.53–2.71) in the targeted intraoperative radiotherapy and 0.95% (CI 0.39–2.31) in the external beam radiotherapy group. The results, however, are confounded by the option of investigators to supplement IORT with external beam if the investigator considered that there were additional risk factors for recurrence on the excision specimen. The main drawback of the technique is that irradiation is delivered before the margins of excision can be assessed on the operative specimen. Intraoperative electrons (3–12 MeV) using a mobile linear accelerator delivering 21 Gy to the 90% isodose are being studied by the Milan group, shielding the chest wall with lead if required [77]. Postoperative brachytherapy after lumpectomy using low-dose rate implants over 4–5 days or high dose rate typically twice daily for 5 days has yielded low LRR [81,82]. In response to the adoption of PBI outside of clinical trials predominantly in the United States and some parts of Europe, consensus guidelines for the use of PBI have been published by ASTRO and GEC, ESTRO [78,83]. While these guidelines may be a pragmatic approach to PBI, they are not based on level I evidence. In the absence of level I evidence, it is important that older patients are not recommended for PBI outside the confines of clinical trials. Patients should be made aware, as the ASTRO guidelines recommend [80], that whole-breast irradiation has a much longer track record of safety and efficacy. Until more level I evidence is published, PBI should remain investigational.

18.4.2 Systemic Treatment for Early Breast Cancer

Primary Endocrine Therapy Surgery is the gold standard for fit elderly women with early breast cancer. However, as already highlighted, alternative approaches, such as PET, may be considered in a specific subset of patients not considered candidates for surgery.

Hundreds of women over the age of 70 with operable breast cancer have been treated in clinical trials comparing surgery plus or minus adjuvant tamoxifen with tamoxifen alone. In all studies, surgery was associated with a significant benefit in terms of local disease control. A systematic review of published data has shown a significant difference in progression-free survival (PFS) between the surgical arm and the PET arm, but only a small, nonsignificant trend for improved overall survival with surgery plus tamoxifen versus tamoxifen alone (overall survival HR 0.86 95% CI 0.73–1.00; $p = 0.06$) [84]. Several factors limit the interpretation of these data, including lack of ER status assessment in most of the studies and the inadequacy of surgery alone for ER-positive breast cancer.

In addition, aromatase inhibitors have shown increased efficacy in comparison with tamoxifen. The ESTEeM (Endocrine–Surgical Therapy for Elderly women with Mammary cancer) trial aimed to assess the role of PET with anastrozole in comparison with surgery with adjuvant anastrozole in women with operable moderately or strongly ER-positive primary breast cancer at aged $\geq$ 75 years. Unfortunately, the study had to close for poor accrual.

On the basis of available data, SIOG highlights the importance of local control in the treatment of early breast cancer and recommends that surgery should not be denied to patients based on age alone [2]. PET may be considered an option for women with an estimated survival, based on age and comorbidity, of 2–3 years, that is, the median duration of response of PET. In this case, an accurate geriatric assessment to define life expectancy and a precise definition of the biological characteristics of disease to define the level of endocrine sensitivity of the tumor are strongly recommended.

Adjuvant Endocrine Therapy   Endocrine therapy is effective in elderly patients with hormone-receptor-positive tumors. Until recently, 5 years of tamoxifen represented the gold standard in adjuvant endocrine therapy, with no age effect on treatment efficacy. Notably, a more recent update of International Breast Cancer Study Group trial IV showed that only 1 year of tamoxifen resulted in a significant and prolonged improvement in disease-free and overall survival that carried over for 21 years in the elderly population [85].

In terms of tolerability, treatment with tamoxifen is associated with an increased risk of endometrial cancer and thromboembolic events, including deep-vein thrombosis, pulmonary embolism, and stroke. These do not translate to a significant excess of deaths from any particular cause [86]. It should be noted that estimates of the risks and benefit from a given treatment, based on results of clinical trials, may not accurately reflect the daily practice experience, due to a healthy selection bias in study participation. A relevant issue in older women may be the concomitant use of drugs that inhibit enzymatic activity of cytochrome 2D6 and thus potentially diminish the effect of tamoxifen (e.g., certain β blockers, antidepressants, antipsychotics) [87].

The adjuvant role of tamoxifen in postmenopausal women has been challenged by the results of clinical trials evaluating the role of aromatase inhibitors. The trials showed that the introduction of an aromatase inhibitor resulted in a reduced risk of tumor relapse, and some initial evidence of overall survival benefit with the strategy of switching to an aromatase inhibitor after 2–3 years of tamoxifen [88]. Older women derive the same benefit from aromatase inhibitors as younger women. A detailed analysis performed by Crivellari et al. explored potential differences in efficacy in elderly women receiving adjuvant tamoxifen or letrozole in the BIG 1–98 trial [89]. Subpopulation Treatment Effect Pattern Plot (STEPP) analysis was used to examine the patterns of differences in disease-free survival (DFS) according to age. The authors found that letrozole was superior to tamoxifen across the age spectrum (interaction of age and treatment, $p = 0.84$).

In the MA.17 trial in which women received letrozole after 5 years of tamoxifen, Muss et al reported no evidence of a heterogeneous effect of letrozole among age groups [90]. No significant difference in DFS or distant DFS was found by three different age groups (<60, 61–69, and ≥ 70 years old). This strategy was associated with a significant advantage in terms of DFS in patients younger than 60 years; however, the interaction between age and treatment was not statistically significant. Chapman et al. investigated the role of competing causes of deaths within MA.17 [91]. During follow-up, 256 deaths were reported (102 from breast cancer, 50 from other malignancies, 100 from other causes, and 4 from unknown causes). Non–breast cancer deaths accounted for 60% of the 252 known deaths (72% for those ≥ 70 years and 48% for those <70 years). Two baseline factors were differentially associated with type of death; cardiovascular disease was associated with a statistically significant increased risk of death from other causes ($p = 0.002$), and osteoporosis was associated with a statistically significant increased risk of death from other malignancies ($p = 0.05$). An increased risk of breast cancer-specific death was associated with lymph node involvement ($p < 0.001$). Increased risk of death from either breast cancer, other malignancy or other causes was associated with older age ($p < 0.001$).

In comparison with tamoxifen, aromatase inhibitors are associated with a higher risk of musculoskeletal disorders [88]. Since bone density decreases with age, older women have a higher risk of developing osteoporosis and complicating fractures. In older patients, hip fractures are associated with a high risk of long-term complications and mortality. In BIG 1–98 the incidence of bone fractures, observed more often in the letrozole group, did not differ by age [89]. Arthralgia and myalgia are reported in different intensity by a substantial proportion of patients receiving aromatase inhibitors. These symptoms might be particularly troublesome for unfit women in whom increase of joint pain might precipitate functional dependence.

Apart from BIG 1–98, which showed that patients on letrozole experienced more cardiovascular events (other than ischemia and cardiac failure) and more severe cardiac events, no significant differences in terms of cardiovascular events were observed in all the other adjuvant trials [88]. Conclusions regarding the relationship between aromatase inhibitors and cardiac risk are limited by the modest number of events reported.

For elderly patients who are considered candidates for endocrine therapy, a patient-profile-based approach should be considered to maximize the therapeutic index of the treatment.

Adjuvant Chemotherapy   Data from the Oxford overview show that the benefit of polychemotherapy progressively decreases with increasing age, with limited data available for patients 70 years or older [92]. However, when the same analysis is restricted to patients with ER-poor disease, a similar benefit is observed across different age groups. We now have mounting evidence that tumor biology, not patient age, determines sensitivity to chemotherapy. In general, patients with endocrine-resistant tumors derive a greater absolute survival benefit compared with patients with endocrine-sensitive tumors. Two independent studies using the SEER database have shown that adjuvant chemotherapy improves overall survival in elderly women with ER-negative tumors [93,94].

In the CALGB 49907 trial, women 65 years or older with stage I, II, IIIA, or IIIB breast cancer were randomized to standard chemotherapy [either cyclophosphamide, methotrexate and fluorouracil (CMF), or cyclophosphamide plus doxorubicin (AC)] or capecitabine [95]. Compared with patients treated with standard chemotherapy, the capecitabine-treated patients were twice as likely to relapse and almost twice as likely to die ($p = 0.02$). Of note, an unplanned subset analysis showed that the major benefit of chemotherapy was in patients with hormone-receptor-negative tumors. Only one phase III trial specifically designed for elderly patients, ≥ 65 years old, has evaluated the additive value of chemotherapy to endocrine therapy [96]. In this study, weekly doses of epirubicin plus tamoxifen improved DFS compared with tamoxifen alone. Unfortunately, this trial was underpowered to conclusively show a benefit.

With regard to choice of chemotherapy, healthy older patients may receive the same regimens as their younger counterparts. However, care is warranted as elderly patients experience greater toxicity, with $\leq 1.5\%$ of patients having treatment-related deaths in a CALGB retrospective analysis [97]. In this study, the two standard regimens were well tolerated, with a similar incidence of severe hematological toxicity and a lower incidence of nonhematological adverse events with AC. A higher percentage of patients completed the due courses of AC than CMF, confirming the existing data of CMF poor compliance in older patients.

Anthracycline-based treatment is associated with a risk of cardiac toxicity. An observational study showed that even in healthy women 66–70 years old treated with anthracycline-containing regimens, the rates of congestive heart failure were significantly higher than with non-anthracycline-containing regimens (HR 1.45) [98]. Of note, there was no reported increase for patients older than 70 years. For patients with cardiac disease with chemosensitive ER-positive tumors or triple-negative tumors, the use of non-anthracycline-containing regimens such as docetaxel and cyclophosphamide (TC) should be considered [99]. This regimen is superior to AC and similar to CMF.

No data are available about the efficacy and safety of adjuvant chemotherapy in elderly women that are unfit to received standard regimens. The CASA trial (IBCSG Trial 32-05 BIG 1–05; Chemotherapy Adjuvant Studies for Women at Advanced Age) aimed to evaluate the role of adjuvant pegylated liposomal doxorubicin in older women with ER-negative breast cancer in whom chemotherapy may be indicated, but where standard regimens used in younger women were felt to be too toxic. Unfortunately, this trial was closed prematurely because of poor recruitment.

Older patients are less likely to be enrolled in clinical trials, especially adjuvant breast cancer trials. The ACTION trial (Adjuvant Cytotoxic Chemotherapy in Older Women, BIG 2–05) was designed to randomize patients aged ≥ 70 years with good performance status and ER-negative or ER-positive high-risk early breast cancer to an AC regimen for four cycles versus a no-treatment option. Unfortunately, this trial also closed prematurely because of poor recruitment. Because of the inclusion of a no-treatment arm, this trial represented a valuable opportunity to study molecular markers of disease progression and response to treatment in this group of patients. This opportunity will again be offered by the ICE trial (Ibandronate with or without Capecitabine in elderly patients with Early breast cancer, BIG 4-04) in which more than 1300 women 65 years or older have been randomized to receive ibandronate plus or minus capecitabine. Patients entered in ICE have been evaluated by the Charlson index and the Vulnerable Elders Survey (VES13), so this study will provide additional information on the value of evaluating comorbidities and function in patients who are candidates to receive adjuvant chemotherapy.

Adjuvant Trastuzumab   Few patients 70 years or older were included in the large adjuvant trials that evaluated trastuzumab, preventing any firm conclusions on the role of this agent in the older population. Trastuzumab is usually well tolerated, but is associated with an age-related risk of cardiac toxicity [100]. Prior to administration of trastuzumab in older patients, management of any preexisting cardiac disease should be optimized. According to SIOG, healthy elderly patients without cardiac disease and with HER2-positive tumors should be considered for trastuzumab treatment. Close cardiac monitoring is essential for older patients receiving trastuzumab in the adjuvant setting [2]. To minimize the risk of cardiac toxicity, non-anthracycline-containing regimens could be considered.

The RESPECT trial (Evaluation of Trastuzumab without Chemotherapy as a Postoperative Adjuvant Therapy in HER2 Positive Elderly Breast Cancer Patients) is currently evaluating the role of trastuzumab without chemotherapy in HER2-positive early breast cancer women age 70–80 years.

18.5   TREATMENT OF METASTATIC BREAST CANCER

The goals of treating metastatic breast cancer in older patients are not different from those in younger patients—maintain quality of life, minimize symptoms from disease, and prolong survival without causing excessive toxicity.

18.5.1   Endocrine Therapy

Endocrine therapy is the treatment of choice in patients with endocrine-sensitive, nonimmediately life-threatening metastatic breast cancer. Several agents are available including tamoxifen, aromatase inhibitors, fulvestrant, and progestins. In the absence of clear evidence of endocrine-resistant disease, the administration of sequential lines of hormonal treatment represents a valuable option. New strategies are under investigation. A randomized phase II trial compared letrozole with or without oral metronomic cyclophosphamide in elderly breast cancer patients [101]. Metronomic scheduling of oral cyclophosphamide with letrozole yielded a superior response rate (87.7%) compared with letrozole alone (71.9%) in the ER-positive subgroup.

18.5.2   Chemotherapy

Chemotherapy is indicated in patients with hormone-receptor-negative disease, hormone-refractory disease, or in case of rapidly progressing disease. Elderly patients with metastatic breast cancer are expected to derive similar benefits from chemotherapy compared to their younger counterparts. Results from a case–control study of patients undergoing chemotherapy for metastatic breast cancer showed no significant differences in time to disease progression and survival for women younger than 50 years, 50–69 years, and 70 years and older [102]. The risk of toxicity is increased in older patients, and therefore preference should be given to chemotherapeutic drugs with safer profiles, such as weekly taxane regimens; newer, less cardiotoxic anthracycline formulations; capecitabine; gemcitabine; and vinorelbine. Choice of chemotherapy drugs and regimens is dependent on individual patient characteristics. This is true particularly in unfit patients. For example, paclitaxel and vinorelbine might be avoided as first choice in the presence of diabetes or peripheral neuropathy, capecitabine and methotrexate doses should be adjusted in case of reduced renal function, and standard anthracyclines should be avoided in women with cardiovascular risk factors.

Oral drugs, such as capecitabine and vinorelbine, appear attractive for elderly patients in order to limit access to the hospital and preserve their functional independence. However, oral administration is associated with several problems, including correct intake of the prescribed dose, interference with food or concomitant medications (e.g., capecitabine with warfarin), and self-reduction or escalation of dose, which may all interfere with the ultimate efficacy of the treatment [103]. Strict follow-up is essential in this population, particularly to avoid overtreatment and debilitating side effects.

18.5.3 Biological Agents

HER2-positive breast cancer is diagnosed in 7–20% of women aged ≥ 70 years in different case series. Data related to the use of trastuzumab in elderly women are limited but retrospective series show that benefits and safety of this agent appear to be conserved in patients 60–70 years old [104]. Retrospective data document age as a risk factor for congestive heart failure in patients receiving trastuzumab, but it may be that this relates more to preexisting cardiac comorbidities than to age alone [105]. Elderly patients without cardiac disease and with HER2-positive tumors should be considered for trastuzumab treatment. Single-agent trastuzumab could be offered to patients who are considered unfit to receive chemotherapy.

Crown et al. evaluated the incidence of diarrhea in patients with solid tumors treated with single-agent lapatinib and found that diarrhoea events in patients 70 years old were similar in severity, onset and resolution compared to younger patients, although some minor differences existed [106]. Patients ≥ 70 years old with breast cancer experienced more grade 3 events compared with younger patients (33% vs. 19%). Geyer et al. found no overall differences in safety or effectiveness of the combination of lapatinib and capecitabine between patients ≥ 65 years and their younger counterparts [107].

Anti-HER2 treatment in combination with endocrine therapy has been shown to be superior to endocrine therapy alone and may represent a valid option for patients with HER2-positive and ER-positive tumors for whom a chemotherapy-based approach in not considered appropriate [108,109]. The addition of trastuzumab to anastrozole and lapatinib to letrozole is associated with an improvement in PFS at the expense of more frequent and more serious adverse events.

Regarding angiogenesis targeted therapy, exploratory subpopulation analyses of the randomized, phase III trials of first-line bevacizumab-containing therapy have been performed to identify differential benefit among clinically relevant subgroups, including the elderly. In E2100, such an analysis suggests that bevacizumab maintained efficacy in patients older than 65 years, but to a lesser extent than younger patients [110]. For patients aged ≥ 65 years in E2100, AVADO, and RIBBON-1, the addition of bevacizumab over chemotherapy alone increased median PFS but not overall survival; a meta-analysis of all three trials showed benefit for PFS in patients <65 years old, PFS HR 0.62 (0.56–0.70); and those aged ≥ 65 years, PFS HR 0.70 (0.56–0.88) [111].

There are limited safety data for older patients treated with bevacizumab, with concern about potential increased risk of vascular events. A pooled analysis of 1745 patients with metastatic breast, colorectal and non–small cell lung carcinomas from five randomized trials showed that patients over the age of 65 years are at increased risk of arterial thromboembolic events, particularly when bevacizumab is given in combination with chemotherapy [112]. Observations in the nonrandomized ATHENA trial assessing safety of bevacizumab in combination with standard (non-anthracycline-based) chemotherapy, suggest that grade ≥ 3 or higher adverse events, particularly hypertension, may be more common in older women [113]. Notably, no excess of arterial or venous thromboembolic events was reported in older compared with younger patients. Safety of first-line bevacizumab combined with paclitaxel by age was explored in a subpopulation analysis in a noninterventional study following approval of bevacizumab, with no age-specific increase in bevacizumab-related toxicity [114]. More data are required for subgroups defined by age and comorbidities.

18.6 CONCLUSIONS

As women are living longer, breast cancer in older women will be an increasingly common diagnosis encountered in clinical practice. Recommendations for management are limited by lack of robust clinical data in this remarkably heterogeneous patient population. Available evidence supports treatment efficacy across the age spectrum, with efficacy determined by disease biology rather than age. Increased toxicity appears to reflect functional status, comordities, and polypharmacy, rather than age per se. Comanagement of older patients by oncologists, surgeons, radiation oncologists, and geriatricians is imperative to provide optimized, individualised care—particularly by incorporation of a functional assessment. The evidence base for modified management strategies in elderly patients is poor. Progress can be achieved through inclusion of older women in clinical trials or detailed observational studies that accurately stratify patient outcomes according to age, functional status, disease stage, and health status.

Elderly patients should be given clear information on disease prognosis, treatment options, and possible related side effects, and should be active participants in their management decisions. Older patients opt for management that maintains functional status and quality of life, with the focus on prevention or minimization of symptoms from the disease and/or from treatment. Misperceptions (e.g., regarding surgical anaesthetic risks, systemic therapy toxicity for limited benefit) must be challenged, and the negative impact of undertreatment on disease outcome must not be underestimated.

REFERENCES

1. Ferlay J, Bray F, Pisani P, Parkin DM. *Cancer Incidence, Mortality and Prevalence Worldwide*, IARC CancerBase No. 5, version 2.0. Lyon, IARCPress GLOBOCAN, 2004.

2. Wildiers H, Kunkler I, Biganzoli L, et al. Management of breast cancer in elderly individuals: Recommendations of the International Society of Geriatric Oncology. *Lancet Oncol* 2007;**8**(12):1101–1115.

3. Carlson RW, Moench S, Hurria A, et al. NCCN Task Force Report: Breast cancer in the older woman. *J Natl Comprehen Cancer Netw* 2008;**6**(Suppl 4):S1–S25.

4. Diab SG, Elledge RM, Clark GM. Tumor characteristics and clinical outcome of elderly women with breast cancer. *J Natl Cancer Inst* 2000;**92**:550–556.

5. Gennari R, Curigliano G, Rotmensz N, et al. Breast carcinoma in elderly women: Features of disease presentation, choice of local and systemic treatments compared with younger postmenopausal patients. *Cancer* 2004;**101**:1302–1310.

6. Poltinnikov IM, Rudoler SB, Tymofyeyev Y, et al. Impact of HER2 Neu overexpression on outcome of elderly women treated with wide local excision and breast irradiation for early breast cancer. *Am J Clin Oncol* 2006;**29**:71–79.

7. Singh R, Hellman S, Heimann R. The natural history of breast carcinoma in the elderly: implications for screening and treatment. *Cancer* 2004;**100**:1807–1813.

8. Lee SJ, Lindquist K, Segal MR, Covinsky KE. Development and validation of a prognostic index for 4-year mortality in older adults. *JAMA* 2006;**295**:801–808.

9. Ravdin PM, Siminoff L, Davis GJ, et al. Computer program to assist in making decisions about adjuvant therapy for women with early breast cancer. *J Clin Oncol* 2001;**19**:980–999.

10. Centers for Disease Control and Prevention (CDC). *Department of Health and Human Services*, CDC, 2008 (available at http://www.cdc.gov/cancer/breast/statistics/age.htm; accessed 4/08/08).

11. Schairer C, Mink PJ, Carroll L, Devesa SS. Probabilities of death from breast cancer and other causes among female breast cancer patients. *J Natl Cancer Inst* 2004;**96**:1311–1321.

12. Satariano WA, Ragland DR. The effect of comorbidity on 3-year survival of women with primary breast cancer. *Ann Intern Med* 1994;**120**:104–110.

13. Claudino W, Quattrone A, Biganzoli L, et al. Moving forward new horizons in oncology: Metabolomics. Available results, current research projects in breast cancer, and future applications *J Clin Oncol* 2007;**25**:2840–2846.

14. Lawton KA, Berger A, Mitchell M, et al. Analysis of the adult human plasma metabolome. *Pharmacogenomics* 2008;**9**:383–397.

15. Yellen SB, Cella DF, Leslie WT. Age and clinical decision making in oncology patients. *J Natl Cancer Inst* 1994;**86**:1766–1770.

16. Husain LS, Collins K, Reed M, Wyld L. Choices in cancer treatment: A qualitative study of the older women's (> 70 years) perspective. *Psychooncology* 2008;**17**:410–416.

17. Ciambrone D. Treatment decision-making among older women with breast cancer. *J Women Aging* 2006;**18**:31–47.

18. Maly RC, Leake B, Silliman RA. Breast cancer treatment in older women: Impact of the patient-physician interaction. *J Am Geriatr Soc* 2004;**52**:1138–1145.

19. Liang W, Burnett CB, Rowland JH, et al. Communication between physicians and older women with localized breast cancer: Implications for treatment and patient satisfaction. *J Clin Oncol* 2002;**20**:1008–1016.

20. Bouchardy C, Rapiti E, Fioretta G, et al. Undertreatment strongly decreases prognosis of breast cancer in elderly women. *J Clin Oncol* 2003;**21**:3580–3587.

21. Louwman WJ, Janssen-Heijnen ML, Houterman S, et al. Less extensive treatment and inferior prognosis for breast cancer patient with comorbidity: A population-based study. *Eur J Cancer* 2005;**41**:779–785.

22. Kesseler HJ, Seton JZ. The treatment of operable breast cancer in the elderly female. *Am J Surg* 1978;**135**:664–666.

23. Hunt KE, Fry DE, Bland KI. Breast carcinoma in the elderly patient: An assessment of operative risk, morbidity and mortality. *Am J Surg* 1980;**140**:339–342.

24. Preece PE, Wood RA, Mackie CR, et al. Tamoxifen as initial sole treatment of localised breast cancer in elderly women: a pilot study. *Br Med J (Clin Res Ed)* 1982;**284**:869–870.

25. Veronesi U, Cascinelli N, Mariani L, et al. Twenty-year follow up of a randomized study comparing breast conserving surgery with radical mastectomy for early breast cancer. *N Engl J Med* 2002;**347**:1227–1232.

26. Fisher B, Anderson S, Bryant J, et al. Twenty-year follow-up of a randomized trial comparing total mastectomy, lumpectomy, and lumpectomy plus irradiation for the treatment of invasive breast cancer. *N Engl J Med* 2002;**347**(16):1233–1241.

27. Clarke M, Collins R, Darby S, et al. Effects of radiotherapy and of differences in the extent of surgery for early breast cancer on local recurrence and 15-year survival: An overview of the randomised trials. *Lancet* 2005;**366**(9503):2087–2106.

28. Measures BCCO. *Analysis of the Mangement of Symptomatic Breast Cancers Diagnosed in 2004*, West Midlands Cancer Investigation Unit, Dec. 2007.

29. Oakley N, Dennison AR, Shorthouse AJ. A prospective audit of simple mastectomy under local anaesthesia. *Eur J Surg Oncol* 1996;**22**:134–136.

30. Fleissig A, Fallowfield LJ, Langridge CI, et al. Post-operative arm morbidity and quality of life. Results of the ALMANAC randomised trial comparing sentinel node biopsy with standard axillary treatment in the management of patients with early breast cancer. *Breast Cancer Res Treat* 2006;**95**:279–293.

31. Veronesi U, Paganelli G, Viale G, et al. A randomized comparison of sentinel-node biopsy with routine axillary dissection in breast cancer. *N Engl J Med* 2003;**349**:546–553.

32. Mansel RE, Fallowfield L, Kissin M, et al. Randomized multicenter trial of sentinel node biopsy versus standard axillary treatment in operable breast cancer: The ALMANAC Trial. *J Natl Cancer Inst* 2006;**98**:599–609.

33. Martelli G, Miceli R, Daidone MG, et al. Axillary dissection versus no axillary dissection in elderly patients with breast cancer and no palpable axillary nodes: Results after 15 years of follow-up. *Ann Surg Oncol* 2010;**18**:125–133.

34. Martelli G, Boracchi P, De Palo M, et al. A randomized trial comparing axillary dissection to no axillary dissection in older patients with T1N0 breast cancer: results after 5 years of follow-up. *Ann Surg* 2005;**242**:1–6.

35. International Breast Cancer Study Group. Randomized trial comparing axillary clearance versus no axillary clearance in older patients with breast cancer: First results of International Breast Cancer Study Group Trial 10–93. *J Clin Oncol* 2006;**24**:337–344.

36. Vlastos G, Verkooijen HM. Minimally invasive approaches for diagnosis and treatment of early-stage breast cancer. *Oncologist* 2007;**12**(1):1–10.

37. Hamazoe R, Maeta M, Murakami A, et al. Heating efficiency of radiofrequency capacitive hyperthermia for treatment of deep-seated tumors in the peritoneal cavity. *J Surg Oncol* 1991;**48**:176–179.

38. Jeffrey SS, Birdwell RL, Ikeda DM, et al. Radiofrequency ablation of breast cancer: First report of an emerging technology. *Arch Surg* 1999;**134**:1064–1068.

39. Singletary SE, Fornage BD, Sneige N, et al. Radiofrequency ablation of early-stage invasive breast tumors: An overview. *Cancer J* 2002;**8**:177–180.

40. Chapgar A, Kuerer HM, Hunt KK, et al. Outcome of treatment for breast cancer patients with chest wall recurrence according to initial stage: Implications for postmastectomy radiation therapy. *Int J Radiat Oncol Phys* 2003;**57**:128–135.

41. Engel J, Eckel R, Aydermir U, et al. Determinants and prognosis of loco regional and distant progression in breast cancer. *Int J Radiat Oncol Phys* 2003;**55**:1186–1195.

42. Punglia RS, Morrow M, Winer EP, et al. Local therapy and survival in breast cancer. *N Engl J Med* 2007;**356**:2399–2405.

43. Pierga J-Y, Girre V, Laurence B, Asselain B, et al. Characteristics and outcome of 1755 operable breast cancers in women over 70 years of age. *Breast* 2004;**13**:369–375.

44. Das IJ, Cheng EC, Freedman G, et al. Lung and heart dose volume analyses with CT simulator in radiation treatment of breast cancer. *Int J Radiat oncol Biol Phys* 1998;42(1):11–19.

45. Korreman SS, Pedersen AN, Nottrup TJ, et al. Breathing adapted radiotherapy for breast cancer: Comparison of free breathing gating with breath-hold technique. *Radiother Oncol* 2005;**76**:311–318.

46. Giordano SH, Kuo YF, Freeman JL, et al. Risk of cardiac death after adjuvant radiotherapy for breast cancer. *J Natl Cancer Inst* 2005;**97**:419–424.

47. Hughes KS, Schnaper LA, Berry D, et al. Lumpectomy plus tamoxifen with or without irradiation in women 70 years of age or older with early breast cancer. *N Engl J Med* 2004;**351**:971–977.

48. Hughes KS, Schnaper LA, Cirrincione C, et al. Lumpectomy plus tamoxifen with or without irradiation in women age 70 or older with early breast cancer. *J Clin Oncol* 2010;**28**: 507.

49. Smith IE, Ross GM. Breast radiotherapy after lumpectomy—no longer always necessary. *N Engl J Med* 2004;**351**:1021–1023.

50. Montgomery DA, Krupa K, Jack WJ, et al. Changing pattern of the detection of locoregional relapse in breast cancer: The Edinburgh experience. *Br J Cancer* 2007;**96**:1802–1807.

51. Tinterri C, Gatzemeier W, Zanini V, et al. Conservative surgery with and without radiotherapy in elderly patients with early-stage breast cancer: A prospective randomised multicentre trial. *Breast* 2009;**18**:373–377.

52. Kunkler I. PRIME II breast cancer trial. *Clin Oncol* 2004;**16**:447–448.

53. Clarke RM, McCulloch PB, Levine MN, et al. Randomized clinical trial to assess the effectiveness of breast irradiation following lumpectomy and axillary dissection for node-negative breast cancer. *J Natl Cancer Inst* 1992;**84**(9):683–689.

54. Forrest AP, Stewart HJ, Everington D, et al. Randomised controlled trial of conservation therapy for breast cancer: 6-year analysis of the Scottish trial. Scottish Cancer Trials Breast Group. *Lancet* 1996;**348**:708–713.

55. Fisher B, Anderson S, Redmond CK, et al. Reanalysis and results after 12 years of follow-up in a randomized clinical trial comparing total mastectomy with lumpectomy with or without irradiation in the treatment of breast cancer. *N Engl J Med* 1995;**333**(22):1456–1461.

56. Mannino M, Yarnold JR. Local relapse rates are falling after breast conserving surgery and systemic therapy for early breast cancer: can radiotherapy ever be safely withheld? *Radiother Oncol* 2009;**90**:14–22.

57. Bartelink H, Horiot JC, Poortmans P, et al. Recurrence rates after treatment of breast cancer with standard radiotherapy with or without additional irradiation. *N Engl J Med* 2001;**345**:1378–1387.

58. Bartelink H, Horiot JC, Poortmans PM, et al. Impact of a higher radiation dose on local control and survival in breast-conserving therapy of early breast cancer: 10-year results of the randomized boost versus no boost EORTC 22881-10882 trial. *J Clin Oncol* 2007;**25**:3259–3265.

59. Huguenin P, Glanzmann C, Lütolf, UM. Acute toxicity of curative radiotherapy in elderly patients. *Strahlenther Onkol* 1996;**172**(12):658–663.

60. Wyckoff J, Greenberg H, Sanderson R, et al. Breast irradiation in the older women: a toxicity study. *J Am Geriatr Soc* 1994;**42**(2):150–152.

61. Prescott RJ, Kunkler IH, Williams LJ, et al. A randomised controlled trial of postoperative radiotherapy following breast-conserving surgery in a minimum-risk older population. The PRIME trial. *Health Technol Assess* 2007;**11**:1–149.

62. Overgaard M, Jensen MB, Overgaard J, et al. Postoperative radiotherapy in high-risk postmenopausal breast cancer patients given adjuvant tamoxifen. Danish Breast Cancer Cooperative Group DBCG 82c randomised trial. *Lancet* 1999;**353**:1641–1648.

63. Cutuli B. Breast cancer irradiation in elderly. *Cancer Radiother* 2009;**13**:615–622.

64. Smith BD, Haffty BG, Hurria A, et al. (2006). Postmastectomy radiation and survival in older women with breast cancer. *J Clin Oncol* 2006;**24**:4901–4907.

65. Truong PT, Lee J, Kader HA, et al. Locoregional recurrence risks in elderly breast cancer patients treated with mastectomy without adjuvant radiotherapy. *Eur J Cancer* 2005;**41**:1267–1277.

66. Kunkler IH, Canney P, van Tienhoven G, Russell NS; corpauMRC/EORTC (BIG 2–04) SUPREMO Trial Management Group (2008). Elucidating the role of chest wall irradiation in 'intermediate-risk' breast cancer: the MRC/EORTC SUPREMO trial. *Clin Oncol (R Coll Radiol)* 2008;**1**:31–34.

67. Smith BD, Haffty BG, Smith GL, et al. Use of postmastectomy radiotherapy in older women. *Int J Radiat Oncol Biol Phys* 2008;**71**:98–106.

68. The START Trialists' Group. The UK Standardisation of Breast Radiotherapy (START) Trial A of radiotherapy hypofractionation for treatment of early breast cancer: A randomised trial. *Lancet Oncol* 2008;**9**:331–341.

69. The START Trialists' Group. The UK Standardisation of Breast Radiotherapy (START) Trial B of radiotherapy hypofractionation for treatment of early breast cancer: A randomised trial. *Lancet* 2008;**371**:1098–1107.

70. NICE. *Early and Locally Advanced Breast Cancer: Diagnosis and Treatment*, Clinical Guideline 80, NICE, London, 2009.

71. Whelan TJ, Pignol J-P, Levine MN, et al. Long-term results of hypofractionated radiation therapy for breast cancer. *N Engl J Med* 2010;**362**:513–520.

72. Smith BD, Bentzen SM, Correa CR, et al. Fractionation for whole breast irradiation: An American Society for Radiation Oncology (ASRO) evidence-based guideline. *Int J Radiat Oncol Biol Phys* 2011;**81**:59–68.

73. Kirova YM, Campana F, Savignoni A, et al. Breast-conserving treatment in the elderly: Long-term results of adjuvant hypofractionated and normofractionated radiotherapy. *Int J Radiat Oncol Biol Phys* 2009;**75**:76–81.

74. Ortholan C, Hannoun-Levi JM, Ferreiro JM, et al. Long-term results of adjuvant hypofractionated radiotherapy for breast cancer in elderly patients. *Int J Radiat Oncol Biol Phys* 2005;**61**:154–162.

75. Coles C, Yarnold J. The IMPORT trials are launched. *Clin Oncol (R Coll Radiol)* 2006;**18**(8):587–590.

76. Vaidya JS, Tobias JS, Baum M, et al. TARgeted Intraoperative radiotherapy (TARGIT): An innovative approach to partial breast irradiation. *Semin Radiat Oncol* 2005;**15**:84–91.

77. Orecchia R, Veronesi U. Intraoperative electrons. *Semin Radiat Oncol* 2005;**15**:76–83.

78. Polgár C, Van Limbergen E, Pötter R, et al. Patient selection for accelerated partial-breast irradiation (ABPI) after breast-conserving surgery: Recommendations of the Groupe Européen de Curiétherapie-European Society for Therapeutic Radiology and Oncology (GEC-ESTRO) breast cancer working group based on clinical evidence. *Radiother Oncol* 2010;**94**(3):264–273.

79. Stewart AJ, Khan AJ, Devlin PM. Partial breast irradiation: A review of techniques and indications. *Br J Radiol* 2010;**83**:369–378.

80. Vaidya JS, Joseph DJ, Tobias JS. Targeted intraoperative radiotherapy versus whole breast radiotherapy for breast cancer (TARGIT-A trial): An international, prospective, randomised, non-inferiority phase 3 trial. *Lancet* 2010;**376**:91–102.

81. Vicini FA, Baglan KL, Kestin LL, et al. Accelerated treatment of breast cancer. *J Clin Oncol* 2001;**19**:1993–2001.

82. Polgár C, Sulyok Z, Fodor J, et al. Sole brachytherapy of the tumor bed after conservative surgery for T1 breast cancer. Five-year results of a phase I/11 study and initial findings of a randomised phase III trial. *J Surg Oncol* 2002;**80**:121–128.

83. Smith BD, Arthur DW, Buchholz TA, et al. Accelerated partial breast irradiation consensus statement from the American Society for Radiation Oncology (ASTRO). *J Am Coll Surg* 2009;**290**(2):269–277.

84. Hind D, Wyld L, Reed MW. Surgery, with or without tamoxifen, *vs* tamoxifen alone for older women with operable breast cancer: Cochrane review. *Br J Cancer* 2007;**96**:1025–1029.

85. Crivellari D, Price K, Gelber RD, et al. Adjuvant endocrine therapy compared with no systemic therapy for elderly women with early breast cancer. 21-year results of International Breast Cancer Study Group Trial IV. *J Clin Oncol* 2003;**21**:4517–4523.

86. Early Breast Cancer Trialists' Collaborative Group. Effects of chemotherapy and hormonal therapy for early breast cancer on recurrence and 15-year survival: An overview of the randomised trials. *Lancet* 2005;**365**:1687–1717.

87. Sideras K, Ingle JN, Ames MM, et al. Coprescription of tamoxifen and medications that inhibit CYP2D6. *J Clin Oncol* 2010;**28**:2768–2776.

88. Biganzoli L. Adjuvant endocrine therapy. In Reed MW, Audisio RA, eds: *Management of Breast Cancer in Older Women*, Springer-Verlag, London, 2010, pp. 231–247.

89. Crivellari D, Sun Z, Coates AS, et al. Letrozole compared with tamoxifen for elderly patients with endocrine-responsive early breast cancer: The BIG 1–98 trial. *J Clin Oncol* 2008;**26**:1972–1979.

90. Muss HB, Tu D, Ingle JN, et al. Efficacy, toxicity, and quality of life in older women with early-stage breast cancer treated with letrozole or placebo after 5 years of tamoxifen: NCIC CTG Intergroup Trial MA17. *J Clin Oncol* 2008;**26**:1956–1964.

91. Chapman JA, Meng D, Shepherd L, et al. Competing causes of death from a randomized trial of extended adjuvant endocrine therapy for breast cancer. *J Natl Cancer Inst* 2008;**100**:252–260.

92. Early Breast Cancer Trialists' Collaborative Group. Polychemotherapy for early breast cancer: An overview of the randomised trials. *Lancet* 1998;**352**:930–942.

93. Elkin EB, Hurria A, Mitra N, et al. Adjuvant chemotherapy and survival in older women with hormone receptor-negative breast cancer: Assessing outcome in a population-based, observational cohort. *J Clin Oncol* 2006;**24**:2757–2764.

94. Giordano SH, Duan Z, Kuo F-Y, et al. Use and outcomes of adjuvant chemotherapy in older women with breast cancer. *J Clin Oncol* 2006;**24**:2750–2756.

95. Muss HB, Berry DA, Cirrincione CT, et al. Adjuvant chemotherapy in older women with early-stage breast cancer. *N Engl J Med*. 2009;**360**:2055–2065.

96. Fargeot P, Bonneterre J, Rochè H, et al. Disease-free survival advantage of weekly epirubicin plus tamoxifen versus tamoxifen alone as adjuvant treatment of operable, node-positive, elderly breast cancer patients: 6-year follow-up results of the French Adjuvant Study Group 08 trial. *J Clin Oncol* 2004;**23**:4622–4630.

97. Muss HB, Woolf S, Berry D, et al. Adjuvant chemotherapy in older and younger women with lymph node-positive breast cancer. *JAMA* 2005;**293**:1073–1081.

98. Giordano SH, Pinder M, Duan Z, et al. Congestive heart failure in older women treated with anthracycline (A) chemotherapy (C). *J Clin Oncol* 2006;**24**(Suppl; Abstract 521).

99. Jones SE, Savin MA, Holmes FA, et al. Phase III trial comparing doxorubicin plus cyclophosphamide with docetaxel plus cyclophosphamide as adjuvant therapy for operable breast cancer. *J Clin Oncol* 2006;**24**:5381–5387.

100. Telli ML, Hunt SA, Carlson RW, et al. Trastuzumab-related cardiotoxicity: Calling into question the concept of reversibility. *J Clin Oncol* 2007;**25**:3525–3533.

101. Bottini A, Generali D, Brizzi MP, et al. Randomized phase II trial of letrozole and letrozole plus low-dose metronomic oral cyclophosphamide as primary systemic treatment in elderly breast cancer patients. *J Clin Oncol* 2006;**24**:3623–3628.

102. Christman K, Muss HB, Case LD, Stanley V. Chemotherapy of metastatic breast cancer in the elderly. The Piedmont Oncology Association experience. *JAMA* 1992;**268**:57–62.

103. Aapro M, Monfardini S, Jirillo A, Basso U. Management of primary and advanced breast cancer in older unfit patients (medical treatment). *Cancer Treat Rev* 2009;**35**:503–508.

104. Brunello A, Monfardini S, Crivellari D, et al. Multicenter analysis of activity and safety of trastuzumab plus chemotherapy in advanced breast cancer in elderly women (> 70 years). *J Clin Oncol*. 2008;**26**(Suppl; Abstract 1096).

105. Giuliani R, Minisini AM, Paesmans M, et al. Is age a risk factor of congestive heart failure (CHF) in patients receiving trastuzumab (H)? Results from two Belgian compassionate use programs in metastatic breast cancer (MBC) patients (pts). *Proc Am Soc Clin Oncol* 2004;**22**(Suppl; Abstract 838).

106. Crown JP, Burris III HA, Boyle F, et al. Pooled analysis of diarrhea events in patients with cancer treated with lapatinib. *Breast Cancer Res Treat* 2008;**112**:317–325.

107. Geyer CE, Forster J, Lindquist D, et al. Lapatinib plus capecitabine for HER2-positive advanced breast cancer. *N Engl J Med* 2006;**355**:2733–2743.

108. Kaufman B, Mackey JR, Clemens MR, et al. Trastuzumab plus anastrozole versus anastrozole alone for the treatment of postmenopausal women with human epidermal growth factor receptor 2–positive, hormone receptor–positive metastatic breast cancer: Results from the randomized phase III TAnDEM study. *J Clin Oncol* 2009;**27**:5529–5537.

109. Johnston S, Pippen J Jr, Pivot X, et al. Lapatinib combined with letrozole versus letrozole and placebo as first-line therapy for postmenopausal hormone receptor–positive metastatic breast cancer. *J Clin Oncol* 2009;**27**:5538–5546.

110. Gray R, Bhattacharya S, Bowden C, et al. Independent review of E2100: A phase III trial of bevacizumab plus paclitaxel versus paclitaxel in women with metastatic breast cancer. *J Clin Oncol* 2009;**27**:4966–4972.

111. O'Shaughnessy J, Dieras V, Glaspy J, et al. Comparison of subgroup analyses of PFS from three phase III studies of bevacizumab in combination with chemotherapy in patients with HER2-negative metastatic breast cancer (MBC). *Cancer Res* 2009;**69**:512s(Suppl; Abstract 207).

112. Skillings JR, Johnson DH, Miller K, et al. Arterial thromboembolic events (ATEs) in a pooled analysis of 5 randomized, controlled trials (RCTs) of bevacizumab (BV) with chemotherapy. *J Clin Oncol* 2005;**23**: 196S.

113. Biganzoli L, Cortes-Funes H, Thomssen C, et al. Tolerability and efficacy of first-line bevacizumab (B) plus chemotherapy (CT) in elderly patients with advanced breast cancer (aBC): Subpopulation analysis of the MO 19391 study. *J Clin Oncol* **27**(Suppl; Abstract 1032).

114. Geberth M, Foerster F, Klare P, et al. Efficacy and safety of first-line bevacizumab (BEV) combined with paclitaxel (PAC) according to age: Subpopulation analysis of a large, multicenter, non-interventional study in patients (Pts) with HER2-negative metastatic breast cancer (MBC). *Cancer Res* **69**(Suppl; abstract 6085).

CHAPTER 19

Colon Cancer

DEMETRIS PAPAMICHAEL

Bank of Cyprus Oncology Centre, Nicosia, Cyprus

RICCARDO A. AUDISIO

St. Helens Teaching Hospital, Merseyside, UK

19.1 INTRODUCTION

Colorectal cancer (CRC) is the third leading cause of cancer death worldwide, representing 10% of cancer diagnoses and deaths [1]. More than 800,000 new cases are diagnosed annually, including 300,000 in the United States and Europe [2]. With a median age at diagnosis of 71 years, CRC is primarily a disease of older individuals [3]. Almost half of all cases occur in patients over 75 years of age, and the incidence increases with advancing age, doubling every 7 years in patients 50 years and over [3,4]. The medical and society burdens of CRC are likely to worsen over the coming decades as the number of older individuals continues to grow. Women and men in the United States 60, 70, and 80 years old can expect to live on average an additional 24 and 20.8, 16.2 and 13.7, and 9.8 and 8.2 years, respectively [5]. On the other hand, survival for patients with CRC continues to improve. A 2005 review of trends in a French population noted an increase in the 5-year survival rate among patients aged 75 years from 1976–1987 to 1988–1999 (47.1% vs. 53.6%, respectively; $p = 0.001$), attributed mainly to an increase in the number of patients being resected for cure and to a decrease in postoperative mortality, rather than to adjuvant chemotherapy, which was used much less frequently in older than younger patients [6].

Older patients are less likely to be included in important clinical trials testing new approaches and treatment strategies; in fact, many of these trials exclude elderly subjects having an upper age limit. In a review of 495 National Cancer Institute–sponsored cooperative group trials in 1997–2000, elderly patients with CRC were significantly underrepresented in phase II/III clinical trials [7]. In trials that *do* include older patients, enrollment of this age group is often low, precluding meaningful conclusions about safety and efficacy. In addition, older participants are generally carefully selected with a good performance status (PS) and minimal comorbidities. This results in data that have limited applicability to real-world patients, creating an information gap for clinicians. Demographic studies confirm that chemotherapy is used less commonly in older

Cancer and Aging Handbook: Research and Practice, First Edition. Edited by Keith M. Bellizzi and Margot A. Gosney.
© 2012 Wiley-Blackwell. Published 2012 by John Wiley & Sons, Inc.

patients with CRC than in younger patients, with close to half of older patients with stage III colon cancer not receiving treatment [8–11]. Although, when it comes to the metastatic setting, most studies, including meta-analyses and reports of pooled study populations going back to even the earliest palliative regimens of 5-fluorouracil (5FU)-based chemotherapy, have reported similar response rates, overall survival (OS) times, times to tumor progression, and dose intensity tolerability for elderly and younger patients [12,13].

19.2 SURGERY FOR CRC IN OLDER PATIENTS

Surgery is the mainstay of treatment for CRC regardless of the patient's age; many older CRC patients are fit for standard therapy, but increasing age, frailty, and comorbidity may question their fitness for certain treatments. Disparity in staging and treatment patterns between younger and older CRC patients have been reported at a cancer registry and national level with lower resection rates for older patients and reduced lymph-node retrieval [14,15].

Under elective conditions, surgery is usually well tolerated, and operative mortality is within acceptable limits, due to modern anaesthetic techniques, as well as accurate selection. However, operative mortality tends to increase with the patient's age, and surgery can be perceived as hazardous in the case of extreme age, comorbidity, and frailty [16]. For this reason it is crucial to define frailty when dealing with oncogeriatric series undergoing surgery; the routine use of assessment tools is warmly recommended.

Different from other cancer sites, CRC most frequently will tend to become a life-threatening surgical emergency if left untreated, and the management of CRC in elderly patients under emergency conditions exposes them to frequent complications with extraordinarily high mortality rates. Every effort should be set in place to prevent this medical catastrophic setting. In the worst-case scenario the use of self-expandable stents is to be considered as a bridge to surgery [17]. Successful stenting allows palliation of the obstructive condition, optimizing nutrition and anemia, offering adequate preabilitation and physiotherapy, and preparing psychological support wherever needed. In any case, a holistic approach to the older CRC patient is mandatory, and the frequent use of neoadjuvant chemoradiation offers a window of opportunity when stenting is not needed.

The Colorectal Cancer Collaborative Group conducted a systematic review of the published and aggregated data, from 28 independent studies and 34,194 patients that compared the outcomes for patients aged 65–74 years, 75–84 years, and 85+ years with those for patients aged <65 years [18]. The findings showed that elderly patients had an increased number of comorbidities, were more likely to present with later-stage disease and to undergo emergency surgery, and were less likely to have curative surgery than younger patients. Overall survival was also reduced in elderly patients, but for cancer-specific survival the age-related differences are much less striking. There is little doubt that, when carefully selected, even very old patients benefit from surgical resection, since a large proportion survive for ≥2 years postsurgery, irrespective of their age. In support of this, the recommendation from an analysis in 9501 rectal cancer patients >80 years of the long-term outcome after surgical intervention states that "age should not detract surgeons from offering optimal therapy to good-risk patients," including octogenarian CRC patients [19,20].

More recently, there has been increasing interest in performing surgery through a laparoscopic approach. There appears to be no statistically significant differences among the younger, middle-aged, and older patients relative to the incidence of conversion, major complications, minor complications, or total laparotomy rate. However, the duration of surgery, stay in the intensive care unit, and postoperative hospitalization may be significantly prolonged in patients older than 70 years [21,22]. With appropriate selection, laparoscopic procedures appear to be a safe option in elderly patients, and the outcome of laparoscopic colorectal surgery in patients aged >70 years is similar to younger patients. Advanced age is no contraindication for laparoscopic colorectal surgery.

From the technical perspective there is no difference in operating on an elderly or a younger patient; however, the response to the intervention may be substantially different, depending on the patient's frailty. This reinforces the need for frailty assessment and the opportunity of developing alternative less invasive procedures. Transanal endoscopic microsurgery (TEMS) for early lesions is a valuable treatment modality that often achieves similar outcomes as abdominal surgery [23].

19.2.1 Liver Metastases from CRC

Despite more recent advances in chemotherapy and the advent of new drugs, the 5-year survival rate for patients with unresected metastatic CRC to the liver ranges from 0–4%. The only treatment capable of achieving a significant long-term survival benefit is hepatic resection. Operative risk associated with liver resection is increased in older patients, due to age-associated reductions in liver volume, diminished hepatic bloodflow, and regenerative capacity. However, several cohort studies enrolling fit elderly patients have not shown age as an independent risk factor for short-term and long-term mortality.

A large UK study reporting on 178 patients aged >70 years undergoing liver resections for metastatic CRC recorded postoperative morbidity and mortality rates of 39% and 5%, respectively [24]. The overall and disease-free survival rates at 1, 3, and 5 years were 86%, 43%, and 32% and 66%, 26% and 16%, respectively. In this study, 34 patients received neoadjuvant chemotherapy. These excellent results are consistent with previously reported series on both older and younger patients. Liver resection of CRC metastases can be performed in selected elderly patients with low mortality and acceptable complication rates. Future research will have to focus on functional status and quality of life after major hepatic surgery in the elderly.

How to select resectable liver metastases versus nonresectable ones requires close collaboration between surgeons and oncologists; since the introduction of effective new compounds, a large number of previously nonresectable cases have now become surgically removable, giving the potential for prolonged survival or even cure.

19.3 RADIOTHERAPY IN THE TREATMENT OF RECTAL CANCER IN OLDER PATIENTS

Approximately a third of CRC patients present with rectal cancer. Relatively recently, the use of the surgical technique total mesorectal excision (TME) has led to a marked reduction in pelvic recurrences [25]. Nevertheless, analysis of 991 treatments in 838 older rectal cancer patients from the Cote d'Or and Calvados tumor registries showed that 54% of patients were able to undergo curative resection; 7%, palliative resection; 12%, bypass laparotomy; 27%, no surgery; 17% were scheduled to receive radiotherapy and 2%, receive chemotherapy [26]. These data clearly demonstrated the insufficient use of radiotherapy either combined with surgery or alone, while chemotherapy was almost never administered. A more detailed analysis by stage shows that approximately 50% of these patients should have been considered eligible for pre- or postoperative radiotherapy. These shortcomings in the approach to the care of the older rectal cancer patient are confirmed by an unpublished report based on the data from 12 cancer registries on the management of rectal cancer in France in 2000 (Anne Marie Bouvier, Guy Lanois, Jean Faivre et le re'seau FRANCIM, unpublished data). Overall, 84.7% of primary rectal tumors were resected, but the resection rates were 89.7% for patients <75 years of age and only 75.1% for patients over 75 years of age. The study showed significant variations in patient management despite access to *Good Clinical Practice Guidelines* and consensus statements, with insufficient access of patients to radiotherapy and research trials (0.8% compared with 7.7% in the younger age group). The variations in relation to radiotherapy were of particular significance because radiotherapy can facilitate R0 resection in initially unresectable cases, prevent local recurrences after good R0 resection and can palliate symptoms such as pain and bleeding. Radiotherapy has also been shown to impact significantly on survival in resectable tumors and is also important for the management of patients with all stages of rectal tumors, from superficial T1 in patients with a 90% cure rate with contact X-ray therapy, to advanced inoperable T4 tumors treated with radiotherapy, combined or not with contact X-ray and/or interstitial brachytherapy [27,28]. The influence of radiotherapy on the treatment of rectal cancer is one of the best evidence-based treatments in oncology. However, there are very few patients in radiotherapy trials who are aged >75 years [27,29–33]. Over the years, the use of radiation together with improved surgical techniques has led to a significant reduction in local recurrence rates and long-term prevention of recurrence [27,29]. All trials involving short-term preoperative radiotherapy, including the Dutch randomized trial in which patients underwent standardized TME resections, showed lower local recurrence rates in the radiotherapy arms, and one can assume that this is likely to be the case in older patients [31]. The available evidence so far suggests that the survival gains from preoperative radiotherapy are the same irrespective of age but that tolerability is not. Data from the Colorectal Collaborative Group clearly indicate that the number of deaths from rectal cancer is reduced as a consequence of preoperative but not postoperative radiotherapy, although the census data for this exclude data from the last 8 years [18]. The analysis also showed there to be an increased number of deaths from other causes within the first year after preoperative radiotherapy and slightly more for postoperative radiotherapy particularly in the older patient group. Acute tolerability to radiotherapy is dose- and volume dependent, and older people are more susceptible than younger patients [34]. Analysis of the data from the Stockholm I trial showed postoperative mortality to be increased in patients aged >75 years [34,35]. However, it was clearly related to a large pelvic and mesenteric target and treatment volume. The reduction of the target volume, to the posterior pelvis only, in the Stockholm II trial was sufficient to eliminate such risk and probably contributed to the demonstration of a survival benefit in addition to the reduction in pelvic recurrences [27]. Subgroup analysis, according to the interval between radiotherapy and surgery, for the Dutch TME trial showed an increase in noncancer-related mortality in older patients, but not in younger patients, depending on the interval between radiotherapy and surgery (Marijnen thesis, 2002, unpublished data) [35–37]. Thus, if carried out according to the protocols used in the Swedish Rectal Cancer trial and the Dutch TME trial, radiotherapy is well tolerated in those patients >75 years and even by those >80 years old (Bengt Glimelius, personal communication). Delivering 5 × 5 Gy over 5 days preoperatively is considered by many not to be ideal, but is at least as effective as the protracted radiotherapy schedule (45–50 Gy over 4–5 weeks and 25–28 fractions of 1.8–2 Gy each) [28,39]. Preoperative combined radiochemotherapy (RTCT) seems slightly superior to preoperative radiotherapy in terms of reduction of pelvic recurrences and RTCT combinations are now the treatment of choice at many centers, with all claiming superiority over radiotherapy alone. However, so far, there is no survival benefit and further studies with new drug combinations are ongoing. In addition, it may be a more appropriate approach for more locally advanced tumors (e.g., T4, circumferential margin involvement), rather than in earlier T3 tumors. There are also very few older patients included in the RTCT trials. In very old and unfit patients for RTCT, 5 × 5 Gy with a delay of 6–8 weeks resulted in marked tumor regressions with a high proportion of R0 resection in patients with primarily inoperable T4 rectal cancer [40]. Thus, both surgery and radiotherapy are important for controlling local recurrence and therefore local failure rates. Both TME and radiotherapy are associated with a slight increase in morbidity, but morbidity will be reduced in the future by improved radiotherapy techniques such as intensity modulated radiotherapy and intensity-modulated proton therapy, which will reduce the radiation burden to normal tissues [41]. Palliative radiation therapy is nearly always feasible except in patients who have previously been heavily irradiated and is likely also to be effective in older patients. Currently, however, there are no trials confirming this.

For the treatment of primary resectable rectal cancer in older patients, therefore, it is appropriate to consider TME with adequate quality assurance and quality control of the procedure. Preoperative radiotherapy should be offered where appropriate using 5 × 5 Gy and immediate surgery (2–3 days) or 40–50 Gy protracted radiotherapy over 4–5 weeks. In both cases, care should be taken in order to reduce the target volume to the posterior pelvis and to use modern treatment planning based on three-dimensional (3D) imaging reconstructions. Preoperative long-course RTCT could be considered more effective than long-course RT alone, but this is uncertain for those aged >75 years and will probably not be tolerated by the very old. Radiotherapy should be used to manage patients with inoperable low rectal tumors (all stages) and similarly in the palliative advanced disease setting in the context of symptom control.

19.4 ADJUVANT CHEMOTHERAPY

It has clearly been demonstrated that adjuvant chemotherapy can reduce the risk from disease recurrence and death in patients with node-positive CRC. On the other hand, the role of adjuvant treatment in patients with stage II disease remains controversial [42].

Sundararajan et al. reported the results of a combined analysis of the Surveillance, Epidemiology, and End Results (SEER) registry and Medicare database, which included 4768 elderly (≥65 years of age) patients [8]. Overall, 52% of these patients were treated with 5FU-based adjuvant chemotherapy. Patients who received treatment had significantly improved survival with a hazard ratio of 0.66. The authors concluded that adjuvant therapy in older patients is associated with reduced mortality, to a degree similar to that achieved in younger patients. Similarly, Jessup et al. evaluated data from 85,934 patients with stage III colon cancer who were registered with the National Cancer Database [43]. The conclusion was that older patients had the same benefit as younger ones, although they were less frequently treated. Neugut et al. used the SEER database to identify stage III, older colon cancer patients treated with 5FU-based adjuvant chemotherapy [44]. More than 30% of older patients who were started on FU-based chemotherapy discontinued treatment early. Mortality rates among such patients were nearly twice as high as in patients who completed 5–7 months of treatment. Finally, a population-based study reported by Bouvier et al. concluded that adjuvant chemotherapy did not have a negative impact on the quality of life of older CRC patients [45]. Several retrospective, older patient-specific pooled analyses were reported supporting the notion that older patients benefit from adjuvant chemotherapy in the same way as their younger counterparts, without significant increase in toxicity [46–48]. Interestingly, Fata et al. reported a trend toward higher disease-free survival (DFS) for patients $\geq$65 years old [46]. Age was not a predictor of DFS or OS, and no significant interaction was observed between age and the efficacy of treatment [47,48]. Dose intensity was similar or slightly lower for older patients [46,47]. The likelihood of dying without cancer recurrence was strongly associated with age [48].

A relatively recently published randomized trial has demonstrated that oral capecitabine is as effective as intravenous 5FU/LV in the adjuvant treatment of stage III colon cancer (X-ACT trial) [49]. A safety analysis of this study evaluated the impact of age on safety and demonstrated a similar favorable safety profile for capecitabine in patients aged <65 years or $\geq$65 years old [49,50]. However, capecitabine dosage should be adapted to renal function in older patients [51]. More recently, an updated analysis of this trial yielded that age was a nonsignificant factor on a multivariate analysis for overall survival [52]. A review of 245 patients registered to an Australian database (BioGrid Australia) who were treated with capecitabine showed a trend for increased toxicity in older patients [53].

In the MOSAIC trial of adjuvant oxaliplatin/5-FU/LV (FOLFOX) versus 5FU/LV age had no impact on the relative benefit of FOLFOX on recurrence-free survival. Older patients had the same benefit from treatment as their younger counterparts [2]. However, this trial had an upper age limit, and only 25 patients older than 75 years of age were included.

A pooled analysis of the ACCENT database was reported at the 2009 meeting of the American Society of Clinical Oncology (ASCO). This analysis used data from 10,499 patients <70 years and 2170 patients $\geq$70 years of age, participating in six phase III adjuvant trials comparing intravenous (IV) FU to combinations with irinotecan, oxaliplatin, or oral FU (capecitabine and UFT/LV) in stage II/III colon cancer [54]. Approximately 75% of patients had stage III disease (74% age <70, 77% age $\geq$70). All outcome measures, namely, OS, DFS, and time to recurrence (TTR), were statistically significantly improved for those in the experimental versus standard arms in the younger patients but not in the older ones; the interaction between age and treatment was statistically significant for all endpoints ($p = 0.01$ for OS, DFS, and TTR). These results were consistent regardless of whether the experimental arm was oxaliplatin-based, irinotecan-based, or oral FU. The authors concluded that older patients do not receive the same benefit from combination treatment and/or oral fluoropyrimidines in the same magnitude as their younger counterparts. The hazard ratio for younger patients was 0.86 (0.79–0.92) for the newer treatment, while in the 2200 older patients, the hazard ratio was 1.14 (0.98–1.32). Disease specific survival was not reported in that analysis, so the issue of death from other causes (which are more often observed in older individuals) was not taken into account.

Because of higher mortality in older patients, two adjuvant trials with FOLFOX ± cetuximab stopped recruiting patients ≥70 years of age because of toxicity. A similar trend was noted in the NSABP C08 trial with adjuvant FOLFOX ± bevacizumab [55].

It is generally believed that older CRC patients with stage III disease should not be denied adjuvant chemotherapy solely on the basis of their chronological age, even though the absolute benefit can be assessed with difficulty, due to the impact of death from other causes in this age group. Infusional 5FU regimens are associated with lower toxicity as compared to bolus regimens, and should be preferred whenever possible. Single-agent capecitabine with appropriate dose modification according to renal function can also be considered as appropriate therapy. Another option is FOLFOX, but it should be underlined that little data exist concerning older patients and should be used very cautiously.

Treatment should ideally be administered for the full 6 months if possible, given the survival benefit observed. Most of the available retrospective data are based on highly selected patients, and extrapolation to the general older patient population should be made with caution.

The multiple regimens available to consider (e.g., 5FU/FA, capecitabine, FOLFOX) also render the decisionmaking process more of a challenge. Therefore, it is difficult to recommend adjuvant therapy for all elderly patients. Although adjuvant therapy trials have included very few patients aged >80 years, the evidence for the elderly patient's ability to tolerate chemotherapy in general suggests that age alone should not exclude any stage III colon cancer patient from consideration for adjuvant therapy. However, there are very little data for those aged >75 years, and therefore age alone may well be a legitimate consideration. Most importantly, the therapeutic decisions with regard to the choice and duration of adjuvant therapy should be reached jointly by patient and physician, taking into account individual preferences and coexistent comorbidities.

19.5 METASTATIC SETTING

19.5.1 5-Fluorouracil-Based Therapy

A pooled analysis of 22 clinical trials assessed the efficacy of 5FU-based treatment in older patients with metastatic colorectal cancer [12]. This analysis included 3825 patients, 629 (16.4%) of whom were over 70 years of age. Overall survival was similar between older and younger patients (10.8 vs. 11.3 months; $p = 0.31$). Similarly, no significant difference was observed in terms of overall response rate (ORR) between age groups (≥70 vs. <70 years: 23.9% vs. 21.1%; $p = 0.14$). Progression-free survival was marginally prolonged in older patients (5.5 months vs. 5.3 months; $p = 0.01$). There was no trend in PFS, OS, or response rate difference between the age groups 70–74, 75–79, and ≥80 years. In all groups, infusional 5FU resulted in significantly improved ORR, OS, and PFS compared with bolus 5FU.

In a similar retrospective review of 658 young (<70 years of age) and 186 older (≥70 years of age) CRC patients, no significant difference was observed between the two age groups in terms of ORR (younger vs. older: 29% vs. 24%; $p = 0.19$) [13]. There was no difference in failure-free survival (FFS) (169 vs. 164 days; $p =$ nonsignificant) or 1-year FFS (19% vs. 18%, respectively; $p =$ nonsignificant). The median OS was slightly shorter in the older age group (350 vs. 292 days, $p = 0.04$); however, disease-specific survival was not assessed. One-year survival was 44% and 48%, respectively. There were four toxic deaths among the younger patients and one toxic death among the older patients. As expected, there were more cancer-unrelated deaths in the older patient population. No significant difference in the incidence of severe (grade III/IV) hematological and nonhematological toxicity was observed between the age groups.

Finally, a pooled analysis of two consecutive trials conducted by the National Institute for Cancer Research in Italy was reported [56]. Of the 215 patients enrolled 82 were over 65 years of age. This study also failed to demonstrate any significant difference in terms of ORR between the two age groups and also toxicity was similar. Overall survival and PFS data were not reported.

19.5.2 Irinotecan-Based Therapy

Combination of 5FU/LV with irinotecan in the first-line treatment of colorectal cancer has been associated with an increase in median OS in randomized trials (59;60). Mitry et al. performed a combined analysis based on individual data of 602 patients included in two phase III trials of irinotecan-free versus irinotecan-based first-line treatment [57]. Univariate and multivariate analyses failed to identify age as an independent prognostic factor for OS. Overall survival was similar between younger (<65 years of age; $n = 402$) and older patients (≥ 65 years of age; $n = 200$) (median OS: 13.21 months vs. 13.80 months; $p = 0.5$), while there was a trend toward higher PFS in favor of the older patient population (median PFS: 4.13 months vs. 5.11 months; $p = 0.05$).

Similarly, an age-specific subgroup analysis of a randomized phase III trial of irinotecan as second-line treatment was reported by Chau et al. [58]. The original study enrolled 339 patients, 72 of whom (21.2%) were ≥ 70 years of age. Patients aged ≥ 70 had similar objective responses (11.1 vs. 9%; $p = 0.585$) and survival (median 9.4 vs. 9 months; $p = 0.74$) compared to younger patients. Moreover, there was no statistically significant difference in the proportion of patients developing irinotecan-specific toxicity (defined as the occurrence of grade 3 or 4 diarrhea, neutropenia, febrile neutropenia, fever, infection, or nausea and vomiting) between the two age groups (<70 vs. ≥ 70: 37.8% vs. 45.8%; $p = 0.218$).

Finally, a combined analysis of 2691 patients participating in randomized trials comparing 5FU/LV versus a irinotecan/5FU/LV combination was reported by Folprecht et al. [59]. This analysis included 2092 younger (<70 years of age) and 599 (≥ 70 years of age) older patients. The test of interaction between age (<70 vs. ≥ 70 years) and treatment arm yielded no significant difference for ORR ($p = 0.33$), PFS ($p = 0.84$), and OS ($p = 0.61$). Significantly greater ORR and PFS were observed with irinotecan-based therapy in both age groups. Overall survival was significantly longer only in the younger patients. In the older patients there was a trend toward higher OS, but this difference failed to reach statistical significance. A trend toward shorter survival during the first treatment weeks was observed in the older patients treated with bolus 5FU/irinotecan regimen (IFL), but this was not the case for older patients receiving infusional 5FU regimens (FOLFIRI). No significant differences were observed in terms of toxicity when age was used as a continuous variable.

19.5.3 Oxaliplatin-Based Therapy

A pooled analysis of three randomized phase III trials in the first- or second-line treatment evaluated 159 older ($\geq$70 years of age) patients treated with oxaliplatin-based regimens (FOLFOX). The relative benefit of FOLFOX did not differ by age for ORR, PFS, and OS [2]. Elderly patients experienced significantly higher hematological toxicity (neutropenia and thrombocytopenia), more fatigue, and significantly less nausea and vomiting.

Similarly, an age-specific retrospective analysis of the OPTIMOX1 trial was reported by Figer et al. [60]. The ORR (59.4% vs. 59%), median PFS (9.0 months vs. 9.0 months; $p = 0.67$), and median OS (20.7 months vs. 20.2 months; $p = 0.57$) were comparable between older (>75) and younger ($\leq$75) patients. Older patients experienced slightly higher grade III/IV toxicity than younger patients: 65% versus 48% ($p = 0.06$), mainly with more neutropenia (41% vs. 24%, $p = 0.03$) and neurotoxicity (22% vs. 11%, $p = 0.06$). Tolerability, however, was manageable and no toxic death occurred in the older patient population.

19.5.4 Single-Agent versus Combination Therapy

The conduct of randomised trials in the setting of older and more frail patients with metastatic CRC appears to be feasible. The FOCUS2 trial evaluated the use of 5FU or capecitabine with or without oxaliplatin with a 2×2 factorial design, as first-line treatment in 460 elderly and/or frail patients with metastatic colorectal cancer [61]. Substitution of capecitabine for 5FU did not improve quality of life (QOL) or efficacy, while it significantly increased grade III/IV toxicity. Addition of oxaliplatin resulted in significantly higher antitumor efficacy without increasing the toxicity. This study has so far been published only in abstract form.

A preliminary analysis of a phase III trial comparing 5FU/LV versus 5-FU/LV/irinotecan as first-line treatment in older colorectal cancer patients was reported by Mitry et al. [62]. According to the authors, this elderly-specific randomized study was a feasible approach. Preliminary results suggested that patients aged >75 years can be treated with standard combination chemotherapy regimens with manageable toxicity.

19.5.5 "Targeted" Therapies

The addition of bevacizumab to irinotecan/5FU/LV chemotherapy as first-line treatment of advanced colorectal cancer resulted in significant prolongation of OS [63]. However, the administration of bevacizumab is associated with an increased risk of arterial thrombotic events (ATEs), especially in patients older than 65 years [64]. The clinical benefit of adding bevacizumab to 5FU-based chemotherapy in older CRC patients was evaluated in a pooled analysis by Kabbinavar et al. [65]. The authors observed a significant prolongation of PFS and OS by the addition of bevacizumab to 5FU-based chemotherapy, similar to the benefit observed in younger patients. In that particular analysis, the risks of toxicity did not exceed that in younger patients.

Of 1953 patients included in the Bevacizumab Regimens: Investigation of Treatment Effects and Safety (BRITE) observational study, 896 patients were $\geq$65 [65–74 ($n = 533$), $\geq$75 ($n = 363$)] and 161 patients were $\geq$80 years of age [66]. A higher rate of ATEs was observed in older patients, which is consistent with previous reports [67].

All other toxicities were comparable to those observed in patients <65 years of age. No difference was observed in terms of PFS between patients aged <65 and ≥65 years. Multivariate analyses revealed that the lower median OS observed in older patients was partly attributed to poorer PS and relative underexposure to active chemotherapy agents and second-line treatment in older individuals. According to the authors, these results indicated that age alone should not be a barrier to using bevacizumab in older colorectal cancer patients, but it should be noted that the inclusion criteria had been very strict, especially regarding cardiovascular comorbidity. In addition, this was conducted in a nonrandomized setting.

There are limited data from studies of anti-EGFR monoclonal antibodies (cetuximab, panitumumab) in older CRC patients. A small study evaluated the efficacy and safety of cetuximab with or without irinotecan in a retrospective cohort of older patients [68]. This study supported the finding that cetuximab has an acceptable toxicity profile and efficacy similar to that observed in younger patients.

Overall, chemotherapy should not be denied to older patients with advanced colorectal cancer. Infusional 5FU has a better toxicity profile compared to bolus regimens. Combination chemotherapy regimens in older individuals (5-FU with irinotecan or oxaliplatin) appear to have an efficacy similar to that in younger patients and should be the treatment of choice whenever possible, although oxaliplatin may be associated with slightly higher toxicity. Capecitabine might be considered in older patients; however, the need for an excellent compliance, the dose adaptation to patient's renal function, and the higher toxicity observed in older patients in a trial with substitution of capecitabine for infusional 5FU in the FOLFOX regimen should be considered. Efficacy and safety, with the exception of ATEs, for bevacizumab in older patients appears to be similar to that in younger ones, and can potentially be integrated to first- and second-line treatment of selected older patients. It should be noted that these data are based on retrospective analyses, which are likely to suffer from selection bias, and prospective studies are clearly needed.

19.6   CONCLUSION

Almost half of colon cancer cases are diagnosed in patients older than 70 years of age. Although chemotherapy in the adjuvant and metastatic setting clearly offers a survival benefit at least in younger individuals, older patients are frequently underrepresented in randomized clinical trials evaluating new cancer treatments, and markedly fewer trials are conducted to address the different risks and objectives in an elderly population. Although first-line treatment strategies such as irinotecan/5FU (FOLFIRI) and oxaliplatin/5FU (FOLFOX) seem feasible in many older patients, it should be noted that much of the data currently available are based on age-specific retrospective analyses from trials. Indeed, some of these trials are likely to suffer from selection bias, as only older patients considered "fit enough" would have entered. Results from clinical trials conducted in younger patients cannot be extrapolated to the general older population. Some older patients tend to have more comorbidities and potentially tolerate surgery, aggressive chemotherapy, radiotherapy, or combined modality treatment less well than their younger counterparts. Thus, prospective, elderly-specific clinical trials should perhaps be the way forward in order to provide an evidence-based decision making process for the management of this specific population.

Overall, as with younger patients, it is important to establish an overall treatment plan for the management of older CRC patients. These patients should receive the most intensive and appropriate treatment thought to be safe and effective according to their biological age and comorbidities. The aim should be to maximize OS while minimizing toxicity to achieve the greatest patient benefit.

REFERENCES

1. Jemal A, Murray T, Ward E et al. Cancer statistics, 2005. *CA Cancer J Clin* 2005;**55**: 10–30.

2. Goldberg RM, Tabah-Fisch I, Bleiberg H, et al. Pooled analysis of safety and efficacy of oxaliplatin plus fluorouracil/leucovorin administered bimonthly in elderly patients with colorectal cancer. *J Clin Oncol* 2006;**24**:4085–4091.

3. Ries LAG, Harkins D, Krapcho M, et al, eds. *Contents of the SEER Cancer Statistics Review, 1975–2003*, National Cancer Institute, Bethesda, MD, 2003 (available at http://seer.cancer.gov/csr/1975_2003/; accessed 9/27/06).

4. Edwards BK, Howe HL, Ries LA, et al. Annual report to the nation on the status of cancer, 1973–1999, featuring implications of age and aging on U.S cancer burden. *Cancer* 2002;**94**:2766–2792.

5. Minino AM, Heron MP, Murphy SL, et al. Deaths: Final data for 2004. *Natl Vital Stat Rep* 2007;**55**:1–119.

6. Mitry E, Bouvier AM, Esteve J, et al. Improvement in colorectal cancer survival: A population-based study. *Eur J Cancer* 2005;**41**:2297–2303.

7. Lewis JH, Kilgore ML, Goldman DP, et al. Participation of patients 65 years of age or older in cancer clinical trials. *J Clin Oncol* 2003;**21**:1383–1389.

8. Sundararajan V, Mitra N, Jacobson JS, et al. Survival associated with 5-fluorouracil-based adjuvant chemotherapy among elderly patients with nodepositive colon cancer. *Ann Intern Med* 2002;**136**:349–357.

9. Potosky AL, Harlan LC, Kaplan RS, et al. Age, sex, and racial differences in the use of standard adjuvant therapy for colorectal cancer. *J Clin Oncol* 2002;**20**:1192–1202.

10. Lemmens VEPP, van Halteren AH, Janssen-Heijnen MLG, et al. Adjuvant treatment for elderly patients with stage III colon cancer in the southern Netherlands is affected by socioeconomic status, gender, and comorbidity. *Ann Oncol* 2005;**16**:767–772.

11. Sargent DJ, Goldberg RM, Jacobson SD, et al. A pooled analysis of adjuvant chemotherapy for resected colon cancer in elderly patients. *N Engl J Med* 2001;**345**:1091–1097.

12. Folprecht G, Cunningham D, Ross P, et al. Efficacy of 5-fluorouracil-based chemotherapy in elderly patients with metastatic colorectal cancer: A pooled analysis of clinical trials. *Ann Oncol* 2004;**15**:1330–1338.

13. Popescu RA, Norman A, Ross PJ, et al. Adjuvant or palliative chemotherapy for colorectal cancer in patients 70 years or older. *J Clin Oncol* 1999;**17**:2412–2418.

14. Damhuis RA, Wereldsma JC, Wiggers T. The influence of age on resection rates and postoperative mortality in 6457 patients with colorectal cancer. *Int J Colorect Dis* 1996;**11**:45–48.

15. Tekkis PP, Smith JJ, Heriot AG, Darzi AW, Thompson MR, Stamatakis JD. Association of Coloproctology of Great Britain and Ireland. A national study on lymph node retrieval in resectional surgery for colorectal cancer. *Dis Colon Rectum* 2006;**49**(11):1673–1683.

16. Damhuis RA, Meurs CJ, Meijer WS. Postoperative mortality after cancer surgery in octogenarians and nonagenarians: Results from a series of 5,390 patients. *World J Surg Oncol* 2005;**3**:71.

17. Sebastian S, Johnston S, Geoghegan T, Torreggiani W, Buckley M. Pooled analysis of the efficacy and safety of self-expanding metal stenting in malignant colorectal obstruction. *Am J Gastroenterol* 2004;**99**(10):2051–2057.

18. Colorectal Cancer Collaborative Group. Surgery for colorectal cancer in elderly patients: A systematic review. *Lancet* 2000;**356**:968–974.

19. Kiran RP, Pokala N, Dudrick SJ. Long-term outcome after operative intervention for rectal cancer in patients aged over 80 years: Analysis of 9,501 patients. *Dis Colon Rectum* 2007;**50**:604–10.

20. Tan KY, Kawamura Y, Mizokami K, Sasaki J, Tsujinaka S, Maeda T, Konishi F. Colorectal surgery in octogenarian patients-outcomes and predictors of morbidity. *Int J Colorect Dis* 2009;**24**(2):185–189.

21. Schwandner O, Schiedeck TH, Bruch HP. Advanced age—indication or contraindication for laparoscopic colorectal surgery? *Dis Colon Rectum* 1999;**42**(3): 356–362.

22. Tan KY, Konishi F, Kawamura YJ, Maeda T, Sasaki J, Tsujinaka S, Horie H. Laparoscopic colorectal surgery in elderly patients: A case-control study of 15 years of experience. *Am J Surg* 2011;**201**(4):531–536. Epub 2010 Jun 3.

23. Tei M, Ikeda M, Haraguchi N, Takemasa I, Mizushima T, Ishii H, Yamamoto H, Sekimoto M, Doki Y, Mori M. Postoperative complications in elderly patients with colorectal cancer: Comparison of open and laparoscopic surgical procedures. *Surg Laparosc Endosc Percutaneneous Tech*. 2009 Dec; **19**(6):488–492.

24. de Liguori Carino N, van Leeuwen BL, Ghaneh P, Wu A, Audisio RA, Poston GJ. Liver resection for colorectal liver metastases in older patients. *Crit Rev Oncol Hematol*. 2008;**67**(3):273–278).

25. Heald RJ, Moran BJ, Ryall RD, et al. Rectal cancer: The Basingstoke experience of total mesorectal excision, 1978–1997. *Arch Surg* 1998;**133**:894–899.

26. Bouvier AM, Launoy G, Lepage C, Faivre J. Trends in the management and survival of digestive tract cancers among patients aged over 80 years. *Aliment Pharmacol Ther* 2005;**22**:233–241.

27. Folkesson J, Birgisson H, Pahlman L, et al. Swedish Rectal Cancer Trial: Long-lasting benefits from radiotherapy on survival and local recurrence rate. *J Clin Oncol* 2005;**23**:5644–5650.

28. Gerard JP, Romestaing P, Ardiet JM, Mornex F. Endocavity radiation therapy. *Semin Radiat Oncol* 1998;**8**:13–23.

29. Swedish Rectal Cancer Trial. Improved survival with preoperative radiotherapy in resectable rectal cancer. *N Engl J Med* 1997;**336**:980–987.

30. Stockholm Colorectal Cancer Study Group. Randomized study on preoperative radiotherapy in rectal carcinoma. *Ann Surg Oncol* 1996;**3**:423–430.

31. Kapiteijn E, Kranenbarg EK, Steup WH, et al. Total mesorectal excision (TME) with or without preoperative radiotherapy in the treatment of primary rectal cancer. Prospective randomised trial with standard operative and histopathological techniques. Dutch ColoRectal Cancer Group. *Eur J Surg* 1999;**165**:410–420.

32. Delaney CP, Lavery IC, Brenner A, et al. Preoperative radiotherapy improves survival for patients undergoing total mesorectal excision for stage T3 low rectal cancers. *Ann Surg* 2002;**236**:203–207.

33. O'Connell JB, Maggard MA, Liu JH, et al. Are survival rates different for youngand older patients with rectal cancer? *Dis Colon Rectum* 2004;**47**:2064–2069.

34. Cedermark B, Johansson H, Rutqvist LE, Wilking N. The Stockholm I trial of preoperative short term radiotherapy in operable rectal carcinoma. A prospective randomized trial. Stockholm Colorectal Cancer Study Group. *Cancer* 1995;**75**:2269–2275.

35. Marijnen CA, Kapiteijn E, van de Velde CJ, et al. Acute side effects and complications after short-term preoperative radiotherapy combined with total mesorectal excision in primary rectal cancer: Report of a multicenter randomized trial. *J Clin Oncol* 2002;**20**:817–825.

36. Marijnen CA, Nagtegaal ID, Kapiteijn E, et al. Radiotherapy does not compensate for positive resection margins in rectal cancer patients: Report of a multicenter randomized trial. *Int J Radiat Oncol Biol Phys* 2003;**55**:1311–1320.

37. Marijnen CA, van de Velde CJ, Putter H, et al. Impact of short-term preoperative radiotherapy on health-related quality of life and sexual functioning in primary rectal cancer: Report of a multicenter randomized trial. *J Clin Oncol* 2005;**23**:1847–1858.

38. Bujko K, Nowacki MP, Nasierowska-Guttmejer A, et al. Long-term results of a randomized trial comparing preoperative short-course radiotherapy with preoperative conventionally fractionated chemoradiation for rectal cancer. *Br J Surg* 2006;**93**:1215–1223.

39. Sebag-Montefiore D, Steele R, Quirke P, et al. Routine short-course pre-op radiotherapy or selective post-op chemoradiotherapy for resectable rectal cancer? Preliminary results of the MRC CR07 randomised trial. *J Clin Oncol* 2006:**18S**(Abstract 3511).

40. Radu C, Berglund K, Påhlman L, Glimelius B. Short-course preoperative radiotherapy with delayed surgery in rectal cancer—a retrospective study. *Radiother Oncol* 2008;**87**:343–349.

41. Ask A, Johansson B, Glimelius B. The potential of proton beam radiation therapy in gastrointestinal cancer. *Acta Oncol* 2005;**44**:896–903.

42. Pallis AG, Mouzas IA. Adjuvant Chemotherapy for colon cancer. *Anticancer Res* 2006;**26**(6C):4809–4815.

43. Jessup JM, Steward A, Greene FL, Minsky BD. Adjuvant chemotherapy for stage III colon cancer: Implications of race/ethnicity, age, and differentiation. *JAMA* 2005;**294**(21):2703–2711.

44. Neugut AI, Matasar M, Wang X, McBride R, Jacobson J, Tsai W, Grann V, Hershman D. Duration of adjuvant chemotherapy for colon cancer and survival among the elderly. *J. Clin Oncol* 2006;**24**(15):2368–2375.

45. Bouvier AM, Jooste V, Bonnetain F, Cottet V, Bizollon M, Bernard M, Faivre J. Adjuvant treatments do not alter the quality of life in elderly patients with colorectal cancer: A population-based study. *Cancer* 2008;**113**(4):879–886.

46. Fata F, Mirza A, Craig G, Nair S, Law A, Gallagher J, Ellison N, Bernath A. Efficacy and toxicity of adjuvant chemotherapy in elderly patients with colon carcinoma: A 10-year experience of the geisinger medical center. *Cancer* 2002;**94**(7):1931–1938.

47. Popescu R, Norman A, Ross P, Parikh B, Cunningham D. Adjuvant or palliative chemotherapy for colorectal cancer in patients 70 years or older. *J Clin Oncol* 1999;**17**(8):2412–2418.

48. Sargent D, Goldberg R, Jacobson S, Macdonald J, Labianca R, Haller D, Shepherd L, Seitz J, Francini G. A pooled analysis of adjuvant chemotherapy for resected colon cancer in elderly patients. *N Engl J Med* 2001;**345**(15):1091–1097.

49. Twelves C, Wong A, Nowacki M, et al. Capecitabine as adjuvant treatment for stage III colon cancer. *N Engl Med* 2005;**352**(26):2696–2704.

50. Scheithauer W, McKendrick J, Begbie S, et al. Oral capecitabine as an alternative to i.v. 5-fluorouracil-based adjuvant therapy for colon cancer: Safety results of a randomized, phase III trial. *Ann Oncol* 2003;**14**(12):1735–1743.

51. Lichtman S, Wildiers H, Chatelut E, et al. International Society of Geriatric Oncology Chemotherapy Taskforce: Evaluation of chemotherapy in older patients—an analysis of the medical literature. *J Clin Oncol* 2007;**25**(14):1832–1843.

52. Twelves C, Scheithauer W, McKendrick J, et al. *Capecitabine versus 5-FU/LV in Stage III Colon Cancer: Updated 5-Year Efficacy Data from X-ACT Trial and Preliminary Analysis of Relationship between Hand-Foot Syndrome (HFS) and Efficacy*, ASCO Gastrointestinal Cancers Symp., 2008, Abstract 274.

53. Field K, Kosmider S, Desai J, et al. *Capecitabine in Colorectal Cancer: A Five-Year Review of Use in Routine Clinical Care*, ASCO Gastrointestinal Cancers Symp 2009; Abstract 402.

54. McClearly N, Meyerhardt J, Green E, et al. Impact of older age on the efficacy of newer adjuvant therapies in >12500 patients (pts) with stage II/III colon cancer: Findings from the ACCENT database. *J Clin Oncol* 2009;**27**(15s): Abstract 4010.

55. Allegra CJ, Yothers G, O'Connell MJ, et al. Initial safety report of NSABP C-08, a randomized phase III study of modified 5-fluorouracil (5-FU)/leucovorin (LCV) and oxaliplatin (OX) (mFOLFOX6) with or without bevacizumab (bev) in the adjuvant treatment of patients with stage II/III colon cancer. *J Clin Oncol* 2008;**26** (Suppl; Abstract 4006).

56. Chiara S, Nobile M, Vincenti M, et al. Advanced colorectal cancer in the elderly: Results of consecutive trials with 5-fluorouracil-based chemotherapy. *Cancer Chemother Pharmacol* 1998;**42**(4):336–340.

57. Mitry E, Douillard J, Van Cutsem E, et al. Predictive factors of survival in patients with a advanced colorectal cancer: An individual data analysis of 602 patients includedin irinotecan phase III trials. *Ann Oncol* 2004;**15**(7):1013–1017.

58. Chau I, Norman A, Cunnigham D, et al. Elderly patients with fluoropyrimidine and thymidylate synthase inhibitor-resistant advanced colorectal cancer derive similar benefit without excessive toxicity when treated with irinotecan monotherapy. *Br J Cancer* 2004;**91**(8):1453–1458.

59. Folprecht G, Seymour M, Saltz L, et al. Irinotecan/Fluorouracil combination in first-line therapy of older and younger patients with metastatic colorectal cancer: combined analysis of 2691 patients in randomized controlled trials. *J Clin Oncol* 2008;**26**(9):1443–1451.

60. Figer A, Perez-Staub N, Carola E, et al. FOLFOX in patients aged between 76 and 80 years with metastatic colorectal cancer: An exploratory cohort of the OPTIMOX1 study. *Cancer* 2007;**110**(12):2666–2671.

61. Seymour M, Maughan T, Wasan H, et al. Capecitabine and oxaliplatinin elderly and/or frail patients with metastatic colorectal cancer: The FOCUS2 trial. *J Clin Oncol* 2007;25(Abstract 9030).

62. Mitry E, Phelip J, Bonnetain F, et al. *Phase III Trial of Chemotherapy with or without Irinotecan in the Front-Line Treatment of Metastatic Colorectal Cancer in Elderly Patients (FFCD 2001-02 Trial): Results of a Planned Interim Analysis*. ASCO Gastrointestinal Cancer Symp. 2008, Abstract 281.

63. Hurwitz H, Fehrenbacher L, Novothy W, et al. Bevacizumab plus irinotecan, fluorouracil and leucovorin for metastatic colorectal cancer. *N Eng J Med* 2004;**350**(23):2335–2342.

64. Scappaticci F, Skillings J, Holden S, et al. Arterial thromboembolicevents in patients with metastatic carcinoma treated with chemotherapy and bevacizumab. *J Natl Cancer Inst* 2007;**99**(16):1232–1239.

65. Kabbinavar F, Hurwitz H, Sarkar S, et al. Addition of bevacizumab to fluorouracil-based first-line treatment of metastatic colorectal cancer: Pooled analysis of cohortsof older patients from two randomized clinical trials. *J Clin Oncol* 2009;**27**(2):199–205.

66. Grothey A, Sugrue M, Purdie D, et al. Bevacizumab beyond first progression is associated with prolonged overall survival in metastatic colorectal cancer. Results from a large observational cohort study (BRiTE). *J Clin Oncol* 2008;**26**(33):5326–5334.

67. Kozloff M, Sugrue M, Purdie D, et al. Safety and effectiveness of bevacizumab and chemotherapy in elderly patients with metastatic colorectal cancer: Results from the BRiTE observational cohort study. *J Clin Oncol* 2008 (Abstract 4026).

68. Bouchahda M, Macarulla T, Spano J, et al. Cetuximab efficacy and safety in a retrospective cohort of elderly patients with heavily pretreated metastatic colorectal cancer. *Crit Rev Oncol Hematol* 2008;**67**(3):255–262.

CHAPTER 20

Lung Cancer

ULRICH WEDDING

Department of Internal Medicine/Palliative Care, Jena University Hospital, Jena, Germany

20.1 INTRODUCTION

Lung cancer is one of the most common malignant tumors and is the leading cause of cancer death in men and in women in Western countries. The majority of patients are diagnosed in an advanced stage of the disease. Treatment options vary considerably according to the stage of the disease. Curative treatment is possible in a limited or regional stage. In advanced stages, treatment is noncurative. Prolongation of life and improvement of symptoms are possible. The treatment of choice is chemotherapy. Differences in tumor biology are increasingly integrated in treatment decisions, with more biological agents becoming available.

20.2 DEFINITION OF TARGET POPULATION

Elderly people or elderly patients are not a well defined group. Some investigators address patients as elderly, when aged ≥65 years, others when they are ≥70 years. Following current recommendations of the European Organization of Research and Treatment of Cancer (EORTC) [1] and the International Society of Geriatric Oncology (SIOG) [2], patients with solid tumors should be considered as elderly when aged ≥70 years.

20.3 EPIDEMIOLOGY

Epidemiological data demonstrate an age-dependent increase in incidence and mortality rates. The following data reflect the situation in the United States. Within the Surveillance, Epidemiology, and End Results (SEER) program, the median age of patients newly diagnosed for lung cancer was 71 years. The median age at death from lung cancer was 72 years. Figures 20.1 and 20.2 demonstrate the age-dependent increase

Cancer and Aging Handbook: Research and Practice, First Edition. Edited by Keith M. Bellizzi and Margot A. Gosney.
© 2012 Wiley-Blackwell. Published 2012 by John Wiley & Sons, Inc.

in incidence (see Fig. 20.1a for male and Fig. 20.1b for female statistics). Incidence rates have increased substantially within the more recent decades, as demonstrated in Figures 20.2 for male and female patients aged 65–74 and 75+ years (see Fig. 20.2a for males aged 65–74, Fig. 20.2b for males aged 75+, Fig. 20.2c for females aged 65–74, and Fig. 20.2d for females aged 75+). The data demonstrate that incidence rates in men aged 64–74 decreased slightly and remained nearly constant in men aged 75+. In female patients however, a substantial increase in incidence rates has occurred since the 1970s in women aged 64–74. Since the year 2000, the rate did not increase further. In women aged 75+, the rates have increased fourfold since the 1970s. The

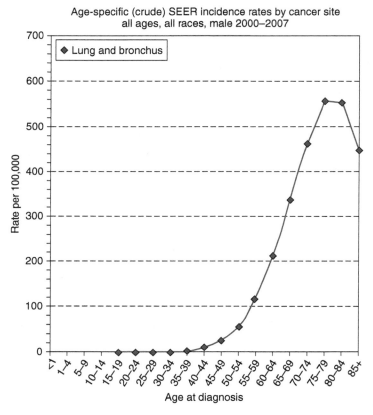

Cancer sites include invasive cases only unless otherwise noted.
Incidence source: SEER 17 areas (San Francisco, Connecticut, Detroit, Hawaii, Iowa, New Mexico, Seattle, Utah, Atlanta, San Jose-Monterey, Los Angeles, Alaska Native Registry, Rural Georgia, California excluding SF/SJM/LA, Kentucky, Louisiana, and New Jersey).
Rates are per 100,000.
Datapoints were not shown for rates that were based on less than 16 cases.

(a)

Figure 20.1 Age-specific SEER incidence rates by age groups in lung cancer, all races: (a) male; (b) female (US data).

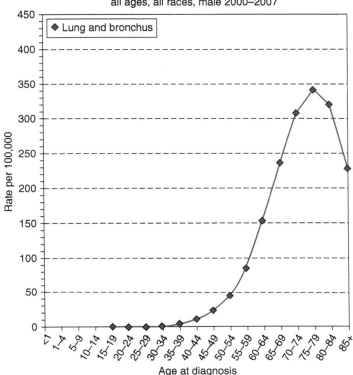

Age-specific (crude) SEER incidence rates by cancer site
all ages, all races, male 2000–2007

Cancer sites include invasive cases only unless otherwise noted.
Incidence source: SEER 17 areas (San Francisco, Connecticut, Detroit, Hawaii,
Iowa, New Mexico, Seattle, Utah, Atlanta, San Jose-Monterey, Los Angeles,
Alaska Native Registry, Rural Georgia, California excluding SF/SJM/LA,
Kentucky, Louisiana, and New Jersey).
Rates are per 100,000.
Datapoints were not shown for rates that were based on less than 16 cases.

(b)

Figure 20.1   (*Continued*)

changes are due mainly to changes in smoking behavior. Figure 20.3 demonstrates
that the 5-year age-adjusted survival rates increased over the more recent decades.
In addition, Figure 20.3 demonstrates that age-adjusted survival rates are worse in
patients aged 65–74 and 75+ years than in those aged 50–64 (see Fig. 20.3a for men
and Fig. 20.3b for women).

20.4 ETIOLOGY

About 90% of lung cancer is caused by smoking of tobacco. Nicotine contains a
variety of different substances. They are able to form DNA adducts causing malignant

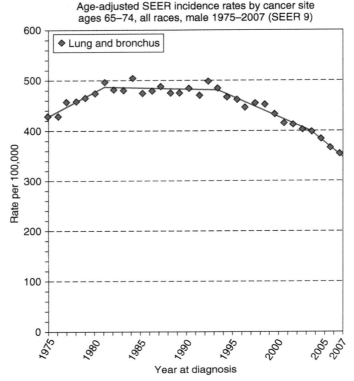

Age-adjusted SEER incidence rates by cancer site
ages 65–74, all races, male 1975–2007 (SEER 9)

Cancer sites include invasive cases only unless otherwise noted.
Incidence source: SEER 9 areas (San Francisco, Connecticut, Detroit, Hawaii,
Iowa, New Mexico, Seattle, Utah, and Atlanta).
Rates are per 100,000 and are age-adjusted to the 2000 US std population
(19 age groups-Census P25-1130). Regression lines are calculated using
the Jointpoint Regression Program Version 3.4.3, April 2010,
National Cancer Institute.

(a)

Figure 20.2 Changes in age-specific SEER incidence rates from 1975 to 2007 in lung cancer, all races: (a) male, age groups 65–74; (b) male, age groups 75+; (c) female, age groups 65–74; (d) female, age groups 75+ (US data).

transformation. Nicotine increases the risk of lung cancer in both active and passive smokers. Compared to nonsmokers, the risk increases with cumulative doses: 5–10 cigarettes/day ≤5–10 fold increase; 20 cigarettes/day 15–20-fold increase. The latency time is about 20–30 years. Other etiological agents are asbestos, radon, and other ionizing rays.

The second most important risk factor is age. Lung cancer incidence rates increase substantially with advancing age.

Family history is also a risk factor. First degree relatives have a 2.5-fold increase risk. However, genetically defined risk factors are thus far unknown.

As nicotine causes other types of cancer as well, including head–neck cancer, bladder cancer, and esophageal cancer, it is important to consider synchronous or metachronous second primaries.

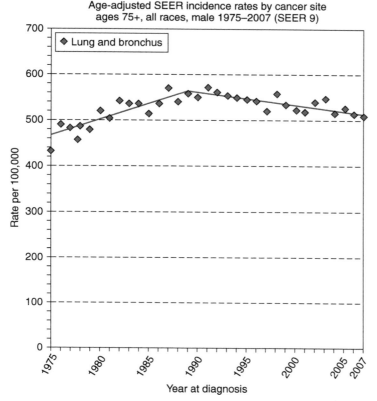

Age-adjusted SEER incidence rates by cancer site
ages 75+, all races, male 1975–2007 (SEER 9)

Cancer sites include invasive cases only unless otherwise noted.
Incidence source: SEER 9 areas (San Francisco, Connecticut, Detroit, Hawaii,
Iowa, New Mexico, Seattle, Utah, and Atlanta).
Rates are per 100,000 and are age-adjusted to the 2000 US std population
(19 age groups-Census P25-1130). Regression lines are calculated using
the Jointpoint Regression Program Version 3.4.3, April 2010,
National Cancer Institute.

(b)

Figure 20.2   (*Continued*)

Currently no data demonstrate that the carcinogenic agents behave differently in
younger versus elderly people, if adjusted for latency rates.

20.5 HISTOLOGY

Lung cancer is classified in different subtypes. The major two categories are small cell
lung cancer (SCLC) and non–small cell lung cancer (NSCLC). The latter is further
classified as squamous cell carcinoma, adenocarcinoma, and large cell carcinoma.

An important subtype of the adenocarcinomas is bronchoalveolar carcinoma. The
median age at diagnosis is younger in patients with SCLC than in patients with NSCLC.
Reasons for earlier occurrence of SCLC compared to NSCLC are unclear.

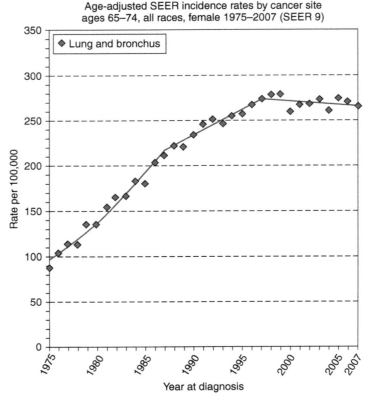

Age-adjusted SEER incidence rates by cancer site ages 65–74, all races, female 1975–2007 (SEER 9)

Cancer sites include invasive cases only unless otherwise noted.
Incidence source: SEER 9 areas (San Francisco, Connecticut, Detroit, Hawaii, Iowa, New Mexico, Seattle, Utah, and Atlanta).
Rates are per 100,000 and are age-adjusted to the 2000 US std population (19 age groups-Census P25-1130). Regression lines are calculated using the Jointpoint Regression Program Version 3.4.3, April 2010, National Cancer Institute.

(c)

Figure 20.2 (*Continued*)

20.6 MOLECULAR BIOLOGY

Typical molecular changes in lung cancer are activation of oncogenes, such as MYC amplification, RAS mutation, EGFR mutation, or inactivation of tumor suppressor genes, such as 3p deletion, p53 mutation, or loss of pRB.

Currently there is no evidence available on any molecular differences between tumors developing in younger and in elderly patients.

20.7 CLASSIFICATION AND STAGING

Table 20.1 reports the classification of NSCLC according to TNM category Table 20.2 shows the UICC stages. Traditionally SCLC was classified as limited or extended

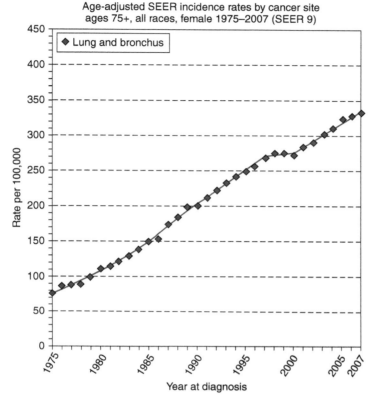

Age-adjusted SEER incidence rates by cancer site
ages 75+, all races, female 1975–2007 (SEER 9)

Cancer sites include invasive cases only unless otherwise noted.
Incidence source: SEER 9 areas (San Francisco, Connecticut, Detroit, Hawaii,
Iowa, New Mexico, Seattle, Utah, and Atlanta).
Rates are per 100,000 and are age-adjusted to the 2000 US std population
(19 age groups-Census P25-1130). Regression lines are calculated using
the Jointpoint Regression Program Version 3.4.3, April 2010,
National Cancer Institute.

(d)

Figure 20.2   (*Continued*)

disease. However, SCLC should now be classified according to TNM categories and
UICC stages as well. Classification and staging (Fig. 20.4) do not change with the
age of the patient. However, in elderly patients the clinical diagnosis of lung cancer
is seldom confirmed by biopsy and histology. In addition, in confirmed cases of lung
cancer, the staging remains unclear in some elderly patients. Chronological age is a
reason for less diagnostic workup [3].

20.8   PROGNOSIS

The 5-year survival rates differ according to the UICC stage of the disease. The main
prognostic factors are performance status and comorbidity.

Age is an adverse prognostic factor in lung cancer. The outcome is worse in
older patients with cancer [4]. In addition, outcome is worse in patients with poor

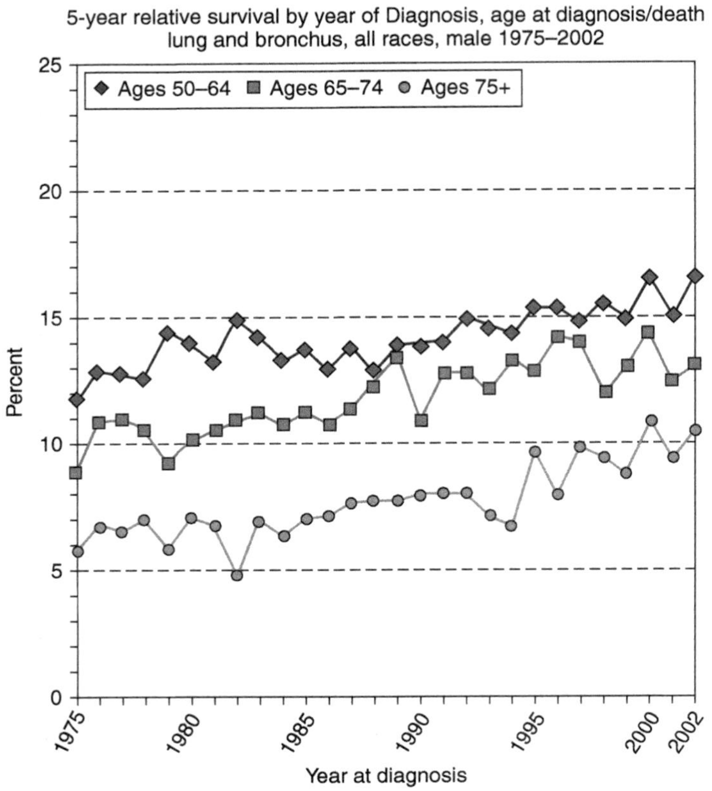

5-year relative survival by year of Diagnosis, age at diagnosis/death
lung and bronchus, all races, male 1975–2002

```
25

        ◆ Ages 50–64   ■ Ages 65–74   ○ Ages 75+

20

15

Percent

10

5

0
    1975      1980      1985      1990      1995      2000  2002
                         Year at diagnosis
```

Cancer sites include invasive cases only unless otherwise noted.
Survival source: SEER 9 areas (San Francisco, Connecticut, Detroit, Hawaii,
Iowa, New Mexico, Seattle, Utah, and Atlanta).
The 5-year survival estimates are calculated using monthly intervals.

(a)

Figure 20.3   Changes in 5-year relative survival rates according to age groups from 1975 to 2007 in lung cancer, all races: (a) male; (b) female (US data).

performance status [5] and in patients with comorbidity [6]. The relative frequency of patients with poor performance status [7–9] and with comorbidity increases with age [10]. Most of the trials reporting outcome in older patients do not adjust for age-associated decline in performance status, comorbidity, or other age-associated changes. It is therefore unclear whether age itself is associated with worse outcome or whether age-associated changes or age-associated undertreatment are reasons for the poorer prognosis of older patients with lung cancer.

20.9   PREVENTION AND EARLY DIAGNOSIS

The best primary prevention is to never start smoking in the first place, or to stop smoking at the earliest possible time. Even if a person is already 60, 70, or 80 years of age, cessation of smoking improves health and possibly survival. Strategies for early diagnosis or screening data and recommendations are described in Chapters 2 and 8.

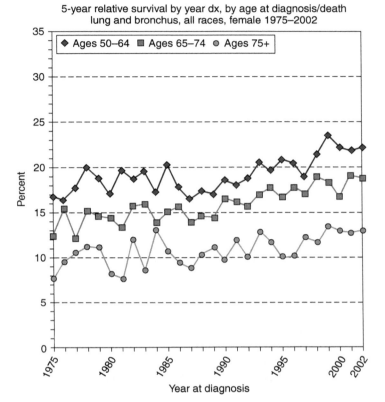

5-year relative survival by year dx, by age at diagnosis/death
lung and bronchus, all races, female 1975–2002

Cancer sites include invasive cases only unless otherwise noted.
Survival source: SEER 9 areas (San Francisco, Connecticut, Detroit, Hawaii, Iowa, New Mexico, Seattle, Utah, and Atlanta).
The 5-year survival estimates are calculated using monthly intervals.

(b)

Figure 20.3 (*Continued*)

20.10 CLINICAL PRESENTATION

About 90% of patients are diagnosed according to symptoms they developed and 10% on incidental findings. For a variety of diseases clinical presentation may change with increasing age of the patient. There are no data available reporting different clinical presentation in younger and elderly patients with lung cancer. The disease might present with symptoms directly caused by the tumor or indirectly caused, such as paraneoplastic syndromes.

20.10.1 General Symptoms

There are no specific clinical signs enabling an early diagnosis in lung cancer patients. Signs of endobronchial growth are cough, hemoptysis, dyspnea, and retention pneumonia; signs of intrathoracic growth (with pleural effusion, pericardial effusion, compression of vena cava) are pain, dysphagia, hoarseness, and Horner's syndrome.

TABLE 20.1   TNM Classification of Lung Cancer According to Seventh Edition TNM Staging of Lung Tumors of the American Joint Committee on Cancer

	Description
T-Category	
Tx	Cytology of sputum or broncho-alveolar lavage demonstrating malignant cells without tumour in bronchoscopy or scans
T0	No primary tumour
Tis	Carcinoma in situ
T1a	Tumour $<= 2$cm
T1b	Tumour > 2cm and $<= 3$cm
	surrounded by lung or visceral pleura, no signs of infiltration of a more proximal bronchus
T2a	Tumour > 3 cm and $<= 5$ cm
T2b	Tumour > 5 cm and $<= 7$ cm
	Invasion of visceral pleura
T3	Tumour > 7 cm
	Tumour < 2 cm to the carina
	Invasion of chest wall, diaphragm, phrenic nerve, mediastinal pleura, parietal pericard
	Separate nodule(s) in the primary lobe
T4	Invasion of heart, great vessels, trachea, oesophagus, spine
	Tumour in the carina
	Separate nodule(s) in a different ipsilateral node
N-Category	
Nx	No staging procedures to exclude regional lymph node involvement
N1	In ipsilateral peribronchial and/or ipsilateral hilar lymph nodes and intrapulmonary nodes
N2	In ipsilateral mediastinal and/or subcarinal lymph nodes
N3	In contralateral mediastinal, contralateral hilar, ipsilateral or contralateral scalenic or supraclavicular lymph nodes
M-Category	
Mx	No staging procedures to exclude distant metastases
M0	No signs of distant metastases
M1a	Intrathoracal metastases, pleural dissemination and or malignant pericardial effusion
M1b	Distant metastases

TABLE 20.2   UICC Classification of Lung Cancer

Stage	TNM
IA	$T_1N_0M_0$
IB	$T_2N_0M_0$
IIA	$T_1N_1M_0$
IIB	$T_2N_1M_0$
	$T_3N_0M_0$
IIIA	$T_3N_1M_0$
	$T_{1-3}N_2M_0$
	$T_4N_{0-1}M_0$
IIIB	$T_4N_2M_0$
	$T_{1-4}N_3M_0$
IV	$T_{1-4}N_{0-3}M_1$

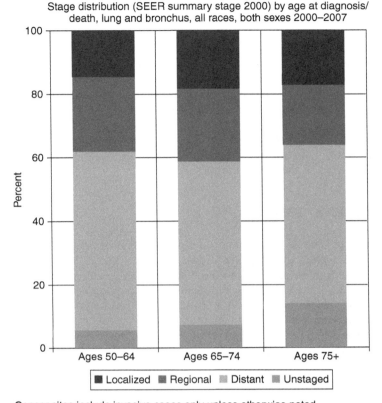

Figure 20.4   Stage distribution according to age groups from 2000 to 2007 in lung cancer, all races, both sexes (US data).

In some patients, symptoms leading to diagnosis are caused by lymph node metastases or distant metastasis, such as swelling of supraclavicular lymph nodes, bone pain in case of skeletal metastases, or dizziness, headache, or neurological deficits in the case of CNS metastases.

20.10.2   Paraneoplastic Syndromes

Some paraneoplastic syndromes are quite typical for patients with lung cancer, including Cushing syndrome, SIADH, hypercalcaemia, and Lambert–Eaton syndrome. There are no data reporting differences in occurrence of paraneoplastic syndromes related to the chronological age of the patient.

Cushing's Syndrome   Clinical signs of Cushing's syndrome occur in 0–2% of all lung cancer patients and in 6% of patients with SCLC.

SIADH   The syndrome of inappropriate secretion of antidiuretic hormone (SIADH) is based on an increased release of antidiuretic hormone (ADH). It occurs in ~10% of patients with SCLC.

Hypercalcemia   About 10% of all lung cancer patients present with hypercalcemia. Hypercalcemia is caused by an increased secretion of parathormone-related peptide. Approximately 10–15% of cases occur in patients without bone metastases. Treatment is application of bisphosphonates, fluid, and diuretics.

Lambert–Eaton Syndrome   Lambert-Eaton syndrome occurs in about 6% of patients with SCLC. Patients present with a muscular weakness especially of the lower extremities and of the pelvic muscles.

20.11   DIAGNOSTIC TESTING

Diagnostic testings serve to judge tumor and patients' characteristics. Only a detailed judgment of both enables treatment decisions.

Diagnostic tests can be divided into basic diagnostics, diagnostics for locoregional staging, diagnostics to exclude distant metastases, diagnostics to judge technical resectability, and diagnostics to judge patient's fitness for treatment. The latter becomes more important the older a patient is.

Figures 20.5 and 20.8 provide algorithms for diagnostic workup. Figure 20.5 focuses on staging procedures, Figure 20.6 focuses on operability [11].

20.11.1   Basic Diagnostics

Basic diagnostics include

- History and physical examination, including weight loss and performance status, as both are major prognostic variables
- Confirmation of the diagnosis via biopsy for histological proof, as a major first step
- Computer tomography of the chest and the upper abdomen, including adrenal glands, as they are often involved in metastatic disease
- Complete blood count, chemistry, and coagulation

Further investigations depend on the location and the suspected stage of the tumor.

20.11.2   Diagnostics for Locoregional Staging

The diagnostic procedures to determine locoregional stage differ according to the assumed stage of the disease. The main issues are whether regional lymph nodes are involved and whether distant metastases are present.

20.11.3   Diagnostics to Exclude Distant Metastases

The risk of distant metastases increases with the T and N categories of the tumor. Major organs involved in distant metastases are brain, bone, liver, and adrenal glands.

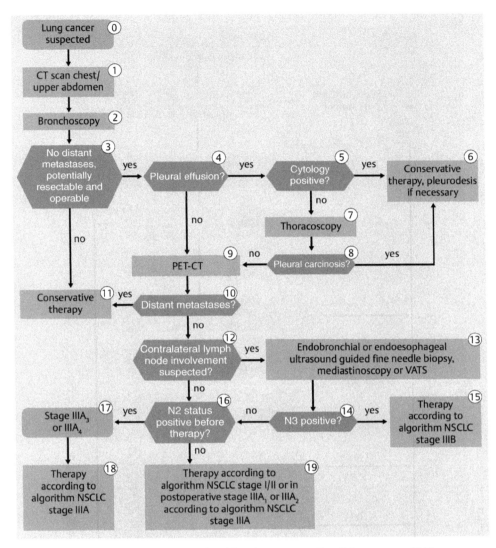

Figure 20.5 Diagnostic algorithm for non–small cell lung cancer [11].

20.11.4 Diagnostics to Judge Technical Resectability

If the tumor is locally or regionally defined surgery might be the treatment of choice. The resectability of the tumor depends upon the site and the local extent.

20.11.5 Diagnostics to Judge Patient's Fitness for Treatment

Most therapeutic procedures are not without side effects. Fitness for treatment differs according to the extent of surgery, the region of radiotherapy, and aggressiveness of the chemotherapy.

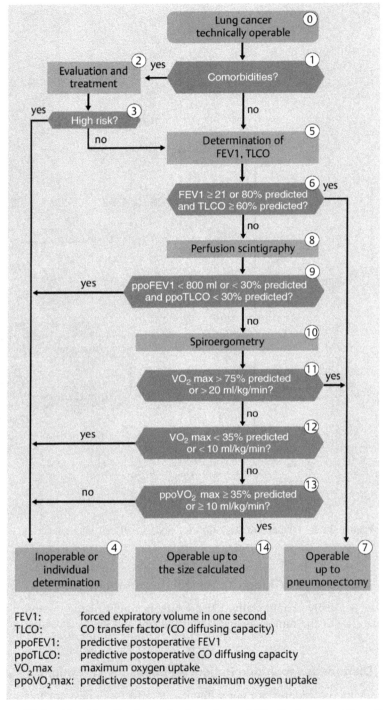

FEV1: forced expiratory volume in one second
TLCO: CO transfer factor (CO diffusing capacity)
ppoFEV1: predictive postoperative FEV1
ppoTLCO: predictive postoperative CO diffusing capacity
VO₂max maximum oxygen uptake
ppoVO₂max: predictive postoperative maximum oxygen uptake

Figure 20.6 Algorithm for the evaluation of operability for lung resections [11].

The major traditional criteria to judge a patient's fitness for treatment are lung function test and ECOG-PS.

20.12 COMPREHENSIVE GERIATRIC ASSESSMENT

Following current recommendations from the European Organization of Research and Treatment of Cancer (EORTC) [1] and the International Society of Geriatric Oncology (SIOG) [2], patients with solid tumors should receive a CGA as a basis for treatment decision, when aged 70 years and older. EORTC recommends at least a minimal dataset to be able to compare patients between different trials [12].

The principles of a comprehensive geriatric assessment (CGA) are presented in Chapter 29. In this section, data on results of a CGA in lung cancer patients are presented.

The Multicenter Italian Lung cancer in the Elderly Study (MILES) included data on CGA activities of daily living (ADLs), instrumental activities of daily living (IADL), and comorbidities, assessed using the Charlson comorbidity scale (CCS). In addition, the trials included the measurement of health related quality of life (HR-QOL), assessed with the EORTC-QLQ-C30. The authors conclude that pretreatment global QOL and IADL scores, but not ADL and comorbidity, have significant prognostic value on survival of elderly patients with advanced non–small cell lung cancer who were treated with chemotherapy. Using these scores in clinical practice might improve prognostic prediction for treatment planning [13].

20.13 COMORBIDITY

Comorbidity is the existence of any additional diseases in the presence of an index case with cancer. Comorbidity is of major prognostic relevance in cancer patients in general and in lung cancer patients in particular. As nicotine use causes not only lung cancer but also cardiovascular and other lung diseases, comorbidities are very common in lung cancer patients. Therefore nicotine abuse might cause the cancer and prevent effective treatment strategies, for example in patients with severe cardiovascular comorbidities or in patients with chronic lung disease, where a standard approach to the resection of the tumor (e.g. via lobectomy or complete resection of a lung) might not be possible.

Nicotine use causes other cancers such as head and neck, bladder, and esophageal cancer.

There have also been reports on the prognostic impact of comorbidities on survival in lung cancer patients.

Read et al. analyzed the role of comorbidities on the 1-year survival rate of patients with different types of tumors and within different tumor stages. The less aggressive the tumors, the more local or regional their stage, and the smaller the size of the tumor, the greater the extent to which the 1-year survival rate was associated with comorbidity and not with the tumor [6].

Age and comorbidity independently influence patient selection for treatment of stage III NSCLC with combined modality therapy [14].

The presence of comorbidity is associated with toxicity in patients with advanced NSCLC treated with pemetrexed/carboplatin or with gemcitabine/carboplatin as first-line therapy of stage IIIB/IV NSCLC [15].

20.14 TREATMENT OPTIONS

Do treatment options differ according to the age of the patient? The database for treatment recommendations with high-level evidence is poor in elderly patients, as such patients are underrepresented in clinical trials. Hutchins and coworkers [1] reported the relative frequency of patients aged >65 years in trials of the South-West Oncology Group (SWOG) and compared it to the relative frequency of cancer patients in the US population. In the SWOG trials, 39% of lung cancer patients were 65 years and older compared to 66% of all cases in the United States [16]. Similar results are reported by Lewis et al. for trials of the US National Cancer Institute (NCI) [17]. The main recommendation therefore is to include elderly patients with lung cancer in clinical trials. Jatoi et al. [18] addressed the issue of how the recruitment of elderly patients in lung cancer trials could be improved. The authors compared four trials of the North Central Cancer Treatment Group. Two had abolished upper age limits and two others were especially assigned to the needs of elderly patients. The latter were better able to recruit elderly patients [18].

Population-based analysis of registry data demonstrate that in elderly patients the tumors are less often confirmed by histology, that stage classification is more often incomplete, and that elderly patients frequently receive less treatment according to guidelines established [19,20].

Owonikoko et al. [3] analyzed the SEER database of the years 1998–2003. They indentified 316,682 patients with lung cancer, 45,912 (14%) were 80 years or older, 103,963 (33%) were aged 70–79 years, and 166,807 (53%) were younger than 70 years. Overall survival rate at 5 years decreased with age and were 7.4%, 12.3%, and 15.5%, respectively. Patients aged 80 years or older were less likely to receive local therapy (no surgery or radiation) than younger patients. Overall outcomes for patients who underwent surgical therapy or radiation were comparable across the three age groups [3].

Figure 20.4 reports the stage of lung cancer at diagnosis according to age based on SEER data. The relative frequency of patients diagnosed in advanced stage increases with advanced age as does the relative frequency of patients with unclassified stage.

20.15 SURGERY

Surgery is the primary treatment of choice for stages I and II and for some subsets of stage IIIA NSCLC. The role of surgery in the elderly population has changed significantly since the mid-1990s. During the 1980s, age was considered a relative contraindication to thoracotomy, and surgical intervention in elderly people was approached with great hesitation. Nevertheless, advances in anesthetic management and surgical techniques have allowed the inclusion of increasing numbers of elderly patients in surgical studies. Yet, age still appears to be a major factor influencing treatment choice, and curative cancer-directed surgery is often omitted in elderly patients.

Mery et al. [21] analyzed the data from 14,555 patients registered in the Surveillance, Epidemiology, and End Results (SEER) database from 1992 to 1997. Age was grouped into the following three categories: <65 years ($n = 5057$; 35%); 65–74 years ($n = 6073$; 42%); and >75 years ($n = 3425$; 23%). Curative surgery was performed in 92% of those aged <65 years, 86% of those aged 65–74 years, and 70% of those >75 years of age. Differences were significant. Survival decreased with age. The median survival times were 71, 47, and 28 months, respectively, for patients <65, 65–74, and >75 years of age ($p < 0.0001$). For the younger patients, lobectomy conferred better survival times after 2 years than did limited resections after 2 years. However, there was no difference in survival between lobectomy and limited resections in terms of survival time for the elderly patients. The statistical difference in long-term survival between those patients undergoing lobectomy and those undergoing limited resections disappeared at age 71 years [21].

Several studies support that the surgical treatment of NSCLC in older people is feasible and that age per se is not a contraindication for various surgical procedures [4]. Pneumonectomy is associated with a higher incidence of postoperative morbidity and mortality in elderly patients. The literature is heterogeneous regarding the effect of age on postoperative morbidity and mortality in lobectomy. So far data do not support the use of more limited surgery compared to lobectomy per se in older patients. In more recent years video-assisted thoracoscopic surgery (VATS) has emerged as a minimally invasive surgical technique. McVay and colleagues reported a series of 159 lung cancer patients aged >80 years (range 80–94) treated with VATS lobectomy, with very low postoperative morbidity (18%) and mortality (1.8%) [22]. However, randomized trial data are missing.

Patients with lung cancer should not be excluded from surgical resection with lobectomy or more limited procedures solely on the basis of their chronological age. New surgical techniques, and improvement in peri- and postoperative management enable surgical resection even in patients considered as inoperable in former times [23].

Figure 20.7 provides an algorithm for the therapy of non–small cell lung cancer stages I/II and T3N1M0 [11].

Figure 20.8 provides an algorithm for the therapy of non–small cell lung cancer stage IIIA (T1–3N2M0) [11].

20.16 RADIOTHERAPY

Radiotherapy is effective in lung cancer. Tumors in older compared to younger patients do not differ in sensitivity to radiotherapy, and radiotherapy may be a treatment option in several different situations.

In patients with resectable tumors, but not considered fit for surgery, definitive radiotherapy might be an option. The largest series was reported by Pignon. They did not find a significant difference in efficacy between younger and older patients. However, age was associated with higher rates of weight loss [24].

Newer techniques of radiation such as three-dimensional (3D) conformal radiotherapy, intensity-modulated radiation therapy, and stereotactic radiotherapy may improve efficacy of radiotherapy further and reduce radiotherapy-related toxicity further. These therefore might be treatment options, especially for elderly patients with comorbidity and functional decline [4].

No randomized comparison between surgery and radiotherapy in elderly patients with lung cancer has been performed.

Currently no data support the use of adjuvant radiotherapy after curative surgery in elderly patients with lung cancer or the use of preoperative or postoperative radiochemotherapy in elderly patients with lung cancer.

In locally advanced disease one treatment option is either sequential or concurrent radiochemotherapy [i.e. radiotherapy plus chemotherapy (RTCT)]. Liang et al. [25]

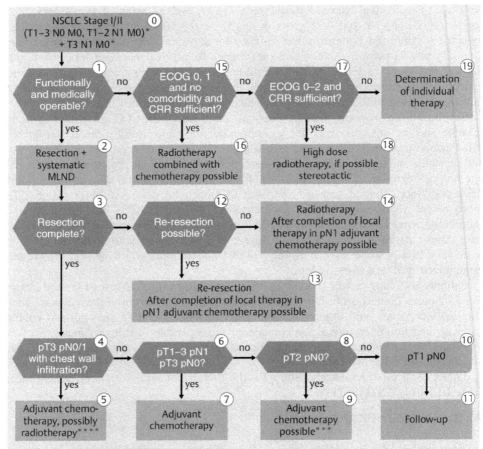

MLND: Mediastinal Lymph Node Dissection; CRR: Cardiorespiratory Reserve.
Operability and resectability are assessed preoperatively by thoracic surgeon and pneumologist. Except for pT1 pN0 all patients will be presented after surgery or in inoperability to an interdisciplinary conference including at least pneumology, oncology, thoracic surgery, radiation oncology, and diagnostic radiology. The next steps (indication radiotherapy; indication chemotherapy) will be defined and documented.

*   after a sensitive mediastinal staging according to diagnosis chapter.
**   pN1 implies a high risk of systemic relapse; after R0 resection patients with pN1 (pT1–3) benefit most from adjuvant chemotherapy, therefore this can be recommended in an individual case also after completion of local therapy in previous R1/2 resection.
***   in exploratory subgroup analysis of adjuvant therapy studies pT2pN0 shows no consistent survival benefit with adjuvant therapy. A recommendation can be made in individual cases.
**** in cases of chest wall infiltration and histologically proven R0 resection the need of radiotherapy of the tumor bed may be discussed because of tumor location or vicinity of tumor to the resection margin.

Figure 20.7 Algorithm for the therapy of non–small cell lung cancer of stages I/II and T3N1M0 [11].

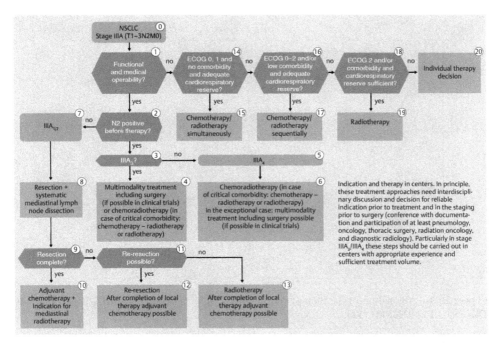

Figure 20.8 Algorithm for the therapy of non–small cell lung cancer of stage IIIA (T1–3N2M0) [11].

report a meta-analysis of 11 trials, including 2043 patients. The results confirmed that concurrent RTCT significantly increases median survival time (16.3 vs. 13.9 months; 95% CI 1.09–1.26), response rate (64.0% vs. 56.3%; 95% CI 1.10–1.72), albeit at the expense of both increased hematological toxicity (neutropenia and thrombocytopenia) and nonhematological toxicity (nausea/vomiting, stomatitis, and esophagitis). Of the 11 trials, [7] systematically excluded patients older than 75 years. In most of the trials the patients had to have an ECOG or WHO-PS of <2 or a Karnofski-PS >70% [25]. However, this is a treatment option in patients without severe comorbidity who have excellent performance status.

Figure 20.9 provides an algorithm for the therapy of non–small lung cancer of stage IIIA/B (T4N0/1M0, T4N2M0, T1–4N3M0) [11].

20.17 MEDICAL TREATMENT

Medical treatment differs for patients with NSCLC or SCLC. A variety of reviews are available for more detailed analysis [4,26,27,53]. Chemotherapy was and is the cornerstone of medical treatment. New molecular defined treatment options have been developed in more recent years, however.

20.17.1 Small Cell Lung Cancer (SCLC)

According to the SEER program, about 30% of patients diagnosed with SCLC are 70 years and older, and about 10% are 80 years and older [3]. Traditionally SCLC is staged

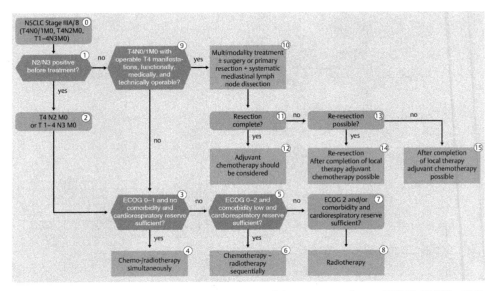

Figure 20.9 Algorithm for the therapy of non–small lung cancer of stage IIIA/B (T4N0–1M0, T4N2M0, T1–4N3M0) [11].

as limited and extended disease. However, staging according to TNM classification is now recommended. As most of the trials used traditional staging, the recommendations described in the following subsections are based on this classification.

Limited Disease　In patients with SCLC, the treatment of choice depends upon the clinical stage. In very limited disease (T1/2, N0/1, M0), primary surgery should be followed by four cycles of combination chemotherapy. A PET/CT scan has to exclude mediastinal lymph node involvement before treatment. Prophylactic cranial irradiation should follow.

In patients with T3/4 and/or N2/3, M0 (limited disease), the treatment of choice is chemotherapy with cisplatin and etoposide. Patients should receive at least four cycles. Continued response has to be confirmed with each cycle. If possible, radiotherapy should be applied simultaneously. However, data on simultaneous chemoradiotherapy are very limited in patients aged 75 years and older. As toxicity increases with age, simultaneous chemoradiotherapy is a treatment option for very selected older patients. In patients with good performance status and lack of comorbidity, a sequential chemoradiotherapy might be employed as an alternative.

Figure 20.10 provides an algorithm for the therapy of preoperative pathologically proven small cell lung cancer in stage cT1/2,N0/1,M0 (very limited disease) [11].

Figure 20.11 provides an algorithm for the treatment of small cell lung cancer in stage T3/4 and/or N2/3,M0 (limited disease) [11].

Extended Disease　In patients with stage M1 disease (tradionally called *extended disease*) the treatment of choice is chemotherapy.

Pelayo Alvarez et al. [28] presented a Cochrane review on the effectiveness of chemotherapy in extensive SCLC compared with best supportive care (BSC) or placebo

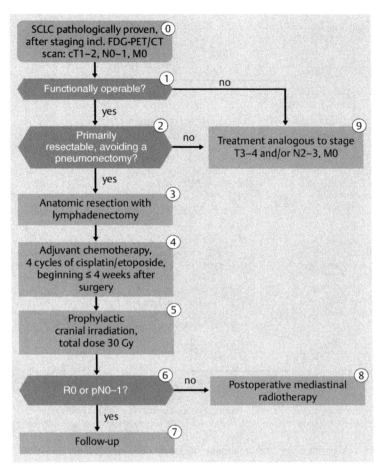

Figure 20.10   Algorithm for the therapy of preoperative pathologically proven small cell lung cancer in stage cT1/2,N0/1,M0 (very limited disease) [11].

treatment. Two studies provided first-line chemotherapy, and treatment prolonged survival. However, patients aged >70 years were excluded from this trial, dating back to the 1970s. Two studies used second-line chemotherapy, and the overall survival and quality of life in these patients was better in the chemotherapy group compared to the group of patients receiving best supportive care alone [28].

Single-agent chemotherapy, such as oral etoposide, is inferior to standard intravenous multidrug chemotherapy in the palliative treatment of patients with SCLC and poor performance status [29].

Cisplatin or carboplatin combined with etoposide is the regimen most commonly used. Other active regimens are adriamycin, cyclophosphamide, vincristine (ACO), and cisplatin/carboplatin plus topoisomerase inhibitors, such as topotecan or irinotecan, or platin plus paclitaxel, or platin plus gemcitabine.

In progressive disease a second-line treatment, such as topotecan, can prolong life and improve symptoms [30].

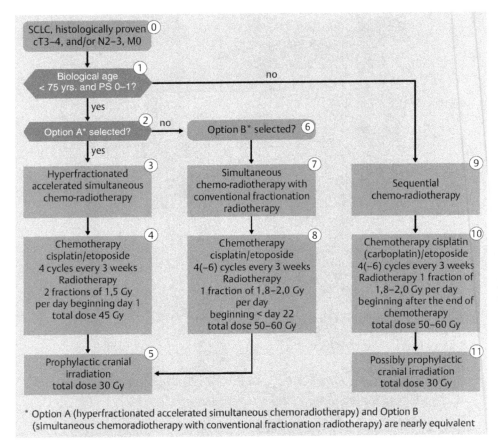

* Option A (hyperfractionated accelerated simultaneous chemoradiotherapy) and Option B
(simultaneous chemoradiotherapy with conventional fractionation radiotherapy) are nearly equivalent

Figure 20.11   Algorithm for the treatment of small cell lung cancer in stage T3/4 and/or N2/3,M0 (limited disease) [11].

Figure 20.12 provides an algorithm for the treatment of small cell lung cancer with distant metastases M1 (extensive disease) [11].

Figure 20.13 provides an algorithm for the treatment of relapsed small cell lung cancer [11].

20.17.2   Non–Small Cell Lung Cancer (NSCLC)

Medical treatment of NSCLC is adjuvant or palliative.

Adjuvant Treatment   A number of trials have been published demonstrating that the application of adjuvant chemotherapy after complete resection of NSCLC in stages II and $IIIA_{1/2}$ improves overall survival. In adjuvant treatment the possible future benefit of improvement in overall survival has to be weighed against possible risks, such as treatment related toxicity and cost. Only a small number of patients will benefit from the treatment. As the risk of toxicity increases with advanced age and the remaining life expectancy decreases, the decision-making between potential benefits and risks will differ between elderly and younger patients.

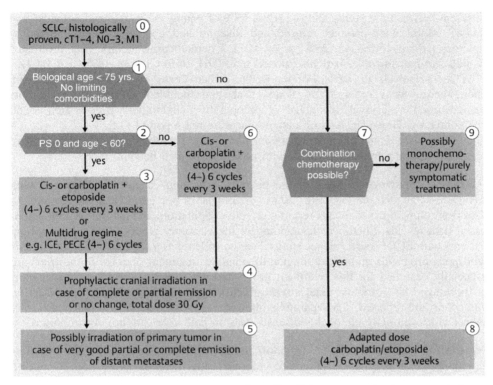

Figure 20.12   Algorithm for the treatment of small cell lung cancer in the stage of distant metastases M1 (extensive disease) [11].

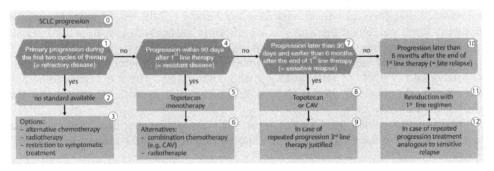

Figure 20.13   Algorithm for the relapse treatment of small cell lung cancer [11].

Different treatment schedules have been suggested. JBR.10 was a phase III randomized trial of adjuvant cisplatin and vinorelbine versus observation after complete resection of stage IB or stage II NSCLC. The main goal of this study was to determine whether adjuvant postoperative chemotherapy conferred a survival benefit compared with observation alone. The chemotherapy regimen used in JBR.10 was vinorelbine 25 mg/m^2 on days 1, 8, 15, and 22 and cisplatin 50 mg/m^2 on days 1 and 8 of a 28-day cycle [31]. Of the 482 patients randomly assigned to JBR.10, 327 were young and 155 were old. Comparing baseline characteristics, only PS remained significantly different between the young and old (PS0: 57% of young vs. 36% of old patients; $p = 0.004$). More older patients refused and discontinued chemotherapy compared to younger patients (40% vs. 23%; $p = 0.01$). Chemotherapy significantly prolonged overall survival for older patients (hazard ratio 0.61; 95% CI 0.38–0.98; p < 0.04).

A meta-analysis of trials evaluating the effectiveness of preoperative adjuvant chemotherapy was reported by Song et al. and included 13 trials. The authors demonstrated a survival advantage of preoperative chemotherapy compared to no chemotherapy. However, data on patient age were not reported [32].

In conclusion, in fit older patients, adjuvant chemotherapy or preoperative chemotherapy is a treatment option with potential survival benefit.

Palliative Treatment Most of the patients with lung cancer are diagnosed with advanced-stage disease (see Fig. 20.4). Treatment is not curative at this stage. As data from clinical trials always report a selected population, an analysis of population-based data reveals a better understanding of the currently practiced treatment option. Patients with ECOG performance status 2 are considered as a separate group of patients with poor prognosis and less tolerance to standard treatment options. Some trials are especially designed for this treatment group and are reported separately. The cohort of those aged 80 years and older are those least represented in clinical trials. Data on this cohort are reported in a separate paragraph. As most patients with advanced lung cancer will eventually die of this disease, data on palliative care are also reported.

Population-Based Analysis Davidoff and coworkers demonstrated that only a limited number of elderly patients (aged 65 years and older) with advanced NSCLC receive chemotherapy. Of the 21,285 patients, identified in the SEER-Medicare database, 25.8% received first-line chemotherapy only. Increasing age and comorbidity and poor performance status were associated with less use of chemotherapy, either single-agent or platinum based regimens. Use of chemotherapy was significantly associated with improved 1-year survival rate, compared to no therapy (27.0% vs. 11.6%). The use of platinum-based combined therapy was significantly associated with improved 1-year survival rate, compared to single-agent chemotherapy (30.1% vs. 19.4%) [33].

Chrischilles et al. analyzed the use of, and toxicity from, chemotherapy in patients with advanced NSCLC in relation to age and comorbidity. The use of chemotherapy decreased with advanced age, as did the rate of adverse events, independent of the level of comorbidity [34].

Elderly patients were the focus of some trials evaluating first-line treatment. Data on maintenance, second-, or even third-line treatment are more limited to subgroup analysis.

First-Line Treatment A Cochrane review published in 2010 confirmed the survival advantage of patients with advanced NSCLC treated with chemotherapy. The authors identified 19 trials, including 2714 patients, comparing either single-agent or combination chemotherapy with supportive care alone [35]. The authors did not find clear evidence of a difference or trend in the relative effect of chemotherapy in patient subgroups defined by age or performance status. Some trials in particular included elderly patients and they are reported in more detail here.

The Elderly Lung Cancer Vinorelbine Italian Group Study (ELVIS) addressed the question as to whether elderly patients with advanced NSCLC benefit from first-line chemotherapy. The trial compared single-agent vinorelbine to supportive care.

In this study, 154 patients aged 70 years and older were randomly assigned to BSC or vinorelbine 30 mg/m^2 on days 1 and 8. The study clearly demonstrated a significant survival advantage for vinorelbine. The differences in median survival were 21 versus 28 weeks, the 6-month survival rates 41% versus 55%, and the 12-month survival rates were 32% vs. 14%. In addition, vinorelbine treatment resulted in improved HR-QOL compared to best supportive care. No treatment discontinuation due to toxicity occurred. There were no treatment-related deaths [36].

The Multicenter Italian Lung cancer in the Elderly Study (MILES) addressed the question as to which single agent is most appropriate for treating elderly patients. The MILES trial compared docetaxel with vinorelbine; 182 NSCLC patients aged 70 years and older were randomized to receive either docetaxel or vinorelbine. The primary endpoint was overall survival. There were no significant differences in overall survival between the two treatment arms. However, there was a trend toward a higher survival in the docetaxel arm. Median survival was 14.3 versus 9.9 months. Progression-free survival, response, and disease-related symptoms were significantly improved in the docetaxel arm compared to the vinorelbine arm. Toxicity rates, except for neutropenia, were not significantly different between the two arms [37].

A 2010 Japanese trial evaluated first-line treatment of advanced NSCLC using a standard carboplatin dose either combined with a 3-weekly paclitaxel or with weekly paclitaxel in patients aged 70 years and older. Patients treated with the weekly regimen had equivalent efficacy but less toxicity compared with those treated with the standard 3-weekly regimen [38].

Figure 20.14 provides an algorithm for the treatment of stage IV/IIIB non–small cell lung cancer [11].

Maintenance Treatment Erlotinib was approved for maintenance treatment after following first-line chemotherapy of advanced NSCLC (see text below).

Second-Line Treatment Most patients develop disease that is resistant to first-line or maintenance treatment. In these patients second-line treatment is an option.

Di Maio et al. analyzed individual patients' data from nine randomized trials of second-line treatment in advanced NSCLC. The primary endpoint was overall survival. The prognosis of patients eligible for second-line treatment for advanced NSCLC is significantly affected by gender, performance status, histology, stage, previous use of platinum, and response to first-line drugs. The median age of the patients was 61 years (range 26–84). Age was initially included (<70 years vs. >70 years), but was not a significant factor for survival [39].

Weiss and colleagues reported a subgroup analysis of patients aged 70 years and older in a trial of second-line treatment for advanced NSCLC. Patients received either docetaxel or pemetrexed. Survival did not differ between younger and older patients. Older patients treated with pemetrexed demonstrated a longer progression-free survival and overall survival compared to those treated with docetaxel; however, this was not significant. The rates of febrile neutropenia was significantly lower in those treated with pemetrexed (2.5 vs. 19%, $p = 0.025$) [40].

A trial reported by Pallis et al. demonstrated that a combination chemotherapy of docetaxel and cisplatin is not superior to single-agent treatment with docetaxel [41].

Other active agents are available. The treatment choice depends on the type of first-line therapy, the histology, EGFR mutation status, the comorbidity, and the performance status of the patient.

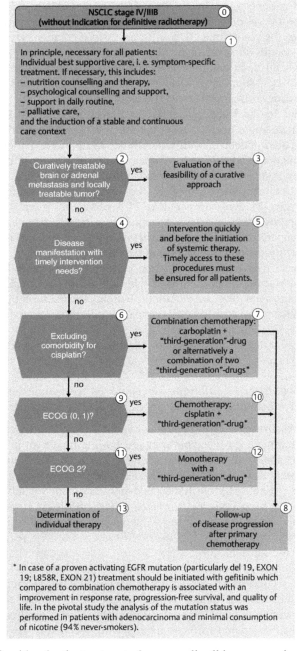

Figure 20.14 Algorithm for the treatment of non–small cell lung cancer in stage IV/IIIB [11].

20.18 MOLECULAR DEFINED TARGETS

An increasing number of molecular targets have been identified within more recent years. Some of them lead to the development of drugs.

20.18.1 EGFR Inhibitors

The epidermal growth factor receptor (EGFR) pathway is activated in more than half of the patients with NSCLC. There are different agents available for inhibiting EGFR (e.g. cetuximab, gefitinib, erlotinib). Data on gefitinib and erlotinib are summarized in a 2011 review [42].

Cetuximab Cetuximab is a monoclonal antibody targeting the epidermal growth factor receptor. Efficacy was evaluated in a prospective randomized controlled trial. Patients in the standard arm were treated with cisplatin and vinorelbine for up to six cycles. In the experimental arm, cetuximab was added and was continued after the end of chemotherapy until disease progression or unacceptable toxicity occurred. The primary endpoint was overall survival. In this trial, 1125 patients were randomly assigned to chemotherapy plus cetuximab or chemotherapy alone. Overall survival was significantly longer in those receiving cetuximab HR 0.871 (95% CI 0.76–0.99; $p = 0.044$). Median survival was 11.3 months in those receiving cetuximab compared to 10.1 months in those treated with conventional chemotherapy [43]. The trial had no upper age limit. However, the median age was 58 years. The forest plot for patients <65 years was 0.85 (0.72–0.99) in favor of the addition of cetuximab, and 0.93 (0.73–1.20) for those aged 65 years and older.

Lin et al. reported a systematic review of trials evaluating the addition of cetuximab to first-line chemotherapy treatment for advanced NSCLC. Four trials were included. The addition of cetuximab to chemotherapy improved overall survival and overall response rate. However, the median age of the patients was 58–66 years.

Gefitinib Patients with non–small cell lung cancer harboring mutations in the epidermal growth factor receptor (EGFR) gene respond well to the EGFR-specific tyrosine kinase inhibitor gefitinib. However, after initial approval in the United States, the FDA changed approval for gefitinib to patients (1) currently receiving and benefiting from gefitinib, (2) patients who previously received and benefited from gefitinib, and (3) previously enrolled patients or new patients in noninvestigational new drug (IND) clinical trials approved by an IRB prior to June 17, 2005 (http://www.cancer.gov/cancertopics/druginfo/fda-gefitinib; accessed 5/09/11). However, approval varies in different countries. In Europe, gefitinib is approved by the EMEA for use in patients with NSCLC who carry activating EGFR mutations.

Common adverse events associated with gefitinib are diarrhea, rash, acne, dry skin, nausea, and vomiting.

A randomized controlled trial comparing single-agent gefitinib versus chemotherapy with cisplatin plus docetaxel in patients with first-line treatment in advanced NSCLC and harboring EGFR mutations excluded patients aged >75 years [44].

Jiang et al. [45] performed a meta-analysis of randomized controlled trials to compare the efficacy, quality of life (QOL), symptom improvement, and toxicities of gefitinib with docetaxel in previously treated advanced NSCLC. Four trials comprising 2257 patients were included. Overall survival and progression-free survival were similar; however, gefitinib showed an advantage over docetaxel in terms of objective response rate, quality of life, and tolerability [45].

Erlotinib Erlotinib is approved in the United States by the Food and Drug Administration (FDA) and in Europe by the EMEA for patients with locally advanced or metastatic NSCLC, previously treated with chemotherapy as a second- or third-line therapy. Elderly patients who are treated with erlotinib have clinical outcomes that are similar to those for younger patients but have a higher rate of grade 3 or 4 toxicity (35% for patients ≥ 70 years vs. 18% for patients <70 years) [46].

The data from the SATURN trial revealed that erlotinib received approval for first-line maintenance treatment of locally advanced or metastatic non–small cell lung cancer (NSCLC) in patients whose disease had not progressed after four cycles of platinum-based chemotherapy [47]. The median age of the patients was 60 years, range 30–83 years. Patients with ECOG-PS >1 were excluded from the trial. In the forest plot, results were significantly different for patients younger than 65 years than for those aged 65 years and older.

20.18.2   VEGF Inhibitors

Malignant tumors require a blood supply to grow, and they stimulate vascular growth. Vascular endothelial growth factor (VEGF) inhibitors prevent vascular growth.

Bevacizumab   Botrel et al. [48] undertook a systematic review and meta-analysis on the efficacy of bevacizumab plus chemotherapy compared to chemotherapy alone in first-line treatment of advanced NSCLC. They identified four trials including 2200 patients. The addition of bevacizumab increased the response rate and progression-free survival; however, the effect on overall survival remained unclear [48].

20.18.3   ALK Inhibitors

Some patients with NSCLC, who are usually younger, former or nonsmokers and have adenocarcinoma, exhibit a fusion of the anaplastic lymphoma kinase (ALK) with the ELM4 gene. About 3% of NSCLC patients have a ELM4-ALK fusion gene. Crizotinib is an inhibitor of ALK. Within a phase I trial, crizotinib demonstrated impressive remissions in the majority of patients [49].

20.19   SPECIAL LUNG CANCER PATIENTS

20.19.1   Patients with Performance Status 2

Performance status (PS), according to the Eastern Cooperative Oncology Group (ECOG), or Karnofski-performance status (KPS) is a major predictor of survival and toxicity. Poor PS is defined as ECOG-PS of 2 or KPS $<= 70$. Poor performance status is an adverse prognostic factor in patients with NSCLC. Shorter survival and higher frequency and severity of toxicity occur in such patients. With increasing age the frequency of patients with poor performance status increases. As chemotherapy is more toxic in patients with poor performance status, special treatment protocols have been developed.

20.19.2   Patients Aged 80 Years and Older

In the United States, 15–20% of all lung cancer patients are 80 years and older. Altundag et al. reported the data of the MD Anderson Cancer Center. Of 13,690 patients seen in the Thoracic Oncology Department between the years 1997 and 2004, 496 (3.6%) patients were 80 years and older; 46 of them had advanced NSCLC and were chemotherapy-naive. These patients were treated at the center and had at least one follow-up visit. They were compared to a younger cohort who were matched with respect to treatment, race, histology, and gender. Platinum regimens were given in 43% versus 79% ($p < 0.0001$), the response rate was 41% versus 47%, the median progression-free survival was 5.5 versus 3.9 months ($p = 0.216$), and the median overall survival was 10.7 versus 9.8 months ($p = 0.43$). Hematologic and nonhematologic toxicities were similar. The authors concluded that selected patients 80 years of age and older may tolerate and benefit from chemotherapy [50].

Oxnard et al. [20] performed a retrospective chart review in 111 patients aged 80 years and older who were treated for lung cancer in a large teaching hospital. Of 70 patients with stage III or IV disease, 36% received cytotoxic chemotherapy and 27% received oral targeted therapy alone; 32% of these patients received the stage-specific treatment as recommended in guidelines. Of the patients who did not receive treatment according to guidelines, 26% electively refused and 74% were not offered therapy [20].

Heskett et al. [51] reported the results of two prospective trials. Patients aged 70 or older who were chemotherapy-naive and had stage IIIB/IV NSCLC, aged 70 with an ECOG-PS of 0 or 1, or patients of any age with PS2 were included. Patients received either three cycles of vinorelbine followed by three cycles of docetaxel or single-agent docetaxel. 21% of patients were aged 80 years or older. The authors concluded that chemotherapy regimens were associated with an encouraging disease control rate (54%) in patients 80 years or older with advanced NSCLC and were well tolerated. Selected octogenarians with advanced NSCLC may benefit from single–agent chemotherapy [51].

The data on patients aged 80 years and older are very limited, but do suggest that some patients with advanced-stage disease might benefit from single-agent chemotherapy.

20.20 CONCLUSIONS AND PALLIATIVE CARE

Most patients with primary or secondary advanced disease will die of their lung cancer. These patients benefit from palliative care. A recent trial reported patients with newly diagnosed metastatic NSCLC who were randomized between standard care including chemotherapy versus chemotherapy and early palliative care. The primary endpoint was quality of life at 12 weeks measured with the functional assessment of cancer therapy–lung (FACT-L) scale. In addition, anxiety and depression were measured with the Hospital Anxiety and Depression (HADS) scale. Patients in the early palliative care group had better quality of life at week 12 (98.0 vs. 91.5; $p = 0.03$), exhibited less anxiety and depression (16% vs. 38%, $p = 0.01$), received less aggressive end-of-life care (16% vs. 38%, $P = 0.01$), and had a longer median survival than did patients in the standard care arm (11.6 months vs. 8.9 months, $P = 0.02$) [52]. Median age of the patients in this trial was 65 years. There is no obvious reason why the results should not be valid for elderly patients as well as for younger patients, although this has to be confirmed. However, they demonstrate that patients should be informed of the possibility of integrating a palliative care physician early in the treatment of their advanced disease.

REFERENCES

1. Pallis AG, Fortpied C, et al. EORTC elderly task force position paper: Approach to the older cancer patient. *Eur J Cancer* 2010;**46**(9):1502–1513.

2. Extermann M, Aapro M, et al. Use of comprehensive geriatric assessment in older cancer patients: Recommendations from the task force on CGA of the International Society of Geriatric Oncology (SIOG). *Crit Rev Oncol Hematol* 2005;**55**(3):241–252.

3. Owonikoko TK, Ragin CC, et al. Lung cancer in elderly patients: an analysis of the surveillance, epidemiology, and end results database. *J Clin Oncol* 2007;**25**(35):5570–7.

4. Pallis AG, Gridelli C, et al. EORTC Elderly Task Force and Lung Cancer Group and International Society for Geriatric Oncology (SIOG) experts' opinion for the treatment of non-small-cell lung cancer in an elderly population. *Ann Oncol* 2009;**21**(4):692–706.

5. Perrone F, Di Maio M, et al. Outcome of patients with a performance status of 2 in the Multicenter Italian Lung Cancer in the Elderly Study (MILES). *J Clin Oncol* 2004;**22**(24):5018–20; author reply 5020–5021.

6. Read WL, Tierney RM, et al. Differential prognostic impact of comorbidity. *J Clin Oncol* 2004;**22**(15):3099–3103.

7. Extermann M, Overcash J, et al. Comorbidity and functional status are independent in older cancer patients. *J Clin Oncol* 1998;**16**(4):1582–7.

8. Repetto L, Venturino A, et al. Performance status and comorbidity in elderly cancer patients compared with young patients with neoplasia and elderly patients without neoplastic conditions. *Cancer* 1998;**82**(4):760–5.

9. Repetto L, Fratino L, et al. Comprehensive geriatric assessment adds information to Eastern Cooperative Oncology Group performance status in elderly cancer patients: an Italian Group for Geriatric Oncology Study. *J Clin Oncol* 2002;**20**(2):494–502.

10. Wedding U, Roehrig B, et al. Comorbidity in patients with cancer: prevalence and severity measured by cumulative illness rating scale. *Crit Rev Oncol Hematol* 2007;**61**(3):269–76.

11. Goeckenjan G, Sitter H, et al. Prevention, diagnosis, therapy, and follow-up of lung cancer: interdisciplinary guideline of the German Respiratory Society and the German Cancer Society. *Pneumologie* 2010;**65**(1):39–59.

12. Pallis AG, Ring A, et al. EORTC workshop on clinical trial methodology in older individuals with a diagnosis of solid tumors. *Ann Oncol* 2011;**22**(8):1922–6.

13. Maione P, Perrone F, et al. Pretreatment quality of life and functional status assessment significantly predict survival of elderly patients with advanced non-small-cell lung cancer receiving chemotherapy: a prognostic analysis of the multicenter Italian lung cancer in the elderly study. *J Clin Oncol* 2005;**23**(28):6865–72.

14. Firat S, Pleister A, et al. Age is independent of comorbidity influencing patient selection for combined modality therapy for treatment of stage III nonsmall cell lung cancer (NSCLC). *Am J Clin Oncol* 2006;**29**(3):252–257.

15. Gronberg BH, Sundstrom S, et al. Influence of comorbidity on survival, toxicity and health-related quality of life in patients with advanced non-small-cell lung cancer receiving platinum-doublet chemotherapy. *Eur J Cancer* 2010;**46**(12):2225–34.

16. Hutchins LF, Unger JM, et al. Underrepresentation of patients 65 years of age or older in cancer-treatment trials. *N Engl J Med* 1999;**341**(27):2061–2067.

17. Lewis JH, Kilgore ML, et al. Participation of patients 65 years of age or older in cancer clinical trials. *J Clin Oncol* 2003;**21**(7):1383–1389.

18. Jatoi A, Hillman S, et al. Should elderly non-small-cell lung cancer patients be offered elderly-specific trials? Results of a pooled analysis from the North Central Cancer Treatment Group. *J Clin Oncol* 2005;**23**(36):9113–9.

19. Ramsey SD, Howlader N, et al. Chemotherapy use, outcomes, and costs for older persons with advanced non-small-cell lung cancer: evidence from surveillance, epidemiology and end results-Medicare. *J Clin Oncol* 2004;**22**(24):4971–8.

20. Oxnard GR, Fidias P, et al. Non-small cell lung cancer in octogenarians: Treatment practices and preferences. *J Thorac Oncol* 2007;**2**(11):1029–1035.

21. Mery CM, Pappas AN, et al. Similar long-term survival of elderly patients with non-small cell lung cancer treated with lobectomy or wedge resection within the surveillance, epidemiology, and end results database. *Chest* 2005;**128**(1):237–245.

22. McVay CL, Pickens A, et al. VATS anatomic pulmonary resection in octogenarians. *Am Surg* 2005;**71**(9):791–793.

23. Linden PA, Bueno R, et al. Lung resection in patients with preoperative FEV1 < 35% predicted. *Chest* 2005;**127**(6):1984–90.

24. Pignon T, Gregor A, et al. Age has no impact on acute and late toxicity of curative thoracic radiotherapy. *Radiother Oncol* 1998;**46**(3):239–48.

25. Liang HY, Zhou H, et al. Chemo-radiotherapy for advanced non-small cell lung cancer: concurrent or sequential? It's no longer the question: A systematic review. *Int J Cancer* 2010;**127**(3):718–728.

26. Honecker F, Wedding U, et al. Chemotherapy in elderly patients with advanced lung cancer. Part I: General aspects and treatment of small cell lung cancer (SCLC). *Onkologie* 2004;**27**(5):500–5.

27. Pallis AG, Shepherd FA, et al. Treatment of small-cell lung cancer in elderly patients. *Cancer* 2010;**116**(5):1192–200.

28. Pelayo Alvarez M, Gallego Rubio O, et al. Chemotherapy versus best supportive care for extensive small cell lung cancer. *Cochrane Database Syst Rev* 2009; Issue 4, No. CD001990.

29. Girling DJ. Comparison of oral etoposide and standard intravenous multidrug chemotherapy for small-cell lung cancer: A stopped multicentre randomised trial. Medical Research Council Lung Cancer Working Party. *Lancet* 1996;**348**(9027):563–566.

30. O'Brien ME, Ciuleanu TE, et al. Phase III trial comparing supportive care alone with supportive care with oral topotecan in patients with relapsed small-cell lung cancer. *J Clin Oncol* 2006;**24**(34):5441–7.

31. Pepe C, Hasan B, et al. Adjuvant vinorelbine and cisplatin in elderly patients: National Cancer Institute of Canada and Intergroup Study JBR.10. *J Clin Oncol* 2007;**25**(12):1553–61.

32. Song WA, Zhou NK, et al. Survival benefit of neoadjuvant chemotherapy in non-small cell lung cancer: An updated meta-analysis of 13 randomized control trials. *J Thorac Oncol* 2010;**5**(4):510–516.

33. Davidoff AJ, Tang M, et al. Chemotherapy and survival benefit in elderly patients with advanced non-small-cell lung cancer. *J Clin Oncol* 2010;**28**(13):2191–7.

34. Chrischilles EA, Pendergast JF, et al. Adverse events among the elderly receiving chemotherapy for advanced non-small-cell lung cancer. *J Clin Oncol* 2010;**28**(4):620–7.

35. Group N-SCLCC Chemotherapy and supportive care versus supportive care alone for advanced non-small cell lung cancer. *Cochrane Database Syst Rev* 2010; Issue 5, No. CD007309.

36. Anonymous. Effects of vinorelbine on quality of life and survival of elderly patients with advanced non-small-cell lung cancer. The Elderly Lung Cancer Vinorelbine Italian Study Group. *J Natl Cancer Inst* 1999;**91**(1):66–72.

37. Gridelli C, Perrone F, et al. Chemotherapy for elderly patients with advanced non-small-cell lung cancer: the Multicenter Italian Lung Cancer in the Elderly Study (MILES) phase III randomized trial. *J Natl Cancer Inst* 2003;**95**(5):362–72.

38. Sakakibara T, Inoue A, et al. Randomized phase II trial of weekly paclitaxel combined with carboplatin versus standard paclitaxel combined with carboplatin for elderly patients with advanced non-small-cell lung cancer. *Ann Oncol* 2010;**21**(4):795–9.

39. Di Maio M, Lama N, et al. Clinical assessment of patients with advanced non-small-cell lung cancer eligible for second-line chemotherapy: a prognostic score from individual data of nine randomised trials. *Eur J Cancer* 2010;**46**(4):735–43.

40. Weiss GJ, Langer C, et al. Elderly patients benefit from second-line cytotoxic chemotherapy: a subset analysis of a randomized phase III trial of pemetrexed compared with docetaxel in patients with previously treated advanced non-small-cell lung cancer. *J Clin Oncol* 2006;**24**(27):4405–11.

41. Pallis AG, Agelaki S, et al. A randomized phase III study of the docetaxel/carboplatin combination versus docetaxel single-agent as second line treatment for patients with advanced/metastatic non-small cell lung cancer. *BMC Cancer* 2010;**10**:633.

42. Cataldo VD, Gibbons DL, et al. Treatment of non-small-cell lung cancer with erlotinib or gefitinib. *N Engl J Med* 2011;**364**(10):947–955.

43. Pirker R, Pereira JR, et al. Cetuximab plus chemotherapy in patients with advanced non-small-cell lung cancer (FLEX): an open-label randomised phase III trial. *Lancet* 2009;**373**(9674):1525–31.

44. Mitsudomi T, Morita S, et al. Gefitinib versus cisplatin plus docetaxel in patients with non-small-cell lung cancer harbouring mutations of the epidermal growth factor receptor (WJTOG3405): an open label, randomised phase 3 trial. *Lancet Oncol* 2010;**11**(2):121–8

45. Jiang J, Huang L, et al. Gefitinib versus docetaxel in previously treated advanced non-small-cell lung cancer: A meta-analysis of randomized controlled trials. *Acta Oncol* 2011;**50**(4):582–588.

46. Wheatley Price P, Ding K, et al. Erlotinib for advanced non-small-cell lung cancer in the elderly: an analysis of the National Cancer Institute of Canada Clinical Trials Group Study BR.21. *J Clin Oncol* 2008;**26**(14):2350–7.

47. Cappuzzo F, Ciuleanu T, et al. Erlotinib as maintenance treatment in advanced non-small-cell lung cancer: a multicentre, randomised, placebo-controlled phase 3 study. *Lancet Oncol* 2011;**11**(6):521–9.

48. Botrel TE, Clark O, et al. Efficacy of bevacizumab (Bev) plus chemotherapy (CT) compared to CT alone in previously untreated locally advanced or metastatic non-small cell lung cancer (NSCLC): Systematic review and meta-analysis. *Lung Cancer* 2011;**74**(1):89–97.

49. Katayama R, Khan TM, et al. Therapeutic strategies to overcome crizotinib resistance in non-small cell lung cancers harboring the fusion oncogene EML4-ALK. *Proc Natl Acad Sci USA* 2011;**108**(18):7535–7540.

50. Altundag O, Stewart DJ, et al. Many patients 80 years and older with advanced non-small cell lung cancer (NSCLC) can tolerate chemotherapy. *J Thorac Oncol* 2007;**2**(2):141–146.

51. Hesketh PJ, Lilenbaum RC, et al. Chemotherapy in patients > or = 80 with advanced non-small cell lung cancer: combined results from SWOG 0027 and LUN 6. *J Thorac Oncol* 2007;**2**(6):494–8.

52. Temel JS, Greer JA, et al. Early palliative care for patients with metastatic non-small-cell lung cancer. *N Engl J Med* 2010;**363**(8):733–42.

53. Honecker F, Wedding U, et al. Chemotherapy in elderly patients with advanced lung cancer. Part II: Treatment of non-small cell lung cancer (NSCLC). *Onkologie* 2004;**27**(6):583–8.

54. Goldstraw P. The revised TNM staging system for lung cancer. *J Thorac Oncol* 2009;**4**(6):671–673.

CHAPTER 21

Prostate Cancer

NICOLAS MOTTET

Urology Service, University Hospital, Saint-Etienne, France

JEAN-PIERRE DROZ

Claude Bernard University, Lyon, France

21.1 INTRODUCTION

According to GLOBOCAN statistics, there were almost 680,000 new cases of prostate cancer worldwide in 2002, with prostate cancer ranking as the fifth most common malignancy in adults and the second most common malignancy in men [1]. In 2002, a total of approximately 220,000 men died from prostate cancer, the most prevalent cancer in men with an estimated (based on 5-year survival) 2,300,000 men worldwide living with the disease. Prostate cancer occurs predominantly in older adults. According to the US Surveillance, Epidemiology, and End Results (SEER) registry, the median age at diagnosis in the years 2000–2007 was 68 years. Respectively 60% and 25.7% of new cases were diagnosed, and over 90% and 71.2% of prostate cancer–specific deaths occurred in men ≥65 years and ≥75 years of age [2]. The overall growth and aging of the world's population is expected to increase the burden of prostate cancer since the proportion of men aged ≥70 years is expected to increase from 0.8% in 2000 to 17.2% by 2050 [3]. The introduction of prostate-specific antigen (PSA) screening has dramatically changed the presentation of the disease, with patients now diagnosed at a younger age and with lower grade/organ-confined disease. However, given the long natural history of prostate cancer, many patients who were not of advanced age at the time of diagnosis are likely to be managed for PSA relapse and disease progression in their old age. These epidemiological statistics illustrate the need for information and guidelines specifically targeting adults with advanced prostate cancer. The International Society of Geriatric Oncology (SIOG) has specifically addressed the issue of decision-making for the management of elderly patients with prostate cancer [4]. The National Cancer Center Network (NCCN) has developed *Senior Adult Oncology Guidelines*, based on classical approaches of geriatric oncology and likely applicable to prostate cancer patients [5,6].

Cancer and Aging Handbook: Research and Practice, First Edition. Edited by Keith M. Bellizzi and Margot A. Gosney.
© 2012 Wiley-Blackwell. Published 2012 by John Wiley & Sons, Inc.

21.2 CLINICAL PRESENTATION

The diagnosis of prostate cancer is usually based on elevated PSA level or abnormal digital rectal examination (DRE). In elderly people, the situation is different as most guidelines do not recommend individual PSA-based screening after 75 years of age because of an expected life expectancy of less than 10 years. Therefore, in this elderly population, most biopsies are performed on the basis of clinical findings such as abnormal DRE or clinical signs of advanced disease in a symptomatic patient. The most frequent clinical presentations are described below.

Patients may be asymptomatic with suspicious findings on clinical examination for other reasons: systematic DRE, systematic ultrasonography (US) of the upper urinary tract showing hydronephrosis, or bone Xray revealing dense ivory-like bone (the "ivory vertebra" sign). High PSA levels when screening is requested by patients themselves or performed inappropriately will also raise suspicion. It is noteworthy that so-called normal PSA levels increase with age [7], even if this finding is controversial [8] and if no data are available for men above 75 years of age.

Symptoms leading to a suspicion of prostate cancer can be local with voiding complications such as dysuria, hematuria, nonspecific voiding dysfunction as with benign prostatic hyperplasia, and chronic or acute urinary retention. The discovery of a firm, indolent, and irregular gland should prompt biopsy. Symptoms may also relate to locoregional disease such as acute renal colic, decreased renal clearance with bilateral ureterohydronephrosis, and enlarged nodes associated with suspicious DRE findings. Finally, the presence of bone pain, localized to the pelvic bone, the femurs, or the spine, typically progressively increased by movements or walking, leading to the discovery of condensed bone lesions, and associated with abnormal DRE findings should also raise suspicion.

Sometimes prostate cancer is suspected when a man presents with impending spinal cord compression, back pain increased by coughing, and radiating pain. Spine Xrays and DRE are recommended. A diagnosis of prostate cancer must also be suspected when a man presents with clearly altered general condition, weight loss, and diffuse bone pain.

In most situations, the prostate is smooth, suggestive of benign prostatic hyperplasia, but elevated PSA levels can lead to suspicion of malignancy. In contrast, a firm and clearly abnormal gland with normal PSA levels should not rule out the diagnosis of cancer. If the benefit of biopsies in symptomatic patients is rarely questionable, the key message concerns asymptomatic patients. The balance between the theoretical, but clinically unproven, benefit gained from a possibly devastating diagnosis, and the lack of benefit, in either clinical outcome or survival, for many asymptomatic patients must always be considered.

21.3 DIAGNOSIS, STAGING, AND PROGNOSTIC FACTORS

21.3.1 Diagnosis

Guidelines on this topic include those published by the European Association of Urology (EAU) [9,10], the American Urological Association [11], and the NCCN [5]. The diagnosis of prostate cancer is based only on prostate biopsy, as neither image nor serum PSA level (except when above several hundred nanograms per milliliter) are specific of the disease; an elevated PSA of ≤ 100 ng/mL can be seen, for instance, in patients with prostate inflammation (such as caused by acute prostatitis). Even if, in some specific uncommon situations, prostate biopsy before treatment can be questionable (patients with very high PSA, unequivocal DRE, and images of bone metastases), the standard of management should be histological confirmation. The method to be used for prostate biopsy—target or random biopsies—is an unresolved question in older men in whom screening and detection of small cancer foci are seldom a priority. These biopsies are obtained through a transrectal approach. Rectal preparation and antibiotic prophylaxis are mandatory. Warfarin and clopidogrel, but not aspirin, must be stopped before the examination. Biopsies are usually performed as outpatient procedures under ultrasound (US) guidance. When a nodule is palpable, DRE guidance is a reasonable alternative, as in patients with a clearly abnormal prostate. When a curative approach is discussed, 10–12 core biopsies must be obtained [10]. When palliation is the goal, less extensive sampling may be considered. Histological data should clarify the following points: number of cores, presence or absence of cancer, length of cancer on each core, and, most importantly, modified Gleason score [12]. This score, which consists of the Gleason grade of the dominant component plus the highest grade, irrespective of its extent, cannot be below 4 (2+2) on biopsies. The presence of high-grade prostate intraepithelial neoplasia is usually of low practical interest in elderly patients.

21.3.2 Staging Procedures

Accurate tumor staging, in particular the determination of whether the tumor is confined to the prostate gland, is essential for treatment decision making. It is based on the TNM staging developed by the American Joint Committee on Cancer and International Union against Cancer, which is the most widely used system worldwide and is now available online [13].

The methods for local staging include DRE, serum PSA level determination, endorectal US, and, in some specific situations, computerized tomography (CT) scan and endorectal magnetic resonance imaging (MRI). Staging methods to evaluate locoregional disease (i.e., lymph node involvement) are based on CT or MRI. Images are never specific, and suspicion is based only on node size (1 cm in the shorter axis). The gold standard for node evaluation is histological examination during lymph node dissection, a situation that is exceptional in the elderly population. The presence of distant metastases is assessed by CT scan, MRI, and bone scan. It must be remembered that bone scan images are not disease-specific, especially in elderly patients with extensive osteoarthritis. If curative treatment is considered, a complete workup is needed to define the actual extent of the disease, especially extension outside the gland. MRI appears to be superior to CT scan for local staging, but not for assessing nodal extension. However, MRI could be of interest as no nephrotoxic vascular injection is required.

21.3.3 Prognostic Factors

The optimal management of patients with prostate cancer requires accurate assessment of the risk of unfavorable outcome. The most widely used prognostic factors are clinical T stage, pretreatment serum PSA level, and Gleason score on prostate biopsy. These factors are the basis of a widely used risk stratification tool developed by D'Amico et al. to evaluate the probability of biochemical relapse 5 years after curative therapy [14]. In patients of the low-risk group (<25% probability of PSA failure after local treatment at 5 years), tumor stage is T1c–T2, serum PSA level <10 ng/mL, and Gleason score ≤6. More recently, the NCCN guidelines have identified a subgroup of patients with stage T1c, Gleason score ≤6, PSA <10 ng/mL, less than three positive cores, each with <50% of cancer component, and PSA density <0.15 ng/mL/g [5]. These patients are at very low risk of long-term relapse, and no immediate active treatment is recommended. This no-treatment scenario, even if still debated for younger men, is probably the primary option for older patients. In the D'Amico classification, patients in the high-risk group (>50% probability of PSA failure at 5 years) have a tumor stage ≥T2c, or a serum PSA level >20 ng/mL, or a Gleason score of ≥8, whereas other patients are classified in the intermediate-risk group (25–50% probability of PSA failure at 5 years). This classification has been widely published and validated.

Prediction of pathological stage (extracapsular extension, seminal vesicle and lymph node invasion), as initially suggested using Partin's tables, was based on DRE, PSA level, and biopsy Gleason score [15]. However, these factors predict only pathological probability, not patient survival, and clearly underestimate node involvement. Prediction of outcome from surrogate markers, mainly PSA relapse-free survival, has been proposed in various scores and nomograms. Most are based on either pretherapeutic data when available, or postsurgery results (pT, pN, Gleason score of the surgical specimen, margins). Some of these scores have been validated by several institutions and therefore might represent useful tools for assessing individual patients [16–18]. However, most consider PSA relapse-free survival, and not overall or specific survival. This is a major limitation as the relationship between PSA recurrence and survival is, at best, weak and very long-term in most cases.

The predictive value of PSA kinetics is also being investigated. There is evidence that, in case of biochemical recurrence after radical prostatectomy or radiation therapy, PSA doubling time (PSA-DT) can identify patients at high risk of dying of the disease [19]. The usual threshold is 12 months, and the lower the PSA-DT, the worse the prognosis. But the calculation of the doubling time is still a matter of debate; it requires several values at several months (years) of distance. Assessment of the predictive value of PSA-DT in 381 older patients undergoing radiation therapy for clinically localized prostate cancer [20] has shown a direct relationship between 10-year specific survival and the D'Amico risk group (ranging from 100% to 55%).

Conversely, the estimated 10-year non-prostate-specific cancer death was respectively 27%, 17%, and 12% in patients at high, intermediate, and low risk. Nearly identical estimates of death due to prostate cancer or from other cause were observed in PSA-relapsing men with a PSA-DT ≤12 months. Despite their old age, the cause of death in these patients with short PSA-DT was nearly exclusively prostate cancer.

21.4 HEALTH STATUS EVALUATION IN ELDERLY PROSTATE CANCER PATIENTS

The experts who developed the SIOG guidelines [4] limited patient assessment to dependence, nutrition, and comorbidities. All three domains are likely to be detected by screening tools, and, for comorbidities, evaluation may allow immediate management. A comprehensive geriatric assessment (CGA) is recommended in frail patients and in some vulnerable patients identified by screening. The ADL (activities of daily living) scale measures the patient's ability to accomplish basic activities of daily living: bathing, dressing, toileting, transfer, continence, and feeding [21]. One ADL impairment is abnormal, except when considering incontinence in these patients with prostate disease. The IADL (instrumental ADL) scale measures the patient's ability to accomplish basic activities that require a higher level of cognition and judgment [22]. Given that the patients are men, only four items of the original IADL scale have been selected: financial management, medication management, use of transportation, and use of the telephone. One IADL impairment is considered abnormal. The CIRS-G (cumulative illness rating system—geriatrics) is a simplified version of the original comorbidity scale, modified to facilitate routine bedside use [23]. Grade 2 comorbidity is controlled by first-line treatment; grade 3, by second-line or multidrug treatment; and grade 4 is uncontrolled. Nutritional status is estimated very simply from the variation of weight during the past 3 months; good nutritional status corresponds to a variation of <5%, risk of malnutrition to a weight loss between 5% and 10% of body weight, and severe malnutrition to a weight loss of >10%.

Elderly patients are divided into four health status groups: fit, vulnerable, frail, and patients too sick for intervention. Fit patients have no serious comorbidity (CISR-G grade 0, 1, or 2), are functionally independent (no dependence in IADL and ADL), and have no malnutrition. Their health status is considered sufficiently good for them to tolerate any form of standard cancer treatment. Vulnerable patients are dependent in one or more IADL (but not in ADL), or they present one uncontrolled comorbid condition (CISR-G grade 3), or a risk of malnutrition. These patients may benefit from additional geriatric intervention and may receive standard cancer treatment after resolution of geriatric problems. Frail patients are dependent in one or more ADL, or have two or more uncontrolled comorbid conditions (i.e., at least two grade 3 or one grade 4 CISR-G comorbidities), or show major malnutrition. Patients in this group should benefit from a geriatric intervention and can be given specific adapted cancer treatment. Patients who are considered too sick for intervention have a very poor health status resulting from a combination of different forms of impairment. These patients are eligible only for end-of-life palliation.

To illustrate the heterogeneity of health statuses among elderly patients, we studied 60 patients with prostate cancer [24]. Median age was 78 years (range 68–92 years). Only 20 patients (33%) were totally independent in ADL and eight in IADL. Only one-third of the patients were well-nourished, whereas 27 were at risk of malnutrition, and 12 were already malnourished. According to the CIRS-G scale, all patients had at least three comorbid conditions, with a median of seven (range 3–12). The median total score was 13 (range 3–25), the median severity index was 1.88 (range 1–2.86), and the median number of severe comorbidities was 1 (0–9). Finally, only four patients were considered fit. However, two-thirds of the patients had advanced disease, and it is important to consider that their prostate cancer management was influenced by health status evaluation findings. Geriatric evaluation is therefore mandatorily incorporated in the decisionmaking process.

21.5 TREATMENT OF LOCALIZED DISEASE

21.5.1 Radical Prostatectomy

The results of a Scandinavian randomized trial of 695 men (mean age 65 years) with localized prostate cancer demonstrate that, compared with conservative management, radical prostatectomy (RP) reduces prostate cancer mortality and the risk of metastases, but there is no, or little, further increase in benefit at ≥ 10 years after surgery [25]. The risk of death and of postoperative complications following RP is a function more of severity of comorbidities than chronological age [26], especially in elderly patients [27]. No randomized trial is available so far about survival benefits in prostate cancer patients detected by screening. In potent men with organ-confined disease, a nerve sparing procedure is the treatment of choice. Lymph node dissection is optional in low-risk patients, but mandatory in those with intermediate or high risk. Neoadjuvant hormonal treatment is pointless as it adds no relapse-free survival benefit [28]. Adjuvant androgen deprivation therapy (ADT) is controversial [29]. Positivity of surgical margins is associated with an increased risk of relapse. However, its impact on specific and overall mortality is still unclear [30]. In patients at high risk after prostatectomy, three trials have shown a benefit of adjuvant radiotherapy over salvage radiotherapy in terms of PSA relapse-free survival [31–33]. However, only one of these trials has tested metastasis-free survival and survival benefits [31]. Furthermore, the criteria for salvage therapy were not predefined, and the patients included were a mixture of pT2–R1, pT3–R1, pT3–R0, and PSA >0.1 ng/mL, thus weakening the strength of the evidence. No specific information on the outcome of elderly patients is given in these trials. Urinary incontinence is a common complication of RP, with reported incidence rates between 3% and 74% [26], and older age has been consistently identified as a risk factor. In 1291 men from the Prostate Cancer Outcome Study undergoing RP between 1994 and 1995, age was significantly associated with the level of urinary control and the frequency of incontinence after surgery [34]. Analysis of 11,522 men from the SEER-Medicare database, who underwent RP between 1992 and 1996, confirmed that long-term incontinence was significantly related to increasing age (24% after 75 years vs. 17–18% before, $p < 0.001$), but also to the severity of comorbidities (from 18% for Charlson 0 to 21% for Charlson ≥ 2, $p = 0.03$) [26]. In clinical practice, it is important to consider that older patients who have a good mobility score and are physically active are likely to suffer a level of incontinence similar to that of younger patients. Conversely, older patients who live a sedentary lifestyle are at higher risk of developing persistent incontinence after surgery. Pre- or post-RP pelvic floor muscle training may accelerate return to continence in older adults, but confirmation from clinical trials is needed. Finally, salvage treatments for elderly patients with disturbing permanent incontinence are the same as those proposed to younger men. Impotence is the second significant side effect of RP, especially when a non-nerve-sparing procedure is used or in older patients [35]. However, the data available are even more imprecise. Finally, age itself is still discussed as a possible prognostic factor for recurrence [36], possibly related to PSA level, Gleason score, and T status [37].

Altogether, it appears reasonable to conclude that older adult patients who are candidates for radical prostatectomy should (1) have poor-risk prostate cancer (i.e., a high risk of prostate cancer–specific death); (2) be in good health, either in the fit or the vulnerable groups (i.e., with high probability of survival at 5–10 years); and (3) have a low risk of incontinence (good pelvic floor tonicity).

21.5.2 External Beam Radiation Therapy (EBRT)

No randomized trial has compared EBRT and watchful waiting, but EBRT offers a nonsignificant difference in survival and quality of life compared to surgery.

Three-dimensional conformal radiotherapy (3D-CRT) is the gold standard of treatment, and intensity-modulated radiotherapy (IMRT), an optimized form of 3D-CRT, has become an increasingly interesting option. However, major changes in the dose and field of irradiation have been proposed according to the risk categories. No patient should receive a dose below 70 Gy, which, even for low-risk patients, has been associated with decreased relapse-free survival [38]. For patients with locally advanced disease (T3/4, N0), EBRT alone is no longer the standard of care and must be combined with ADT, based on the results of randomized clinical trials showing a clear overall survival benefit at 10 years using either a neoadjuvant concomitant [39] or a concomitant adjuvant treatment [32]. The duration of ADT has been specifically addressed in a noninferiority trial, and a clear benefit has been seen with the 3-year treatment modality compared to the 6-month arm [40]. A retrospective analysis of 527 patients with nonmetastatic prostate cancer has shown the absence of relationship between age (four groups, <60, 60–69, 70–74, and ≥75 years) and risk of acute or late genitourinary or gastrointestinal toxicity after EBRT [41]. A population-based study of 31,643 patients (aged 65–85 years) with nonmetastatic prostate cancer and treated with EBRT and/or brachytherapy has shown improved 5-year and 8-year survival rates in patients with stage T3/4 disease receiving adjuvant ADT, but no survival advantage for men with T1/2 disease [42]. These findings are consistent with clinical practice guidelines. However, the survival advantage associated with combining EBRT and ADT in high-risk prostate cancer patients may apply only to those with no or minimal comorbidities (i.e., fit patients), as suggested by a 2008 study by D'Amico et al. [43]. With modern irradiation techniques, long-term toxicity is usually low, with <5% expected severe toxicities. The most frequent toxic events are hematuria (5%), stricture (6%, including 2% grade 3/4), urinary incontinence (5%, including 0.5% grade 3/4), proctitis (8%), and diarrhea (3.7%). After more than 2 years of follow-up, the impotence rate is around 50%. The outcome, in terms of cancer control and treatment-related late comorbidity, of older patients undergoing EBRT is similar to that of younger patients. However, a discordant trial suggests that age itself might be an independent predictor of time to death from prostate cancer, with patients >75 years of age having a decreased specific survival compared to younger patients [44].

21.5.3 Brachytherapy

Brachytherapy is indicated in patients with clinical stage T1b–T2a-b tumors, N0, M0, Gleason score ≤6, and PSA level ≤10 ng/mL, with a prostate volume of <50 mL, and good International Prostate Symptom Score (IPSS) [9,10]. This technique appears to be suitable for the treatment of older prostate cancer patients. Nevertheless, the survival benefit in older adult patients with low-risk localized disease is not established. Complications of brachytherapy appear to be slightly less severe than those associated with EBRT or RP, but evidence from the SEER database suggests that urinary, bowel, and erectile complications significantly increase with both age and severity of comorbidities [45]. Results from a multivariate analysis have shown that the Charlson comorbidity index is a stronger predictor of brachytherapy complications than chronological age. However, the place of brachytherapy in older adults is questionable as indications for brachytherapy are almost the same as for watch-and-wait management.

21.5.4 Comparison of Surgery, EBRT, and Brachytherapy

No randomized trial has compared the three treatment modalities. The same team has repeatedly reported a retrospective cohort analysis, with nearly similar rates of biochemical relapse-free survival at 8 years for RP and EBRT (72% and 70%, respectively, $p = 0.010$). The slightly higher relapse rate reported with EBRT was attributed to the higher number of high-risk patients in this group and to insufficient dose (<72 Gy). Age (<65 vs. ≥65 years) was not an independent predictor of treatment relapse ($p = 0.78$) [46]. In a study of 10,472 localized prostate cancer patients, no overall survival difference between surgery, EBRT, and brachytherapy has been reported [47]. After adjusting for age, comorbidities, stage, and biopsy Gleason score, a specific survival benefit has been observed for RP. This nonrandomized retrospective trial has not been published yet, and results must be interpreted with caution.

Regarding quality of life (QOL) or overall side effects, results from the Prostate Cancer Outcome Study have demonstrated that urinary incontinence is significantly more common with surgery (14–16%) than with EBRT (4%), while bowel urgency and painful hemorrhoids are significantly worse with EBRT (29% and 20%, respectively) than with surgery (19% and 10%, respectively) [48]. Similar differences between surgery and EBRT have been observed by different investigators, with better urinary stress continence after radiation therapy (EBRT or brachytherapy), and better bowel and urinary functions after surgery. Sexual function is always impaired, although to a lesser extent when using brachytherapy. Quality of life has also been shown to vary with the number of physical symptoms, and it is statistically significantly better in the treated group than in nontreated patients [49].

21.5.5 Alternative Local Treatment Modalities: HIFU and Cryotherapy

Minimally invasive high-intensity focused ultrasound (HIFU) has emerged as a potential therapeutic option in patients with clinically localized, low-, or intermediate-risk prostate cancer, and prostate volume <50 mL [50]. However, this treatment remains experimental [10]. Longer follow-up and comparison with established therapies are required to confirm HIFU efficacy before it can be recommended as standard care. HIFU could then become an option for older patients with localized prostate cancer who are unable to undergo curative surgery or radiation therapy but who require potentially curative intervention. It might also be an option for salvage treatment of local relapses in previously irradiated patients with persistent N0M0 disease.

Cryosurgery consists of inserting cryoneedles into the tumor under transrectal US guidance. The ideal candidates for cryosurgery are patients at low or intermediate risk [10], with a prostate volume of ≤40 mL. A randomized trial comparing EBRT and cryosurgery in 244 patients with clinically localized low and intermediate prostate cancer has been published [51]. After a median follow-up of 100 months, no difference in disease progression at 36 months, overall, or disease-specific survival has been reported. However, patient numbers were too small to draw significant clinical conclusions.

21.5.6 Androgen Deprivation Therapy Alone

Following more recent results obtained with EBRT and ADT, the place of the combination modality should be clarified, compared to ADT alone. Two prospective randomized clinical trials conducted in locally advanced N0M0 patients have been presented [52,53]. Both have evidenced a clear benefit in disease-specific survival and metastasis-free survival. Of note, no increased cardiac death rate has been reported in patients treated with the combination compared to EBRT alone.

In patients unfit to undergo aggressive local treatment or who refuse intervention, the issue of systematic, immediate ADT is raised. This has been examined by the EORTC 30891 trial, in which newly diagnosed T1–4, N0–2, M0 patients were randomized to either immediate or deferred ADT [54]. After a median follow-up of 7.8 years, the conclusion is that immediate ADT provides a small but statistically significant benefit in overall survival, but not in disease-specific survival. Most deaths are related to prostate cancer or cardiovascular disease. The many side effects of the therapy and the marginal survival benefit to be expected from it highlight the need for a straightforward, in-depth discussion with every patient before treatment initiation. Only a subgroup of patients might potentially benefit from immediate treatment, namely, patients above 70 years of age, with PSA >50 ng/mL, and PSA DT <1 year.

21.5.7   Other Issues Related to Treatment of Localized Disease

Potential Relationship between Relapse and Survival   It must be highlighted that most available data on treatment efficacy are related to biological relapse-free survival, except for RP, where survival data are available. Biological relapse is still discussed as a surrogate endpoint for overall or specific survival [55]. It might be associated with decreased survival. But relapsing patients represent a heterogeneous population with regard to the risk of secondary progression or death. Some parameters, such as early relapse (<15 months after initial treatment), low PSA DT (<12 months), and high Gleason score, have been associated with decreased survival [56]. Those parameters could be used to identify relapsing patients at high risk of death, who could potentially be candidates for salvage treatment. A PSA-DT of >15 months at relapse has a specific survival rate at 15 years of 90%, while it is as low as 30% when the PSA-DT is <9 months, and 0% when it is <3 months.

Watch-and-Wait Policy   Two strategies are available for patients not receiving immediate treatment: "watchful waiting" (also "watch and wait" policy) and "active surveillance." These strategies have very different objectives. The rationale for watchful waiting is based on the assumption that many patients who die while having prostate cancer do not actually die of the cancer. Once they have troublesome symptoms from the disease, they can be effectively managed by palliative modalities. Nevertheless, this requires careful clinical follow-up so that the patients receive ad hoc treatment as soon as they become symptomatic. This watchful waiting strategy should also be considered in patients for whom the risk of disease progression is present for only a short period of time (i.e., patients who have a small chance of survival because of advanced age and/or the presence of comorbidities). On the other hand, suitable candidates for active surveillance are patients who have very low-risk tumors (low Gleason score, PSA level, and clinical stage), who might be cured by immediate active treatment. Treatment is postponed until signs of progression occur while the patient is still potentially curable. Caution is recommended when offering active surveillance, especially to older patients, because Gleason undergrading is frequent in men of advanced age, especially in those who have high PSA levels [57]. However, the same holds true for patients of all ages, and an easy way to increase reliability is simply to repeat the biopsies. Of course, delayed treatment is always possible for patients who require more explanation, or those who express a personal preference for avoiding or postponing the side effects of definitive therapy.

The advantages of watchful waiting and active surveillance include avoiding the side effects of definitive therapy, maintenance of QOL, and reducing the risk of unnecessary treatment for small, indolent tumors. Disadvantages include the risk of developing progressive disease or metastases that would be difficult to treat in patients with poor expected survival. Increased anxiety and frequent medical examinations might also be of concern but, given that this is a shared decision with detailed explanations, this drawback might not be as important as expected [58]. Active surveillance is becoming an increasingly safe solution as the results from multiple prospective cohorts become available [59]. However, in the specific scope of older adult treatments, the periodic biopsies required for active surveillance must be discussed more extensively than in younger men [5]. The decision between watchful waiting and active surveillance in older adult patients should not be based solely on chronological age, but rather on the estimated individual risk of dying of prostate cancer or of other causes.

Tailoring the Treatment to the Patient Evidence suggests that, in both the United States [60] and Europe [61], only a minority of older adults with localized prostate cancer receive curative therapy. The 2010 EAU guidelines recommend that "as a standard, an assessment of the patient's life expectancy, overall health status and tumor characteristics is necessary before any treatment decision can be made." It is also stated that "life expectancy, rather than patient age, should be the factor considered in treatment selection" [10].

Results of a retrospective cohort study from the SEER database, which included 14,516 men with localized prostate cancer detected by screening and receiving conservative management, have shown that within a 10-year follow-up period, the risk of dying from prostate cancer increases with increasing Gleason score, regardless of age at diagnosis [62]. Survival is clearly improved for patients with a Gleason score ≤ 7, with a 10-year specific survival rate of 90% for T1c/2 disease between 75 and 79 years of age, and around 85% after 80 years. For patients with a Gleason score > 7, overall specific survival is clearly decreased to $< 80\%$. Non–prostate cancer survival at 10 years is 40% for patients aged between 75 and 79 years, and around 20% after 80 years. These specific survival results are clearly better than those observed in non-screened patients [63], highlighting the effect of the time bias induced by detection and the importance of clarifying the survival prognosis of each individual patient before engaging him with any form of active treatment, especially for patients in the low- and probably in the intermediate-risk groups. This is especially important as a specific survival benefit of active local disease treatment over watchful waiting has been described only in patients younger than 65 years [25], in a cohort of nonscreening-detected patients. This benefit is seen after 10 years of follow-up and remains stable thereafter. One might therefore expect the cutoff age for seeing such a benefit to be lower in screening-detected patients.

The influence of comorbidity on survival has been studied by Tewari et al. [64], who have shown that the risk of non–prostate cancer mortality is 3 times higher in patients with severe comorbidity (Charlson score ≥ 2) than in those with mild comorbidity

(Charlson score 0–1). In a Swedish nationwide cohort of 6849 men aged 70 years or older [65], with a Gleason score <8 and serum PSA values <20 ng/mL, the prostate cancer specific death rate at 10 years was 3.6% in the group receiving surveillance and watchful waiting, 2.4% after prostatectomy, and 3.3% after EBRT. When adjusting for risk category, Charlson score, and socioeconomic status, there was a significantly lower risk of specific death after surgery or EBRT compared to surveillance. The rate of non–prostate cancer death was 19% in the surveillance group, versus 8.5% with prostatectomy and 14.2% with EBRT, highlighting the impact of initial selection for the different treatment modalities. In a multivariate analysis, Charlson score >2 and lower socioeconomic status were both associated with decreased nonspecific survival. Alibhai et al have evaluated treatment efficacy in men older than 65 years with localized prostate cancer by using a decision model integrating patient age, co-morbidity, Gleason score, patient preferences, and treatment efficacy data [66]. Their results show that prostatectomy and EBRT significantly improve life expectancy and quality-adjusted life expectancy in older men with mild comorbidity and moderately or poorly differentiated prostate cancer. They conclude that "curative therapy should be seriously considered in men up to age 80 years who have high-grade disease." A population-based cohort study of men aged 75–84 years with clinically localized prostate cancer has shown that aggressive treatment (RP or EBRT) was more likely to induce urinary, bowel, and erectile dysfunction than conservative management [67]. The adjusted disease-specific mortality ratio was 0.43 (95% CI 0.15–1.28), which is in favor of aggressive treatment. However, the absolute 5-year disease-specific survival difference between groups was small (98% vs. 92%) since most deaths were due to other causes. When offering patients aged >75 years aggressive treatment associated with uncertain survival benefits, a balance between expected survival and possible adverse treatment effects should be presented. As with the Swedish cohort of men older than 70 years, an observational study of 44,630 US patients aged 65–80 years with localized, well-, or moderately differentiated prostate cancer has suggested a significant overall survival advantage for patients receiving curative treatment, including men aged 75–80 years [68]. The survival benefit was again attributed to a reduction in non–prostate cancer mortality. Results of a Canadian population-based cohort of 6183 men aged >70 years have demonstrated that 40% of the patients selected for RP did not have sufficient life expectancy to warrant attempting curative therapy, and 70% of those who received radiation therapy died before the 10-year cutoff point [69]. These findings highlight the need for more stringent selection criteria for radiation therapy and prostatectomy, including accurate health status assessment. This suggests that treatment decisions in older adults should balance the risk of dying of prostate cancer with the risk of dying from another cause (i.e., severity and number of comorbidities that contribute to the patient's health status in general).

21.6   TREATMENT OF ADVANCED DISEASE

Androgen deprivation therapy (ADT) is the standard treatment of metastatic prostate cancer [70]. It has a major impact on symptoms, particularly on pain, but only a non-significant impact on survival. To date, there is no proven benefit of complete androgen blockade, and no clear advantage of early ADT in patients with increased PSA [54]. Whereas there is no evidence of ADT efficacy in older patients, the treatment produces important side effects, such as the metabolic syndrome and its cardiovascular consequences [71] and osteoporosis [72]. The two problems have very different impacts on patient health. The metabolic syndrome adds a competitive risk of death from associated comorbidities to the risk of death from prostate cancer. This cannot be measured precisely but only estimated. Osteoporosis is mainly a risk of functional impairment (fracture) for which a direct proportionality relationship has been established. The metabolic syndrome is clearly an important problem in patients with only rising PSA, which is a very slowly progressing disease, but becomes of very little importance in patients with castration-resistant prostate cancer (CRPC), for whom the median survival is around 18 months. This problem has not yet been specifically addressed in guidelines, but its management likely follows the same rules as for choosing curative treatments in elderly cancer patients; the death risk associated with the metabolic syndrome must be balanced with the estimated death risk from other causes. Osteoporosis is an important issue in all CRPC patients since it has significant negative effects on quality of life and possibly on survival. Clear recommendations have been made for the prevention of osteoporosis in prostate cancer patients [9]. Additionally, zoledronic acid is indicated for the treatment of hormone-refractory prostate cancer metastatic to the bone [73].

The use of chemotherapy has become a standard of care for CRPC patients. Two randomized trials have demonstrated the effect of docetaxel on overall survival and quality of life [74,75]. The most important trial is the randomized study TAX 327 comparing standard palliative treatment (MP) and a combination of low-dose prednisone with either 3-weekly or weekly docetaxel (74). Both docetaxel arms have shown a significantly better palliative effect than MP, but the 3-weekly schedule only significantly increased overall survival. This study included subgroup analyses, particularly of patients aged <65 years or ≥65 years, which demonstrated that age had no impact on outcome. It also demonstrated that toxicity did not vary with age. Patients treated with the weekly schedule had less grade 3/4 neutropenia (and neutropenic fever) but more fatigue. However, only the 3-weekly schedule has been approved for CRPC. More recently, the Tropic study has compared mitoxantrone plus prednisolone versus cabazitaxel plus prednisolone after failure of first-line docetaxel chemotherapy [76]. Results have demonstrated the superiority of the experimental arm over the standard arm, with improved overall survival (15.1 vs. 12.8 months, respectively). Other treatment modalities can also be used in the palliative setting. Bone surgery is indicated in patients with fractures or spinal cord compression. Transurethral resection of the prostate and ureteric bypass are mandatory when compression occurs. External radiotherapy has shown good clinical efficacy on painful bone metastases. None of these treatments is contraindicated by patient age.

Radiopharmaceuticals are also useful for the treatment of painful lesions in older patients with CRPC. Two randomized trials have demonstrated the superiority of strontium [77] and samarium [78] over respectively localized radiation therapy alone or placebo in patients with painful localized metastases. Samarium administration can be repeated, and this approach has been shown to induce no clinically significant platelet toxicity. As yet, no study has specifically examined this strategy in older adults, but the toxicity profile of radiopharmaceuticals appears suitable for use in this patient population. There are no published data on the effect of radiopharmaceuticals in patients previously treated with chemotherapy, although this approach might be useful in frail patients with pain who are not suitable for adapted chemotherapy.

21.7 PRACTICAL GUIDELINES

Specific guidelines for the management of elderly prostate cancer patients have been elaborated only relatively recently and are often a merge between urological guidelines for prostate cancer [5,10,11] and either an evaluation of life expectancy [10] or a more in-depth evaluation of patient health status. The two approaches have been integrated into practical guidelines proposed by the SIOG [4,79].

Table 21.1 summarizes the screening tools used for evaluating patient health status. It is noteworthy that subdividing health status into different groups is insufficient; a comprehensive geriatric assessment (CGA) is mandatory to diagnose health status impairment and propose geriatric interventions. But individual evaluation of life expectancy is clearly not appropriate; this criterion is used only in public health sciences for examining populations. The phrase to be used here is "evaluation of an individual's chance of survival." Therefore, treatment decision is based on a pertinent evaluation and balance of patient's chance of survival related to general health status and related to cancer. The solution of the problem is simple in the case of metastatic disease, but difficulties are more important for localized disease. The first step must be to assess disease extension since the difference between local and locally advanced disease is the most important factor influencing outcome. Factors like T stage and, more importantly, Gleason score and serum PSA level, are taken into account for placing the patient in the low-, intermediate-, or high-risk group. This allows for assessment of the individual's chance of survival from prostate cancer. If his chance of survival related to general health status is high, he should be offered curative treatment, particularly in high-risk disease. Given that the two major complications of prostatectomy are incontinence and impotence, RP should be used only in case of local, poor-risk prostate cancer in healthy men who are estimated to have a low risk of incontinence, namely, fit men with good pelvic floor tonicity. EBRT is the curative treatment likely offered to all other patients who are not candidates for prostatectomy. The major complications

TABLE 21.1 Health Status Evaluation and Decision Making

Heath Status Evaluation/ Groups	Fit	Vulnerable	Frail	Terminal Illness
Co−morbidity CISR-G [23]	Grades 0/1/2	At least one grade 3	Several grade 3 or one grade 4	Multiple
	AND	OR	OR	AND/OR
Dependence ADL [21] IADL [22]	No abnormality No abnormality	No abnormality ≥1 abnormality	At least one or more ADL abnormality	Dependence
	AND	OR	OR	AND/OR
Malnutrition	Weight loss <5%	Weight loss 5−10%	Weight loss >10%	Malnutrition
Geriatric intervention	None	One domain	Multiple domains	Multiple domains
Cancer treatment	Standard	Standard after geriatric intervention	Adapted treatment	Palliative treatment

are impotence and, more importantly, rectitis, even if its incidence decreases with improved technology. In patients who have a good chance of survival related to health status but poor cancer-related survival prognosis, neoadjuvant or adjuvant androgen deprivation can be associated with EBRT to improve cancer outcome. Brachytherapy induces complications such as rectitis, and its indication is limited by prostate size. Moreover, it is likely to be inactive in poor-risk and probably also in intermediate-risk disease. The same question may be raised about alternative treatments such as HIFU or cryotherapy, which are less aggressive but also less effective in poor and even intermediate-risk prostate cancers. These techniques may be helpful in case of failure of EBRT when salvage treatment is indicated and likely to influence outcome.

21.8 CONCLUSION

Finally, given that half of the patients with newly diagnosed prostate cancer are older than 70 years, specific studies must be performed to refine the decisionmaking in this group. The objective is to eventually increase their chance of survival and their quality of life.

ACKNOWLEDGMENTS

The authors thank Marie-Dominique Reynaud for revision of the manuscript.

REFERENCES

1. Parkin DM, Bray F, Ferlay J, Pisani P. Global cancer statistics 2002. *CA Cancer J Clin* 2005;**55**:74–108.
2. Altekruse SF, Kosary CL, Krapcho M, Neyman N, Aminou R, Waldron W et al. *SEER Cancer Statistics Review, 1975–2007*, National Cancer Institute. Bethesda, MD, 2010 (http://seer.cancer.gov/csr/1975_2007/, based on 11/09 SEER data submission, posted to SEER website, 2010).
3. US Census Bureau, International Data Base. (http://www.census.gov, 2010).
4. Droz JP, Balducci L, Bolla M, Emberton M, Fitzpatrick JM, Joniau S et al. Management of prostate cancer in older men: Recommendations of a working group of the International Society of Geriatric Oncology. *BJU Int.* 2010;**106**(4):462–9.
5. NCCN Guidelines on Prostate Cancer (see http://www.nccn.org/professionals/physician_gls/PDF/prostate.pdf, 2010).
6. NCCN Guidelines on Senior Adult Oncology (see http://www.nccn.org/professionals/physician_gls/PDF/senior.pdf, 2010).
7. Morgan TO, Jacobsen SJ, McCarthy WF, Jacobson DJ, McLeod DG, Moul JW. Age-specific reference ranges for prostate-specific antigen in black men. *N Engl J Med* 1996;**335**(5): 304–310.
8. Catalona WJ, Southwick PC, Slawin KM, Partin AW, Brawer MK, Flanigan RC, et al. Comparison of percent free PSA, PSA density, and age-specific PSA cutoffs for prostate cancer detection and staging. *Urology* 2000;**56**(2):255–260.
9. Heidenreich A, Aus G, Bolla M, Joniau S, Matveev VB, Schmid HP, et al. EAU guidelines on prostate cancer. *Eur Urol* 2008;**53**(1):68–80.

10. European Association of Urology. Online Guidelines on Prostate Cancer (see http://www.uroweb.org/gls/pdf/Prostate%20Cancer%202010%20June%2017th.pdf, 2010).

11. American Association Urology. *Guideline for the Management of Clinically Localized Prostate Cancer, 2007* (available at http://www.auanet.org/content/guidelines-and-quality-care/clinical-guidelines/main-reports/proscan07/content.pdf, 2010).

12. Epstein JI, Allsbrook WC, Jr., Amin MB, Egevad LL. The 2005 International Society of Urological Pathology (ISUP) Consensus Conference on Gleason Grading of Prostatic Carcinoma. *Am J Surg Pathol* 2005;**29**(9):1228–1242.

13. TNM online (see http://www3.interscience.wiley.com/cgibin/mrwhome/104554799/HOME, 2010).

14. D'Amico AV, Moul J, Carroll PR, Sun L, Lubeck D, Chen MH. Cancer-specific mortality after surgery or radiation for patients with clinically localized prostate cancer managed during the prostate-specific antigen era. *J Clin Oncol* 2003;**21**(11):2163–2172.

15. Partin AW, Kattan MW, Subong EN, Walsh PC, Wojno KJ, Oesterling JE, et al. Combination of prostate-specific antigen, clinical stage, and Gleason score to predict pathological stage of localized prostate cancer. A multi-institutional update. *JAMA* 1997;**277**(18):1445–1451.

16. Han M, Partin AW, Zahurak M, Piantadosi S, Epstein JI, Walsh PC. Biochemical (prostate specific antigen) recurrence probability following radical prostatectomy for clinically localized prostate cancer. *J Urol* 2003;**169**(2):517–523.

17. Kattan MW, Zelefsky MJ, Kupelian PA, Cho D, Scardino PT, Fuks Z et al. Pretreatment nomogram that predicts 5-year probability of metastasis following three-dimensional conformal radiation therapy for localized prostate cancer. *J Clin Oncol* 2003;**21**(24):4568–4571.

18. Kattan MW, Potters L, Blasko JC, Beyer DC, Fearn P, Cavanagh W et al. Pretreatment nomogram for predicting freedom from recurrence after permanent prostate brachytherapy in prostate cancer. *Urology* 2001;**58**(3):393–399.

19. D'Amico AV, Moul JW, Carroll PR, Sun L, Lubeck D, Chen MH. Surrogate end point for prostate cancer-specific mortality after radical prostatectomy or radiation therapy. *J Natl Cancer Inst* 2003;**95**(18):1376–1383.

20. D'Amico AV, Cote K, Loffredo M, Renshaw AA, Schultz D. Determinants of prostate cancer-specific survival after radiation therapy for patients with clinically localized prostate cancer. *J Clin Oncol* 2002;**20**(23):4567–4573.

21. Katz S, Ford AB, Moskowitz RW, Jackson BA, Jaffe MW. Studies of illness in the aged. The Index of ADL: A standardized measure of biological and psychosocial function. *JAMA* 1963;**185**:914–919.

22. Lawton MP, Brody EM. Assessment of older people: self-maintaining and instrumental activities of daily living. *Gerontologist* 1969;**9**(3):179–186.

23. Linn BS, Linn MW, Gurel L. Cumulative illness rating scale. *J Am Geriatr Soc* 1968;**16**(5):622–626.

24. Terret C, Albrand G, Droz JP. Geriatric assessment in elderly patients with prostate cancer. *Clin Prostate Cancer* 2004;**2**(4):236–240.

25. Bill-Axelson A, Holmberg L, Filen F, Ruutu M, Garmo H, Busch C, et al. Radical prostatectomy versus watchful waiting in localized prostate cancer: the Scandinavian prostate cancer group-4 randomized trial. *J Natl Cancer Inst* 2008;**100**(16):1144–1154.

26. Begg CB, Riedel ER, Bach PB, Kattan MW, Schrag D, Warren JL, et al. Variations in morbidity after radical prostatectomy. *N Engl J Med* 2002;**346**(15):1138–1144.

27. Sanchez-Salas R, Prapotnich D, Rozet F, Mombet A, Cathala N, Barret E, et al. Laparoscopic radical prostatectomy is feasible and effective in "fit" senior men with localized prostate cancer. *Br J Urol Int* 2010;**106**(10):1530–6.

28. Shelley MD, Kumar S, Wilt T, Staffurth J, Coles B, Mason MD. A systematic review and meta-analysis of randomised trials of neo-adjuvant hormone therapy for localised and locally advanced prostate carcinoma. *Cancer Treat Rev* 2009;**35**(1):9–17.

29. Wong YN, Freedland S, Egleston B, Hudes G, Schwartz JS, Armstrong K. Role of androgen deprivation therapy for node-positive prostate cancer. *J Clin Oncol* 2009;**27**(1):100–105.

30. Boorjian SA, Karnes RJ, Crispen PL, Carlson RE, Rangel LJ, Bergstralh EJ, et al. The impact of positive surgical margins on mortality following radical prostatectomy during the prostate specific antigen era. *J Urol* 2010;**183**(3):1003–1009.

31. Thompson IM, Tangen CM, Paradelo J, Lucia MS, Miller G, Troyer D, et al. Adjuvant radiotherapy for pathological T3N0M0 prostate cancer significantly reduces risk of metastases and improves survival: Long-term followup of a randomized clinical trial. *J Urol* 2009;**181**(3):956–962.

32. Bolla M, van PH, Collette L, van CP, Vekemans K, Da PL, et al. Postoperative radiotherapy after radical prostatectomy: A randomised controlled trial (EORTC trial 22911). *Lancet* 2005;**366**(9485):572–578.

33. Wiegel T, Bottke D, Steiner U, Siegmann A, Golz R, Storkel S, et al. Phase III postoperative adjuvant radiotherapy after radical prostatectomy compared with radical prostatectomy alone in pT3 prostate cancer with postoperative undetectable prostate-specific antigen: ARO 96-02/AUO AP 09/95. *J Clin Oncol* 2009;**27**(18):2924–2930.

34. Stanford JL, Feng Z, Hamilton AS, Gilliland FD, Stephenson RA, Eley JW, et al. Urinary and sexual function after radical prostatectomy for clinically localized prostate cancer: The Prostate Cancer Outcomes Study. *JAMA* 2000;**283**(3):354–360.

35. Parsons JK, Marschke P, Maples P, Walsh PC. Effect of methylprednisolone on return of sexual function after nerve-sparing radical retropubic prostatectomy. *Urology* 2004;**64**(5):987–990.

36. Xu DD, Sun SD, Wang F, Sun L, Stackhouse D, Polascik T, et al. Effect of age and pathologic Gleason score on PSA recurrence: Analysis of 2911 patients undergoing radical prostatectomy. *Urology* 2009;**74**(3):654–658.

37. Barlow LJ, Badalato GM, Bashir T, Benson MC, McKiernan JM. The relationship between age at time of surgery and risk of biochemical failure after radical prostatectomy. *Br J Urol Int* 2010;**105**(12):1646–1649.

38. Kupelian P, Kuban D, Thames H, Levy L, Horwitz E, Martinez A, et al. Improved biochemical relapse-free survival with increased external radiation doses in patients with localized prostate cancer: The combined experience of nine institutions in patients treated in 1994 and 1995. *Int J Radiat Oncol Biol Phys* 2005;**61**(2):415–419.

39. Roach M, III, Bae K, Speight J, Wolkov HB, Rubin P, Lee RJ, et al. Short-term neoadjuvant androgen deprivation therapy and external-beam radiotherapy for locally advanced prostate cancer: long-term results of RTOG 8610. *J Clin Oncol* 2008;**26**(4):585–591.

40. Bolla M, de Reijke TM, Van TG, Van den Bergh AC, Oddens J, Poortmans PM, et al. Duration of androgen suppression in the treatment of prostate cancer. *N Engl J Med* 2009;**360**(24):2516–2527.

41. Jani AB, Parikh SD, Vijayakumar S, Gratzle J. Analysis of influence of age on acute and chronic radiotherapy toxicity in treatment of prostate cancer. *Urology* 2005;**65**(6):1157–1162.

42. Zeliadt SB, Potosky AL, Penson DF, Etzioni R. Survival benefit associated with adjuvant androgen deprivation therapy combined with radiotherapy for high- and low-risk patients with nonmetastatic prostate cancer. *Int J Radiat Oncol Biol Phys* 2006;**66**(2):395–402.

43. D'Amico AV, Chen MH, Renshaw AA, Loffredo M, Kantoff PW. Androgen suppression and radiation vs. radiation alone for prostate cancer: A randomized trial. *JAMA* 2008;**299**(3):289–295.

44. D'Amico AV, Cote K, Loffredo M, Renshaw AA, Chen MH. Advanced age at diagnosis is an independent predictor of time to death from prostate carcinoma for patients undergoing external beam radiation therapy for clinically localized prostate carcinoma. *Cancer* 2003;**97**(1):56–62.

45. Chen AB, D'Amico AV, Neville BA, Earle CC. Patient and treatment factors associated with complications after prostate brachytherapy. *J Clin Oncol* 2006;**24**(33):5298–5304.

46. Kupelian PA, Elshaikh M, Reddy CA, Zippe C, Klein EA. Comparison of the efficacy of local therapies for localized prostate cancer in the prostate-specific antigen era: A large single-institution experience with radical prostatectomy and external-beam radiotherapy. *J Clin Oncol* 2002;**20**(16):3376–3385.

47. Stephenson RA. Comparison of overal survival in localized prostate cancer with prostatectomy, EBRT and brachytherapy. *J Urol* 2010;**183**(4):113.

48. Potosky AL, Davis WW, Hoffman RM, Stanford JL, Stephenson RA, Penson DF, et al. Five-year outcomes after prostatectomy or radiotherapy for prostate cancer: The prostate cancer outcomes study. *J Natl Cancer Inst* 2004;**96**(18):1358–1367.

49. Johansson E, Bill-Axelson A, Holmberg L, Onelov E, Johansson JE, Steineck G. Time, symptom burden, androgen deprivation, and self-assessed quality of life after radical prostatectomy or watchful waiting: The Randomized Scandinavian Prostate Cancer Group Study Number 4 (SPCG-4) clinical trial. *Eur Urol* 2009;**55**(2):422–430.

50. Crouzet S, Rebillard X, Chevallier D, Rischmann P, Pasticier G, Garcia G, et al. Multicentric oncologic outcomes of high-intensity focused ultrasound for localized prostate cancer in 803 patients. *Eur Urol* 2010;**58**(4):559–66.

51. Donnelly BJ, Saliken JC, Brasher PM, Ernst SD, Rewcastle JC, Lau H, et al. A randomized trial of external beam radiotherapy versus cryoablation in patients with localized prostate cancer. *Cancer* 2010;**116**(2):323–330.

52. Warde P, Mason MD, Sydes MR, Gospodarowicz MK, Swanson G, Kirkbride P, et al. Intergroup randomized phase III study of androgen deprivation plus radiation therapy in locally advanced prostate cancer. *J Clin Oncol* 2010;**28**:18s.

53. Mottet N, Peneau M, Mazeron J, Molinie V, Richaud P. Impact of radiotherapy combined with androgen deprivation (ADT) versus ADT alone for local control in clinically locally advanced prostate cancer. *J Clin Oncol* 2010;**28**:15s.

54. Studer UE, Whelan P, Albrecht W, Casselman J, de RT, Hauri D, et al. Immediate or deferred androgen deprivation for patients with prostate cancer not suitable for local treatment with curative intent: European Organisation for Research and Treatment of Cancer (EORTC) Trial 30891. *J Clin Oncol* 2006;**24**(12):1868–1876.

55. Collette L, Burzykowski T, Schroder FH. Prostate-specific antigen (PSA) alone is not an appropriate surrogate marker of long-term therapeutic benefit in prostate cancer trials. *Eur J Cancer* 2006;**42**(10):1344–1350.

56. Freedland SJ, Humphreys EB, Mangold LA, Eisenberger M, Dorey FJ, Walsh PC, et al. Death in patients with recurrent prostate cancer after radical prostatectomy: Prostate-specific antigen doubling time subgroups and their associated contributions to all-cause mortality. *J Clin Oncol* 2007;**25**(13):1765–1771.

57. Isariyawongse BK, Sun L, Banez LL, Robertson C, Polascik TJ, Maloney K, et al. Significant discrepancies between diagnostic and pathologic Gleason sums in prostate cancer: The predictive role of age and prostate-specific antigen. *Urology* 2008;**72**(4):882–886.

58. Steineck G, Helgesen F, Adolfsson J, Dickman PW, Johansson JE, Norlen BJ, et al. Quality of life after radical prostatectomy or watchful waiting. *N Engl J Med* 2002;**347**(11):790–796.

59. Klotz L, Zhang L, Lam A, Nam R, Mamedov A, Loblaw A. Clinical results of long-term follow-up of a large, active surveillance cohort with localized prostate cancer. *J Clin Oncol* 2010;**28**(1):126–131.

60. Bubolz T, Wasson JH, Lu-Yao G, Barry MJ. Treatments for prostate cancer in older men: 1984–1997. *Urology* 2001;**58**(6):977–982.

61. Houterman S, Janssen-Heijnen ML, Hendrikx AJ, van den Berg HA, Coebergh JW. Impact of comorbidity on treatment and prognosis of prostate cancer patients: A population-based study. *Crit Rev Oncol Hematol* 2006;**58**(1):60–67.

62. Lu-Yao GL, Albertsen PC, Moore DF, Shih W, Lin Y, DiPaola RS, et al. Outcomes of localized prostate cancer following conservative management. *JAMA* 2009;**302**(11):1202–1209.

63. Albertsen PC, Hanley JA, Fine J. 20-year outcomes following conservative management of clinically localized prostate cancer. *JAMA* 2005;**293**(17):2095–2101.

64. Tewari A, Johnson CC, Divine G, Crawford ED, Gamito EJ, Demers R, et al. Long-term survival probability in men with clinically localized prostate cancer: A case-control, propensity modeling study stratified by race, age, treatment and comorbidities. *J Urol* 2004;**171**(4):1513–1519.

65. Stattin P, Holmberg E, Johansson JE, Holmberg L, Adolfsson J, Hugosson J. Outcomes in localized prostate cancer: National Prostate Cancer Register of Sweden follow-up study. *J Natl Cancer Inst* 2010;**102**(13):950–958.

66. Alibhai SM, Naglie G, Nam R, Trachtenberg J, Krahn MD. Do older men benefit from curative therapy of localized prostate cancer? *J Clin Oncol* 2003;**21**(17):3318–3327.

67. Hoffman RM, Barry MJ, Stanford JL, Hamilton AS, Hunt WC, Collins MM. Health outcomes in older men with localized prostate cancer: Results from the Prostate Cancer Outcomes Study. *Am J Med* 2006;**119**(5):418–425.

68. Wong YN, Mitra N, Hudes G, Localio R, Schwartz JS, Wan F, et al. Survival associated with treatment vs. observation of localized prostate cancer in elderly men. *JAMA* 2006;**296**(22):2683–2693.

69. Jeldres C, Suardi N, Walz J, Saad F, Hutterer GC, Bhojani N, et al. Poor overall survival in septa- and octogenarian patients after radical prostatectomy and radiotherapy for prostate cancer: A population-based study of 6183 men. *Eur Urol* 2008;**54**(1):107–116.

70. Sharifi N, Gulley JL, Dahut WL. Androgen deprivation therapy for prostate cancer. *JAMA* 2005;**294**(2):238–244.

71. Keating NL, O'Malley AJ, Smith MR. Diabetes and cardiovascular disease during androgen deprivation therapy for prostate cancer. *J Clin Oncol* 2006;**24**(27):4448–4456.

72. Shahinian VB, Kuo YF, Freeman JL, Goodwin JS. Risk of fracture after androgen deprivation for prostate cancer. *N Engl J Med* 2005;**352**(2):154–164.

73. Saad F, Gleason DM, Murray R, Tchekmedyian S, Venner P, Lacombe L, et al. A randomized, placebo-controlled trial of zoledronic acid in patients with hormone-refractory metastatic prostate carcinoma. *J Natl Cancer Inst* 2002;**94**(19):1458–1468.

74. Berthold DR, Pond GR, Soban F, de WR, Eisenberger M, Tannock IF. Docetaxel plus prednisone or mitoxantrone plus prednisone for advanced prostate cancer: Updated survival in the TAX 327 study. *J Clin Oncol* 2008;**26**(2):242–245.

75. Petrylak DP, Tangen CM, Hussain MH, Lara PN, Jr., Jones JA, Taplin ME, et al. Docetaxel and estramustine compared with mitoxantrone and prednisone for advanced refractory prostate cancer. *N Engl J Med* 2004;**351**(15):1513–1520.

76. De Bono JS, Oudard S, Ozguroglou M, Hansen S, Machiels JH, Shen L, et al. Cabazitaxel or mitoxantrone with prednisone in patients with metastatic castration-resistant prostate cancer (mCRPC) previously treated with Docetaxel: final results of a multinational phase III trial (TROPIC). *J Clin Oncol* 2010;**28**:15s.

77. Porter AT, McEwan AJ. Strontium-89 as an adjuvant to external beam radiation improves pain relief and delays disease progression in advanced prostate cancer: Results of a randomized controlled trial. *Semin Oncol* 1993;**20**(3 Suppl 2): 38–43.

78. Serafini AN, Houston SJ, Resche I, Quick DP, Grund FM, Ell PJ, et al. Palliation of pain associated with metastatic bone cancer using samarium-153 lexidronam: A double-blind placebo-controlled clinical trial. *J Clin Oncol* 1998;**16**(4):1574–1581.

79. Droz JP, Balducci L, Bolla M, Emberton M, Fitzpatrick JM, Joniau S, et al. Background for the proposal of SIOG guidelines for the management of prostate cancer in senior adults. *Crit Rev Oncol Hematol* 2010;**73**(1):68–91.

CHAPTER 22

Ovarian Cancer

CLAIRE FALANDRY

Geriatrics Unit, Lyon University, Hospices Civils de Lyon, Pierre-Bénite, France

GILLES FREYER

Department of Medical Oncology, Lyon University, Hospices Civils de Lyon, Pierre-Bénite, France

ERIC PUJADE-LAURAINE

Department of Oncology, Descartes University of Paris, Paris

22.1 INTRODUCTION

Since the 1970s, management of advanced ovarian cancer was largely improved through the succession of both an extensive debulking surgical step and adjuvant chemotherapy. This allowed overall survival rates to improve, with the median survival exceeding the 35 months in most published series [1]. Nevertheless the reported overall survival rates of elderly patients, in population-based studies or even in randomized trials, are far lower. These differences may be explained by frequent suboptimal management in the former, but also by excessive toxicities, leading to dose limitations or treatment termination. In this context, standard treatment feasibility needed to be explored in elderly-specific populations and specific conclusions to be drawn. An extensive effort has already been made, in order to explore both surgical and chemotherapic management in elderly populations. Nevertheless, highly variable populations have been depicted, starting with age definition (from >60 to >75 and even >80). This has led to different conclusions that are difficult to translate into real-life practice.

22.2 DEMOGRAPHICS

Ovarian cancer is the leading cause of death from gynecological cancer in the Western world [2]. Incidence and mortality increase with age, with incidence peaking between 75 and 79 years and mortality between 80 and 84 years. About half of the cases appear in women over the age of 65 years [3]. Age has been long recognized as an independent prognostic factor for ovarian cancer [4,5], and differences in survival rates have increased with treatment and management improvements [6–8].

Cancer and Aging Handbook: Research and Practice, First Edition. Edited by Keith M. Bellizzi and Margot A. Gosney.
© 2012 Wiley-Blackwell. Published 2012 by John Wiley & Sons, Inc.

Advanced FIGO stages III and IV repredsent the vast majority of ovarian cancer at diagnosis and this proportion increases with age [9,10]. This can be explained by an asymptomatic disease at early stages and a delay in clinic examinations. Histoprognostic features of ovarian cancer in the elderly subject are generally worse than in their younger counterparts: more advanced stages, mixed histology, less differentiated tumors.

22.3 TREATMENT STRATEGIES

22.3.1 From Theory to Real-Time Practice

The main improvements in ovarian cancer management since the 1950s can be summarized as a surgical step—seeking to achieve the smallest tumor residue—and development of platinum-based polychemotherapy. The current accepted standard of care for patients newly diagnosed with advanced stage ovarian cancer is optimal surgical debulking (i.e., no macroscopic residual disease) performed either upfront or in a delayed fashion by a trained gynecologic oncologist [11,12], and six cycles of platinum–taxane-based chemotherapy given either in adjuvant or neoadjuvant setting. Both surgery and chemotherapy outcomes have been studied in an elderly population. In both cases, some contradictions arise when comparing trial results—usually promoting standard treatment options—and real-time practice, as it has been analyzed from the SEER (Surveillance, Epidemiology, and End Results) program data and a study from the German AGO (Arbeitsgemeinschaft Gynaekologische Onkologie) collaborative group on "nonenrolled" patients. Significantly, as in many oncogeriatric fields, elderly patients are either excluded from medical trials or selected within restrictive inclusion criteria favoring biased results and conclusions and also justifying some hesitations in applying standard treatment to vulnerable cancer patients. Indeed, in a SWOG (SouthWest Oncology Group) retrospective analysis of 16,396 patients enrolled in 164 trials during the 1990s, increasing age appeared to be a limitation to trial enrolment [13]. In ovarian cancer, patients older than 65 years accounted for 30% of trial-included patients while representing more than 48% of the overall population of patients. In a survey from the US Food and Drug Administration comparing patients enrolled in registration trials for new drugs to SEER cancer demographics, only 9% of cancer patients older than 75 years were included in clinical trials, while representing 31% of the overall ovarian cancer patients [14]. Factors interfering with elderly patients' inclusion in clinical trials have been extensively reviewed and include physician's perceptions; fear of time consumption; restrictive inclusion criteria, notably on comorbid conditions; or functional status or lack of social support [15,16]. The "nonenrolled" cohort of ovarian cancer patients of AGO were older than their "enrolled" counterparts (mean aged 66.7 vs. 57.2 years), and cancer management differed mainly on surgical debulking [17].

22.3.2 Surgery

Indeed, elderly ovarian cancer patients often undergo less radical surgery than do their younger counterparts, even with equivalent comorbidities [18]. According to a meta-analysis published by Bristow et al. in 2002, maximal cytoreductive surgery was, during the platinum era, one of the more powerful determinants of survival in advanced ovarian carcinoma [19]. In addition to age itself, reduced debulking contributes to the poorer outcome in elderly patients [20].

Nevertheless, according to many published series, age itself should not interfere with optimal surgical management. For some authors, in optimal surgical conditions, maximal debulking rates do not decrease with age [18,21–23]. In a retrospective cohort published by Bruchim et al. comparing management of 46 patients 70 years or older to 143 younger patients, only 54.3% of elderly patients underwent primary debulking surgical interventions, compared to 84.5% of the younger group ($p = 0.001$), but age was not a limiting factor for optimal debulking in patients who underwent surgery (53% vs. 54% in old vs. young groups, respectively) [22]. The same conclusions were drawn by Uyar et al. in a multiinstitutional review of ovarian cancer management (131 elderly patients ≥ 70 years) and Wright et al. in a retrospective series (129 younger patients <70 and $46 \geq 70$) [18,21]. In both studies age had no impact on postoperative complication rates, and Wright found that younger and older groups had the same duration of hospital stay and survival [21]. For both the Bruchim and Uyar studies, age had a significant impact on platinum-based chemotherapy with higher rates of treatment-related toxicities (mainly hematological), dose reductions, and treatment delays in the older group [18,22]. Such nonsignificant differences between elderly and nonelderly patients' outcomes after surgery can be explained by significant improvements in surgical techniques and perioperative intensive care during the 1980s, which yielded a decrease in perioperative mortality from 8.9% to <3.2% in preplanned surgical conditions [24].

Some controversies appeared from other series. As suggested by a GOG (Gynecologic Oncology Group) retrospective analysis of six clinical trials; even in standardized surgical procedures and on relatively selected patients, advancing age is associated with larger volumes of residual disease [5]. In a retrospective study from Cloven et al., patients aged >80 years undergoing debulking surgery had 38% risk of major postoperative morbidity and 11% of death-prolonged hospitalization, but most of them were discharged to home and were able to receive postoperative chemotherapy [25]. Moreover, optimal debulking of <1 cm had a major impact on overall survival (32.5 months vs. 3.5 months) but was achieved in only 25% of the patients despite aggressive surgical effort. In a retrospective study on 85 octogenarians treated between 1991 and 2006 and published by Moore et al. in 2006, 86% presented with advanced disease, 80% had cytoreductive surgery, and 74% were left with <1 cm residual disease. But death prior to hospital discharge and within 60 days of surgery occurred in 13% and 20% of patients. Among patients who underwent surgery, 13% were unable to receive planned adjuvant therapy, 22% were treated with single-agent platinum, and 37% completed fewer than three cycles of chemotherapy. This led the authors to conclude that patients over 80 years may not tolerate combination surgery and chemotherapy and that the high proportion of postoperative complications and deaths argues for a more prudent approach to management in this group of patients [26]. Similar conclusions can be drawn from the population-based experience of Diaz-Montes et al. Short-term outcomes of 168 women aged 80 years and older operated from 1990 to 2000 for ovarian cancer were compared to 2249 younger patients' postoperative outcomes in a statewide hospital discharge database. Octogenarian patients were significantly more likely to have a longer hospital stay (median 10 days vs. 7 days, $p < 0.0001$) and a 2.3-fold higher 30-day mortality rate (5.4% vs. 2.4%, $p = 0.036$) [27]. According to the SEER cancer statistic reviews, age remains the most predictive factor for suboptimal surgical management. Optimal surgical procedures were performed in 43.7% of patients <60, 29.5% between 60 and 79 years, and 21.7% ≥ 80 years between 1973 and

1999 [3]. Similar rates (respectively 21% and 40%) have been observed in two successive phase II trials from the French GINECO (Groupe d'Investigateurs Nationaux pour l'Etude des Cancers de l'Ovaire et du sein) group, designed for analyzing the feasibility of two chemotherapy regimen, the first from 1998 to 2000 and the second from 2000 to 2003 [28,29].

Reasons for this suboptimal surgical treatment include fear of more advanced cancers at time of diagnosis, presence of comorbidities, and some nonmedical factors such as socio-economic or racial origins [30,31]. Elderly people also are more often cared for by nononcologists such as general surgeons and obstetricians/gynecologists [32] or in emergency situations [27] for cancer complications (occlusion, perforation, infection), and are less likely to undergo surgery at a university hospital [27].

Controversial results after surgery and surgeons' frequent reluctance to undertake maximal cytoreductive surgery in vulnerable elderly patients led some teams to consider other management strategies, including secondary surgery. Non-elderly-specific trials evaluated the place of a secondary cytoreduction after either a nonmaximal primary surgery (EORTC 55865 trial [33]) or after a maximal primary debulking effort (GOG trial [34]). According to as yet unpublished data, neoadjuvant chemotherapy followed by interval debulking surgery does not seem to worsen prognosis compared to primary debulking surgery followed by chemotherapy [35]. Moreover, delayed cytoreductive surgery yielded lower complication rates [35]. Although elderly people represented only a minority of those included in these trials, it is tempting to consider this treatment as an alternative for vulnerable elderly patients with high initial tumor burden.

Preoperative Assessment   In the context of high perioperative morbidity and mortality risks, another challenging question is the place of preoperative assessment. The elderly patients should not be considered as a uniform group but as a highly heterogeneous population, in which medical and functional assessments play a central role.

In the large field of surgical management of elderly patients, because of higher risks of postoperative morbimortality and longer hospital stays, some authors have considered the need for specific preoperative geriatric assessment tools. Some retrospective analyses have identified some covariates of interest, and low serum albumin levels before surgery are significantly associated with suboptimal cytoreduction in univariate analyses and with death in multivariate analyses, along with increasing age [36]. Comorbidities also impact on perioperative morbidity and mortality, as well as the surgeon's specialty, who undertakes the surgery [27].

Since commonly used preoperative assessments are not validated in geriatric cancer populations [37] Audisio et al. developed PACE (preoperative assessment of cancer in the elderly), a specific screening assessment [38] combining indices from geriatric and anesthesia fields [the screening tool CGA for (comprehensive geriatric assessment), BFI (brief fatigue index), and ASA and Satariano indicies]. Its validation included 389 older patients, although inclusion was restricted to patients having a MMS score ≥ 18 for ethical reasons, rendering it difficult to extend to mild to moderate cognition deficits. Some components of this mixed screening tool were predictive of 30-day morbidity and mortality and length of hospital postoperative stay: IADL (instrumental activities of daily living) score <8, PS (performance status) >1, and moderate to severe fatigue (BFI) score (>3), leading the authors to conclude that this screening tool should be used for future studies.

22.3.3 Chemotherapy

As with surgical management, some differences appear in the literature between dogma and real practice. During the first randomized trials of the platinum era, elderly people were either excluded or selected on restrictive inclusion criteria. Nevertheless, some subgroup analyses were published, concluding that the chemotherapy protocols have similar risk/benefit ratios [39], with perhaps slightly increased hematotoxicity but decreased gastrointestinal secondary events, better quality of life during chemotherapy [40], and the same efficacy [41,42]. In a subgroup analysis of the AGO-OVAR3 trial, which recruited 103 patients over 70 years (median age 73), there was no difference between elderly and younger patients in terms of paclitaxel, carboplatin, or cisplatin dose intensity, as well as chemotherapy tolerance and patients quality of life. Febrile neutropenia was more common in older subjects (5% vs. 1%, $p = 0.005$), and treatment was more often prematurely discontinued [43]. Despite these increased limiting toxicities, in Eisenhaurer's analysis of 108 patients older than 65 years, compared to 184 younger ones, treated between 1998 and 2004 at the Memorial Sloan-Klettering Cancer Center, elderly patients demonstrated similar rates of initial response, platinum resistance, PFS, and OS to younger patients [42]. Hershman et al. also concluded, from a population-based analysis of the SEER program database, that even if only half of patients over age 65 years were treated with platinum-based therapy, survival should improve by 38% in this group, with benefit rates similar to those described among younger patients, justifying an increasing effort to treat elderly patients in much the same way as younger ones [41].

Some controversies appeared from series of older and more frail patients. In Uyar's analysis of treatment patterns by decades in elderly patients at a multiinstitutional level, 36% of patients aged 70–79 years and 41% of patients aged >80 treated with platinum-based chemotherapy required dose reductions or termination of therapy [18]. In Bruchim's retrospective cohort comparing cancer management of 46 patients over age 70 years to 143 younger ones, elderly patients had significantly more hematological toxicities (75% vs. 36.3%; $p = 0.001$) and were more likely to have dose reductions and treatment delays (60% vs. 22.4%; $p < 0.001$, and 46.6% vs. 19.1%; $p = 0.004$, respectively) [22]. In Ceccaroni's retrospective analysis of 148 patients over 70 years treated between 1990 and 2000 (median age 73) in Italian cancer centers, treatment delays over 7 days were often required (16.9% of the cases) [44]. Villella drew the same conclusion while comparing treatment delays of 31 patients >70 years to 44 <55 treated between 1996 and 2001 at the Columbia University College of Physicians and Surgeons [45]. In Kurtz' subgroup analysis of elderly patients (>70) included in the GINECO and GCIG (Gynecologic Cancer InterGroup) CALYPSO randomized clinical trial, which compared a carboplatin + pegylated liposomal doxorubicin to a carboplatin + paclitaxel standard in platinum-sensitive relapse, elderly patients represented 16% of the included population (median age 73) and had the same treatment tolerance, except for an excess in grade >2 neuropathies, due largely to carboplatin–paclitaxel combinations [46].

These controversies show the need to be circumspect with previous results, as they may be biased by either selective inclusion criteria or investigators' reluctance to include elderly people in clinical trials. Factors influencing these biases were analyzed and found that clinicians often looked only at chronological age, rather than geriatric covariates [47]. While adjuvant chemotherapy with six cycles of carboplatin–paclitaxel [48,49] is still presented as the standard in the elderly, real practice is different.

Population-based studies, mainly from the SEER program, showed a higher rate of monotherapies or even abstention from therapy in patients aged >65. According to the analysis of Sundarajan et al. using 1992–1996 SEER program data, abstention reached 17% of patients over 65 years. Compared to the 65–69 age group, the odds ratios by age group for receiving therapy within 4 months of diagnosis were 0.96 for 70–74 years, 0.65 for 75–79 years, 0.24 for 80–84 years, and 0.12 for patients over 85 years of age, showing a dramatic decrease of chemotherapy use after 80 years. Reasons for suboptimal treatment include age itself [50] and fear of comorbidities and also some nonmedical factors such as socioeconomic or racial origin [51]. As previously explained, extensive surgical management itself seems to compromise chemotherapy feasibility in vulnerable elderly people [18,22], leading some authors to consider either delayed surgical treatment or even surgical abstention [26].

Influence of Geriatric Parameters on Chemotherapy Tolerance and Cancer Survival   Since the subgroup analyses of large randomized trials frequently reflect only a partial and biased picture of the real treatment tolerance in elderly people, since 1997 GINECO dedicated a specific program to elderly ovarian cancer patients. Its first purpose was to analyze the feasibility of some "standard" chemotherapies in the light of geriatric assessment, with as large inclusion criteria as possible [performance status (PS) ≤3, absence of severe disease limitation, no cognitive exclusion criteria except patient's inability to understand and accept treatment procedures]. In the first study conducted between 1998 and 2000, 83 patients aged ≥70 years (median age 76) with stage III or IV ovarian carcinoma received six courses of a 3-weekly carboplatin-cyclophosphamide (CC) combination. Chemotherapy feasibility, defined as the probability of receiving six courses without premature arrest of treatment due to severe toxicity, tumor progression, death, or patient's or investigator's decision, was 72%. No deaths occurred as a result of chemotherapy toxicity, and those that occurred were generally manageable [29]. Three factors appeared to have a poor prognostic value. Two of these emerged from the geriatric assessment: (1) symptoms of depression and (2) if the number of daily medications taken was greater than six. The final factor was FIGO stage IV. Symptoms of depression in this study were simply reported by the investigator at inclusion of the patient, but were linked neither to the PS nor to the mini–mental status in the statistical analysis [29].

The second study, performed between 2000 and 2003 in the same GINECO centers and in the same population of patients, evaluated the feasibility of a 3-weekly carboplatin AUC 5–paclitaxel 175 mg/m^2 (CP) combination. Chemotherapy feasibility rate, defined as previously, was 68.5 %. Respective toxicities of the two chemotherapy regimen are presented in Table 22.1. Interestingly, despite similar inclusion criteria, patients' characteristics were slightly different. There were notably an increased rate of surgical debulking (40% vs. 21% of tumor residue ≤1 cm), a trend toward younger patients with better performance status in the CP study. This could be explained by investigator's concern that this combination had a higher risk of toxicity to vulnerable patients.

Data from these two trials ($n = 155$ patients) were pooled in a retrospective multivariate analysis. Among risk factors for a poor outcome, the *depression* item was evaluated by the hospital anxiety and depression scale (HADS) [52]. With a cutoff of 15, this scale can discriminate between two populations with different prognoses (12 months for higher scores, >35 months for HADS <15). Initial stage IV and

TABLE 22.1   Evolution of Patient Characteristics at Inclusion in Three Successive Elderly-Specific Trials from GINECO

Patient Characteristics	CC Group (1998–2000)	CP Group (2000–2003)	Carboplatin Group (2008–2010)
		Number (%)	
	83 (100)	72 (100)	111 (100)
Age (years)			
Median	76	75	78
≥80	20 (24)	18 (25)	45 (41)
Extremes	70–90	70–89	70–93
Performance status			
0–1	47 (56)	53 (74)	63 (57)
2–3	36 (44)	19 (26)	48 (43)
≥1 dependence on ADL	—	—	61 (55)
≥1 dependence on IADL	—	38 (68)	93 (75)
Depression			
Simple investigator's assessment	19 (23)	5 (9)	20 (18)
HADS ≥15	—	16 (22)	41 (37)
≥4 comedications	35 (42)	19 (26)	76 (69)

lymphopenia at study entry were also significantly associated with poor survival. Surprisingly, despite patient characteristics favoring the CP group of patients, survival curves were strictly comparable and, in the prognostic analysis, paclitaxel use appeared to be an independent poor prognostic factor for survival (HR = 2.42, $p = 0.001$) [28]. With the limit of a cautious interpretation of a retrospective analysis of a relatively small population, those data cast doubt on the usefulness of combining paclitaxel with platinum in elderly patients with advanced ovarian carcinoma. This finding did not seem to be linked to unexpected toxicities or premature treatment interruption, but there was a nonsignificant trend toward a reduced chemotherapy feasibility in the CP group as compared to the CC group (68.5% vs. 72 %). These results were discussed by Zola et al. in an editorial, in which they concluded that, according to available results at that time, "there (was) no evidence for not treating elderly ovarian cancer patients with the standard treatment or excluding them from randomised clinical trials" [52].

More recently, Pignata et al. reported the MITO-5 (Multicentre Italian Trial in Ovarian cancer) study, a phase II trial of 26 stage IC—IV ovarian cancer patients. It assessed the tolerance of a weekly carboplatin + paclitaxel schedule: carboplatin AUC 2 + paclitaxel 60 mg/m^2 on days 1, 8, 15 every 4 weeks. They included elderly patients, a median age of 77, a significant proportion of who had some ADL and/or IADL dependences, although most had a performance status of 0 or 1 [53]. Only three limiting toxicities were observed (heart rhythm, prolonged hematological toxicity, liver transaminase increase), and four individuals developed grade 1 peripheral neuropathy. Thus this weekly schedule appears currently to be an alternative to the usual carboplatin–paclitaxel standard regimen.

22.4 TOWARD CROSSTALK BETWEEN ONCOLOGICAL AND GERIATRIC ASSESSMENTS

Given these analyses of controversies between current standards, which until quite recently were promoted for elderly people; and elderly-specific studies, which highlight some excessive toxicities using these same standards, it seems reasonable to conclude that different issues have been addressed. On one hand, subgroup analyses from large randomized trials included fit patients selected on restrictive inclusion criteria; on the other hand, elderly-specific trials favoring large inclusion criteria provided conclusions about more vulnerable populations. Biases exist in both kinds of studies, illustrating that the two subgroups of patients have different geriatric profiles. Indeed, the GINECO study included from 2008 to 2010 111 patients in a third phase II study that evaluated prospectively the prognostic value of psychologic and geriatric covariates in elderly advanced ovarian cancer patients treated by six courses of a carboplatin AUC 5 monotherapy. Despite very close inclusion criteria, patients' characteristics at inclusion differed largely from the two previous studies, resulting in an older and more vulnerable population (Table 22.1). Two main reasons may explain this trend. On one hand, one can expect some competition of this study with large randomized studies, that either increased or excluded age limitations and allowed inclusion of some "young and fit" elderly patients; on the other hand, and investigators' may have been concerned that such monotherapy could reduce the patient's response to treatment.

Advanced ovarian cancer must be seen as a rapidly symptomatic and fatal condition that justifies some rapid and aggressive treatment. Nevertheless, in a very old or dependent population, initial maximal cytoreduction and carboplatin–paclitaxel may be excessive [26,28]. Therefore, different clinical strategies should be proposed, favoring maximal efficacy in fit elderly individuals but optimal efficacy/tolerance ratios in vulnerable ones (Fig. 22.1). In future elderly-specific studies such as GINECO's trials,

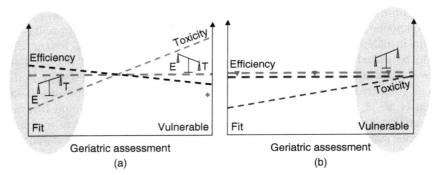

Geriatric assessment
(a)

Geriatric assessment
(b)

Figure 22.1 A model promoting different treatment strategies for ovarian cancer management in the elderly based on geriatric assessment: (a) standard treatment; (b) alternate treatment. Many studies and notably subgroup analyses of large randomized studies showed that standard treatments may be manageable in fit elderly, with globally the same efficacy (or slightly decreased for surgical debulking; see *on left panel) and manageable increase in toxicities. Nevertheless, these toxicities appear excessive in the very old or vulnerable elderly patients, leading to an unfavorable benefit/risk ratio. For this population of vulnerable elderly, a slight decrease in treatment efficiency may be preferred to standard treatment, in order to avoid treatment-linked morbimortality and preserve favorable benefit/risk ratio. Among alternate treatments previously proposed are delayed cytoreduction and carboplatin monotherapy.

the result will be two distinct groups of patients being explored by different trials, in which patients should be categorized into "fit" and "vulnerable" groups.

22.5 CONCLUSION

Despite demographics showing higher incidence and mortality rates over the age of 70 years, ovarian cancer clinical trials have long restricted elderly patients' trial inclusion on either established inclusion criteria or even age limit. This led to a paradox—currently accepted standards have been established on trial-included patients with a median age between 50 and 55, when median age is actually over 65 years in the Western world. In addition, many contradictions appear during analysis of published trials on ovarian cancer in elderly individuals, since populations of interest have been highly heterogeneous and rarely characterized by geriatric parameters. The future challenge for oncologists will be to explore this heterogeneity and to disentangle it on the basis of oncogeriatric assessment. This may reduce current barriers to elderly patients entering into clinical trials.

REFERENCES

1. Spriggs DR. Ovarian cancer as a chronic disease: A new treatment paradigm. Highlights of a roundtable discussion. *Cancer Control* 2001;**8**(6 Suppl 1):5–7; discussion 8–18.
2. Jemal A et al. Cancer statistics, 2005. *CA Cancer J Clin* 2005;**55**(1):10–30.
3. Ries LA. Ovarian cancer. Survival and treatment differences by age. *Cancer* 1993; **71**(2 Suppl):524–529.
4. Alberts DS et al. Analysis of patient age as an independent prognostic factor for survival in a phase III study of cisplatin-cyclophosphamide versus carboplatin-cyclophosphamide in stages III (suboptimal) and IV ovarian cancer. A Southwest Oncology Group study. *Cancer* 1993;**71**(2 Suppl):618–627.
5. Thigpen T et al. Age as a prognostic factor in ovarian carcinoma. The Gynecologic Oncology Group experience. *Cancer* 1993;**71**(2 Suppl):606–614.
6. Chan JK et al. Ovarian cancer in younger vs older women: A population-based analysis. *Br J Cancer* 2006;**95**(10):1314–1320.
7. Barnholtz-Sloan JS et al. Ovarian cancer: Changes in patterns at diagnosis and relative survival over the last three decades. *Am J Obstet Gynecol* 2003;**189**(4):1120–1127.
8. Chan JK et al. Stages III and IV invasive epithelial ovarian carcinoma in younger versus older women: What prognostic factors are important? *Obstet Gynecol* 2003; **102**(1):156–161.
9. Young R, Fuks Z, Hoskins W. Cancer of the ovary. In De Vita VT Jr, Hellman S, Rosenberg SA, eds. *Cancer Principles in Practice of Oncology*, Lippincott, Philadelphia 1989, pp. 1162–1196.
10. Yancik R. Ovarian cancer. Age contrasts in incidence, histology, disease stage at diagnosis, and mortality. *Cancer* 1993;**71**(2 Suppl):517–523.
11. Delgado G, Oram DH, Petrilli ES. Stage III epithelial ovarian cancer: The role of maximal surgical reduction. *Gynecol Oncol* 1984;**18**(3):293–298.
12. Venesmaa P, Ylikorkala O. Morbidity and mortality associated with primary and repeat operations for ovarian cancer. *Obstet Gynecol* 1992;**79**(2):168–172.

13. Hutchins LF et al. Underrepresentation of patients 65 years of age or older in cancer-treatment trials. *N Engl J Med* 1999;**341**(27):2061–2067.

14. Talarico L, Chen G, Pazdur R. Enrollment of elderly patients in clinical trials for cancer drug registration: A 7-year experience by the US Food and Drug Administration. *J Clin Oncol* 2004;**22**(22):4626–4631.

15. Townsley CA, Selby R, Siu LL. Systematic review of barriers to the recruitment of older patients with cancer onto clinical trials. *J Clin Oncol* 2005;**23**(13):3112–3124.

16. Villella J, Chalas E. Optimising treatment of elderly patients with ovarian cancer: improving their enrollment in clinical trials. *Drugs Aging* 2005;**22**(2):95–100.

17. Harter P et al. Non-enrolment of ovarian cancer patients in clinical trials: Reasons and background. *Ann Oncol* 2005;**16**(11):1801–1805.

18. Uyar D et al. Treatment patterns by decade of life in elderly women (> or = 70 years of age) with ovarian cancer. *Gynecol Oncol* 2005;**98**(3):403–408.

19. Bristow RE et al. Survival effect of maximal cytoreductive surgery for advanced ovarian carcinoma during the platinum era: A meta-analysis. *J Clin Oncol* 2002;**20**(5):1248–1259.

20. Wimberger P et al. Impact of age on outcome in patients with advanced ovarian cancer treated within a prospectively randomized phase III study of the Arbeitsgemeinschaft Gynaekologische Onkologie Ovarian Cancer Study Group (AGO-OVAR). *Gynecol Oncol* 2006;**100**(2):300–307.

21. Wright JD, Herzog TJ, Powell MA. Morbidity of cytoreductive surgery in the elderly. *Am J Obstet Gynecol* 2004;**190**(5):1398–1400.

22. Bruchim I, Altaras M, Fishman A. Age contrasts in clinical characteristics and pattern of care in patients with epithelial ovarian cancer. *Gynecol Oncol* 2002;**86**(3):274–278.

23. Ben-Ami I et al. Perioperative morbidity and mortality of gynecological oncologic surgery in elderly women. *Int J Gynecol Cancer* 2006;**16**(1):452–457.

24. Lichtinger M et al. Major surgical procedures for gynecologic malignancy in elderly women. *South Med J* 1986;**79**(12):1506–1510.

25. Cloven NG et al. Management of ovarian cancer in patients older than 80 years of Age. *Gynecol Oncol* 1999;**73**(1):137–139.

26. Moore KN et al. Ovarian cancer in the octogenarian: Does the paradigm of aggressive cytoreductive surgery and chemotherapy still apply? *Gynecol Oncol* 2008;**110**(2):133–139.

27. Diaz-Montes TP et al. Surgical care of elderly women with ovarian cancer: A population-based perspective. *Gynecol Oncol* 2005;**99**(2):352–357.

28. Trédan O et al. Carboplatin cyclophosphamide or carboplatin pacitaxel in elderly with advanced ovarian cancer? Analysis of two consecutive trials from the GINECO. *Ann Oncol* 2007;**18**(2):256–262.

29. Freyer G et al. Comprehensive geriatric assessment predicts tolerance to chemotherapy and survival in elderly patients with advanced ovarian carcinoma: A GINECO study. *Ann Oncol* 2005;**16**(11):1795–1800.

30. Chan JK et al. Racial disparities in surgical treatment and survival of epithelial ovarian cancer in United States. *J Surg Oncol* 2008;**97**(2):103–107.

31. Vercelli M et al. Relative survival in elderly European cancer patients: Evidence for health care inequalities. The EUROCARE Working Group. *Crit Rev Oncol Hematol* 2000;**35**(3):161–179.

32. Hightower RD et al. National survey of ovarian carcinoma. IV: Patterns of care and related survival for older patients. *Cancer* 1994;**73**(2):377–383.

33. van der Burg ME et al. The effect of debulking surgery after induction chemotherapy on the prognosis in advanced epithelial ovarian cancer. Gynecological Cancer Cooperative Group of the European Organization for Research and Treatment of Cancer. *N Engl J Med* 1995;**332**(10):629–634.

34. Rose PG et al. Secondary surgical cytoreduction for advanced ovarian carcinoma. *N Engl J Med* 2004;**351**(24):2489–2497.

35. Vergote I et al. Timing of debulking surgery in advanced ovarian cancer. *Int J Gynecol Cancer* 2008;**18**(Suppl 1):11–19.

36. Alphs HH et al. Predictors of surgical outcome and survival among elderly women diagnosed with ovarian and primary peritoneal cancer. *Gynecol Oncol* 2006;**103**(3):1048–1053.

37. Audisio RA et al. The surgical management of elderly cancer patients; recommendations of the SIOG surgical task force. *Eur J Cancer* 2004;**40**(7):926–938.

38. Audisio RA et al. Shall we operate? Preoperative assessment in elderly cancer patients (PACE) can help. A SIOG surgical task force prospective study. *Crit Rev Oncol Hematol* 2008;**65**(2):156–163.

39. Giovanazzi-Bannon S et al. Treatment tolerance of elderly cancer patients entered onto phase II clinical trials: An Illinois Cancer Center study. *J Clin Oncol* 1994;**12**(11):2447–2452.

40. Le T et al. Quality of life evaluations in patients with ovarian cancer during chemotherapy treatment. *Gynecol Oncol* 2004;**92**(3):839–844.

41. Hershman D et al. Effectiveness of platinum-based chemotherapy among elderly patients with advanced ovarian cancer. *Gynecol Oncol* 2004;**94**(2):540–549.

42. Eisenhauer EL et al. Response and outcomes in elderly patients with stages IIIC-IV ovarian cancer receiving platinum-taxane chemotherapy. *Gynecol Oncol* 2007;**106**(2):381–387.

43. Hilpert F et al. Feasibility, toxicity and quality of life of first-line chemotherapy with platinum/paclitaxel in elderly patients aged $\geq$ 70 years with advanced ovarian cancer—a study by the AGO OVAR Germany. *Ann Oncol* 2007;**18**(2):282–7.

44. Ceccaroni M et al. Gynecological malignancies in elderly patients: Is age 70 a limit to standard-dose chemotherapy? An Italian retrospective toxicity multicentric study. *Gynecol Oncol* **2002**;85(3):445–450.

45. Villella JA et al. Comparison of tolerance of combination carboplatin and paclitaxel chemotherapy by age in women with ovarian cancer. *Gynecol Oncol* 2002;**86**(3):316–322.

46. Kurtz JE et al. Can elderly patients with recurrent ovarian cancer (ROC) be treated with a platinum-based doublet? Results from the CALYPSO trial. *J Clin Oncol* 2010;**28**:15s.

47. Moore DH et al. An assessment of age and other factors influencing protocol versus alternative treatments for patients with epithelial ovarian cancer referred to member institutions: A Gynecologic Oncology Group study. *Gynecol Oncol* 2004;**94**(2):368–374.

48. Begg CB, and Carbone PP. Clinical trials and drug toxicity in the elderly. The experience of the Eastern Cooperative Oncology Group. *Cancer* 1983;**52**(11):1986–1992.

49. Higgins RV et al. Is age a barrier to the aggressive treatment of ovarian cancer with paclitaxel and carboplatin? *Gynecol Oncol* 1999;**75**(3):464–467.

50. Maas HA et al. The influence of age and co-morbidity on treatment and prognosis of ovarian cancer: A population-based study. *Gynecol Oncol* 2005;**97**(1):104–109.

51. Sundararajan V et al. Variations in the use of chemotherapy for elderly patients with advanced ovarian cancer: A population-based study. *J Clin Oncol* 2002;**20**(1):173–178.

52. Zola P, Ferrero A. Is carboplatin-paclitaxel combination the standard treatment of elderly ovarian cancer patients? *Ann Oncol* 2007;**18**(2):213–4.

53. Pignata S et al. A phase II study of weekly carboplatin and paclitaxel as first-line treatment of elderly patients with advanced ovarian cancer. A Multicentre Italian Trial in Ovarian cancer (MITO-5) study. *Crit Rev Oncol Hematol* 2008;**66**(3):229–236.

PART VI

CANCER SURVIVORSHIP AND AGING

CHAPTER 23

Theoretical Perspectives from Gerontology and Lifespan Development

THOMAS O. BLANK

Human Development and Family Studies, University of Connecticut, Storrs, CT

23.1 INTRODUCTION

It is widely recognized that one's risk of cancer increases with age [1–5]. Over 70% of new cancer cases are diagnosed in men and women over the age of 65. As life extension for many cancers becomes more common, many who are "young" at time of diagnosis and treatment grow to be older cancer survivors. Thus it is valuable to explore the nexus of gerontological theories and concepts of successful aging with psychooncological models of adjustment to further elucidate positive and negative health outcomes in older adults and to aid in working with older persons with cancer so as to optimize their lives. In trying to merge these sets of theories and models, it is important to begin with basic points of correspondence.

The major goal of oncology is to optimize the cancer experience by using best practices and treatment approaches in a way that be allows for high quality of life despite the threat of the cancer. To be able to do so effectively, oncologists must be aware of the components of individuals and their contexts that will facilitate or constrain adaptation and optimal functioning postcancer. Models from gerontology and aging can contribute to the goal of "best practices" related to older persons dealing with cancer as newly diagnosed patients and, increasingly, with the vast number of older cancer survivors.

In parallel fashion, a major goal of gerontology is to enable older persons to experience what is variously labeled as optimal aging, successful aging, or positive aging, aging with a sense of well-being [6–9]. Some usages of such terms (especially successful aging, as described by Rowe and Kahn [7]) almost explicitly exclude older cancer survivors from the opportunity to be successful agers, because the model includes absence of impairment and/or chronic illness as one of its key criteria. Fortunately, other approaches much more clearly see positive or successful aging as *taking into account* chronic diseases and even impairments and coping with those and integrating them with broader self-identity [6,8–10]. Thus, part of the reason to understand how

Cancer and Aging Handbook: Research and Practice, First Edition. Edited by Keith M. Bellizzi and Margot A. Gosney.
© 2012 Wiley-Blackwell. Published 2012 by John Wiley & Sons, Inc.

older persons deal with challenging life events such as cancer is to enhance optimal, positive aging.

This chapter focuses primarily on social gerontological and psychology of aging theories as they relate to psychosocial aspects of cancer among that large and growing group of older cancer survivors.

23.2 AN OVERARCHING PERSPECTIVE

From birth to death, life is a complicated balancing act of gains and losses, being and doing, becoming and changing, change and stability, action and reaction, and giving and receiving. We are constantly changing the world and being changed by it. Each person brings to these interrelated dualities varying skills and competencies and capabilities—and, as with physical balance, as one gets older (and especially very old), the balancing act becomes more difficult to manage. One may be in danger of "falling," losing that balance. The reasons can be literally physical; they can be cognitive, or self-identity; or they can be social and interpersonal. Some threats to balance in later life are societal, in terms of attitudes toward and opportunities available for older persons. Maintaining balance requires more and more adjustment. Sometimes deliberate choices are made, as we shall see in lifespan and gerontological theories. Sometimes it is certainly less conscious, as one "naturally" exercises more caution to avoid the circumstances that could provide pitfalls, the broken sidewalks, loose rugs, and flights of stairs of everyday life. Experiencing cancer can be one of those flights of stairs, an unexpected and unfamiliar challenge, calling forth activation of existing resources and mechanisms to maintain some kind of balance or to regain balance when it has caused one to fall.

Current social, psychological, and lifespan developmental theory provides us, as researchers and clinicians, with tools to understand and explain the nature of the shifting challenges and opportunities, the dynamically changing sets of personal and social resources, and the skills of aging and older people. They lead us to the recognition of both undeniable losses and challenges that make dealing with cancer more difficult for older persons and the equally important factors that are likely to make it easier for them to deal with it than younger persons. The balancing act and how it affects the experience of cancer as a psychosocial phenomenon have direct implications for practice.

The cancer experience can produce physical, social, psychological, and existential/spiritual changes. These, in turn, require the individual to make adaptations and cope with both the situation and his or her reactions. Interestingly, the reactions of those who have had cancer range broadly, from considering it as one's biggest life event, with life altering import, to seeing it as just another in a lifetime of events, not something that is greatly anxiety provoking beyond the time of diagnosis and treatment or likely to change one's view of self or the world. Also, the significantly altered pathway can be one that narrows and constricts the individual's future or one that opens the door to becoming a fuller, more positive person; this pathway can be predominantly negative and distressing or positive and enhancing.

Many factors can lead to these divergent pathways in response to cancer. Age and aging certainly are one source of the divergent experiences. Old age may provide a particularly acute set of challenges of decline in physical systems that frame the experience very differently from a younger person [4,11–15]. The problematic nature of an aging body is very important for understanding cancer and for the interplay of aging processes and the cancer experience; aging affects every phase of the cancer trajectory, from screening and prevention issues to treatment decisions and survivorship. Indeed, some studies specifically addressing older cancer survivors have found significant levels of distress and depression even many years after treatment, at least sometimes more than non-cancer-related older comparisons [4,16–18]. Yet, many studies show that older persons, on average, report *less* psychological impact than younger ones [19–21]. Thus, it is critically important to tease out how aging with cancer is different both from cancer at younger ages and from aging without a cancer experience.

To realize the goals of this chapter, the author will first describe two broad perspectives: the life course perspective and lifespan development/psychology of aging and will then present several specific examples of current theories prominent in psychology and aging and social gerontology that apply those perspectives in a way that may clarify the variability across individuals and the patterns of aging and quality of life that are directly applicable to older cancer survivors.

23.3 BASIC APPROACHES AND CONCEPTS OF LIFESPAN DEVELOPMENTAL PSYCHOLOGY AND LIFECOURSE PERSPECTIVES

Lifespan development and lifecourse perspectives are at distinctly different levels of understanding. The lifecourse perspective is primarily a sociological approach, with an emphasis on how social structures and life events frame and affect individuals as they move through their time on earth [22,23]. An especially important component is akin to the well-known real estate description of the three most important factors in the value of a home—location, because it alerts us to the major importance of one's placement in both time and space. In other words, experiencing cancer is very different in the early twenty-first century from what it was in the past or will be in the future, and it is a different experience if one is old or younger at this time. Likewise, it is very different in the United States and its healthcare and political climate than in other countries. The equally influential lifespan developmental approach [26-29] is much more individualistically oriented, concerned with how one's cognitive and emotional processing affects one's experiences and behaviors and the meaning that one gives to a specific experience, such as cancer [6,24,25]. It also is concerned with placement, in this case in relation to the developmental processes throughout individual lives and the psychological (and physical) status and characteristics of the individual.

However, both perspectives share critical elements that will frame the remainder of this chapter:

1. Both are contextual, in the sense that they emphasize that every experience, judgment, and action is embedded in a specific situation, which provides parameters for what those experiences, judgments, and actions are [23,25]. What people do and how they feel about their actions are not random or independent, but, rather, are partly constrained and partly facilitated by the characteristics of that specific situation. A central tenet of the approach espoused in this chapter is that life is intrinsically lived "in relation to." The "to" can be in many directions and facets—in relation to one's own physical characteristics and capabilities and one's desires, to other individuals, social

structures, cultural norms and beliefs, historical events, and, most importantly, the history of the person him/herself—past experiences, choices, challenges, and triumphs, and as extended to the future in terms of future goals and desired lives. They are "in relation to" the context and the full life experience of the individual *and* the history and structure of the social and cultural systems of which the person is a part. Each of these relationships is critical individually in its influence on individual thoughts, emotions, and actions; even more importantly, they interact with each other in an intricate dance of forces and pressures, providing opportunities for accomplishment and yet placing obstacles in the way of what the individual feels to be successful and desirable. In many ways, life is a balancing act of a range of forces from within the individual and that person's social and societal context.

2. Reality is fluid and dynamic—the network of forces acting on the person continually changes. The author will expand on this shortly, but the essential element is that life is an ongoing balancing act among all these changing elements, with the result that in order to "stay the same," one has to constantly change and adapt (cope), while in most cases, one is changing in response to the changing environment and progressing along different lines of development according to how one's context is changing. As part of this dynamic nature, a simultaneous and interlinked process of narrowing/constriction and broadening/facilitating are the dialectic of all development.

3. This fluidity and seamlessness of reality leads to a third aspect, the importance of specific life events to produce sometimes dramatic changes in one's life [22,23,30]. The idea here is that throughout life one experiences a relatively small number of events (say, one or two dozen) that can "push" one's trajectory of development in a different way, leading to a different path. These events require action and thought on the part of the person and, to some degree, a decision as to whether to "go with the flow" and change or try to resist the flow and remain the same. These are the points in life that, as they accumulate, result in a life that is different from what the individual could possibly have predicted, especially because many of these events are not self-chosen. Cancer, of course, has the potential to be one of these non-self-chosen but defining events.

4. A fourth piece of the lifecourse/lifespan development approach that is critical for applying this to cancer and aging is that every life event (indeed, every experience, even the most trivial and prosaic) has aspects to it that are losses and others that are gains [6,10,25,31]. The most positive new direction in life at the minimum means abandoning other directions, and often it requires expenditure of energy and loss of some resources. Fortunately for us as human beings, every loss or challenge, no matter how devastating, can also provide us with new insights and perspectives and new, unexpected directions toward growth, because the ways one has dealt with that event can form a foundation for such gain [32–35]. This notion of posttraumatic or positive life change is well established in understanding a range of life experiences, specifically those including cancer [36–39]. It is a reflection of the old folk adage that "when life hands you a lemon, make lemonade" or that "every cloud has a silver lining" (with the addition that every blue sky has the potential to be a loss or a negative).

5. Finally, this approach includes a view of life, including life in old age, to incorporate an element of agency on the part of the individual [6,25,40,41]. That individual is constantly in motion, incorporating and reacting to ongoing experiences and the constraints and opportunities afforded by contexts and experiences, constructing a life as it follows the twists and turns of both planned-for and accidental events. This view

of active engagement in tasks of living is not new; nor is it only to be found in a lifespan/lifecourse approach. Indeed, it is a central part of the well-known model of Erik Erikson [42] as an expanding set of challenges to the individual as one's world expands and then, possibly, contracts, as well as theories by Alfred Adler [43] and others.

23.4 DEFINITIONAL ISSUES AND CASE EXAMPLES

One important definitional issue for a chapter in this book is that of aging [44]. What do we mean by "age" and "aging" when considering how cancer and aging interrelate? Aging clearly includes a range of processes, from relatively systematic biological and physiological changes at every level from molecular to whole body, to changes in one's personality and identity. Often, however, it is reduced to the individual's membership in an age category; "cancer and aging" means looking at cancer in old people. Our society often looks at aging not just in relation to cancer but to all health, economics, and so on; chronological age is often used to categorize and compare groups of individuals. Thus, for example, how does one approach treating a newly diagnosed cancer patient aged 82 years versus one aged 42 or 62 years? Many studies in both cancer research and gerontology/psychology of aging proceed in exactly this way, comparing "old" (e.g., ≥65) to "young" (e.g., ≤65). It is probably obvious that this is not a particularly useful way to proceed. People of the same age can differ dramatically on how they function, how healthy they are, how they think and react, and what their social circumstances are. Thus, other ways of defining age may be more useful. One alternative is functional age—what one can do independently, how capable one is, which can be in terms of cognitive processing, specific physical activities, and perhaps in relation to cancer, how well one would be able to withstand treatment rigors. Another is social age, which has to do with how the person is integrated into society (working or retired, place in family system), and still another is subjective age. An interesting example of subjective age is a qualitative study by Esbensen et al. of older cancer survivors (all >65 years at time of the study), in which several specifically indicated that the diagnosis of cancer was the signal that they were old; it changed their subjective age from middle age [45]. Each way of defining age has its merits and limitations, and so it is important to attend to which is being used in specific research and recommendations. The lifecourse/lifespan developmental approach instead emphasize the fluidity of age, that "aging" is a continual movement through time. For our purposes the part of that movement through time is in the latter parts of a typical lifespan, but the focus is the process, not a specific way station in terms of chronological age.

A related important factor that relates back to the emphasis on location and placement in time is that of cohort [22,23]. This is critical for understanding older persons and cancer. Anyone who is now 80 was born in 1930, whereas anyone who is now 40 was born in 1970. While obvious, this is often ignored in discussing age and aging in relation to any event, certainly including cancer. Those who are 80 have literally grown up in a different world from those born later (or earlier, of course). They have experienced different individual events, to be sure, but perhaps even more importantly, they have experienced different societal events. One of many societal events relevant to this chapter is that the attitudes toward both aging ("60 is the new 40"!) and cancer have changed dramatically since the 1980s or 1970s. Thus, being diagnosed with cancer at 80 and not 40 in 2010 is different in terms of not only age but also cohort. It will simply be experienced differently because of the historical record.

As an illustrative exercise, let us think of three men recently diagnosed with early-stage prostate cancer. Ernie is 82. He has diabetes, has a pacemaker, and walks with a walker. His wife of 57 years died 3 years ago; he has four children in their 40 s and early 50s. Jim is 51 and in otherwise good health. He works in marketing. He recently remarried and now has two adolescent stepchildren living with him and a 26-year-old son living with his exwife. Carl is also 51 and in otherwise good health. He is a gay man who has never married. He works on a loading dock of a mattress manufacturer. His father died of prostate cancer at age 66, and his older brother was diagnosed with it 5 years ago at age 54.

Obviously, the experience of these three men will be extremely different. Ernie comes from a different cohort and has a very different backdrop of personal health. Jim and Carl are identical in age (and cohort), yet they are living very different lives, with varying job demands, family responsibilities, and, very importantly, familial history related to prostate cancer. The contexts of their experiences are dramatically different, and thus they present both different kinds of challenges and potential losses and different kinds of opportunities for potential gains. These differences, and how and why they will matter from treatment through survivorship, can be arranged in a matrix that has two major dimensions, each with two categories (obviously, this is highly simplified). One dimension is personal versus "extrapersonal" (other people, environments) factors (basically, lifespan developmental vs. lifecourse), while the other is factors that are challenges and negative versus resources or factors that may have positive impact on well-being. Each of these will be very briefly addressed, culminating in presentation of a perspective that incorporates elements of several current gerontological theories that fit within the lifespan developmental/lifecourse paradigm.

23.5 A MATRIX OF FACTORS INFLUENCING WELL-BEING OF OLDER CANCER PATIENTS AND SURVIVORS

23.5.1 The Personal, Intraindividual Side of Normal Aging

Physical Aging It is well known and perhaps obvious that as people get older their bodies age, and these aging processes have considerable impact on how cancer is experienced as well as treated [4,13,14,46–49]. For purposes of this chapter we will very briefly summarize the physical aging processes that impact cancer patients and survivors as they age. These processes are primarily negative, and they include both primary, or normal, aging and secondary, or disease-driven, aging. They greatly affect the balancing act of dealing with both regular aspects of life and, especially, ability to deal with particularly stressful life events. Normal aging processes can be summarized as a "big four" of losses or changes, each of which applies in multilevel, systemic fashion from intracellular to organ systems to body behaviors and activities [50,51]. In functional terms they are (1) loss of speed, or generalized slowing, including slowing in nerve conduction, reaction time, metabolism, and up to macrolevel slowing of cognitive processing, speech, movement, and readiness to receive new information; (2) loss of flexibility, or hardening, from wrinkling to musculature, blood vessel restriction, and balance and, psychologically, lessened ability to assimilate new information or process it efficiently; (3) loss of acuity, or *dulling*, which is pervasive across all senses; and (4) loss of stamina or energy, an apparent result of which is lessened reserve capacity or ability to "bounce back" when the body is assailed by internal or external threats. The result of these patterns of loss means that without considerable effort an older person will have lower functional status than when younger and in comparison to younger individuals with average performance for their ages. These obviously have implications for cancer affliction and for how one's cancer will be treated and the level of health and well-being that will result.

Disease-driven processes, or secondary aging, are often added to these primary effects, and they are also likely to be involved in how older persons deal with cancer; most major diseases (of course, including cancer) are age-related, such that they are identified primarily with older age. Most older adults have at least one, and regularly several, chronic disease conditions that form a backdrop of comorbidity for their cancer experience. These have both direct effects, such as limited mobility or function, and indirect effects, such as leading to deteriorating sleep patterns or nutrition, which, in turn, lower stamina and energy even more than primary aging. They also interact with the primary aging processes.

A model developed by Lawton and Nahemow [52]. is useful in understanding the implications of these changes. They indicate that functioning is the result of the interaction of two factors: personal competence or capabilities and the demands (or facilitating factors) in the environment. Persons can be more or less capable of manipulating environments, whereas environments can be more or less receptive to efforts by individuals to manipulate and control them. When those are in relative balance (or good fit), the individual functions well and responds positively in an emotional sense. When they are out of balance (with the environment experienced as either too demanding or too unchallenging), the individual responds with frustration and lack of motivation to attempt to influence the environment. The losses that we have just considered make it likely that as persons age they become less environmentally capable of effecting their desired impacts on the environment. Individuals may respond in several ways: by attempting to increase their capabilities (say, by engaging in an exercise program to improve muscle strength to increase ability to move around), by moving to a new, less demanding environment (e.g., moving to assisted living), by changing the existing environment (using assistive technologies), by changing "themselves" by obtaining and using prosthetics (such as better eyeglasses, hearing aids, or even dental implants), or, finally, by changing their social environment to enable them to manage in the existing environment with their existing capacities (asking family members for help). Some of these approaches involve selecting different environments, and many are compensatory for the lost skills. These will be clarified later in considering more current formulations.

Together, the physiological and concurrent cognitive changes provide a negative, loss-driven context for cancer and aging [50,51,53,54]. Physical aging constrains the capacity of the individual to marshal resources to deal with the tumor and with subsequent decisions, treatment regimens, and side effects. Tumor dynamics are also likely to be different (but that is not a focus of this chapter). At the same time, it should be noted that considerable research has shown that many individuals progressing well into what we term "old age" (remembering again that chronological age is not a very good marker) can continue to perform and function well because their capabilities, although lower than before, are still sufficient to be above the threshold needed for performance [50,51,53]. Also, it is important to remember that these facets are dynamically in flux, sometimes in a downward spiral but other times responding to treatments, to personal choices such as exercise or dietary change. It is also critically important for providers to place these losses in a bigger picture of the interplay of gains and losses even into very old age and the very large differences in impact of losses from individual to individual and from context to context. Just like the leaves of trees in fall, which show the loss to come but in so doing are allowing the tree itself from the pressure to grow, but instead marshal its resources and preserve itself, so persons as they age and experience physical losses may use those losses to free themselves from the need to grow and allowing the possibilities of preservation and maintenance. It is equally important to recognize the loss inherent in the negative changes and the gain allowed by those very changes.

Personality and Personal Resources While the physical factors of biological aging and comorbid diseases appear unremittingly negative, on a more positive side, older persons usually have personal resources to bring to bear, and there is at least some evidence that some of these personal resources increase with age. These range from coping and adaptive skills to orientations to the world, and they will be described more below in presenting the socio-emotional selectivity and selection, optimization, and compensation (SOC) theories. They can also be captured in observations that older persons may have developed effective coping strategies in dealing with previous life experiences and that they may have developed wisdom, an ability to place their current situation in a broader, more favorable context [42,55]. There is also evidence of an important role for religion and spirituality in maintaining or enhancing well-being through the cancer experience, which may have developed as one's faith has matured [56–58]. The remainder of the chapter focuses on those resources and how they may be expressed as one ages and, especially, as one integrates cancer into his or her aging experience.

23.5.2 The Social, Interpersonal, and Lifecourse Side of Cancer and Aging

Individual aging obviously does not happen in a vacuum. Ever-widening circles of others, beginning with one's family and friends, including one's healthcare providers, and culminating in the influences of macrosocial forces such as economic, healthcare, and social policies and programs, all provide static contexts at a point in time and, as noted earlier, dynamically change over time as anyone, older or younger, deals with cancer. We obviously do not have time to include this wide range of factors in this chapter, but it is worthwhile to provide a framework for the individual processes already noted.

One frame derives from the importance of a relatively small number of life events in altering the trajectory for the person from then on [6,28,30,35]. These life events, and their timing, fit in different ways into the social structure, providing a robust frame for an experience such as a cancer diagnosis and treatment. An expectable life event is normative. That does not mean that it is necessary or universal, but that it is typical. Normative events include education, marriage, children, and retirement. There are also many types of nonnormative events. Some are rare or even unique, some are specific to a cohort or to a specific historical time (war, economic upturn or downturn), and some are nonnormative not because they are unusual but because they occur at an unexpected time (an offtime life event). The pattern of normative and nonnormative life events, ultimately unique to each individual, forms a critically important backdrop to subsequent life experiences and how they are interpreted.

Cancer, at any age, is usually categorized as a nonnormative event. However, for quite a few older people, some cancers, especially breast cancer and prostate cancer, may almost feel normative. As illustrated by the brief description of Carl in Section 23.4, because of the strong indication of familial cancer, *not* getting cancer may be nonnormative, and getting it only when old would be offtime. Even without family history, these cancers have almost taken on a nature of being common and expectable, especially with media attention to celebrity after celebrity who has been diagnosed. Older persons may develop expectations that include cancer. Then, when it occurs, it is not experienced as "threatening" or, indeed, as a major life event. This is not to say that it is not distressing or problematic, at least initially, but insofar as it is interpreted as expectable or "normative," it is a less intense experience. In our three brief descriptions, for both Ernie and Carl this may be the case. On the other hand, John would be highly likely to see it as an unexpected, and potentially life-threatening, life event, high on his list of such events. Thus, he is likely to struggle more with it. Perhaps in that struggle he will ascertain the gain that is embedded in and part of the loss or threat more than the other men. Indeed, this is what we find with younger compared to older persons who have been diagnosed with cancer [19–21,59,60].

23.6 OVERVIEW OF RELEVANT THEORIES AND CONCEPTS

For the remainder of this review, we will briefly describe an interrelated set of models that have been developed since the 1980s or 1990s in psychology of aging and lifespan development and, to a lesser extent, lifecourse. Those who are interested can then pursue the much more detailed descriptions of the models contained in the references. Despite their differences, all of the approaches see personality as primarily a process of adaptation to changing life circumstances using a changing set of personal resources. They see personality as expressed in action, especially in ways of influencing the world or responding to the ways in which the world influences the person. Whereas they see older people as responding to the losses that may be increasingly besetting them by redirecting remaining energy toward conservation, what they see as most relevant to sustaining their sense of self and their important relationships to others. Older persons are actively managing their balance, shifting in new directions and exerting considerable energy toward maintaining their balance in areas important to them. Adaptation, use of coping strategies, and development of a new meaning for one's life and a new normal are key aspects to how one deals with a cancer diagnosis and the potentially changed trajectory of one's life. Thus these models have direct relevance for cancer and aging, even though they have seldom been applied (a few exceptions will be reviewed as well). So, the discussion here will barely scratch the surface of these models and concepts and explore how they can help in the concrete reality of living with, working with, and enabling the well-being of older persons with cancer so that they can live their lives with dignity, positive identity, and meaning.

The basis for this set of theories is the nature of aging already described. All recognize, and some especially emphasize, the social and, especially, physical losses as a person ages (especially in extreme old age). As already noted, these losses form a backdrop for every experience and choice that the individual makes. They may increasingly result in a poor "goodness of fit" between the person and his or her environmental demands [52]. They can constrict the range of choices and actions of the individual. As a result, the individual is likely to take steps to make alterations like those noted in that previous discussion. We should note that it is critically important to remember what was discussed previously about the dialectic interplay of gain and loss and the gain inherent in the losses themselves [25,31]. Losses can even *enable* gains, as when loss of a role such as retirement allows one to be less driven and focused on "success" so that one can finally focus on what one sees as important—family, leisure, intellectual or artistic pursuits, and so on, or when a narrowing of information processing attention can enable one to ignore the irrelevant or irritating and focus on the relevant and satisfying in life.

The SOC (selection–optimization–compensation) theory states that the nature of how individuals relate to their environments systematically changes as they age [31,61,62]:

1. They provide conceptual rationales and empirical evidence for the notion that older persons are more selective than younger ones; that is, they select *away* from many circumstances and situations, by not engaging in activities that may be too strenuous or peripheral to their needs and, alternatively, select *toward* activities that are more important to them.

2. Once they have done so, they take steps to optimize their ability to perform those activities, such as rehearsal of skills.

3. Finally, especially when their capabilities cannot meet the demands, they pursue compensatory actions; as already noted, this may be achieved by having other people provide for them (thus, choosing some dependency vs. independence in the service of meeting basic needs) or obtaining compensatory devices.

Brandstadter and colleagues add to this approach by directly addressing goals, on one hand and coping strategies on the other hand [63,64]. Goals are seen as critically important to living one's life in a satisfying and functional way. People use "tenacious goal pursuit" in their efforts to change the environment in such a way as to fulfill the goals; they actively try to assimilate the environment. As people age, some goals may no longer seem attainable. Thus, what they are likely to do is to either set different, perhaps less lofty, goals (similar to selection) or shift from a focus on goal pursuit to one of accommodating their own views and actions to fit with the environment and what it offers. As noted before, this may be advantageous toward mental health and well-being and a real gain that is embedded in the loss of ability to attain goals that are not as relevant to their lives as they might be. In a somewhat overlapping vein, Heckhausen and Schulz emphasize that persons throughout life have a need for what they term *primary control*—to have a direct effect on one's environment [40,65]. As the losses of aging accumulate and primary control becomes increasingly difficult, older persons turn toward secondary control, which is control over their reactions to the environmental circumstances rather than continued (presumably ineffectual) attempts to control the environment. All of these approaches place emphasis on the importance of emotional regulation in later life [40,66].

This set of approaches shares an intellectual connection, whether implicitly or explicitly, with Jung and other theorists who have emphasized that older persons approach the world in a more interior-focused way than when they were younger [64,65,67]. In other words, they are less *extraverted* (focusing on the external environment and how to manipulate it) and more *introverted* (focusing on their internal lives and feelings, as well as thinking about the "big picture" and how they fit into it). They are also consonant with Erikson's theory of lifespan development [42]. At the same time, they also fit with continuity theory, which emphasizes that as people age, they may feel threats to a sense of continuity in their past lives and yet feel an even greater need than earlier to have that sense of continuity of self as they contemplate the end of their lives and strive for the integrity (integrality) that Erikson, for example, identified as essential to being satisfied with the one life that one was given [68,69]. These theorists indicate that persons shift their coping strategies toward ones that can be in the service of maximizing continuity.

The socioemotional selectivity theory developed by Laura Carstensen and explicated and tested by her and her colleagues incorporates many ideas already reviewed, but it places much greater emphasis on the explicit recognition of time, in this case, time *left* in one's life; this is directly relevant to considering cancer at all ages and, especially, cancer and aging [70–72]. They describe similar strategic changes and adaptations as the other theorists; in fact, they stress in particular that older persons will select not only physical environments and tasks but also their relationships with others, increasingly on the basis of the degree to which those support regulation of emotion and maintenance of self. They contrast tasks and relationships focused on information and novelty with those focused on self-preservation and emotional satisfaction. The former are particularly relevant in circumstances that are future-oriented, since they support learning new skills and knowing new things, while the latter are much more present-oriented and concerned with conserving energy and maintaining the current status.

Carstensen and other researchers have shown that older persons' approaches to social cognitions, social choices, and relationship patterns generally and consistently shift toward present-oriented, emotionally satisfying choices and relationships [8,70–74]. For example, Ryff and her colleagues have found that older persons systematically shift from emphases on personal growth and purpose in life to positive relations and self-acceptance [8,74].

Again, while rooted in "loss" to some degree, this narrowing of focus is a gain in the sense of approaching emotion-laden events in a more personally satisfying, less stressful way. That, in itself, is important to understanding and dealing with cancer and aging—to know that older cancer survivors will often be more focused on emotion management and emotional support. But their emphasis on perceived time remaining rather than chronological age makes this particular theory even more important for clinical approaches to all cancer patients and survivors. They have postulated that when time remaining comes to the forefront, younger persons will perform like older ones; conversely, when older persons focus on a longer time perspective, they will perform more like typical younger ones. The expected shift of focus was seen in a few studies with those with cancer and other potentially terminal diseases [75,76]. The Pinquart et al. study, in particular, is very interesting. They found that younger survivors' approaches varied across time in relation to their sense of their cancer as life threatening, initially making the "elder shift" in relationships, but then returning to more youth-like patterns after treatment; and *then*, those who experienced a recurrence shifted again to the older pattern whereas those with a clean follow-up report did not. This appears to show that younger persons with cancer may, indeed, become "old" in terms of personality and patterns of orientation to the world in a way similar to the shift of already elderly participants who felt that having cancer put them into the elderly category for the first time [45].

Finally, in a similar vein, Costanzo et al. have specifically examined their optimal aging model in relation to long-term cancer survivors [77]. They found that cancer had long-term negative impacts on affect and aspects of mental health, with decreases in environmental mastery, positive relations with others, and self-acceptance, and yet also a considerable amount of maintenance of personal growth, autonomy, and spirituality. Furthermore, as we have noted before in relation to other studies, the effects were stronger for younger than older survivors.

23.7   LESSONS AND IMPLICATIONS FOR PROFESSIONALS

What lessons may be taken from this for those who provide care to older persons with cancer? In a very important sense, the dictum is the same as it is for *all* cancer patients and survivors—to meet each individual where he or she is psychologically and socially, to find out what that person's goals are (for treatment *and* for life), and then to enable her/him as best as possible to meet those goals. Obtaining both histories of experiences and goals and indications of current goals and satisfactions would enable providers to see into the world of the cancer survivor. That knowledge allows for a goodness of fit between what is provided and what is needed. One difference with aging, which can never be ignored, is the reality of physical and sometimes social losses that narrow the framework of the individual's life. But that is only a part of a story that includes both gains and losses throughout old age. Thus, with older cancer survivors, what the goals are, what the person can bring to those goals in terms of physical and social functioning and resources, and the broader contexts for those goals (one's social networks, e.g., or how healthcare is constructed) are all different from the experience of younger cancer survivors. Thus, what is needed from others, including healthcare providers, are all likely to be different because of what we have discussed—the passage of time through the lifespan, the structures of the lifecourse, the life experiences of the person, and even the amount of time that person sees on the horizon of the rest of her/his life. As a result, there are systematic differences between young and old cancer patients and survivors far beyond just their years or just their physical differences.

A different lesson to be drawn from lifespan development and lifecourse is equally important. Because of the nuances and idiosyncrasies of one's development through life, the role of cohort factors, and the importance of all the dynamic aspects of the context of the cancer experience, diversity is the rule, not the exception. Gerontologists describe how people become more different from each other, not more similar, as they age. Thus, every effort must be made to treat every newly diagnosed person, every patient in treatment, every person transitioning out of treatment, and every long term survivor as the individual she or he is.

23.8   CONCLUSIONS

Thus, what is essential is to ascertain that starting point related to treatment choices, how treatment effects will be responded to, and how interactions with caregivers, both formal and informal, will be sought out and framed. The theories and concepts reviewed can serve to help identify those starting points for each individual and to apply that identification to the goals of best practice of gerontology and of oncology.

Then one can enable and encourage the kinds of gains that we have reviewed while minimizing the negative impact of losses. At the same time, it is also important to avoid pressuring individuals toward "growth" or "involvement" beyond what fits with their orientation and their self-identity [78]. A final and important point is to recognize that even as advancing age interacts with complicated and serious health problems such as cancer and its treatment, most people *do* age quite well, and most older cancer survivors maintain high quality of life and have lives that are personally enriching and meaningful to self and also exert a positive influence on the well-being of other people.

REFERENCES

1. Jemal A, Siegel R, Xu J, Ward E. Cancer statistics 2010. *CA Cancer J Clin* 2010;**60**(5):277–300.
2. Yancik R, Ries LAG. Cancer in older persons: An international issue in an ageing world. *Semin Oncol* 2004;**31**:128–136.
3. Surveillance, Epidemiology, and End Results (SEER) Program. Prevalence database: *US Estimated Complete Prevalence Counts on 1/1/2004*, National Cancer Institute, DCCPS, Surveillance Research Program, Statistical Research and Applications Branch, (www.seer.cancer.gov; released 4/07, based on the 11/06 SEER data submission.)
4. Hunter CP, Johnson KA, Muss HB. *Cancer in the Elderly*, Marcel Dekker, New York, 2000.
5. Edwards BK, Howe HL, Ries LA, et al. Annual report to the nation on the status of cancer, 1973–1999, featuring implications of age and aging on U.S. cancer burden. *Cancer* 2002;**94**:2766–2792.
6. Hill RD. *Positive Aging*, Norton, New York, 2006.
7. Rowe JW, Kahn RL. *Successful Aging*, Dell, New York, 1999.
8. Ryff CD, Singer B. Contours of positive human health. *Psychol Inquiry* 1998;**9**:1–28.
9. Vaillant GE. *Aging Well*, Little, Brown, New York, 2003.
10. Lazarus RS, Lazarus BN. *Coping with Aging*, Oxford Univ. Press, New York, 2006.
11. Hewitt M, Rowland JH, Yancik R. Cancer survivors in the United States: age, health, and disability. *J Gerontol A Biol Sci Med Sci* 2003;**58**:82–91.
12. Institute of Medicine. *Cancer in Elderly People: Workshop Proceedings*, National Academies Press, Washington, DC, 2007.
13. Lichtman SM, Balducci L, Aapro M. Geriatric oncology: A field coming of age. *J Clin Oncol* 2007;**25**:1821–1823.
14. Balducci L. Cancer in the older person. *Generations* 2007;**30**:45–50.
15. Rowland JH, Yancik R. Cancer survivorship: The interface of aging, comorbidity, and quality care. *J Natl Cancer Inst* 2006;**98**:504–505.
16. Cohen H. Cancer survivorship and aging: A double whammy. *Lancet Oncol* 2006;**7**:882–883.
17. Deimling GT, Bowman KF, Sterns S, Wagner LJ, Kahana B. Cancer-related health worries and psychological distress among older adult, long term cancer survivors. *Psychooncology* 2006;**15**:306–320.
18. Nelson CJ, Weinberger MI, Balk E, Holland J, Breitbart W, Roth AJ. The chronology of distress, anxiety, and depression in older prostate cancer patients. *Oncologist* 2009;**14**:891–899.
19. Blank TO, Bellizzi KM. After prostate cancer: Predictors of well-being among long-term prostate cancer survivors. *Cancer* 2006;**106**:2128–2135.

20. Hinz A, Krauss O, Hauss JP, Hoeckel, M, Kortmann RD, Stolzenburg JU, Schwarz R. Anxiety and depression in cancer patients compared with the general population. *Eur J Cancer Care* 2010;**19**:522–529.

21. Schroevers MJ, Ranchor AV, Sanderman R. Role of age at the onset of cancer in relation to survivors' long-term adjustment: A controlled comparison over an eight-year period. *Psychooncology* 2004;**13**:740–752.

22. Elder GH. The life course and human development. In Lerner RM, ed. *Handbook of Child Psychology*. Vol. 1: *Theoretical Models of Human Development*, Wiley, New York, 1998, pp. 939–991.

23. Settersten RA. *Invitation to the Life Course: Toward a New Understanding of Later Life*, Baywood, Amityville, NY, 2002.

24. Lamb ME, Freund AM, Lerner RM. *Handbook of Life-Span Development*. Vol. 2: *Social and Emotional Development*, Wiley, New York, 2010.

25. Baltes PB, Lindenberger U, Staudinger UM. Lifespan theory in developmental psychology. In Damon W, Lerner RM, eds. *Handbook of Child Psychology*, Vol. 1, 6th ed., Wiley, New York, pp. 569–664.

26. Lerner RM. *Concepts and Theories of Human Development*, 3rd ed., Psychology Press, New York, 2001.

27. Rowland JH. Developmental stage and adaptation: Adult model. In Holland JC, Rowland JH, eds. *Handbook of Psycho-oncology*, Oxford Univ. Press, New York, 1989, pp. 25–45.

28. Ram N, Morelli S, Lindberg C, Carstensen LL. From static to dynamic: The ongoing dialectic about human development. In Schaie KW, Abeles RP, eds., *Social Structures and Aging Individuals: Continuing Challenges*, Springer, New York, 2008, pp. 115–130.

29. Riegel KF. *Foundations of Dialectical Psychology*, Academic Press, New York, 1979.

30. Cohen, LH. *Life Events and Psychological Functioning: Theoretical and Methodological Issues*, Sage, Beverly Hills, CA, 1988.

31. Baltes PB. Theoretical propositions of life-span developmental psychology: On the dynamics between growth and decline. *Devel Psychol* 1997;**23**:611–626.

32. Park CL, Lechner SC, Antoni MH, Stanton AL. *Medical Illness and Positive Life Change*, American Psychological Association, Washington, DC, 2008.

33. Park CL, Cohen LH, Murch R. Assessment and prediction of stress-related growth. *J Personality* 1996;**64**:71–105.

34. Tedeschi RG, Calhoun LG. *Trauma and Transformation: Growing in the Aftermath of Suffering*, Sage, Thousand Oaks, CA, 1995.

35. Updegraff JA, Taylor SE. From vulnerability to growth: Positive and negative effects of stressful life events. In Harvey JH, Miller D, eds. *Loss and Trauma: General and Close Relationship Perspectives*, Brunner-Routledge, Philadelphia, 2000, pp. 3–28.

36. Bellizzi KM, Blank TO. Understanding the dynamics of post-traumatic growth in breast cancer survivors. *Health Psychol* 2006;**25**:47–56.

37. Bower JF, Meyerowitz BE, Desmond KA, Bernaards CA, Rowland JH, Ganz PA. Perceptions of positive meaning and vulnerability following breast cancer: Predictors and outcomes among long-term breast cancer survivors. *Ann Behav Med* 2005;**29**:236–245.

38. Cordova MJ, Cunningham LC, Carlson CR, Andrykowski MA. Posttraumatic growth following breast cancer: A controlled comparison study. *Health Psychol* 2001;**20**:176–185.

39. Bellizzi KM, Miller MF, Arora NK, Rowland JH. Positive and negative life changes of cancer experienced by survivors of non-Hodgkin's lymphoma. *Ann Behav Med* 2007;**38**:188–199.

40. Heckhausen J. *Developmental Regulation in Adulthood*, Cambridge Univ. Press, New York, 1998.

41. McAdams DP, Olson BD. Personality development: Continuity and change over the life course. *Annu Rev Psychol* 2010;**61**:517–542.

42. Erikson E, Erikson J, Kivnick H. *Vital Involvement in Old Age*, Norton, New York, 1986.

43. Adler A. *What Life Should Mean to You*, Grossett & Dunlap, New York, 1931.

44. Schaie KW. A general model for the study of developmental problems. *Psychol Bull* 1965;**64**:92–107.

45. Esbensen BA, Swane CH, Hallberg IR, Thome B. Being given a cancer diagnosis in old age: A phenomenological study *Int J Nurs Stud* 2008;**45**:393–405.

46. Cohen H. The cancer aging interface: A research agenda. *J Clin Oncol* 2007;**25**:1945–1948.

47. Rao AV, Demark-Wahnefried W. The older cancer survivor. *Crit Rev Oncol Hematol* 2006;**60**:131–143.

48. Given CW, Given B, Azzouz F, Stommel M, Kozachik S. Comparison of changes in physical functioning of elderly patients with new diagnoses of cancer. *Med Care* 2000;**38**(5):482–493.

49. Repetto L, Comandini D, Mammoliti S. Life expectancy, co-morbidity and quality of life: The treatment equation in the older cancer patients. *Crit Rev Oncol Hematol* 2001;**37**:147–152.

50. Spirduso W, Francis K, MacRae P. *Physical Dimensions of Aging*, 2nd ed., Human Kinetics, Champaign, IL, 2005.

51. Whitbourne SK. *The Aging Individual: Physical and Psychological Perspectives*, 2nd ed., Springer, New York, 2002.

52. Lawton MP, Nahemow L. Ecology and the aging process. In Eisdorfer C, Lawton MP, eds. *Psychology of Adult Development and Aging*, American Psychological Association, Washington, DC, 1973, pp. 619–674.

53. Craik FIM, Salthouse TA. *Handbook of Aging and Cognition*, 2nd ed., Lawrence Erlbaum, Mahwah, NJ, 2000.

54. Park DC, Schwarz N. *Cognitive Aging: A Primer*, Taylor & Francis, Philadelphia, 2000.

55. Scheibe S, Kunzmann U, Baltes PB. Wisdom, life longings, and optimal development. In Blackburn JA, Dulmus CA, eds. *Handbook of Gerontology*, Wiley, New York, 2007, pp. 117–142.

56. Thomas LE, Eisenhandler SA. *Aging and the Religious Dimension*, Auburn House, Westport, CT, 1994.

57. Koenig HG. *Aging and God: Spiritual Pathways to Mental Health in Midlife and Later Years*, Haworth, New York, 1994.

58. Krause N. Religion and health in later life. In Birren JE, Warner KW, eds. *Handbook of the Psychology of Aging*, 6th ed., Elsevier, New York, 2006, pp. 499–518.

59. Eton DT, Lepore SJ. Prostate cancer and health-related quality of life: A review of the literature. *Psychooncology* 2002;**11**:307–326.

60. Institute of Medicine/National Research Council (IOM/NRC). *From Cancer Patient to Cancer Survivor: Lost in Transition*, National Academies Press, Washington, DC, 2006.

61. Baltes PB. On the incomplete architecture of human ontogeny: Selection, optimization, and compensation as a foundation for developmental theory. *Am Psychol* 1997;**52**:366–380.

62. Freund AM, Baltes PB. The orchestration of selection, optimization, and compensation: An action-theoretical conceptualization of a theory of developmental regulation. In Perrig WJ, Grob A, eds. *Control of Human Behavior, Mental Processes, and Consciousness*. Lawrence Erlbaum, Mahwah, NJ, 2000, pp. 35–58.

63. Brandstadter J, Renner G. Tenacious goal pursuit and flexible goal adjustment: Explication of age-related analysis of assimilative and accommodative strategies of coping. *J Personality Soc Psychol* 1990;**65**:58–67.

64. Brandstadter J. Adaptive resources in later life: Tenacious goal pursuit and flexible goal adjustment. In Csikszentmihalyi M, Csikszentmihalyi IS, eds. *A Life Worth Living: Contributions to Positive Psychology*, Oxford Univ. Press, New York, 2006, pp. 143–164.

65. Heckhausen J, Schulz R. Life-span theory of control. *Psychol Rev* 1995;102:284–304.

66. Hooker K, Choun S, Hall B. Personality and emotion in later life. In Cavanaugh JC, Cavanaugh CK, eds. *Aging in America*. Vol. 1: *Psychological Aspects*, Praeger, Santa Barbara, CA, 2010.

67. Jung CG. *Essential Jung*, Princeton Univ. Press, 1983.

68. Atchley RC. *Continuity and Adaptation in Aging*, Johns Hopkins Univ. Press, Baltimore, 2000.

69. Tobin, SS. *Preservation of Self in the Oldest Years*, Springer, New York, 1999.

70. Carstensen LL, Isaacowitz DM, Charles ST. Taking time seriously: A theory of socioemotional selectivity. *Am Psychol* 1999;54:165–181.

71. Carstensen LL, Fung HH, Charles ST. Socioemotional selectivity theory and the regulation of emotion in the second half of life. *Motiv Emotion* 2003;27:103–123.

72. Fung HH, Siu TM. Time, culture, and life-cycle changes of social goals. In Miller TW, ed. *Handbook of Stressful Transitions across the Lifespan*, Springer, New York, 2010, pp. 441–464.

73. Blanchard-Fields F. Age differences in everyday problem-solving effectiveness: Older adults select more effective strategies for interpersonal problems. *J Gerontol B Psychol Sci Soc Sci* 2007;62:61–4.

74. Ryff C D, Essex MJ. Psychological well-being in adulthood and old age. In Schaie K W, Lawton M P, eds., *Annual Review of Gerontology and Geriatrics*, Vol. 11. Springer, New York, 1992.

75. Kausar R, Akram M. Cognitive appraisal and coping of patients with terminal vs. nonterminal diseases. *J Behav Sci* 1999;9:13–28.

76. Pinquart M, Silbereisen RK. Socioemotional selectivity in cancer patients. *Psychol Aging* 2006;21:419–423.

77. Costanzo E, Ryff CD, Singer B. Psychosocial adjustment among cancer survivors: Findings from a national survey of health and well-being. *Health Psychol* 2009;28:147–156.

78. Holland J, Lewis S. *Human Side of Cancer: Living with Hope, Coping with Uncertainty*, HarperCollins, New York, 2000.

CHAPTER 24

Adaptation and Adjustment to Cancer in Later Life: A Conceptual Model

GARY T. DEIMLING

Department of Sociology, Case Western Reserve University, Cleveland, OH

BOAZ KAHANA

Department of Psychology, Cleveland State University, Cleveland, OH

KAREN BOWMAN

Department of Sociology, Case Western Reserve University, Cleveland, OH

24.1 INTRODUCTION

The title of this chapter, Adaptation and Adjustment to Cancer by Older Adults, begs the questions of what we mean by "adaptation" and "adjustment" to cancer and what are the key conceptual categories and measures that define adaptation and adjustment. To address this question, we propose a conceptual model that includes the factors that are most relevant to the adaptation and adjustment of older adults who have been diagnosed with and treated for this disease. This conceptual model is then used to organize a review of research findings from both the oncology and aging literatures. We also integrate research findings from our own National Cancer Institute study on the quality of life of older-adult, long-term cancer survivors.

24.2 ADJUSTMENT AND ADAPTATION TO CANCER

24.2.1 Definition

Although there is no generally accepted distinction of what constitutes adjustment as opposed to adaptation to cancer, adjustment is typically conceptualized and measured as an outcome of the cancer experience. In contrast, adaptations often are represented by other factors or the process that influence these outcomes. For example early research by Andrykowski and colleagues [1] on life after cancer operationalized adjustment in terms of outcome measures such as psychological distress, life outlook, interpersonal

Cancer and Aging Handbook: Research and Practice, First Edition. Edited by Keith M. Bellizzi and Margot A. Gosney.
© 2012 Wiley-Blackwell. Published 2012 by John Wiley & Sons, Inc.

relationships, and spiritual and religious satisfaction. They note that cancer is "a traumatic event.... with the potential to produce long-lasting changes of both a positive as well as negative nature" [2, p. 827]. Much of the research that is reviewed throughout this chapter takes a similar multidimensional approach to adjustment and treats it as an outcome of cancer-related stressors. In most research adjustment is treated as a *static outcome*, defined and/or measured at one point in time in the cancer experience. Brennan [2] notes, however, that the term adjustment "suggests the completion of change from one state to another, yet research has often focused on adjustment as were merely the endpoint of coping with the global threat of cancer rather than the processes of change occurring within the individual" [2, p. 1]. This suggests that adjustment is a better operationalized as the change over time in individuals who have been diagnosed and treated for cancer. An example of this approach is represented in research by Hassey-Dow and Lafferty [3]. That study operationalized adjustment outcomes as changes over time in the overall health, psychological adjustment, and social and sexual adjustment. Deshields et al. [4] presents emotional adjustment in terms of standard measures of psychological distress, with better adjustment represented by lower levels of distress. However, as in much of the longitudinal research, data on the average change for the sample over time are reported, not the magnitude of change for individuals. Also similar to most research, change is examined from some point during the illness process (e.g., from the end of treatment) to one or more points in time after the end of treatment.

Perhaps the most desirable approach to examining adjustment to cancer is represented by Tartaro and colleagues [5], who use a *prospective, longitudinal design* collecting data from a point in time prior to diagnosis to later points in time. Similar to other research, their study conceptualizes adjustment outcomes to include tradition distress outcome measures such as depression, anxiety, and social impairment.

24.2.2   Adaptation in Contrast to Adjustment

In contrast to adjustment, which is based on psycho-social quality of life outcomes, adaptation focuses on the factors and processes that influence these outcomes. For example, Dow and Lafferty [3] treated "adaptation" as distinct from "adjustment" by viewing factors such as the meaning of cancer, worry about the future, and changes in personal relationships as elements of adaptation. Treating adaptation as a process that mediates or moderates the impact of illness stressors on adjustment outcomes is an outgrowth of the stress–coping paradigm in which stressors either do or do not culminate in distress outcomes depending on the adaptation that takes place. The model proposed later in this chapter provides a template based on this orientation toward adaptation.

24.3   A CONCEPTUAL MODEL OF ADJUSTMENT TO CANCER

In order to structure the discussion of the impact of cancer on older adults, a conceptual model of the cancer adaptation/adjustment process is proposed that incorporates important conceptual categories specifically relevant to later life. This model, based on the broader stress and coping paradigm, takes a relative inclusive approach considering an array of cancer and other personal and health factors relevant for older adults that may engender the need for adaptation, that is, the *stressor factors*. It also includes a range of factors that may mediate and/or moderate the impact of cancer and other life stressors as they may contribute to quality of life outcomes. These are viewed as aspects of the adaptation process.

The range of quality of life outcomes that reflect adjustment to cancer is similarly broad with outcomes ranging from those that reflect physical health and functioning, as well as mental or emotional health, and social and spiritual well-being. The model also takes a lifecourse approach that considers factors that affect and define adjustment to cancer that are relevant from midlife through the earlier phases of older adulthood [the "young old" (elderly)] into the later years of life [the "old old" (elderly)]. The model presented is an elaboration of the model that was originally develop to guide our research at the Quality of Life-After Cancer (QOL-AC) project (R01-CA-798975; see also Deimling and Kahana [6], Principal Investigators 1998–2003; Deimling et al. [7], Principal Investigators 2003–2012), which was conducted at Case Western Reserve University/University Hospitals of Cleveland.

Our study employed a longitudinal survey research design (six waves of in-person interviews over a 12-year period) to examine a broad range of quality-of-life (QOF) outcomes among a sample of 472 older adult (over age 60), long-term ($\geq$5 years since diagnosis) selected randomly from among tumor registry patients who met the sample design criteria. The sample included survivors of the three most common survivable cancers among older adults: breast, colorectal, and prostate cancer. The original sample design called for inclusion of equal numbers of men and women in the gender-specific and gender-common cancers and oversampled African-Americans who ultimately constituted approximately 40% of the sample.

24.3.1 Application of the Stress–Coping Paradigm

The conceptual orientation that overlays the model is derived from the traditional stress–coping paradigm, primarily the work of Lazarus and Folkman [8] and Pearlin [9]. The stress–coping paradigm has a long history in the study of health. In its most general form, this paradigm identifies significant life events as having the potential to be both acute and chronic stressors. Applied to cancer survivorship, specific cancer-related and noncancer stressors are viewed as potentially having direct and/or indirect effects on a range of adjustment outcomes, operationalized in this research as dimensions of QOL. For example, at the time of cancer occurrence, it is clear that the effects of treatments such as surgery, radiation, and chemotherapy are acute stressors along with the obvious threat of loss of life. However, cancer also is a chronic stressor because the side effects of the illness and treatment are often long-term, and new health problems resulting from the disease or treatment that are referred to as *late effects* may emerge even decades after treatment. These, along with the continuing threat to life represented by recurrence or a new cancer, may continue throughout the remainder of life. Thus the stress paradigm, which incorporates both acute and chronic stressors, is a useful approach to studying the adjustment to cancer. Prior research by Ensel and Lin [10] demonstrated the usefulness of this approach in the study of long-term health outcomes, documenting the power of "distal" stressors on current health and indicating the vulnerability of older adults to stressors that occurred in the more distant as well as the recent past.

However, the stress paradigm does not assume that all stressors, health-related or others, will result in negative distress outcomes. In fact, it posits that coping and other resources can buffer or ameliorate the impact of serious stressors. There are numerous factors such as personal dispositions, proactive behaviors, and social resources that can moderate the effects of the significant acute and chronic stressors that cancer and its treatment represent. Thoits [11] points out that individuals can be "activists on behalf of their own well-being ... and purposefully engage in problem solving, and/or actively reconstructing the meaning of their life experiences in order to sustain their sense of self worth and alleviate anxiety and tension" [11, p. 58]. She asserts that traumas in earlier life may enhance both physical and emotional well-being not so much by inoculating them from stress, but by motivating them to make personal changes. Research on cancer survivors has begun to take this approach [2], and Tedeschi and Calhoun [12] frame the positive outcomes of traumatic stress in terms of phenomena such as personal strengths, new possibilities, and appreciation of life. All of these are viewed as important aspects of the adaptation process.

24.3.2 The Cancer Survivorship Model

The cancer survivorship (i.e., adaptation/adjustment) model presented in Figure 24.1 reflects the complexity and range of factors that are likely to culminate in either the successful or unsuccessful adaptation of older adults to being diagnosed with and

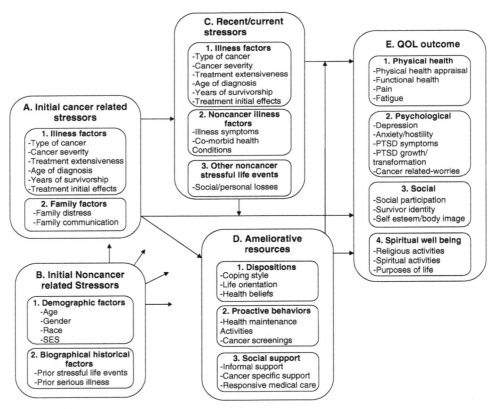

Figure 24.1 The cancer survivorship model: (a) initial cancer-related stressors; (b) initial non-cancer-related stressors; (c) recent/current stressors; (d) ameliorative resources; (e) QOL outcomes.

treated for cancer. The model comprises five categories of factors: (a) initial cancer-related stressors, (b) initial (prior) non-cancer-related stressors, (c) recent/current stressors, (d) ameliorative resources, and (e) quality-of-life outcomes. Categories (a)–(d) are viewed as having direct and/or indirect effects on a range of outcomes, (e). Factors listed in categories (c) and (d) are also viewed as factors that have the potential to ameliorate or exacerbate the effects of stressors and are treated as moderators in the model. In the sections that follow the model is unpacked to explain how each category of factors is involved in the adjustment challenges that older adults face in response to cancer and it treatment into long-term survivorship. Given the space limitations of this chapter, not all of the factors identified in the model will be discussed. We have selected those factors for which there is the most existing research and/or those that have been the focus of our own research.

24.4 STRESSORS

24.4.1 Initial/Past Cancer-Related Stressors

The first group of factors, (a) identifies the cancer-related stressors that may drive the adaptation process and have either direct or indirect effects on adjustment outcomes, (e). They include characteristics of the disease such as the specific type of cancer, the severity of disease at diagnosis (stage), as well as the characteristics of treatment including the type, and extensiveness of therapies employed (surgery, radiation, chemotherapy, hormone therapy, etc.). Two chronological factors are also included: age at diagnosis and the number of years of survivorship. These two factors are important in that they reflect the lifecourse stage in which the adaptation process began and the passage of time during which the process continued.

Ramsey and colleagues [13] found that the type of cancer can differentiate the functional problems experienced by survivors, and the psychosocial oncology literature links severity of disease to long-term adjustment of cancer survivors. For example, Ell and colleagues [14], in a study of breast, colorectal, and lung cancer survivors, most of whom were older adults, found that the physical symptoms experienced, (a surrogate measure of disease severity and prognosis) were associated with psychological adjustment problems. While our own research has not found differences by cancer type after controlling for gender, we did find that the cancer symptoms experienced during treatment continue to be related to psychological distress among older adult survivors many years later [15]. We also found that type of treatment, specifically, having received chemotherapy, is associated with greater depression among the long-term survivors in our study.

Since the 1990s there has been an increasing recognition of the family relevant issues that affect adjustment to cancer. Like any serious illnesses, especially those that occur in later life, cancer happens to families. In fact, family members have been referred to as "secondary survivors" who are profoundly affected by the diagnosis of cancer in a loved one [16]. For example, Benyamini and colleagues [17] found that those close to the survivor, including family members, experience a range of distress outcomes, and that these are longlasting effects.

Our research on older adult survivors and family members [18] has indicated that survivors' reports of family distress and communication problems during illness are significant predictors of later adjustment problems among survivors. That analysis also documented that cancer stage at diagnosis is a predictor of the distress that family members experience. This suggests that family members may interpret cancer stage as an indicator of prognosis or potential survival, with later stage cancer increasing the associated distress.

24.4.2   Prior Non-Cancer-Related Stressors

The second category (Fig. 24.1b) recognizes that individuals who have experienced cancer are likely to have also experienced other noncancer life stressors. Pearlin's [9] sociological formulation of the general stress model alerts us to the impact that an individual's sociodemographic characteristics may have as potential chronic stressors. For example, being older, female, a member of a racial or ethnic minority, or having less education or lower income may confer another form of jeopardy that survivors face. Older cohorts of adults, particularly older minority individuals, are likely to have less education along with lower incomes, which provide them with fewer potential financial or medical resources, which, in turn, might impact the adjustment process. Further, women and minorities are also to have more comorbidities and related functional deficit [19], which may play a role as additional stressors.

Chronological age, both during the illness and during the survivorship period, is also an important factor. In research comparing younger and older cancer patients/survivors, age was found to be associated with poorer physical functioning and global QOL, but better emotional and social functioning [20]. With regard to education, Clough-Gorr and colleagues [21] found that less educated individuals reported greater decline in mental health over a 5-year period after a cancer diagnosis. In our own research, we also found that older age, rather than being a psychosocial stressor, was associated with lower levels of anxiety and hostility [15], and lower levels of stress appraisal [22]. However, greater education was associated with a higher level of stress appraisal and cancer worry. With regard to race, our research found that race (being African-American) was associated with less depression, anxiety, and cancer worry [23]; lower likelihood of viewing cancer as a stressful experience [22]; but poorer physical functioning [19].

Also particularly important for older adults are prior serious stressful life events that may add to the vulnerability of older adult patients and survivors. The stress paradigm suggests that prior or chronic stressors such as these may interact with acute, current stressors [24] such as continuing cancer-related factors. In our research [15] on older adult survivors, nearly three-fourths of the respondents had experienced one or more traumatic life events earlier in their lives. The most prominent was the death of a loved one due to accident, homicide, or suicide, but other nonnormative stressors such as incarceration of a family member were also mentioned. Our analysis also found that noncancer stressful life events were significantly correlated with greater anxiety, hostility, and the posttraumatic stress disorder (PTSD) subscales for hyperarousal, and avoidance among survivors.

24.4.3   Recent/Current Stressors and Ameliorative Resource

The third and fourth components (Fig. 24.1c,d) of the model include factors that may either exacerbate or ameliorate the impact of cancer-relevant and life stressors. The factors listed in group (c) alert us to the importance that continuing cancer/treatment-related symptoms (e.g., edema, weakness, loss of function, fatigue, pain, scarring) may have and how they combine with other non-cancer-related illness symptoms and co-morbid health conditions to increase the vulnerability of survivors as they age. Our own research [15] also found that continuing cancer or treatment-related symptoms are significant predictors of greater hostility, depression and the hyperarousal dimension of PTSD. We also found these symptoms to be related to more stressful appraisals of the cancer experience by survivors [22].

Of potential importance are recurrences of the initial cancer and new cancers. With increasing age the likelihood of a second cancer also increases [25]. In our own research on older adult long-term survivors, approximately 25% of respondents have experienced a second or third cancer. Additionally, older adults are likely to experience a broad range of increasing illness symptoms, any of which may represent a serious stressor, especially if symptoms are similar to cancer symptoms previously experienced.

The second important category of current stressors are those represented by the comorbid conditions and their symptoms that are likely among older adults but are not directly related to cancer or its treatment. It is this group of stressors that are likely to increase as the survivor ages, and have the potential to amplify the impact of cancer on QOL [26–28]. Moreover, the impact of these chronic health stressors may be further exacerbated by other personal/social losses common in later life. In research specifically on older adults, Andersen and colleagues [29] point to the importance of other comorbid health conditions as exacerbating the impact of cancer in older adults. Our research on older long-term survivors has shown that comorbidities and illness symptoms not attribute to cancer by survivors are the two most powerful predictors of functional difficulties, with nearly twice the impact that cancer-related factors have on this outcome [19]. They are also significant predictors of pain and weakness [30].

The model also suggests that other life stressors not linked to health may have an impact on adjustment to cancer and/or may amplify the effect of cancer and other health factors. With increasing age, other stressful life events are likely to accumulate, such as the recent death of a spouse or lifelong friends, illnesses among adult children and grandchildren, or divorce among their adult children. Our research [15] documents the role that current, non-cancer-related life events have as significant predictors of psychological distress, including anxiety, indicating the need to control for the effects of these noncancer factors when examining the impact of cancer on older adults adjustment.

The factors listed in Figure 24.1d are those that may ameliorate the impact of cancer and noncancer stressors, past and recent. These factors, particularly coping, play a prominent role in the cancer literature, and our conceptualization considers these factors as representing the *adaptation* elements of the model. Included in this category are personal dispositions such as coping style, health beliefs, life orientations such as optimism, and proactive behaviors such as health maintenance activities. Social support can include informal support from family, friends, and other cancer survivors, and the support provided by responsive medical care and cancer-specific services. As portrayed in the model, these resources may have direct effects on QOL outcomes or, alternatively, may moderate the impact of cancer-linked and non-cancer-linked stressors common among older adults.

Dunkel-Schetter and colleagues [31], in some of the early research on coping with cancer, found that the most prominent form of coping among cancer patients was distancing. Seeking support, positive focus, and cognitive escape-avoidance were the next most frequently employed coping strategies, which were used about equally, while behavioral escape–avoidance was the least used strategy. Using a similar conceptualization, Hack and Degner [32] found that acceptance/resignation at baseline (≤6 months after diagnosis) was associated with depression and anxiety three years later. McCaul and his colleagues [33] examined coping and adjustment to breast cancer in older women soon after diagnosis and found that the most Frequently utilized coping strategy at both baseline and follow-up was active behavioral coping, followed by active cognitive coping. The coping strategy used least was avoidance coping. Furthermore, Moorey and colleagues [34] demonstrated that coping with cancer varies by illness severity, with earlier-stage cancer patients in treatment reporting higher levels of fighting spirit and lower levels of helplessness, anxious preoccupation, and fatalism when compared with more advanced stage patients.

With regard to age, Aldwin and colleagues [35] found that in the general population the use of all types of coping decreases with advancing age from early midlife through the "old-old" (elderly) (85+). Significant declines were noted for instrumental action, social support, cognitive reframing, and interpersonal hostile coping. They suggest that part of the decline seen among the oldest adults is that they may have a more matter-of-fact approach to illness and physical limitations. They also indicate that the oldest adults are more likely to accept conditions that are beyond their control compared those who are younger.

Our research on long-term cancer survivors [23,36] found that denial is not a prominent form of coping among older adults. We also found planning and acceptance to be the most common coping strategies among these survivors. Moreover, the older the survivors in our sample, the less likely they were to use planning, denial, venting, or seeking social support. Regarding the relationship between coping and distress, in our research denial was found to be associated with greater anxiety and depression. Survivors who used denial as a coping strategy also continued to worry more about cancer.

Research has also shown that coping styles vary according to whether an individual has an optimistic or pessimistic life orientation. For example, Schou and colleagues [37] found that dispositional optimism is significantly positively correlated with "fighting spirit" and negatively associated with hopelessness. Our research [23], also documented the important role that optimism plays as a predictor being associated with lower levels of anxiety, depression, and cancer-related worry. This replicates the previous findings of Carver and colleagues [38]. These results demonstrate the importance of controlling for the effects of personal/dispositional characteristics in the analysis of the stressor–distress relationship and considering these factors as part of the adaptation process.

24.5 QUALITY-OF-LIFE OUTCOMES AS INDICATORS OF ADJUSTMENT TO CANCER

The last conceptual category in our model (Fig. 24.1e) displays a broad range of *quality-of-life (QOL) outcomes*. It is this category that most directly operationalizes adjustment to cancer. Included are such diverse QOL aspects as health outcomes (long-term and late health effects, the presence of pain, fatigue, and functional difficulties), psychological outcomes (traditional measures of distress, PTSD and posttraumatic growth), and aspects of social life such as social participation, identity, and spirituality. These conceptual categories, while not exhaustive, reflective the breadth of the literature on adjustment to cancer. An extensive literature documents that many cancer patients and survivors experience diminished quality of life from the physical health problems, psychological distress, and social life disruption that can be associated with cancer (see Bloom [39] for a comprehensive review).

24.5.1 Physical Health

The outcome with perhaps the most direct link to cancer is physical health QOL. With long-term survival of many cancers becoming the norm, there has been a shift in focus on research since the mid-1990s from the outcome of treatment in terms of survival/death to the health legacy of the disease itself and the treatment that made survival possible [39]. This refocuses our emphasis from survival to survivorship and directs us to examine the ways that cancer and/or its treatment produce or complicate the treatment of other later life illnesses. The long-term health effects of cancer range from those that minimally impact activities of daily living to those that may impair major organ systems. The cancer literature shows that effects such as decreased general functioning may persist for up to 20 years [40]. Looking at the most common survivable cancers among older adults research on breast, prostate, and colorectal cancer is instructive. Among breast cancer survivors lymphedema and shoulder morbidity are typical late effects [41] and may progress in prevalence and severity over time [42]. Prostate cancer survivors report that late effects of radiation range from difficulty or frequency of urinating to diarrhea [43] and rectal complications [44]. For men treated for this form of cancer, urinary problems can continue well into the second decade after treatment [45] and represent a lifelong risk [46]. Among colorectal cancer survivors, functional limitations persisted regardless of cancer stage or duration of time since diagnosis [13].

With regard to age, King and colleagues [47] in a study of breast cancer patients reported worse physical functioning among older compared to younger patients. Sweeney and colleagues [48], comparing older female survivors with a range of cancers with similarly aged individuals with no history of cancer, found survivors to have more functional limitations. Ganz and colleagues [49] found older breast cancer survivors to demonstrate poorer health outcomes compared to younger survivors. Finally, in a population-based sample of survivors with a range of cancers, Keating and colleagues [50] found that older adult survivors reported worse physical health than did similarly aged participants in their study who did not have a history of cancer.

In our research [51], we found that functional difficulties among cancer survivors increased with advancing age, similar to age-related declines shown in the general population. Importantly, we also found that initial and continuing cancer-related factors are statistically significant predictors of functioning decades after diagnosis. These cancer-related factors include specific types of treatment such as radiation and chemotherapy. We also found that stage at diagnosis, a surrogate measure for disease severity and continuing cancer-related symptoms, to be important predictors of functional difficulties. Taken together, these cancer factors were found to explain significant variation in functioning over and above what is explained by demographic factors, comorbidities, and non-cancer-related symptoms.

Pain and fatigue are also likely to be ongoing issue for cancer patients/survivors and have special significance for older adults, who, because of age-related comorbidities such as arthritis and cardio-pulmonary problems, are already at risk. Research has documented that pain is one of cancer's most frequent and problematic symptoms and is often underreported and undertreated among older and minority patients [52] and that it does not dissipate over time [13].

While the persistence of pain among survivors is problematic in its own right, if that pain affects broader physical functioning, its impact on quality of life may be even greater. Bosompra and colleagues [53] found that pain is an important part of the "disablement process" among survivors. While they generally found pain intensity and frequency levels to be low, both were predictors of functional status. Our research [30] found that older adult cancer survivors do experience pain, and to a lesser extent they report weakness and a lack of energy and that these are associated with more functional difficulties. However, in our analysis it was also clear that health problems and symptoms unrelated to cancer explain a major portion of the pain and weakness that older long-term survivors report and that the cancer–pain link may diminish with the passage of time.

In terms of fatigue, research has revealed that chronic fatigue can be over twice as high among cancer survivors compared to the general population and that its presence increases with advancing age [54]. Among breast cancer survivors fatigue was reported 3 times as frequently as in a matched comparison sample [55]. Other research has found that fatigue was present in over three-fourths of cancer patients and that its severity did not decrease over time [56]. Importantly, Mast [57] found that low to moderate levels of fatigue that persisted were also related to comorbidities that are typically greater among older adult cohorts. In our own research, weakness and energy level, two factors related to fatigue were prominent among older adult survivors [23]. While the independent effect of age was not significantly related to weakness, age was a significant predictor of energy level. The data further indicated that the key factors predicting weakness and energy level were the comorbidities and noncancer symptoms that survivors reported.

24.5.2   Psychological or Emotional Health

A second category of QOL outcomes are the psychological distress outcomes. These are suggested by the general stress paradigm and also have been extensively examined in the psycho-oncology literature. They include a broad range of general mental health outcomes such as depression and anxiety along with the more extreme responses to stress such as posttraumatic stress disorder (PTSD). Beyond these more general distress outcomes, there has been a more recent increase in attention to cancer specific outcomes such as cancer-related health worries.

In terms of general psychosocial outcomes, early research by Cella and Tross [58] identified the range of psychological late effects, including general anxiety, avoidance, and death anxiety. Other research has found reduced emotional QOL in long-term survivors [59]. Importantly, Thomas and colleagues [60] noted that anxiety rates among long-term survivors do not differ greatly from those of patients with active disease, suggesting that time does not diminish these threats to QOL.

Specific to aging and cancer, Zabora and colleagues [61] found clinical levels of distress in about one-third of breast, prostate, and colon cancer survivors, and Ganz and colleagues [49] found older survivors reporting poorer psychosocial QOL compared to younger survivors. This is similar to earlier research by Vinokur and colleagues revealing that those over age 60 reported lower levels of emotional well-being compared to those younger survivors during the period shortly after treatmen [62]. In contrast, King and colleagues [47] found that older patients reported better socioemotional functioning when compared to younger breast cancer patients soon after treatment. Comparing both younger and older cancer survivors to those similarly aged individuals who have not had cancer, both Hewitt and colleagues [63] and Arndt [64] found less difference between older adults than between younger adults. In our own research on older adults, increasing age within this group was found to be associated with lower levels of anxiety and hostility, although unrelated to depression or PTSD symptoms [15]. Finally, in terms of change over time, Clough-Gorr et al. [21] found that among older adults breast cancer survivors' mental health did not change over the 5-year period after diagnosis, which is consistent with our findings in relative stability over time [30].

Looking specifically at depression, an important QOL outcome for older adults, research generally confirms that depression is common among cancer patients [65] and higher than in the general population [66]. In our own research on older adult survivors [23], approximately 24% of our sample scored above the cutoff for clinical levels of depression (scores of ≥ 16 on the CES-D). This is substantially higher than rates of clinical depression in the general population over age 65, which range from 8% to 17% [67]. Strommel and colleagues [68] found that depression is predicted by a number of cancer factors such as cancer site and stage, as well as age-related factors such as comorbidities, and physical functioning. In our research [15,23] significant predictors of depression among older adult long-term survivors included having received chemotherapy and the persistence of cancer-linked symptoms.

Psychosocial oncology has included the extreme or traumatic stress framework for a number of years [69,70]. Andrykowski and colleagues [71] found that PTSD symptoms did not decline in the year following breast cancer treatment. Smith and colleagues [72,73] noted that this type of symptom can be reactivated by the anniversary of the cancer treatment events, visits to the physician or hospital or fatigue. They also documented that presence of nonpathological but "unacceptable" levels of PTSD-like symptoms that often occur as survivors approach the anniversary of the completion of treatment. Specifically with regard to older adults, in our own research [15] very few long-term survivors reached the criterion for a clinical diagnosis of PTSD. However, subclinical levels of PTSD symptoms were found to be correlated with depression and anxiety. However, they did not appear to either increase or decrease with advancing age.

Looking at the other side of the impact of trauma, the psychooncology literature has more recently begun to look at the positive mental health outcome of cancer survivorship such as the possibility of post-traumatic growth [12] and an interest in identity formation in terms of posttraumatic transformation is also emerging [74] Underlying alternative orientations to psychological sequelae of cancer is the recognition that trauma brings about significant changes in the self [75] that may involve changes in life outlook resulting from efforts to integrate suffering into a renewed self-understanding [76]. Our research [74] with older survivors has found that the younger survivors within this group reported altered decision-making as a form of posttraumatic transformation.

Another QOL outcome that has become prominent is cancer-related worry. After treatment, concerns about recurrence are likely to replace these fears [77], along with the distress associated with continued testing and monitoring [78,79]. With the passage of time and normal aging, worries about recurrence may be reduced to some degree while concerns about another cancer may increase [80]. Also with increasing age, older adults are likely to experience a broad range of illness symptoms that could be perceived as serious threats, especially if they are similar to cancer symptoms previously experienced [17,81]. Thus, for older survivors, continuing cancer-related fears/worries/concerns may replace stressors that they previously experienced related to diagnosis, treatment and their survival prognosis. In our own research [23], over half of these long-term survivors continued to report fears of recurrence and concerns that the symptoms they are experiencing may represent a recurrence or new cancer. We found that these concerns were linked to depression and anxiety. However, with this group of older adults, age was not significantly associated with any of the distress outcomes.

24.5.3 Social Quality of Life

The model also proposes that cancer can affect the *social QOL* of older adult survivors in as much as impaired physical functioning may interfere with the survivor's ability to participate in meaningful social activities [82]. Both the gerontological [83,84] and oncology literatures [85] document the important link between functional decline and social activity restrictions in older adults, and these have been found to increase with advancing age. Other research with cancer survivors has shown that deficits in physical functioning can lead to dependence on others, which may affect their sense of autonomy, independence, and feelings of helplessness [86]. These feelings may, in turn, translate into changes in role functioning. Importantly, Ferrell and colleagues [87,88] found a relatively strong association between participation restrictions and anxiety, depression, and role functioning. In our research with older survivors [82], advancing age had an indirect effect on social participation restrictions through functional difficulties.

Other aspects of social QOL proposed in the model are those linked to the individual's social identity. Cancer is one form of life-threatening illness that has the potential to alter the salience of specific identities, and replace primary identities with those related to the illness [75]. Giles and Johnston [89], recognizing the potential of cancer to impact core identities, indicate that the loss of identity experienced by cancer survivors may be similar to that of dementia, another illness common to later life.

One way that sex-specific cancers common among older adults, such as prostate and breast cancer, can affect core elements of the self is through gender identity. Gray and colleagues [90] note that for men, prostate cancer "challenges the way they experience their masculinity." Thorne and Murray [91] point out that women diagnosed with breast cancer are presented with "a confusing array of ideologies," and that the resulting impact on the gender-related social construction of this disease may impact how they make decisions about treatment options.

Alternatively, cancer can be viewed as an opportunity for personal growth, and improved well-being and can motivate reintegration of the self or self-transformation as noted earlier. Zebrack [92] provides a quote from a survivor who states that "for a long time now, maybe four or five years, cancer has felt like it's been part of a quilt . . . one of those patches is cancer," [92, p. 238]. This comment suggests that with the passage of time and normal aging, the cancer experience can be integrated into larger life experiences. In our research [23] on identity and survivorship, we found that most older survivors view being a survivor as an important part of who they are and do not see themselves as being a "victim" or "less whole" as a result of cancer. Further, they are not overly concerned about how others view them as a result of having cancer.

It appears that, at least for older adults, cancer has lost much of its stigma and may in fact be normative given the likelihood that their age peers have experienced this disease.

The last category of QOL outcomes in our model is one proposed by Ferrell [87,88] in their multi-dimensional model of adjustment to cancer, *spiritual well-being*. Brady and colleagues [93] found support for the inclusion of spirituality as a QOL measure in psychooncology, and Carver and colleagues [38] found the use of religion to be one of the most prominent adaptation strategies among cancer survivors. Visser and colleagues [94] note that changes in self-image, relationship changes, and uncertainty that are part of the cancer experience may "threaten an individuals sense of meaning to life" [94, p. 565] and that spirituality is part of a search for connectedness and meaning.

Many of the studies of spirituality or religion/religiosity examine their relationships to what are referred to in our model as *stressors* and/or *QOL outcomes* [95]. Research has consistently shown that spirituality and/or religiosity are associated with lower levels of psychological distress, and that this relationship persists when the effects of sociodemographic and cancer/illness factors are controlled [96].

In our unpublished analyses we found that 54% of older survivors considered themselves to be religious or very religious and 30% indicated that their religiosity increased after having had cancer. However, neither of these factors was found to be associated with any of the cancer characteristics such as extensiveness of treatment, stage at diagnosis, or number of years since diagnosis. Nor was either of these religiosity measures correlated with psychosocial outcomes such as anxiety, depression, cancer-related worry, or life satisfaction among our older adult survivors. However, being female or being African-American was correlated with religiosity.

It is also possible that religiosity may have a moderating influence on the relationship between cancer stressors and distress outcomes. In terms of our model, taking this approach to religiosity would place it in the category of an ameliorative resource, similar to coping, and as such part of the adaptation process. Our future research we plan to examine the possibility of these more complex relationships.

24.6 SUMMARY AND IMPLICATIONS FOR FUTURE RESEARCH

The conceptual model proposed in this chapter attempts to integrate the many approaches to understanding the adaptation and adjustment to cancer that have emerged since the 1980s. During this period there has been an exponential growth in research on life after a diagnosis of cancer. In many ways, the impact of cancer on the individual and that person's family is universal and not necessarily age-linked. However, in many other ways older adults demonstrate either increased vulnerability or greater resilience to this illness, suggesting that these may be two sides of the same coin.

Looking first at the vulnerability side of the coin, it is clear that older adults experience greater vulnerability because they often have significantly more comorbidities. These comorbidities bring with them additional illness symptoms and functional challenges that add to the continuing cancer-linked symptoms and functional difficulties. This is especially true for women and minorities such as African-Americans. Older adults may also experience symptoms that are not readily ascribed to one or more comorbidities and thus may be interpreted as either a cancer recurrence or the onset of a new cancer. This is even more problematic for the oldest survivors who have less formal education and, therefore, perhaps a less sophisticated understanding of illness symptoms. Older adults may also have less inclination to ask their healthcare practitioners questions about these symptoms. All of these issues translate into greater risks to older adults' physical health QOL compared to younger cohorts.

Looking at the resilience side of the coin, many of the studies of psychological and emotional well-being QOL reviewed above suggest that older adults are not more disadvantaged. The research presented here and a more extensive review provided in Avis and Deimling [97] indicate that older adults, compared to younger adults, or those relatively older within the group of older adults do not report higher levels of distress outcomes such as anxiety and cancer worry. The findings for depression are mixed, with some studies showing that older cohorts may be at greater risk in terms of this threat to QOL. However, this may not be due to cancer but rather to increases in depression that are associated with other aspects of aging such as increased comorbidities, functional decline, and social activity limitations.

In terms of the adaptation process, the research on coping suggests that older adults are likely to employ specific forms of coping that are associated with better adjustment outcomes, such as planning and acceptance, and that these are linked to lower levels of distress and may be a source of greater resilience. However, there is evidence that coping overall may decline with age. Older adults also report higher levels of religiosity or spirituality, which also may be a moderating resource.

What complicates our understanding of the role that age or aging has on the adaptation process and adjustment to cancer is the fact that most research does not report age differences in general or age differences within the cohort of older adults studied. Yet, much of the research on QOL after cancer is conducted with breast, colorectal, and prostate cancer survivors, many of whom are older adults.

What we have not seen in research is an approach that treats age or membership in specific age cohorts as either a moderating factor between cancer stressors and distress outcomes. In fact, we have not conceptualized it in our model as a moderator, but rather as a factor that directly impacts other factors in the model. Future research and conceptual modeling should consider this approach, and we plan to conduct this type of analysis in the near future.

Another factor that makes it difficult to develop generalizations about the impact of age or aging on adjustment to cancer is the fact that most studies lack a prospective longitudinal design and typically do not provide either a noncancer comparison (control) group, or a younger cohort for age comparison [97]. Even with the obvious desirability of such comprehensive designs, the cost and complexity of this approach render them rare. This suggests that additional meta-analysis of the increasingly diverse research on cancer survivorship is needed. Hopefully, the conceptual integration that our proposed model employs will be used to identify the key conceptual categories for this type of analysis.

Finally, the message of this chapter is that "age matters." However, how it matters is very complex, and with the exception of the generalizations noted above, many questions still remain to be answered. The scholars from the fields of both oncology and gerontology, many of whom have contributed to other chapters of this book, are in an exciting place and time in cancer and aging research, where our respective expertise and knowledge are being brought to bear on this important topic for both fields. It's our hope that this chapter has raised questions and provides the framework that will motivate future applications of the complex research designs and methodologies to directly address the adaptation and adjustment of older adults to cancer.

ACKNOWLEDGMENT

This chapter was prepared with the support of NIH Grant CA-798975. The authors wish to thank Cory Cronin, Sherri Brown and Holly Renzhofer, predoctoral fellows, for their invaluable assistance in the preparation of this manuscript.

REFERENCES

1. Andrykowski MA, Curran SL, Studts JL, Cunningham L, Carpenter JS, McGrath PC, Loan DA, Kenady DE. Psychosocial adjustment and quality of life in women with breast cancer and benign breast problems: A controlled comparison. *J Clin Epidemiol* 1996;**49**:827–834.

2. Brennan J. Adjustment to cancer—coping or personal transition? *Psychooncology* 2001;**10**:1–18.

3. Dow KH, Lafferty P. Quality of life, survivorship, and psychosocial adjustment of young women with breast cancer after breast-conserving surgery and radiation therapy. *Oncol Nurs Forum* 2000;**27**;1555–1564.

4. Deshields T, Tibbs T, Fan MY, Bayer L, Taylor M, Fisher E. Ending treatment: The course of emotional adjustment and quality of life among breast cancer survivors immediately following radiation therapy. *Support Care Cancer* 2005;**13**:1018–1026.

5. Tartaro J, Roberts J, Nosarti C, Cryford T, Luecken L, David A. Who benefits? Distressing, adjustment and benefit-finding among breast cancer survivors. *J Psychosoc Oncol* 2005;**23**:45–64.

6. Deimling GT, Kahana B. *Quality of Life of Older Adult Long Term Cancer Survivors*, proposal to the National Cancer Institute, RO1-CA798975 (funded 10/01/98).

7. Deimling GT, Bowman KF, Kahana B. *Quality of Life of Older Adult Long-Term Cancer Survivor*. A proposal to the National Cancer Institute, 2R01-CA798975 (funded 10/01/03).

8. Lazarus R, Folkman S. *Stress Appraisal and Coping*, Springer, New York, 1984.

9. Pearlin LI. The sociological study of stress. *J Health Soc Behav* 1989;**30**:241–256.

10. Ensel WM, Lin N. Age, the stress process, and physical distress: The role of distal stressors. *J Aging Health* 2000;**12**(2):139–168.

11. Thoits P. Stressor and problem-solving: The individual as psychological activist. *J Health Soc Behav* 1994;**35**:143–159.

12. Tedeschi RG, Calhoun LG. *Trauma & Transformation: Growing in the Aftermath of Suffering*. Sage, Thousand Oaks, CA, 1995.

13. Ramsey S, Andersen M, Etzioni R, Moinpour C, Peacock S, Potosky A, et al. Quality of life in survivors of colorectal carcinoma. Cancer 2000;**88**:1294–1303.

14. Ell KO, Nichimoto RH, Mantell JE, Hamovitch MB. Psychological adaptation to cancer: A comparison among patients, spouses, and nonspouses. *Family Syst Med* 1988;**6**:335–348.

15. Deimling GT, Schaefer M, Kahana B, Bowman KF, Reardon J. Racial differences in the health of older adult long-term cancer survivors. *J Psychosoc Oncol* 2002;**24**:77–94.

16. Rowland JH. Psycho-Oncology and breast cancer: A paradigm for research and intervention. *Breast Cancer Res Treat* 2004;**31**:315–324.

17. Benyamini Y, McClain CS, Levanthal EA, Levnthal H. Living with the worry of cancer: Health perceptions and behaviors of elderly people with self, vicarious, or no history of cancer. *Psychooncology* 2003;**12**(2):161–172.

18. Bowman KF, Rose JH, Deimling GT. Appraisal of the cancer experience by family members and survivors in long-term survivorship. *Psychooncology* 2006;**15**:834–845.

19. Deimling GT, Arendt JA, Kypriotakis G, Bowman KF. Functioning of older, long-term cancer survivors: The role of cancer and comorbidities. *J Am Geriatr Soc* 2009;**57**:S289–S292.

20. Arndt V, Merx H, Stegmaier C, Ziegler H, Brenner H. Quality of life in patients with colorectal cancer 1 year after diagnosis compared with the general population: A population-based study. *J Clin Oncol* 2004;**22**:4829–4836.

21. Clough-Gorr KM, Ganz PA, Silliman RA. Older breast cancer survivors: Factors associated with change in emotional well-being. *J Clin Oncol* 2007;**25**:1334–1340.

22. Bowman KF, Smerglia VL, Deimling GT. A stress model of cancer survivorship in older long-term survivors. *J Mental Health Aging* 2004;**10**:163–182.

23. Deimling GT, Bowman KF, Sterns S, Wagner LJ, Kahana B. Cancer-related health worries and psychological distress among older adult, long-term cancer survivors. *Psychooncology* 2006;**15**:306–320.

24. Dohrenwend B. Integrating perspectives of traumatic stress and everyday stress research. Keynote address given at the International Society for Traumatic Stress Studies, Montreal, Nov. 1997.

25. American Cancer Society. *Cancer Facts & Figures 2007,* American Cancer Society, Atlanta, 2002.

26. Havlick RJ, Yanicik R, long S, et al. The National Institute on Aging and the National Cancer Institute SEER collaborative study on comorbidity and early diagnosis of cancer in the elderly. *Cancer* 1994;**74**:2101–2106.

27. Rowland JH, Yancik R. Cancer survivorship: The interface of aging, co-morbidity and quality care. *J Natl Cancer Inst* 2006;**98**:504–505.

28. Karlamangla A, Tinetti M, Guralnik J, et al. Co-morbidity in older adults: Nosology of impairment, diseases, and conditions. *J Gerontol* 2007;**62A**:296–300.

29. Anderson B, Kiecolt-Glaser J, Glaser R. A biobehavioral model of cancer stress and disease course. *Am Psychol* 1994;**49**:389–404.

30. Diemling GT, Bowman KF, Wagner LJ. The effects of cancer-related pain and fatigue on functioning on older adult, long-term cancer survivors. *Cancer Nurs* 2007;**30**:421–433.

31. Dunkel-Schetter C, Feinstein L, Taylor S, et al. Patterns of coping with cancer. *Health Psychol* 1992;**11**:79–87.

32. Hack TF, Degner LF. Coping responses following breast cancer diagnosis predict psychological adjustment three years later. *Psychooncology* 2004;**13**:235–247.

33. McCaul KD, Sandgren AK, King B, O'Donnell S, Branstetter A, Foreman G. Coping and adjustment to breast cancer. *Psychooncology* 1999;**8**:230–236.

34. Moorey S, Frampton M, Greer S. The cancer coping questionnaire: A self-rating scale for measuring the impact of adjuvant psychological therapy on coping behaviour. *Psychooncology* 2003;**12**:331–344.

35. Aldwin CM, Sutton KJ, Chiara G, Spiro A. Age differences in stress, coping, and appraisal: Findings from the normative aging study. *J Gerontol Psychol Sci* 1996;**51B**:P179–P188.

36. Deimling GT, Wagner LJ, Bowman KF, Sterns S, Kercher K, Kahana B. Coping among older-adult, long-term cancer survivors. *Psychooncology* 2005;**15**(2):143–159.

37. Schou I, Ekeberg Ø, Ruland CM, Sandvik L, Kårasen R. Pessimism as a predictor of emotional morbidity one year following breast cancer surgery. *Psychooncology* 2004;**13**:309–320.

38. Carver CS, Pozo C, Harris SD, et al. How coping mediates the effect of optimism on distress: A study of women with early stage breast cancer. *J Personality Soc Psychol* 1993;**65**:375–390.

39. Bloom JR. Surviving and thriving? *Psychooncology* 2002;**11**:89–92.

40. Vecht CJ. Cancer pain: A neurological perspective. *Curr Opin Neurol* 2000;**13**:649–653.

41. Hojris J, Andersen J, Overgaard M, Overgaard J. Late treatment-related morbidity in breast cancer patients randomized to postmastectomy radiotherapy and systemic treatment versus systemic treatment alone. *Acta Oncol* 2000;**39**:355–372.

42. Johnansson S, Svenson H, Denkamp J. Timescale of evolution of late radiation injury after postoperative radiotherapy of breast cancer patients. *Int J Radiat Oncol Biol Phys* 2000;**48**:745–450.

43. Perez CA, Michalski JM, Purdy JA, Wasserman TH, Williams K, Lockett MA. Three-dimensional conformal therapy or standard irradiation in localized carcinoma of prostate: Preliminary results of a nonrandomized comparison. *Int J Radiat Oncol Biol Phys* 2000;**47**:629–637.

44. Storey MR, Pollack A, Zagars G, Smith L, Antolak J, Rosen I. Complications from radiotherapy dose escalation in prostate cancer: Preliminary results of a randomized trial. *Int J Radiat Oncol Biol Phys* 2000;**48**:635–642.

45. Gardener BG, Zietman AL, Shipley WU, Skowronski UE, McManus P. Late normal tissue sequelae in the second decade after high dose radiation therapy with combined photons and conformal protons for locally advanced prostate cancer. *J Urol* 2002;**167**:123–126.

46. Jung H, Beck-Bornholdt HP, Svoboda V, Alberti W, Herrmann T. Quantification of late complications after radiation therapy. *Radiother Oncol* 2001;**61**:219–222.

47. King MT, Kenny P, Shiell A, Hall J, Boyages J. Quality of life three months and one year after first treatment for early stage breast cancer: Influence of treatment and patient characteristics. *Quali Life Res* 2000;**9**:789–800.

48. Sweeney C, Schmitz KH, Lazovich D, et al. Functional limitations in elderly female cancer survivors. *J Natl Cancer Inst* 2006;**98**:521–529.

49. Ganz PA, Guadagnoli E, Landrum MB, et al. Breast cancer in older women: quality of life and psychological adjustment in the 15 months after diagnosis. *J Clin Oncol* 2003;**21**:4027–4033.

50. Keating NL, Nørredam M, Landrum MB, Huskamp HA, Meara E. Physical and mental health status of older long-term cancer survivors. *J Am Geriar Soc* 2005;**53**(12):2145–2152.

51. Deimling GT, Sterns S, Bowman KF, Kahana B. Functioning and activity participation restrictions among older adults, long-term cancer survivors. *Cancer Investig* 2007;**25**:106–116.

52. Bernebei R, Garmbassi G, Lapane K, et al. Management of pain in elderly patients with cancer. *JAMA* 1998;**279**(23):1877–1882.

53. Bosompra K, Ashikaga T, O'Brien PJ, Nelson L, Skelly J. Swelling, numbness, pain, and their relationship to arm function among breast cancer patients: A disablement process model perspective. *Breast J* 2002;**8**(6):338–348.

54. Fossa SD, Dahl AA, Loge J. Fatigue, anxiety, and depression in long-term survivors of testicular cancer. *J Clin Oncol* 2003;**21**(7):1249–1254.

55. Servaes P, Verhagen S, Bleijenberg G. Determinants of chronic fatigue in disease-free breast cancer patients: A cross-sectional study. *Ann Oncol* 2002;**13**(4):589–598.

56. Berglund G, Bolund C, Fornander T, Rutqvist LE, Sjoden PO. Late effects of adjuvant chemotherapy and postoperative radiotherapy on quality of life among breast cancer patients. *Eur J Cancer* 1991;**27**(9):1075–1081.

57. Mast ME. Correlates of fatigue in survivors of breast cancer. *Cancer Nurs* 1998;**21**(2):136–142.

58. Cella D, Tross S. Psychological adjustment to survival from Hodgkin's disease. *J Consult Clin Psychol* 1986;**54**(5):616–622.

59. Holzner B, Kemmler G, Kopp M, Moschen R, Schweigkofler H, Dünser M, Margreiter R, Fleischhacker W, Sperner-Unterweger B. Quality of life in breast cancer patients—not enough attention for long-term survivors? *Psychomatics* 2001;**42**:117–123.

60. Thomas SF, Glynne-Jones R, Chait I, Marks DF. Anxiety in long-term cancer survivors influences the acceptability of planned discharge from follow-up. *Psychooncology* 1997;**6**:190–196.

61. Zabora J, BrintzenhofeSzoc K, Curbow B, Hooker C, Piantadosi S. The prevalence of psychological distress by cancer site. *Psychooncology* 2001;**10**:19–28.

62. Vinokur AD, Threatt BA, Vinokur-Kaplan D, Satariano WA. The process of recovery from breast cancer for younger and older patients: Changes during the first year. *Cancer* 1990;**65**:1242–1254.

63. Hewitt M, Rowland JH, Yanik R. Cancer survivors in the United States: Age, health and disability. *J Gerontol Med Sci* 2003;**58**:82–91.

64. Arndt V, Merx H, Sturmer T, Stegmaier C, Ziegler H, Brenner H. Age-specific detriments to quality of life among breast cancer patients one year after diagnosis. *Eur J Cancer* 2004;**40**:673–680.

65. Gotay CC, Muraoka MY. Quality of life in long-term survivors of adult-onset cancers. *J Natl Cancer Inst* 1998;**90**:656–667.

66. Sellick SM, Crooks DL. Depression and cancer: an appraisal of the literature for prevalence, and practice guideline development of psychological interventions. *Psychooncology* 1999;**8**:315–333.

67. Blazer D. Depression in late life: Review and commentary. *J Gerontol A Biol Sci Med Sci* 2003;**58**:M249–M265.

68. Strommel M, Kurtz ME, Kurtz JC, et al. A longitudinal analysis of the course of depressive symptomatology in geriatric patients with cancer of the breast, colon, lung, or prostrate. *Health Pyschol* 2004;**23**:564–573.

69. Rowland J. Psycho-oncology and breast cancer: A paradigm for research and intervention. *Breast Cancer Res Treat* 1994;**31**:315–324.

70. Welch-McCaffery D, Hoffman B, Leigh S, Loescher L, Meyskins F. Surviving adult cancers. Part 2: Psychosocial implications. *Ann Int Med* 1989;**111**:517–524.

71. Andrykowski MA, Cordova MJ, McGarth PC, Sloan DA, Kenday DE. Stability and change in posttraumatic stress disorder symptoms following breast cancer treatment: A 1-year follow-up. *Pyschooncology* 2000;**9**:69–78.

72. Smith MY, Redd WH, Peyser C, Vogl D. Post-traumatic stress disorder in cancer: a review. *Psychooncology* 1999;**8**:521–537.

73. Smith K, Lesko. Psychosocial problems in cancer survivors. *Oncology* 1988;**2**(1):33–44.

74. Kahana, B, Kahana, E, Diemling, Sterns, S. Determinants of altered life perspectives among older long-term cancer survivors. *Cancer Nurs* (in press).

75. Zebrack BJ. Cancer survivor identity and quality of life. *Cancer Pract* 2000;**8**(5):238–242.

76. Arman M, Rehnsfield A. The hidden suffering among breast cancer patients: A qualitative metasynthesis. *Qual Health Res* 2003;**13**:510–527.

77. Ferrell BR, Grant MM, Funk BM, Otis-Green SA, Garcia NJ. Quality of life in breast cancer survivors: Implications for developing social services. *Oncol Nurs Forum* 1998;**25**(5):887–895.

78. Burish TG, Tope DM. Psychological techniques for controlling the adverse side effects of cancer chemotherapy: Findings from a decade of research. *J Pain Symptom Manage* 1992;**7**(5):287–301.

79. Glanz K, Lerman C. Psychological impact of breast cancer: A critical review. *Ann Behav Med* 1992;**14**(3):204.

80. Mullens AB, McCaul KD, Erickson SC, Sandgren AK. Coping after cancer: Risk perceptions, worry and health behaviors among colorectal cancer survivors. *Psychooncology* 2004;**13**(6):367–376.

81. Easterling DV, Leventhal H. Contribution of concrete cognition to emotion-neutral symptoms as elicitors of worry about cancer. *J Appl Psychol* 1989;**74**(5):787–796.

82. Deimling GT, Sterns S, Bowman KF, Kahan B. Functioning and activity participation restrictions among older adult, long-term cancer survivors. *Informa Healthcare* 2007;**25**:106–116.

83. Duke J, Leventhal H, Brownlee S, Leventhal E. Giving up and replacing activities in response to illness. *J Gerntol B Psychol Sci Soc Sci* 2002;**57**:367–376.

84. Fukukawa Y, Nakashima C, Tsuboi S, Niino N, Ando F, Kosugi S, Shimokata H. The impact of health problems on depression and activities in middle-aged and older adults: age and social interactions as moderators. *J Gerontol B Psychol Sci Soc Sci* 2004;**59**:19–26.

85. Fialka-Moser V, Crevenna R, Korpan M, Quittan M. Cancer rehabilitation. *J Rehab Med* 2003;**35**:153–162.

86. Luoma M, Hakamies-Blomqvist L. The meaning of quality of life in patients being treated for advanced breast cancer: A qualitative study. *Psychooncology* 2004;**13**:729–739.

87. Ferrell B, Dow K, Grant M. Measurement of the quality of life in cancer survivors. *Qual Life Res* 1995;**4**:523–531.

88. Ferrell B, Grant M, Funk B, Otis-Green S, Garcia N. Quality of life in breast cancer: Part I: Physical and social well being. *Cancer Nurs* 1997;**20**:398–408.

89. Giles B, Johnston G. Identity loss and maintenance: Commonality of experience in cancer and dementia. *Euro J Cancer Care* 2004;**13**:436–442.

90. Gray RE, Fitch MI, Fergus KD, Mykhalovskiy E, Church K. Hegemonic masculinity and the experience of prostate cancer: A narrative approach. *J Aging Ident* 2002;**7**(1):43–62.

91. Thorne SE, Murray C. Social constructions of breast cancer. *Health Care Women Int* 2000;**21**:141–159.

92. Zebrack BJ. Cancer survivor identity and quality of life. *Cancer Pract* 2000;**8**(5):238–242.

93. Brady MJ, Peterman AH, Fitchett G, Mo M, Cella D. A case for including spirituality in quality of life measurement in oncology. *Psychooncology* 1999;**8**:417–428.

94. Visser A, Garssen B, Vingerhoets A. Spirituality and well-being in cancer patients: A review. *Psychooncology* 2010;**19**:565–572.

95. Salsman JM, Segerstrom SC, Breechting EH, Carlson CR, Andrykowski MA. Posttraumatic growth and PTSD symptomatology among colorectal cancer survivors: A 3-month longitudinal examination of cognitive processing. *Psychooncology* 2009;**18**:30–41.

96. Schnoll RA, Harlow LL, Brower L. Spirituality, demographic and disease factors, and adjustment to cancer. *Cancer Pract* 2000;**8**(6):298–304.

97. Avis NE, Deimling GT. Cancer survivorship and aging. *Cancer Suppl* 2008;**113**(12):3519–3529.

CHAPTER 25

Long-Term and Late Physical and Psychosocial Effects of Cancer in Older Adults

KERRI M. CLOUGH-GORR

Section of Geriatrics, Boston University Medical Center, Boston, MA
Institute of Social and Preventative Medicine (ISPM), University of Bern, Bern, Switzerland
National Institute for Cancer Epidemiology and Registration (NICER), ISPM University of Zürich, Zürich, Switzerland

REBECCA A. SILLIMAN

Section of Geriatrics, Boston University Medical Center, Boston, MA

25.1 INTRODUCTION

With improvements in cancer screening and treatment over the past several decades, the risk of cancer mortality following diagnosis has steadily decreased. This has resulted in an increasing number of cancer survivors in the United States, nearly 11.4 million, the majority (60%) of whom are 65 years of age or older [1]. Notably, despite advances in early detection and treatment, the overall burden of cancer is expected to increase because of aging of the US population, heralding a growth in the number of older cancer survivors estimated to double over the ensuing decades [2]. Even though cancer treatment ends, the risks of side effects and longer-term complications may persist. For older survivors as compared to younger ones, the functional consequences of cancer and its treatment have a greater impact related to the interaction of cancer treatment sequelae, coexisting diseases, and age-related disabilities. This is particularly important since both comorbidities and functional impairments increase with age and appear to be more prevalent in older cancer survivors [3]. For older cancer patients, survivorship beyond recovery from treatment means living with the potential of long-term complications in conjunction with the common diseases and disabilities of aging.

Cancer survivorship in older adults is complex and involves many aspects of care. Long-term and late effects of cancer treatment can come from any of the three main types of cancer treatment (surgery, radiation therapy, and chemotherapy, including hormonal therapy) and may vary significantly by age, type of cancer, and type and intensity of treatment [4]. Primary cancer treatments can result in a wide range of physical and psychological long-term and late effects. Because older cancer survivors

Cancer and Aging Handbook: Research and Practice, First Edition. Edited by Keith M. Bellizzi and Margot A. Gosney.
© 2012 Wiley-Blackwell. Published 2012 by John Wiley & Sons, Inc.

are living longer after cancer treatment, identification, prevention, and management of long-term and late effects is an important part of cancer care. This chapter explores both the physical and psychosocial long-term and late effects of cancer in older adults. We will discuss their consequences in some of the most common cancers and consider literature-based recommendations for managing and minimizing them.

25.2   PHYSICAL LATE AND LONG-TERM CANCER EFFECTS

It is important to distinguish between long-term and late effects of cancer treatment. Long-term effects are those that are persistent from the time of treatment, while late effects are those toxicities that are absent or subclinical at the conclusion of therapy that become apparent later. Their unmasking is thought to be due to organ senescence or the failure of compensatory mechanisms (such as occur with aging). They present months to years after treatment [5]. In practice, it is often difficult to identify the point when symptoms first appear; thus the distinction between long-term and late effects may be unclear [6]. In addition, cancer treatment may cause both long-term and late effects. Since the 1990s documentation of cancer-related physical effects has expanded, coinciding with several major national initiatives focusing on survivorship [3,4,6–8]. The list of cancer-related long-term and late physical effects is long and will not be fully addressed herein (Table 25.1 provides a summary for older cancer survivors). We will instead focus primarily on a few that are common and clinically important to the survivorship experience of older cancer patients.

Breast cancer survivors who have had surgery to remove lymph nodes (or radiation therapy to the lymph nodes) may develop lymphedema (abnormal buildup of lymph fluid that causes swelling) in the arm on the treated side. This is one of the most common complications of breast cancer and varies in the time onset following treatment. Symptoms may persist for years [9,10]. Lymphedema is difficult to manage, especially in older women because it can vary between dormant, acute, and transient states interacting with age-related conditions over the course of survivorship. One study demonstrated that persistent lymphedema is common in older breast cancer survivors and affects physical function and general mental health [11]. Although lymphedema is not life-threatening, when persistent, it has long-term physical consequences (e.g., cosmetic disfiguration, physical discomfort, limited arm movement leading to loss of functional ability, increased risk of infection) [12–15]. These symptoms may be particularly problematic when coupled with age-associated conditions such as osteoarthritis of the shoulder or hand.

Likewise, treatment of prostate cancer, one of the most common cancers in older men, can also result in long-term and late effects that may considerably impact health and quality of life for older survivors. Prostate cancer is of particular concern not simply because of burgeoning numbers of survivors but also because most men live with rather than die from prostate cancer. This means that large numbers of prostate cancer survivors may experience very long periods of living with the substantial repercussions of treatment. For example, studies have shown that sexual, urinary, and/or bowel function problems, which vary by treatment type, are still common years after treatment, affecting quality of life [16,17]. Furthermore, a 2008 review found a strong link between androgen ablation therapy and subtle but significant cognitive declines in men with prostate cancer [18]. Other studies have shown that treatment choices are not

TABLE 25.1 Possible Long-Term and Late Physical Effects of Cancer in Older Patients by Cancer Treatment Type

Treatment	Long-Term Side Effects	Late Side Effects
Chemotherapy	Fatigue	Cataracts
	Neuropathy	Liver problems
	Cognitive problems	Lung disease one loss
	"Chemobrain"	Osteoporosis
	Heart failure	Reduced lung capacity
	Kidney failure	Second primary cancers
	Liver problems	
Radiation therapy	Fatigue	Cataracts
	Skin sensitivity	Cavities and tooth decay
		Heart problems
		Hypothyroidism
		Lung disease
		Intestinal problems
		Cognitive problems
		Second primary cancers
Surgery	Scars	Lymphedema
	Chronic pain	
Hormonal therapy	Hot flashes	Thromboembolic disease
	Sexual dysfunction	Cataracts
	Fatigue	Bone loss
	Joint and muscle pain	Osteoporosis
		Heart problems
		Diabetes
		Second primary cancers

Sources: Data from Arriagada et al. [4], Aziz [5], and Hewitt et al. [8].

always informed by pretreatment dysfunction (which impacts long-term/late effects) and that men who regretted their treatment choice had poorer scores on every measure of generic and prostate cancer–related quality of life [19,20]. Treatment modality and preexisting dysfunction are the most common predictors of quality of life in men with prostate cancer [16,19,21]. Further evidence regarding treatment-specific outcomes in conjunction with potential impact on quality of life for older men surviving decades after an original diagnosis is needed to improve medical decision-making from treatment through survivorship.

Peripheral neuropathy is a common debilitating chemotherapy-related effect, with an estimated prevalence of 30–40% [22,23]. Peripheral neuropathy symptoms differ in different patients. The type of symptom is closely related to the type of chemotherapy. Unfortunately, diagnostic criteria are inconsistently applied [24]. Thus, prevalence estimates may underrepresent the true burden of cancer-related peripheral neuropathy in older survivors. This will become increasingly important as the number of older adults receiving chemotherapy increases. Because there is insufficient evidence to support a standard approach to diagnosis and treatment, management emphasizes minimizing symptoms and their consequences [7,24]. Peripheral neuropathy can be a serious problem for older adults. For example, in a patient with gait instability due to painful hip osteoarthritis and macular degeneration, a peripheral neuropathy may precipitate falls and lead to fractures.

Similar to peripheral neuropathy, cancer-related fatigue in older adults has not been well studied. Questions remain regarding its definition, measurement, underlying mechanisms, and treatment. A 2008 review noted that fatigue is one of the most common physical late effects of cancer treatment [25]. A study of long-term older breast, colorectal, and prostate cancer survivors showed that >40% of survivors reported symptoms of fatigue attributable to their cancers [26]. Other studies have noted prevalence rates ranging anywhere within 50–96% during active treatment and beyond [27,28]. Untreated fatigue can have dramatic effects on the lives of older cancer survivors because it leads to reduced physical activity [29]. A review of the literature related to fatigue and physical activity in older adults with cancer suggests that older cancer patients with higher levels of physical activity during treatment have lower levels of fatigue, higher levels of physical function, and higher quality of life during and after cancer treatment [29]. A second review of clinical trials of exercise interventions showed similar findings [30].

The consistently positive results across exercise studies, with lack of significant deleterious effects of exercise in cancer patients, suggests that exercise intervention may be beneficial to older adults with cancer not only for treating fatigue but also for other long-term/late effects such as osteoporosis (if including weight bearing exercises). Bone health and fracture prevention have also become important health issues among cancer survivors. Osteoporosis is a common problem among cancer survivors, particularly for older women who underwent chemotherapy premenopausally for breast cancer and for men treated with hormone deprivation therapy for prostate cancer [4,5,8]. Older cancer survivors at risk for bone loss should undergo preventive or therapeutic intervention addressing factors such as physical deconditioning, poor nutrition, and vitamin D deficiency.

Cancer survivors are also at greater risk for recurrence and for developing multiple primary malignancies (MPMs). In fact, one of the most serious late physical effects is the diagnosis of a new cancer. The National Cancer Institute's Surveillance, Epidemiology, and End Results (SEER) program estimates that the risk of developing second or MPM varies from 1% to 16%, depending on primary cancer site and is increasing [31,32]. As with first primary cancers, the incidence of MPM increases with age, and nearly 7% of older cancer survivors are affected [33–35]. Breast cancer survivors represent one of the largest groups of survivors with MPM; the most common site is contralateral breast cancers, followed by prostate and colorectal cancers [34]. These rankings may reflect both the high incidence and survival rates for the first primary cancer, but not necessarily greater risks for a subsequent cancer. Radiation therapy has been linked to higher contralateral breast cancer risk, lung cancer, soft tissue sarcoma, and esophageal cancer [35–39]. Endometrial cancer is associated with previous tamoxifen therapy [4,40]. Risk of leukemia after a primary cancer has been associated with both chemotherapy and radiation therapy [32,41,42].

The growing numbers of older adults surviving cancer makes physical long-term and late effects of their cancer treatments more relevant than ever in geriatric oncology care. Considering not just length but also quality of survival in relation to cancer-related treatment effects is important in the care of older cancer survivors.

25.3 LONG-TERM AND LATE PSYCHOSOCIAL EFFECTS

A cancer diagnosis threatens older patients' emotional well-being from treatment through recovery into survivorship as well as their physical health. As we saw in the previous section, there is an association between symptoms, long-term and late physical effects, and quality of life. The psychosocial effects of cancer are strongly influenced by an older person's personality and coping mechanisms. It is common for persons diagnosed with cancer to develop anxiety and depression during the first years after diagnosis. However, the psychological impact of cancer diagnosis in older cancer patients may be relatively shortlived and less detrimental than in younger patients [27]. Nonetheless, depression and anxiety, when they do occur, can persist much longer seriously affecting quality of life [6,43–45]. Some studies suggest that cancer survivors have poorer general health status, more fatigue, more difficulties with cognitive function, higher rates of depression, and worse quality of life than those without cancer [46–48]. However, there is inconsistency in the quality-of-life (QOL) evidence for older survivors, likely relating to differences in comparison groups (e.g., older vs. younger, with or without cancer), types of measures used, timing of measurement (e.g., at diagnosis, 1–2 years or 5 years postdiagnosis), variability, and selectiveness of study populations (e.g., specific cancers, randomized control trial participants, no comparisons, small sample size), and control for confounders (e.g., age, comorbidities) [3,46,49–52]. Additionally, and no less importantly, interpretation and conclusions about older cancer survivors and quality of life are intimately connected to type and stage of cancer, time since diagnosis, and particular aspects of quality of life (i.e., physical vs. psychosocial domains).

Social support has been shown to provide many benefits associated with the overall health and well-being of older adults. A social network provides a reservoir for social engagement and buffers the impact of major life events by providing emotional and instrumental social support in times of crisis. Social support from family, friends, partners, community, and physicians is associated with better sense of hope and better emotional health, especially among people with cancer [53–55]. A study of long-term older breast cancer survivors found that women with higher levels of social support, and positive ratings regarding the quality of medical interactions with their physicians, were less likely to have poor emotional health 5 years after diagnosis [49]. Intervention studies have consistently demonstrated the beneficial effects of psychosocial support on changing of attitudes from pessimism to optimism [56–58]. In general, the greater the social resources available to an older survivor, the better that individual's chances of managing negative long-term and late cancer effects.

Up to half of all cancer patients report some type of psychological disorder, especially depression, at some point over the course of the cancer experience, which is also common among older adults in general [59–61]. Depression in older adults is a known risk factor for morbidity and poor quality of life [59,62,63]. The prevalence of depression in older cancer survivors has been estimated to range from around 10% to almost 60%, which is higher than estimates among healthy community-dwelling older adults (3–9%) or among those living in nursing homes (10–25%) [6,46,48,64]. Given that depression may manifest itself as a result of cancer and its treatment, higher prevalence rates among older cancer survivors are not surprising. In fact, late-life depression often affects individuals with other medical and/or psychosocial problems, but disentangling interactions with age-related impairments can be quite difficult [59]. A study of older married female cancer survivors has demonstrated that survivorship was associated with higher depressive symptoms that were indirectly related to general health impairments [65]. However, depression in older cancer survivors may be confounded by the overlap of depressive disorder and cancer symptoms, variation in measurement method (e.g., variety of scales, measurement of severity or not), lack of precancer and/or baseline measurement, and insufficient differentiation of other comorbidities, thus complicating a true estimation of its impact. Furthermore, the possible effects and interactions between long-term and late depression and other common cancer effects that often occur simultaneously and known to be related to depression, such as pain and fatigue, are critical to consider but incompletely understood [26,59,65–67].

The interplay between physical and psychosocial long-term and late effects is complex, and particularly important in older adults. First, they share many risk factors (e.g., advancing age, increased comorbidity, decreased physical function, lack of financial resources and/or social supports) [27]. Moreover, physical effects related to disability in older cancer survivors are often themselves causes of psychological effects (e.g., depression). This can result in worsening of psychosocial effects and subsequent decreases in general mental health, emotional well-being, and/or quality of life over survivorship. For example, cognitive dysfunction (e.g., difficulty with attention, concentration, memory) is more prevalent in older cancer survivors than in the general population and has been associated with decreased survival [48,68]. Cognitive impairment can adversely affect physical function and independence in activities of daily living (ADLs; e.g., dressing, preparing a meal, walking, housework). As a result, older cancer survivors with cognitive impairment have greater self-care needs, which may or may not be able to be met. For older adults, being able to live independently is directly related to the ability to perform ADLs. Decreased survival may possibly be related to the cascading effects of decreased physical function, disruption of ADLs, and overall reduced quality of life emanating from cognitive dysfunction and unmet care needs. A 2009 study of long-term cancer survivors showed that factors affecting functional ability are important determinants of quality of life [69]. The literature suggests, albeit not completely without contradiction, that older cancer survivors are likely to be more physically affected by cancer rather than psychologically [27]. In fact, some studies report that older cancer survivors' mental health is similar to or better than that of older adults in the general population, suggesting resilience or successful adaptation despite the physical effects [4,6,27,46]. In general, the physical health status of older long-term cancer survivors is worse than in comparable persons without a cancer diagnosis, and the burden of physical illness related to cancer diagnosis can be greater than that of cancer-specific mental illness [46,70].

In older cancer survivors, cancer treatment may exacerbate existing comorbidities or age-related conditions and/or result in new ones that will unfavorably affect their quality of life over anticipated longer periods of survivorship. Older adults and their care providers face a combined challenge of aging and cancer, which often includes comorbid conditions and varying levels of functional disability and social loss. Clearly, the complex relation of physical and psychosocial late and long-term effects of cancer in older survivors is important and requires further study [71]. These concerns affect both patient and provider, and evidence-based intervention attempts that address these needs ought to be ongoing priority areas for geriatric and psychosocial oncology research and clinical care.

25.4   AGE-RELATED COMPLICATIONS

Many older cancer survivors are at risk for developing physical and psychosocial long-term and late effects of cancer treatment. These may interact with other aging-related conditions and lead to premature morbidity and mortality. Risk factors for long-term or late effects in older adults vary by diagnosis, type of treatment received, age at treatment, comorbidities, time since treatment, and genetic vulnerability, as well as psychological, social, and environmental factors that influence functioning [6].

The benefits of cancer treatment in older adults generally (not always) outweigh the risks of long-term and late effects which include developing a subsequent cancer and effects on quality of life. Yet long-term effects (e.g., neuropathies with related weakness, numbness, or pain, fatigue, cognitive difficulties, elevated anxiety, or depression) and/or late effects of treatment (e.g., musculoskeletal complications, late-onset cardiovascular complications) can be exacerbated by and/or worsen underlying conditions common in older popoulations [6]. Population studies have reported that long-term cancer survivors are more likely to experience physical limitations than those without a history of cancer [6,46,72]. Studies of older survivors, however, have shown that they are more likely to attribute their health problems to aging rather than their cancers [46,73]. In fact, frequent problems such as pain, fatigue, and weakness reported by older cancer survivors are more likely to be attributed to age-related rather than to cancer-related factors [26]. However, older survivors fare worse than older adults without cancer [27,46,74]. For many older persons, cancer occurs against a backdrop of other chronic conditions associated with aging. Commonly occurring underlying comorbidities can interact with long-term and/or late treatment effects and seriously complicate survivorship. For example, older cancer patients with underlying neural damage (common in diabetes) may be at particular risk for more severe chemotherapy-induced peripheral neuropathy [75]. Similarly, chemotherapy-related neuropathy in older adults who are depressed and/or have dementia may present complications with medication management and/or adherence. Treatment decisionmaking for older patients with depression and/or cognitive impairment concomitant with other comorbidities and long-term and/or late cancer effects requires consideration of the risks and benefits, both physical and psychosocial. Cognitive impairment is associated with more severe depression and comorbidities as well as negative impact on functional status [68]. One study showed that older cancer patients with cognitive impairment had significantly lower mean survival time (considering age, tumor stage, and site) than controls without cognitive impairment, despite comparable treatment [76]. Depression and dementia are important underlying conditions that can interact with treatment or long-term/late effects complicating decisionmaking for patient, caregiver(s), and physician alike.

Older women are at special risk for cancer-related health problems [50]. Long-term effects such as fatigue, lymphedema of the arm, or osteoporosis are not life threatening, but when symptoms persist in conjunction with other debilitating medical conditions, they can have long-term physical and psychosocial consequences such as physical discomfort or pain, limited mobility leading to loss of functional ability, and/or impaired quality of life [12–15,77].

Long-term and late cancer effects can be sources of progressive disability leading to disruption in performance of ADLs in older cancer survivors. A study of the National Health Interview Survey data showed that the prevalence of functional limitations was higher in long-term cancer survivors than in controls, varying by cancer type (e.g., ranging from 44.9% in lymphoma survivors to 88.8% in lung cancer survivors) [78]. Another population-based study of older female cancer survivors showed an increased prevalence of functional limitations for 5-year survivors accompanied by increased risk of difficulty performing ADLs [79]. Long-term and late effects such as pain and/or fatigue are predictors of functional difficulties in older cancer survivors [26,80]. Importantly, older adults with functional limitations are at increased risk of morbidity and mortality [79]. Moreover, functional limitations that can result from cancer or its treatment may limit participation in social activities and as a result negatively affect quality of life over survivorship [69].

Common geriatric syndromes (e.g., dementia, delirium, depression, falls), the availability of social support, and the nutritional status of older adults may negatively impact survivorship as well. For instance, dementia, poor nutritional status, and lack of adequate social support have all been reported as predictors for poorer survival in older adults with cancer [81]. Furthermore, MPM in older survivors may not be only late sequelae of cancer treatment but also due to the effects of aging and combinations of other influences (e.g., lifestyle factors, environmental exposures, host factors) [8,33,34,82]. Importantly, long-term and late effects of treatment in older adults in combination with common conditions of aging often have considerable consequences, not just for aging individuals but simultaneously for heathcare systems, families, and other caregivers. Over the last several decades cancer trends have been changing contemporaneously with our knowledge of aging. Many studies have identified aging-related issues, especially the presence of comorbidities among older survivors as priority areas to be addressed in geriatric oncology care and by research on cancer and aging [27].

The changes and challenges of aging can play a significant role in the survivorship experience of older adults. The combined effects of cancer and aging are of concern to graying populations worldwide (a larger proportion in industrialized countries aging; greater numbers in developing countries). Improved understanding of aging, cancer, and their intersection, as well as their potential implications, will be central to the survivorship of older adults.

25.5 PREVENTION AND MANAGEMENT OF LONG-TERM AND LATE EFFECTS

As explored throughout this chapter, age- and cancer-related long-term and late effects can combine to influence important outcomes (e.g., survival, physical function, quality of life) of older cancer survivors. Major areas of concern for older survivors are worries about recurrence, MPM, and the combination long-term and late effects of cancer treatments and existing comorbidities [4,8,83]. With the number of cancer survivors expected to increase in the United States with the aging of the baby boom cohort, follow-up cancer care will play a key role in healthcare of older adults. The prevention and proper management of late and long-term effects may mitigate negative outcomes and hence will be essential to the quality of extended survivorship in older adults with cancer. In fact, one of the greatest challenges of treating the large and growing population of older cancer survivors is to determine the best methods for providing adequate long-term survivorship care.

Follow-up survivorship care consists of periodic routine visits, surveillance for recurrence and new primary cancers, and monitoring of long-term and late cancer effects, as well as providing psychosocial support. Cancer survivorship care is different from regular primary care because older cancer patients often require treatment by multiple specialists in addition to their primary care provider, making coordination of their care a challenge. For many older survivors, their complex healthcare needs are not always met [8]. Development and utilization of comprehensive survivorship care plans, although lacking evidence especially in older adults, are a recommended method for overcoming difficulties related to insufficient continuity of care over the course of survivorship. Cancer survivorship care plans are documents describing the patient's cancer treatment history with accompanying guidelines for follow-up care for both patient and provider(s). The following core elements of survivorship care plans are recommended by the Institute of Medicine: cancer treatment history, potential long-term/late treatment effects with recommended surveillance, links to resources that provide psychosocial support, information on general health and wellness, and a clear timeline for follow-up care, including surveillance for cancer spread, recurrence, or multiple cancers [8]. These core items are intended to improve communication between all providers involved in the full spectrum of care and to educate and empower the patient [84]. Research and evaluation of cancer survivorship care plans are needed to provide evidence examining their impact on long-term follow-up care with regard to health outcomes as well as patient and provider satisfaction.

Primary prevention (e.g., tobacco avoidance and cessation, healthy diet, weight control, physical activity) is the main strategy for reducing the burden of MPM related to lifestyle factors. Systematic surveillance can detect recurrences and new second cancers when they are treatable with more favorable prognoses. In the example of breast cancer, mammography surveillance has been shown to have a protective association with mortality in older survivors [85,86]. Unfortunately, there are many barriers to receiving optimal surveillance (e.g., fragmented and/or poorly coordinated care, insufficient patient information, limited access to care), and the consequences of underutilization of surveillance, as noted above, can be considerable. Despite guidelines for surveillance across cancer types, evidence shows that follow-up cancer care is not being provided as recommended and that racial/ethnic and income differences often account for significant variation in surveillance practices [8,87–89]. New strategies are needed to increase use of surveillance and decrease disparities in follow-up cancer care.

Cancer survivors are also at risk for other important health problems (e.g., cardiovascular disease, diabetes, osteoporosis, and functional decline, to name only a few). The health problems that older cancer survivors experience may be due directly to effects of cancer and/or its treatment, unhealthy behaviors (such as smoking, obesity, and lack of physical exercise), genetics, and/or risk factors that contributed to the first cancer. Except for lifestyle-related factors, few of these risk factors are modifiable.

A review of nearly 40 studies on lifestyle behaviors (e.g., physical exercise, diet, smoking) in cancer survivors found discrepancies between older and more recent studies [90]. Older studies with limited sample sizes, follow-up, and cancer types suggested healthy lifestyle behaviors to be more prevalent in cancer survivors than in comparison subjects, whereas more rigorous (e.g., large sample sizes, longer-term follow-up) recent studies found few differences. These review findings are supported by a 2006 population-based study in Massachusetts where cancer survivors had similar rates of lifestyle risk factors, including smoking, obesity, and decreased physical activity as respondents without cancer [91]. The lack of differences in lifestyle behavior does not support other studies suggesting that cancer survivors report heightened interest in modifying lifestyle behaviors [90], and more relevant to the topic of this chapter is the fact that few of the aforementioned studies addressed older cancer survivors specifically. Furthermore, there is scant evidence for the efficacy of rehabilitation in older cancer patients, which may have potential to prevent, reduce, or promote recovery of disability [7]. This all underscores the importance of studying the long-term and late effects of cancer in older survivors, focusing on potentially modifiable risk factors, as well testing interventions designed to minimize loss of functioning over time [92].

Studies of lifestyle factors such as physical exercise, diet, and smoking suggest that intervention may be beneficial [90]. Exercise intervention in cancer patients is beneficial both during and after treatment [30]. Exercise is associated with improved general heath, physical function, health-related biomarkers (e.g., blood pressure, heart rate), and quality of life among cancer survivors. Collectively, physical exercise intervention trials have shown that along with physical benefits, intervention subjects also had better self-reported health-related quality of life [30]. Nonetheless, specific benefits of exercise, similar to long-term and late cancer treatment effects, may vary according to stage of disease, type cancer treatment, and age, as well as the existing lifestyle of the older adult [93]. Data from trials and cohort studies suggest that maintaining weight and remaining physically active after a cancer diagnosis may also improve cancer-specific survival [94–96]. Dietary factors such as low-fat and/or high-vegetable-content diets may also improve survival in cancer patients [97,98]. Unfortunately, the benefits in older populations and the specific impact of diet and exercise on overall survival have yet to be determined [93]. Thus, although lifestyle factors have known physiological and psychological benefits, further study is required to understand the specific benefit and potential application in older cancer survivors.

Taken on the whole, the evidence suggests, albeit not surprisingly, that lifestyle factors not only are related to primary cancer control and prevention but are also prime targets in reducing the impact of long-term and late effects of cancer treatment in older adults. Therefore, despite gaps in knowledge, there is considerable evidence demonstrating the benefits of healthy diets, regular exercise, and smoking cessation for reducing risk for many common pre- or postcancer comorbidities (e.g., recurrence, second cancers, cardiovascular disease, diabetes, osteoporosis) as well common cancer-related side effects (e.g., fatigue, depression) for which cancer survivors are especially prone [92]. The potential for lifestyle behavior interventions to have a positive impact should be further explored in the context of older cancer survivors.

25.6 CONCLUSIONS

As survival after a cancer diagnosis continues to improve, identification of the long-term and late-stage effects of cancer and its therapy will continue to be critical for survivors of all ages [6,32]. Currently much of the data on late and long-term cancer effects is based on treatments no longer in use and/or from studies that do not include older adults [99]. Studies of late health effects require long-term follow-up, which is particularly challenging in recruiting and retaining older adults. As newer types of cancer treatment are developed, additional research will be needed to assess their impact, especially on older cancer survivors [4,83].

Both cancer survivors and healthcare providers know that recovery from initial treatment is not the end of the cancer experience [8]. As discussed in this chapter, recovering from the physical and psychosocial trauma of cancer may take longer than recuperating from treatment itself and may be amplified in older survivors because of interactions with the aging process. As increasing numbers of older cancer patients experience prolonged survival, they are likely to have ongoing needs related to both their cancer and the accumulating conditions associated with aging. A major challenge for survivorship care of older cancer survivors will be to ensure attention to their long-term cancer-related needs as an integral part of their regular healthcare for the duration of their lives.

The majority of people who are diagnosed with and survive cancer are older adults. Although they represent the largest number of survivors and their numbers are projected to grow even larger in the future, there are few clinical guidelines specific to the unique characteristics of older cancer patients [7]; the survivorship experience of older adults with cancer is relatively unstudied. We have very little evidence regarding the impact of long-term and late-stage effects of cancer in older cancer patients who are living a decade or two postdiagnosis. A research emphasis on older adult cancer survivors is critically needed.

REFERENCES

1. Horner MJ, Ries LAG, Krapcho M, et al. *SEER Cancer Statistics Review, 1975–2006*, National Cancer Institute, Bethesda, MD, 2008.

2. Edwards BK, Howe HL, Ries LA, et al. Annual report to the nation on the status of cancer, 1973–1999, featuring implications of age and aging on U.S. cancer burden. *Cancer*. May 15 2002;**94**(10):2766–2792.

3. Hewitt M, Rowland JH, Yancik R. Cancer survivors in the United States: Age, health, and disability. *J Gerontol A Biol Sci Med Sci* 2003;**58**(1):82–91.

4. Arriagada R, Averbeck D, Dahl AA, et al. OECI Workshop on late side-effects of cancer treatments. *Eur J Cancer* 2009;**45**(3):354–359.

5. Aziz NM. Late effects of cancer treatments. In Chang AE, Ganz PA, Hayes DF, et al., eds. *Oncology: An Evidence-Based Approach*, Springer Science + Business Media, New York, 2006, pp. 1768–1790.

6. Stein KD, Syrjala KL, Andrykowski MA. Physical and psychological long-term and late effects of cancer. *Cancer* 2008;**112**(11 Suppl):2577–2592.

7. Cancer in elderly people: Workshop Proceedings Organization: National Cancer Policy Forum (U.S.). The National Academies Press, 2007, Washington, DC.

8. From Cancer Patient to Cancer Survivor–Lost in Transition: An American Society of Clinical Oncology and Institute of Medicine Symposium Organization: Institute of Medicine, National Research Council. Institute of Medicine (IOM). The National Academies Press 2005, Washington DC.

9. Soran A, D'Angelo G, Begovic M, et al. Breast cancer-related lymphedema—what are the significant predictors and how they affect the severity of lymphedema? *Breast J* 2006; **12**(6):536–543.

10. Kornblith AB, Herndon JE, 2nd, Weiss RB, et al. Long-term adjustment of survivors of early-stage breast carcinoma, 20 years after adjuvant chemotherapy. *Cancer* 2003;**98**(4):679–689.

11. Clough-Gorr KM, Ganz PA, Silliman RA. Older breast cancer survivors: Factors associated with self-reported symptoms of persistent lymphedema over 7 years of follow-up. *Breast J* 2010;**16**(2):147–155.

12. Kwan W, Jackson J, Weir LM, Dingee C, McGregor G, Olivotto IA. Chronic arm morbidity after curative breast cancer treatment: Prevalence and impact on quality of life. *J Clin Oncol* 2002;**20**(20):4242–4248.

13. Paskett ED, Stark N. Lymphedema: Knowledge, treatment, and impact among breast cancer survivors. *Breast J* 2000;**6**(6):373–378.

14. Passik ML, Newman ML, Brennan M. Predictors of psychological distress, sexual dysfunction and physical functioning among women with upper extremity lymphedema related to breast cancer. *Psychooncology* 1995;**4**(4):255–263.

15. Erickson VS, Pearson ML, Ganz PA, Adams J, Kahn KL. Arm edema in breast cancer patients. *J Natl Cancer Inst* 2001;**93**(2):96–111.

16. Stanford JL, Feng Z, Hamilton AS, et al. Urinary and sexual function after radical prostatectomy for clinically localized prostate cancer: The Prostate Cancer Outcomes Study. *JAMA* 2000;**283**(3):354–360.

17. Gore JL, Kwan L, Lee SP, Reiter RE, Litwin MS. Survivorship beyond convalescence: 48-month quality-of-life outcomes after treatment for localized prostate cancer. *J Natl Cancer Inst* 2009;**101**(12):888–892.

18. Nelson CJ, Lee JS, Gamboa MC, Roth AJ. Cognitive effects of hormone therapy in men with prostate cancer: a review. *Cancer* 2008;**113**(5):1097–1106.

19. Chen RC, Clark JA, Manola J, Talcott JA. Treatment "mismatch" in early prostate cancer: Do treatment choices take patient quality of life into account? *Cancer* 2008;**112**(1):61–68.

20. Clark JA, Wray NP, Ashton CM. Living with treatment decisions: Regrets and quality of life among men treated for metastatic prostate cancer. *J Clin Oncol* 2001;**19**(1):72–80.

21. Talcott JA, Manola J, Clark JA, et al. Time course and predictors of symptoms after primary prostate cancer therapy. *J Clin Oncol* 2003;**21**(21):3979–3986.

22. National Cancer Institute. *Chemotherapy-Induced Peripheral Neuropathy*, NCI, Bethesda, MD, Feb. 23, 2010.

23. Hausheer FH, Schilsky RL, Bain S, Berghorn EJ, Lieberman F. Diagnosis, management, and evaluation of chemotherapy-induced peripheral neuropathy. *Semin Oncol* 2006;**33**(1):15–49.

24. Stubblefield MD, Burstein HJ, Burton AW, et al. NCCN task force report: Management of neuropathy in cancer. *J Natl Compr Canc Netw* 2009;**7**(Suppl 5):S1–S26; quiz S27–S28.

25. Fossa SD, Vassilopoulou-Sellin R, Dahl AA. Long term physical sequelae after adult-onset cancer. *J Cancer Surviv* 2008;**2**(1):3–11.

26. Deimling GT, Bowman KF, Wagner LJ. The effects of cancer-related pain and fatigue on functioning of older adult, long-term cancer survivors. *Cancer Nurs* 2007;**30**(6):421–433.

27. Avis NE, Deimling GT. Cancer survivorship and aging. *Cancer* 2008;**113**(12 Suppl): 3519–3529.

28. Respini D, Jacobsen PB, Thors C, Tralongo P, Balducci L. The prevalence and correlates of fatigue in older cancer patients. *Crit Rev Oncol Hematol* 2003;**47**(3):273–279.

29. Luctkar-Flude MF, Groll DL, Tranmer JE, Woodend K. Fatigue and physical activity in older adults with cancer: A systematic review of the literature. *Cancer Nurs* 2007;**30**(5):E35–E45.

30. Knols R, Aaronson NK, Uebelhart D, Fransen J, Aufdemkampe G. Physical exercise in cancer patients during and after medical treatment: A systematic review of randomized and controlled clinical trials. *J Clin Oncol* 2005;**23**(16):3830–3842.

31. Hayat MJ, Howlader N, Reichman ME, Edwards BK. Cancer statistics, trends, and multiple primary cancer analyses from the Surveillance, Epidemiology, and End Results (SEER) Program. *Oncologist* 2007;**12**(1):20–37.

32. Travis LB. The epidemiology of second primary cancers. *Cancer Epidemiol Biomarkers Prev* 2006;**15**(11):2020–2026.

33. Luciani A, Ascione G, Marussi D, et al. Clinical analysis of multiple primary malignancies in the elderly. *Med Oncol* 2009;**26**(1):27–31.

34. Mariotto AB, Rowland JH, Ries LA, Scoppa S, Feuer EJ. Multiple cancer prevalence: A growing challenge in long-term survivorship. *Cancer Epidemiol Biomarkers Prev* 2007;16(3):566–571.

35. Ng AK, Travis LB. Second primary cancers: An overview. *Hematol Oncol Clin North Am* 2008;**22**(2):271–289, vii.

36. Clarke M, Collins R, Darby S, et al. Effects of radiotherapy and of differences in the extent of surgery for early breast cancer on local recurrence and 15-year survival: An overview of the randomised trials. *Lancet* 2005;**366**(9503):2087–2106.

37. Hill-Kayser CE, Harris EE, Hwang WT, Solin LJ. Twenty-year incidence and patterns of contralateral breast cancer after breast conservation treatment with radiation. *Int J Radiat Oncol Biol Phys* 2006;**66**(5):1313–1319.

38. Neugut AI, Robinson E, Lee WC, Murray T, Karwoski K, Kutcher GJ. Lung cancer after radiation therapy for breast cancer. *Cancer* 1993;**71**(10):3054–3057.

39. Roychoudhuri R, Evans H, Robinson D, Moller H. Radiation-induced malignancies following radiotherapy for breast cancer. *Br J Cancer* 2004;**91**(5):868–872.

40. Fisher B, Costantino JP, Wickerham DL, et al. Tamoxifen for prevention of breast cancer: Report of the National Surgical Adjuvant Breast and Bowel Project P-1 Study. *J Natl Cancer Inst* 1998;**90**(18):1371–1388.

41. Campone M, Roche H, Kerbrat P, et al. Secondary leukemia after epirubicin-based adjuvant chemotherapy in operable breast cancer patients: 16 years experience of the French Adjuvant Study Group. *Ann Oncol* 2005;**16**(8):1343–1351.

42. Park MJ, Park YH, Ahn HJ, et al. Secondary hematological malignancies after breast cancer chemotherapy. *Leuk Lymphoma* 2005;**46**(8):1183–1188.

43. Glanz KL et al. The psychological impact of breast cancer: A critical review. *Ann Behav Med* 1992;**14**(3):204–212.

44. Kornblith AB, Powell M, Regan MM, et al. Long-term psychosocial adjustment of older vs younger survivors of breast and endometrial cancer. *Psychooncology* 2007;**16**(10):895–903.

45. Zebrack BJ, Yi J, Petersen L, Ganz PA. The impact of cancer and quality of life for long-term survivors. *Psychooncology* 2008;**17**(9):891–900.

46. Keating NL, Norredam M, Landrum MB, Huskamp HA, Meara E. Physical and mental health status of older long-term cancer survivors. *J Am Geriatr Soc* 2005;**53**(12):2145–2152.

47. Wedding U, Pientka L, Hoffken K. Quality-of-life in elderly patients with cancer: A short review. *Eur J Cancer* 2007;**43**(15):2203–2210.

48. Rao AV, Demark-Wahnefried W. The older cancer survivor. *Crit Rev Oncol Hematol* 2006;**60**(2):131–143.

49. Clough-Gorr KM, Ganz PA, Silliman RA. Older breast cancer survivors: Factors associated with change in emotional well-being. *J Clin Oncol* 2007;**25**(11):1334–1340.

50. Deimling GT, Sterns S, Bowman KF, Kahana B. The health of older-adult, long-term cancer survivors. *Cancer Nurs* 2005;**28**(6):415–424.

51. Pasetto LM, Falci C, Compostella A, Sinigaglia G, Rossi E, Monfardini S. Quality of life in elderly cancer patients. *Eur J Cancer* 2007;**43**(10):1508–1513.

52. Reeve BB, Potosky AL, Smith AW, et al. Impact of cancer on health-related quality of life of older Americans. *J Natl Cancer Inst* 2009;**101**(12):860–868.

53. Ebright PR, Lyon B. Understanding hope and factors that enhance hope in women with breast cancer. *Oncol Nurs Forum* 2002;**29**(3):561–568.

54. Koopman C, Hermanson K, Diamond S, Angell K, Spiegel D. Social support, life stress, pain and emotional adjustment to advanced breast cancer. *Psychooncology* 1998;**7**(2):101–111.

55. Maunsell E, Brisson J, Deschenes L. Psychological distress after initial treatment of breast cancer. Assessment of potential risk factors. *Cancer* 1992;**70**(1):120–125.

56. Andersen BL. Psychological interventions for cancer patients to enhance the quality of life. *J Consult Clin Psychol* 1992;**60**(4):552–568.

57. Classen C, Butler LD, Koopman C, et al. Supportive-expressive group therapy and distress in patients with metastatic breast cancer: A randomized clinical intervention trial. *Arch Gen Psychiatry* 2001;**58**(5):494–501.

58. Targ EF, Levine EG. The efficacy of a mind-body-spirit group for women with breast cancer: A randomized controlled trial. *Gen Hosp Psychiatry* 2002;**24**(4):238–248.

59. Spoletini I, Gianni W, Repetto L, et al. Depression and cancer: An unexplored and unresolved emergent issue in elderly patients. *Crit Rev Oncol Hematol* 2008;**65**(2):143–155.

60. de Jonge P, Ormel J, Slaets JP, et al. Depressive symptoms in elderly patients predict poor adjustment after somatic events. *Am J Geriatr Psychiatry* 2004;**12**(1):57–64.

61. Krishnan KR, Delong M, Kraemer H, et al. Comorbidity of depression with other medical diseases in the elderly. *Biol Psychiatry* 2002;**52**(6):559–588.

62. Geerlings SW, Beekman AT, Deeg DJ, Twisk JW, Van Tilburg W. The longitudinal effect of depression on functional limitations and disability in older adults: An eight-wave prospective community-based study. *Psychol Med* 2001;**31**(8):1361–1371.

63. Penninx BW, Geerlings SW, Deeg DJ, van Eijk JT, van Tilburg W, Beekman AT. Minor and major depression and the risk of death in older persons. *Arch Gen Psychiatry* 1999;**56**(10):889–895.

64. Massie MJ. Prevalence of depression in patients with cancer. *J Natl Cancer Inst Monogr* 2004;**32**:57–71.

65. Townsend AL, Ishler KJ, Bowman KF, Rose JH, Peak NJ. Health and well-being in older married female cancer survivors. *J Am Geriatr Soc* 2009;**57**(Suppl 2):S286–288.

66. Rao A, Cohen HJ. Symptom management in the elderly cancer patient: Fatigue, pain, and depression. *J Natl Cancer Inst Monogr* 2004;**32**:150–157.

67. Soltow D, Given BA, Given CW. Relationship between age and symptoms of pain and fatigue in adults undergoing treatment for cancer. *Cancer Nurs* (2010);**33**(4):296–303.

68. Extermann M. Older patients, cognitive impairment, and cancer: An increasingly frequent triad. *J Natl Compr Canc Netw* 2005;**3**(4):593–596.

69. Deimling GT, Arendt JA, Kypriotakis G, Bowman KF. Functioning of older, long-term cancer survivors: The role of cancer and comorbidities. *J Am Geriatr Soc* 2009;**57**(Suppl 2): S289–S292.

70. Lazovich D, Robien K, Cutler G, Virnig B, Sweeney C. Quality of life in a prospective cohort of elderly women with and without cancer. *Cancer* 2009;**115**(18 Suppl):4283–4297.

71. Given B, Given CW. Cancer treatment in older adults: Implications for psychosocial research. *J Am Geriatr Soc* 2009;**57**(Suppl 2):S283–S285.

72. Ness KK, Wall MM, Oakes JM, Robison LL, Gurney JG. Physical performance limitations and participation restrictions among cancer survivors: A population-based study. *Ann Epidemiol* 2006;**16**(3):197–205.

73. Heidrich SM, Egan JJ, Hengudomsub P, Randolph SM. Symptoms, symptom beliefs, and quality of life of older breast cancer survivors: A comparative study. *Oncol Nurs Forum* 2006;**33**(2):315–322.

74. Mao JJ, Armstrong K, Bowman MA, Xie SX, Kadakia R, Farrar JT. Symptom burden among cancer survivors: Impact of age and comorbidity. *J Am Board Fam Med* 2007; **20**(5):434–443.

75. Hildebrand J. Neurological complications of cancer chemotherapy. *Curr Opin Oncol* 2006; **18**(4):321–324.

76. Robb C, Boulware D, Overcash J, Extermann M. Patterns of care and survival in cancer patients with cognitive impairment. *Crit Rev Oncol Hematol* 2010; **74**(3):218–224.

77. Maunsell E, Brisson J, Deschenes L. Arm problems and psychological distress after surgery for breast cancer. *Can J Surg* 1993;**36**(4):315–320.

78. Schootman M, Aft R, Jeffe DB. An evaluation of lower-body functional limitations among long-term survivors of 11 different types of cancers. *Cancer* 2009;**115**(22):5329–5338.

79. Sweeney C, Schmitz KH, Lazovich D, Virnig BA, Wallace RB, Folsom AR. Functional limitations in elderly female cancer survivors. *J Natl Cancer Inst* 2006;**98**(8):521–529.

80. Luciani A, Jacobsen PB, Extermann M, et al. Fatigue and functional dependence in older cancer patients. *Am J Clin Oncol* 2008;**31**(5):424–430.

81. Pallis AG, Fortpied C, Wedding U, et al. EORTC elderly task force position paper: Approach to the older cancer patient. *Eur J Cancer* 2010; **46**(9):1502–1513.

82. Khuri FR, Kim ES, Lee JJ, et al. The impact of smoking status, disease stage, and index tumor site on second primary tumor incidence and tumor recurrence in the head and neck retinoid chemoprevention trial. *Cancer Epidemiol Biomarkers Prev* 2001;**10**(8):823–829.

83. Yancik R, Ries LA. Cancer in older persons: An international issue in an aging world. *Semin Oncol* 2004;**31**(2):128–136.

84. Ganz PA, Casillas J, Hahn EE. Ensuring quality care for cancer survivors: Implementing the survivorship care plan. *Semin Oncol Nurs* 2008;**24**(3):208–217.

85. Lash TL, Clough-Gorr K, Silliman RA. Reduced rates of cancer-related worries and mortality associated with guideline surveillance after breast cancer therapy. *Breast Cancer Res Treat* 2005;**89**(1):61–67.

86. Lash TL, Fox MP, Buist DS, et al. Mammography surveillance and mortality in older breast cancer survivors. *J Clin Oncol* 2007;**25**(21):3001–3006.

87. Earle CC, Neville BA. Under use of necessary care among cancer survivors. *Cancer* 2004;**101**(8):1712–1719.

88. Ellison GL, Warren JL, Knopf KB, Brown ML. Racial differences in the receipt of bowel surveillance following potentially curative colorectal cancer surgery. *Health Serv Res* 2003;**38**(6 Pt 2):1885–1903.

89. Keating NL, Landrum MB, Guadagnoli E, Winer EP, Ayanian JZ. Factors related to underuse of surveillance mammography among breast cancer survivors. *J Clin Oncol* 2006;**24**(1):85–94.

90. Stull VB, Snyder DC, Demark-Wahnefried W. Lifestyle interventions in cancer survivors: Designing programs that meet the needs of this vulnerable and growing population. *J Nutr* 2007;**137**(1 Suppl):243S–248S.

91. Fairley TL, Hawk H, Pierre S. Health behaviors and quality of life of cancer survivors in Massachusetts, 2006: Data use for comprehensive cancer control. *Prev Chronic Dis* 2010;**7**(1):A09.

92. Demark-Wahnefried W, Morey MC, Sloane R, Snyder DC, Cohen HJ. Promoting healthy lifestyles in older cancer survivors to improve health and preserve function. *J Am Geriatr Soc* 2009;**57**(Suppl 2):S262–S264.

93. Demark-Wahnefried W, Pinto BM, Gritz ER. Promoting health and physical function among cancer survivors: Potential for prevention and questions that remain. *J Clin Oncol* 2006;**24**(32):5125–5131.

94. Meyerhardt JA, Heseltine D, Niedzwiecki D, et al. Impact of physical activity on cancer recurrence and survival in patients with stage III colon cancer: Findings from CALGB 89803. *J Clin Oncol* 2006;**24**(22):3535–3541.

95. Courneya KS. Exercise in cancer survivors: An overview of research. *Med Sci Sports Exer* 2003;**35**(11):1846–1852.

96. Galvao DA, Newton RU. Review of exercise intervention studies in cancer patients. *J Clin Oncol* 2005;**23**(4):899–909.

97. Meyerhardt JA, Niedzwiecki D, Hollis D, et al. Association of dietary patterns with cancer recurrence and survival in patients with stage III colon cancer. *JAMA* 2007;**298**(7):754–764.

98. Rock CL, Demark-Wahnefried W. Nutrition and survival after the diagnosis of breast cancer: A review of the evidence. *J Clin Oncol* 2002;**20**(15):3302–3316.

99. Aziz NM. Long-term cancer survivors: Research issues and care needs in a key phase of the survivorship spectrum. *Am J Hematol* 2009;**84**(12):782–784.

PART VII

END-OF-LIFE CARE

CHAPTER 26

Palliative Care for Cancer Patients and Their Families

CARDINALE SMITH

Division of Hematology/Medical Oncology and Department of Geriatrics and Palliative Medicine, Mount Sinai School of Medicine, New York, NY

DIANE MEIER

Department of Geriatrics and Palliative Medicine, Mount Sinai School of Medicine, New York, NY

26.1 INTRODUCTION

Palliative care is medical care focused on the relief from suffering and support for the best possible quality of life for patients and their families facing serious, life-threatening illness [1]. Palliative care is given concurrently with other disease-modifying, life-prolonging, and curative therapy. Palliative medicine specialists focus on helping patients and their families cope with a variety of care needs, including symptom control; psychosocial support; physician–patient communication; addressing care goals in relation to the patient's condition, prognosis, values, and preferences; and with transitions in care. Cancer patients often experience significant symptom distress either from the illness itself or from the associated treatments. As such, palliative care should be given throughout the trajectory of cancer care whether during early-stage disease, in which the focus is on cure, or in more advanced disease, when the focus is on maximizing quality of life. Currently, national and international organizations have clinical guidelines that recommend palliative care be routinely integrated into comprehensive cancer care [2–5].

The proportion of the population over the age of 65 is growing, particularly in the United States. Data show that the risk of developing cancer for those aged >65 years is 11 times greater than those aged <65 years [6,7]. Additionally, more than half of all diagnosed cancers and approximately 70% of all cancer deaths in the United States occur in individuals >65 years of age [6,7]. Moreover, it is estimated that by 2030, 70% of all cancers will occur in the elderly. Thus, the integration of palliative care into comprehensive cancer care will become even more important as the population ages [6].

Cancer and Aging Handbook: Research and Practice, First Edition. Edited by Keith M. Bellizzi and Margot A. Gosney.
© 2012 Wiley-Blackwell. Published 2012 by John Wiley & Sons, Inc.

26.2 WHOLE-PATIENT ASSESSMENT

The initial palliative care patient assessment involves evaluating all aspects of the impact of cancer and its treatments on the patient and family. Although there are many assessment tools in use for clinical and research purposes, none are considered standard [8]. The assessment should include an evaluation of the medical, psychological, social, spiritual, and practical needs of patients. Since the needs of each patient are vastly different, the assessment should be performed with an interdisciplinary team (physician, nurse, social worker, nutritionist, etc.). This assessment can begin with the standard history and physical exam, should include the impact of the cancer diagnosis on patient's quality of life, patient's expectations of therapy, and goals of care. In elderly patients it is important to include a comprehensive geriatric assessment that includes evaluating functional status, comorbid medical conditions, cognition, detailed medication review, and nutritional status [9]. The comprehensive geriatric assessment and its components are thoroughly detailed elsewhere in this book.

26.3 COMMUNICATION

Breaking bad news is often a main component of communicating with cancer patients and their families. Despite this, however, few oncologists report receiving formal training in breaking bad news or having the opportunity to observe interviews where bad news was being delivered during training. In an American Society of Clinical Oncology (ASCO) survey conducted in 1998, 38% of oncologists reported breaking bad news was a traumatic experience with a patient [10]. Similarly, in a survey conducted at the 2004 ASCO meeting, oncology fellows reported being more likely to have observation and feedback on bone marrow biopsies than on goals of care discussions [11]. This lack of training can have a negative impact on cancer patients and providers. Poor communication skills have been associated with decreased patient participation in decisionmaking [12], missed opportunities to respond empathically to patient concerns, ignored patient wishes to discuss health-related quality-of-life (QOL) issues, and an increased likelihood of receiving anticancer treatment at the end of life [13]. Alternatively, effective communication has been shown to influence desirable outcomes such as patient satisfaction, compliance with treatments, decreased patient distress, and shared decision-making in cancer care [14,15].

There are existing protocols to help deliver bad news and address goals of care (Table 26.1) [16,17]. These protocols can be applied to most situations of breaking bad news, including a new diagnosis of cancer, cancer recurrence, progression of disease, and transition to hospice. While there are no studies validating the effectiveness of these protocols, they represent best practices and are consistent with patient preferences [18]. Moreover, these protocols can provide a framework for organizing the discussion and allow the physician to focus on the patient or family's responses. When communicating with patients and families it is important to use open-ended questions such as "What do you hope to achieve at this point in your illness?" or "What are your hopes and fears?" or "What is important in your life?" [17]. It is important to avoid language with unintended consequences such as "There is nothing more we can do for you" or "Do you want everything done for you?" [17]. Instead, try saying "We will do everything to give you the best quality of life" or "We will manage your symptoms very aggressively." Additionally, it is important to avoid jargon or euphemisms, and

TABLE 26.1   Protocol for Breaking Bad News and Addressing Goals of Care

Recommendation	Comments
Create the proper setting	• Prior to the meeting determine the most appropriate participants (family members, and other healthcare providers). • Allow adequate time • Determine what to say prior to the meeting.
Clarify what the patient and family already know	• "What have you been told about your medical situation so far?" • This allows you to correct any misinformation and tailor the conversation based on their prior knowledge.
Explore hopes and expectations of patient and family	• Allows you to distinguish between attainable and unattainable goals
Suggest realistic goals	• Suggest attainable goals based on the present clinical scenario and how they can best be achieved • Review appropriateness of disease- modifying treatments • Try to explain using simple language why unrealistic goals can not be met
Use empathic responses	• Very important to allow silence and to listen • Let patient and family express emotions • Once emotions are expressed use a connector such as "I can see how upsetting this is to you."
Make a plan and follow through	• Summarize the plan to ensure that your interpretation of the conversation and decisions is in concordance with patient and family and how the plan of care will meet their goals • Make a plan for continued follow-up • Inform the patient and family how to contact you if they have further questions or concerns • Continue to review and revise the plan as needed

Source: Adapted from Buckman [16] and The Education on Palliative and End-of-life Care Project [17].

instead use plain, simple language. Once the goals of care have been established, a care plan can be formulated that includes the patients' and families' desires for treatment.

26.4 ADVANCE CARE PLANNING

Advance directives allow competent patients to express their wishes for future medical care at times of reduced capacity. They consist of two main components: (1) the healthcare proxy or durable power of attorney for healthcare and (2) treatment directives [19]. The proxy directive authorizes another individual to make medical decisions on behalf of the patient if the patient is unable to do so. Treatment directives provide the medical treatment wishes of the patient facing a life-threatening illness or reduced decisional capacity. Treatment directives often address issues such as do-not-resuscitate (DNR) orders, wishes for life-prolonging treatments such as artificial nutrition and hydration, and the use of antibiotics. They should be used as a guide to provide or withhold medical treatments.

Advance directives are particularly important in the elderly cancer patient as they can help avoid confusion and conflict and ensure that patient's wishes for medical care be followed. The SUPPORT trial (Study to Understand Prognoses and Preferences for Outcomes and Risks of Treatment), a pivotal two-phase study that enrolled nearly 10,000 patients at five major US hospitals, demonstrated that physicians knew when their patients preferred to avoid cardiopulmonary resuscitation only 47% of the time and that 46% of the DNR orders were written within 48 h of death [20]. More recently it has been demonstrated that more than a quarter of elderly adults with a terminal illness may require surrogate decisionmaking at the end of life [21]. Advance directives appear to have a significant effect on the outcomes of decisionmaking, with concordance between patient preferences for care and the care actually received before death being very high [21].

Advance directives are also associated with some limitations [19,22]. These limitations include the inability of directives to accurately describe the complexity of medical problems and what medical care the patient wants in real time, lack of patient understanding of the definition of ventilation and other medical terms, and existing directives not traveling with the patient during institutional transfers. In an attempt to address some of these issues, a new form of advance directive, medical or physician orders for life-sustaining treatment (MOLST or POLST), was developed in Oregon and is currently in use or under development in over 30 states [23]. POLST is appropriate for people who already have an advanced chronic illness and a prognosis measured in 1–2 years. It specifically addresses medical decisions and options that are likely to arise in the near future, including cardiopulmonary resuscitation, antibiotics for infections, artificial food and fluids, and whether the patient would want to be rehospitalized. Additionally, it can be transported with the patient across care settings. POLST appears to be associated with better receipt of medical care reflecting patient treatment preferences (decreased hospitalization and life-sustaining treatments) when compared to traditional practices, improved surrogate understanding of patient goals and preferences, and an improved prevalence, clarity, and specificity of preferences documented [24–26].

26.5 ROLES OF FAMILY AND CAREGIVER IN PALLIATIVE CARE

Caregivers are often family members or friends with a close emotional or personal relationship. The majority of caregivers are women; approximately one-third are over the age of 65 and are in poor health themselves [27]. Caregivers serve a crucial role in the management of patients with cancer. Caregivers provide emotional support; act as an advocate for the cancer patient by assisting with communication, decisionmaking, implementation of treatment plans; and help with activities of daily living. It is important to note that the task of the caregiver can change over time and the requirements placed on the caregiver vary by the stage of illness and setting of care. In early-stage disease the caregiver may be involved primarily with emotional support and practical needs. As the disease progresses and the cancer patient becomes more debilitated, the physical and emotional requirements of the caregiver become more arduous. The role of the caregiver, while extremely important for the impact of illness on the cancer patient as well as the caregiver, is often overlooked by healthcare providers.

Palliative care has been shown to improve caregiver well-being and family satisfaction primarily through a focused interdisciplinary team approach to the patient–family unit [28]. It is essential to assess the needs of the caregiver. It is often obvious who the caregiver is; however, the patient should be asked to identify the person whom they consider to be in the primary support role. Encouraging caregivers to network with other families and linking them with formal resources can help augment informal sources of social support [29]. Caregivers can be encouraged to search for national caregiver groups and disease-specific organizations online.

26.6 SYMPTOM MANAGEMENT

Whether disease- or treatment-related, the assessment and treatment of symptoms is important because symptoms can directly influence the elderly cancer patients' quality of life and survival. Currently there is no gold standard for symptom assessment in palliative care [30]. Although several tools exist, the most commonly used is the Edmonton symptom assessment system (ESAS), which consists of nine visual analog scales or numerical rating scales that evaluate a combination of the most common physical and psychological symptoms [31]. The ESAS has been validated for internal consistency, criterion validity, and concurrent validity [32].

Symptom management in the elderly cancer patient has not been extensively studied. The lack of age-specific assessment guidelines and evidence-based guidelines for symptom management for elderly cancer patients has been recognized by the National Cancer Institute as being a limitation in the ability to provide quality care to this population [33]. Nevertheless, the literature suggests that the elderly patient has a higher number of reported symptoms, which include pain, constipation, fatigue, dyspnea, nausea, and vomiting. The management of pain and constipation will be discussed elsewhere. Sections 26.6.1–26.6.3 discuss the evaluation, management, and treatment of the other commonly reported symptoms. When possible, the nonpharmacologic and pharmacologic management will be discussed.

26.6.1 Fatigue

Fatigue is a subjective sensation, which manifests with a wide array of impaired physical, cognitive, and affective functioning. The prevalence of cancer-related fatigue (CRF) is reported to be greater than 50% in advanced cancer patients as well as those undergoing chemotherapy and radiation [34,35]. It is also commonly reported in long-term cancer survivors [36]. Although the exact mechanism is unknown, it is hypothesized that there are two components: a peripheral component that causes negative energy balance leading to fatigue and a central component wherein cancer or therapy for cancer causes fatigue via neuroendocrine dysfunction [37].

It is first important to modify any potential reversible etiology (medications, metabolic and electrolyte disturbances) that may be contributing. Nonpharmacologic interventions for CRF include having the patient prioritize, pace, and delegate activities; schedule activities at times of peak energy; postpone nonessential activities; take naps that do not interrupt night-time sleep; avoid caffeine in the evening; attend to one activity at a time; and engage in distractions such as music, games, reading, and socializing [38,39]. Exercise has been shown to be associated with significant improvement in CRF. A systematic review evaluating randomized controlled trials (RCTs) evaluating the effects of physical exercise on CRF demonstrated that exercise interventions involving moderately intense (55–75% of heart rate), aerobic exercise (e.g., walking, cycling) 10–90 min in duration 3–7 days per week are effective at either reducing or stopping the progression of CRF in cancer patients during and after therapy [40]. Although none of these trials exclusively examined CRF in the elderly, more than half included patients >65 years of age. A significant age-related finding was reported in a study in which age was a negative predictor of exercise adherence for participants 75 years and older [41]. Exercise appears to be beneficial in elderly patients, but the feasibility of exercise in different patient subgroups still needs to be evaluated in future trials [42].

Several pharmacologic agents have been and are currently being evaluated to improve CRF. Thus far, the only active agents associated with improvements in CRF have been psychostimulants (such as methylphenidate, dexamphetamine, and other congeners) and corticosteroids. Again, none of these trials exclusively examined CRF in the elderly, but this population was included in the clinical trials. A meta-analysis showed a small but significant improvement in CRF with methylphenidate over placebo; however, it was not possible to determine optimal dosing [43]. In clinical practice starting doses are usually 2.5–5 mg taken at 8 A.M. and noon with a maximum dose of 20 mg per day. Adverse events related to methylphenidate include tremulousness, tachycardia, and insomnia. Modafinil, which is licensed for the treatment of narcolepsy, is a novel psychostimulant that has been shown in a RCT of patients actively on chemotherapy to improve CRF in those with severe baseline fatigue [44]. Corticosteroids have been shown to be beneficial for some patients with CRF; however, side effects limit their long-term use [45]. Steroids may be most helpful for patients with CRF who are in the terminal phase of advanced cancer.

26.6.2 Dyspnea

Dyspnea is the subjective sensation of difficulty breathing. The prevalence is reported to range be between 21% and 90%, depending on the type and stage of cancer [46–48]. Dyspnea most commonly occurs in those with primary lung cancer or pulmonary metastasis [49], but also occurs in cancer patients without direct cardiac or pulmonary involvement. Diffusion capacity, gas exchange, and lung volumes are all reduced in the elderly, and they are notably susceptible to dyspnea [50]. Patient self-report is the best way to diagnose and manage dyspnea. The goal of treatment is symptomatic relief of the patient's expression of dyspnea rather than the correction of objective variables (tachypnea, low oxygen saturation).

It is important to identify the underlying cause and treat it if possible. The causes of dyspnea other than those related directly to the cancer itself are shown in Table 26.2 along with potential treatment modalities. Nonpharmacologic techniques include elevating the head off the bed, avoiding irritants, opening windows, and using a fan to circulate air. Data suggest that the use of oxygen is indicated only in cases of hypoxemia [51–53]. Opioids are the mainstay of pharmacologic management, and several randomized controlled trials including elderly cancer patients have demonstrated their benefit [54,55]. In opioid-naive patients, a starting dose of morphine sulfate 2.5–5 mg orally or its equivalent intravenously or subcutaneously every 4 h can be effective. In those patients already on opioid therapy, an increase of 25% in the baseline dose may provide relief [56].

26.6.3 Nausea and Vomiting

Nausea is defined as the subjective sensation of an unpleasant need to vomit. Vomiting is the expulsion of gastric contents via the mouth. The prevalence in patients with

TABLE 26.2 Treatment of Specific Causes of Dyspnea

Cause of Dyspnea	Potential Treatment

Airway obstruction	Radiation therapy
	Interventional bronchoscopic procedures
	  • Endobronchial stents
	  • Photodynamic therapy
	  • Cryotherapy

Anemia	Transfusion

Anxiety	Benzodiazepines
	  • Lorazepam 0.5–2 mg PO every 4–6 h
	  • Diazepam 5–10 mg PO/IV every 6–8 h
	  • Clonazepam 0.25—2 mg PO every 12 h

Ascites	Paracentesis
Bronchospasm	Bronchodilators
COPD exacerbation	Oxygen, bronchodilators, steroids (inhaled, PO, IV)
Pericardial effusion	Pericardiocentesis, Pericardial window
Pleural effusion	Thoracentesis
Pneumonia	Antibiotics, antivirals, or antifungals
Pneumothorax	Chest tube
Pulmonary edema	Diuretics
Pulmonary embolus	Anticoagulation

Treatment related
  • Radiation pneumonitis
  • Pulmonary toxicity from chemotherapy
	Corticosteroids

cancer is estimated to range within 30–70% depending on the etiology [57,58]. The most common etiologies in patients with cancer are chemotherapy-induced nausea and vomiting (CINV), and radiation induced, opioid induced, bowel obstruction and constipation. Emesis may be a particular problem in the elderly because they are more likely to experience adverse effects of chemotherapy and radiation, may have declining organ function, and are more likely to suffer some degree of cognitive impairment [59].

The pathophysiology of nausea and vomiting is complex and involves the chemoreceptor trigger zone, the cortex, peripheral pathways, and the vestibular apparatus. Each pathway has associated receptors against which pharmacologic agents can be targeted. Nonpharmacologic measures include avoiding strong smells or other nausea triggers; eating small, frequent meals; relaxation techniques [60]; and acupuncture and acupressure [61]. Progressive muscle relaxation and guided mental imagery during periods of chemotherapy have also shown beneficial effects [60,62]. The most commonly used pharmacologic approach is based on identifying the etiology and administering the most potent antagonist targeted toward the implicated receptors. This strategy has been shown to be effective in ≤90% of patients [63]. While there is a paucity of data exclusively on the elderly, potential drug interactions should be identified, especially since the elderly often have increased comorbidities and are more likely to be on multiple pharmacologic agents. Additionally, thought should be given to selection of the appropriate route of administration of the antiemetic to ensure maximum efficacy. A list of antiemetics, routes of administration, and their properties can be found in Table 26.3.

Classification of CINV includes acute (occurring within 24 h of chemotherapy), delayed (occurring >24 h after chemotherapy), refractory (not responsive to optimal antiemetic therapy), breakthrough (occurring despite antiemetic preventive therapy), and anticipatory (conditioned response to prior chemotherapy that occurs before the administration of the next chemotherapy dose) [64]. Chemotherapy is commonly classified into four levels of emetogenic potential (minimal, low, moderate, and high) [65]. There are well-established guidelines for prophylaxis and treatment of CINV based on the risk stratification of chemotherapy; however, none of these guidelines have specific recommendations for prophylaxis of CINV in the elderly [66–68]. It should be noted that one trial evaluating palonsetron, a $5HT_3$ antagonist, and dexamethasone found equivalent therapeutic rates for the acute, delayed, and overall phases of CINV between elderly and nonelderly patients with no significant differences in toxicity [69].

26.7 THE TERMINAL PHASE

Death is a natural process that will occur for every patient. This can be a time of significant difficulty for patients and their families. The most commonly encountered symptoms in the terminal phase include fatigue, anorexia, delirium, pain, dyspnea, and dry mouth. These symptoms result from a variety of physiologic changes that occur in the last hours to days of life, and a summary of these changes as well as potential treatment strategies can be found in Table 26.4. Delirium can be a particularly distressing symptom for families and often requires pharmacologic intervention. Neuroleptic agents are the mainstay of pharmacologic treatment, and of these agents, haloperidol is the agent of choice, as compared to other antipsychotic agents, it has lower sedating properties, is less anticholinergic, and has fewer adverse cardiovascular effects. Delirium in patients with cancer commonly requires the use of more than one agent [85]. The pharmacologic agents commonly used in the management of delirium can be found in Table 26.5. It is important to prepare patients and families for the typical and normal signs and symptoms of impending death so that they know what is expected to happen. Only medications essential to providing comfort should be continued. While patients and families may still be focused on glucose or blood pressure control, such preventive measures must be taken into the context of the patient's life expectancy. Discontinuation of such medications often involves a detailed discussion about the risks and adverse effects outweighing the probable lack of benefit. The least invasive rate of medication administration should be attempted initially using the most invasive route only when absolutely necessary.

26.8 HOSPICE CARE

The hospice provides a type of palliative care that focuses only on patients at the end of life and is not given simultaneously with other forms of life-prolonging or curative therapies. It aims to provide patients with a life expectancy of <6 months with the best quality of life and comfort. Hospice services include medications, durable medical

TABLE 26.3 **Antiemetics Commonly Used to Treat Nausea and Vomiting**

Receptor Site of Action	Drug Name	Dosage/Route	Adverse Effects
Dopamine antagonists (D_2)	Chlorpromazine	10-25 mg PO every 4 h, 25–50 mg IM/IV every 4 h, or 50–100 mg rectally every 6 h	Dystonia, akathisia, sedation and postural hypotension
	Haldol	0.5-2 mg PO, IV/SQ every 6 h (up to 20 mg/dy)	Dystonia and akathisia
	Metoclopramide	10-20 mg PO, IV/SQ before meals and at bedtime or every 6 h	Dystonia, akathisia, abdominal cramping in obstruction
	Prochlorperazine	10-20 mg PO every 6 h, 5–10 mg IV every 6 h or 25 mg rectally every 6 h	Dystonia, akathisia, and sedation
	Trimethobenzamine	250 mg PO every 6–8 h or 200 mg rectally every 6–8 h	Dystonia, akathisia, and sedation
Histamine antagonists (H_1)	Cyclizine	25-50 mg PO/SQ or rectally every 8 h	Dry mouth, sedation, skin irritation at SQ sites may occur
	Diphenhydramine	25-50 mg PO/IV/SQ every 6 h	Sedation, dry mouth, and urinary retention
	Promethazine (also has activity on D_2 and ACH)	12.5–25 mg PO,IV every 4–6 h or 25 mg rectally every 6h	Dry mouth, dystonia, akathisia, and sedation
Acetylcholine antagonists (ACH)	Glycopyrrolate	0.2 mg IV/SQ every 4–6 h	Dry mouth, blurred vision, confusion, urinary retention, ileus
	Hycosamine	0.125-0.25 mg PO/SL every 4h or 0.25-0.5 mg IV/SQ every 4 h	Dry mouth, blurred vision, confusion, urinary retention, ileus
	Scopolamine	0.1-0.4 mg IV/SQ every 4 h or 1.5 mg transdermal patch every 72 h	Dry mouth, blurred vision, confusion, urinary retention, ileus
Serotonin antagonists[a] ($5HT_3$)	Dolasetron	100 mg PO/IV daily	Headache, prolongation of the QTc interval
	Granisetron	1 mg PO daily or twice a day or 1 mg IV daily	Headache, constipation, weakness
	Ondansetron	4-8 mg PO/IV or dissolvable tablet IV every 4–8 h	Headache, constipation, weakness
	Palonosetron	0.25 mg IV on day 1 of chemotherapy[b]	Headache, constipation, prolongation of the QTc interval
Substance P antagonist	Aprepitant	125 mg PO or 115 mg IV on day 1 of chemotherapy 80 mg PO on day 2 and 3[b]	Headache, infusion site pain, metabolized by CYP3A4 caution with drug interactions

(continued)

TABLE 26.3 (*Continued*)

Receptor Site of Action	Drug Name	Dosage/Route	Adverse Effects
Corticosteroids	Dexamethasone	2-10 mg PO/IV every 6 h	Hyperglycemia, GI Bleeding, insomnia, psychosis
Cannabinoids	Dronabinol	2-20 mg PO daily in divided doses	Dizziness, euphoria in the young and dysphoria in the elderly, paranoid reaction, somnolence
Benzodiazepines	Lorazepam[c]	0.5-2 mg PO/IV every 4–6 h	Sedation, respiratory depression
Somatostatin analogue	Octreotide[d]	100 mcg every 8–12 h IV/SQ or 100mcG/h as continuous IV infusion	Bradycardia, headache, malaise, hyperglycemia

[a]Constipation is reported in about 10% of patients. In elderly patients, who have a higher risk of constipation, supplement with a laxative should be considered.
[b]Have not been shown to be effective in terminating nausea or vomiting once it occurs and should not be used for this purpose.
[c]Best used for anticipatory nausea and vomiting.
[d]Efficacious for patients with bowel obstruction.

TABLE 26.4 Physiologic Changes in the Terminal Phase

Decreased oral intake	• Studies have shown no benefit to parenteral or enteral nutrition in dying patients with metastatic cancer
	• Most common complaint is dry mouth
	• Can use lollipop sponges dipped in cold fluids such as water, lemon flavored drink, or sorbet
Respiratory changes	• Breathing becomes shallow and frequent with periods of apnea
	• This can be natural part of the dying process and family or caregivers should be prepared for these changes
Loss of ability to swallow	• Manifests as a gurgling noise "the death rattle"
	• Treat with antichiolinergic medications
	Scopolomine (transdermal, IV, SC)
	Glycopyrrolate (IV, SC)
	Atropine (ophthalmic drops given orally)

equipment, continuous around-the-clock access to care and support, and bereavement services for families. Most hospice care is delivered at home; however, it is also provided in other facilities such as inpatient hospice facilities, nursing homes, assisted-living facilities, and hospitals. The majority of patients enrolled in hospice are >65 years of age, and about 40% of patients are admitted with a diagnosis of cancer [70].

TABLE 26.5   Pharmacologic Therapy of Delirium

Drug Name	Dosage/Route	Comments
Haloperidol	0.5-5 mg PO/IV/IM/SC every 6–12 h	Most commonly used agent. Can prolong QT interval.
Chlorpromazine	12.5–50 mg PO/IV/IM every 8–12 h	Has similar efficacy to haloperidol, but more sedating, anticholinergic and hypotensive effects.
Lorazepam	0.5-2 mg PO/SL/IV every 4–8 h and titrate as needed	Most commonly used as a second agent in combination with haloperidol. Can also be used as a continuous infusion for refractory cases where deep sedation is needed. May worsen delirium in the elderly. Caution with liver failure.
Risperidone	Start at 0.5–1 mg/day PO and titrate up to 4–6 mg/day	In one study shown to have no differences in side effects when compared to haloperidol[95]. Limited use as only available in oral route.
Olanzapine	5 mg PO qhs and titrated to effect (max 20 mg/day)	Risk factors for a poor response to olanzapine in cancer patients are: • Age >70 • History of dementia • CNS metastases • Hypoxia • Hypoactive delirium
Midazolam	1 mg/hour IV and titrated to effect	Most commonly used for refractory cases where sedation is needed.

Cancer patients and their families have improved outcomes in a hospice. In a study comparing survival of hospice to nonhospice patients, hospice care prolonged the lives of some terminally ill cancer patients [71]. Additionally, there is high satisfaction among families with the hospice care received, with approximately 75% rating the care as excellent. Hospice care has also been associated with lower costs when provided earlier in the dying process [72]. Despite these proven benefits, most referrals to hospice occur late in the dying process. Median length of stay in hospice is 21.3 days, and this has remained relatively constant [70]. On average, nearly 16% of Medicare patients are being treated with chemotherapy within 2 weeks of their death, 16% are being referred to hospice within 3 days of their death, and this trend appears to be significantly increasing over time [73]. Late referrals are associated with greater unmet needs, more concerns, and lower satisfaction among caregivers [74].

There are several reasons for late referral of cancer patients to hospice. First, physicians are inadequately trained in communication skills and prognostication. Additionally, physicians tend to overestimate substantially the survival of patients with advanced cancer by a factor of 5 [75]. Moreover, patients with metastatic cancer have been found to overestimate their survival, which may lead them to choose aggressive therapy rather than focusing on symptom control and maximizing quality of life [76,77]. This has been partly attributed to unrealistic expectations created by physicians and poor patient–physician communication [78].

26.9 SUMMARY

Palliative care is an essential component of comprehensive cancer care and is particularly important in the elderly, who bear the burden of this illness. Palliative care focuses on the family and patient as a unit and uses an interdisciplinary team approach to manage complex physical and psychosocial symptoms. The beneficial effects of palliative care have been well documented. Most recently, early palliative care integration in patients with metastatic lung cancer demonstrated a significant improvement in quality of life, depression, and a 2.7-month survival benefit [79]. While providing palliative care is essential for patients with cancer, certain issues specific to the elderly population must be addressed. Most clinical trials and research on symptom management and quality of life is not focused exclusively on the elderly. While the elderly are included in most trials, the ability to detect differences in this patient population compared to their younger counterparts is often very difficult. Future efforts should be aimed at evaluating elderly patients individually for their palliative cancer care needs.

REFERENCES

1. Morrison RS, Meier DE. Clinical practice. Palliative care. *N Engl J Med* 2004;**350**(25): 2582–2590.
2. Ferris FD, Bruera E, Cherny N, et al. Palliative cancer care a decade later: Accomplishments, the need, next steps—from the American Society of Clinical Oncology. *J Clin Oncol* 2009;**27**(18):3052–3058.
3. Levy MH, Back A, Benedetti C, et al. NCCN clinical practice guidelines in oncology: Palliative care. *J Natl Comprehen Cancer Netw* 2009;**7**(4):436–473.
4. Institute of Medicine. *Improving Palliative Care for Cancer: Summary and Recommendations*, IMI, Washington, DC, 2001.
5. WHO. Pain relief and palliative care. In *National Cancer Control Programmes: Policies and Managerial Guidelines*, 2nd ed., World Health Organization, Geneva, Switzerland, 2002, pp. 83–91.
6. Yancik R. Cancer burden in the aged: An epidemiologic and demographic overview. *Cancer* 1997;**80**(7):1273–1283.
7. Yancik R, Ganz PA, Varricchio CG, Conley B. Perspectives on comorbidity and cancer in older patients: Approaches to expand the knowledge base. *J Clin Oncol* 2001;**19**(4):1147–1151.
8. Richardson A, Medina J, Richardson A, Sitzia J, Brown V. *Patients' Needs Assessment Tools in Cancer Care: Principles & Practice*, King's College London, 2005.
9. Repetto L, Comandini D. Cancer in the elderly: Assessing patients for fitness. *Crit Rev Oncol Hematol* 2000;**35**(3):155–160.
10. American Society of Clinical Oncology. Cancer care during the last phase of life. *J Clin Oncol* 1998;**16**(5):1986–1996.
11. Buss MK, Lessen DS, Sullivan AM, Von Roenn J, Arnold RM, Block SD. A study of oncology fellows' training in end-of-life care. *J Support Oncol* 2007;**5**(5):237–242.
12. Beach WA, Easter DW, Good JS, Pigeron E. Disclosing and responding to cancer "fears" during oncology interviews. *Soc Sci Med* 2005;**60**(4):893–910.
13. Detmar SB, Muller MJ, Wever LD, Schornagel JH, Aaronson NK. The patient-physician relationship. Patient-physician communication during outpatient palliative treatment visits: An observational study. *JAMA* 2001;**285**(10):1351–1357.

14. Baile WF, Aaron J. Patient-physician communication in oncology: Past, present, and future. *Curr Opin Oncol* 2005;**17**(4):331–335.

15. Zachariae R, Pedersen CG, Jensen AB, Ehrnrooth E, Rossen PB, von der Maase H. Association of perceived physician communication style with patient satisfaction, distress, cancer-related self-efficacy, and perceived control over the disease. *Br J Cancer* 2003;**88**(5):658–665.

16. Baile WF, Buckman R, Lenzi R, Glober G, Beale EA, Kudelka AP. SPIKES—a six-step protocol for delivering bad news: Application to the patient with cancer. *Oncologist* **5**(4):302–311.

17. The EPEC Project. *Education on Palliative Care and End-of-life Care*, 2010 (available at http://www.epec.net; accessed 8/02/10).

18. Parker PA, Baile WF, de Moor C, Lenzi R, Kudelka AP, Cohen L. Breaking bad news about cancer: Patients' preferences for communication. *J Clin Oncol* 2001;**19**(7):2049–2056.

19. Fischer GS, Arnold RM, Tulsky JA. Talking to the older adult about advance directives. *Clin Geriatr Med* 2000;**16**(2):239–254.

20. SUPPORT Principal Investigators. A controlled trial to improve care for seriously ill hospitalized patients. The study to understand prognoses and preferences for outcomes and risks of treatments (SUPPORT). *JAMA* 1995;**274**(20):1591–1598.

21. Silveira MJ, Kim SY, Langa KM. Advance directives and outcomes of surrogate decision making before death. *N Engl J Med* 2010;**362**(13):1211–1218.

22. Teno J, Lynn J, Wenger N, et al. and SUPPORT Investigators. Advance directives for seriously ill hospitalized patients: Effectiveness with the patient self-determination act and the SUPPORT intervention. Study to understand prognoses and preferences for outcomes and risks of treatment. *J Am Geriatr Soc* 1997;**45**(4):500–507.

23. *Physician Orders for Life-Sustaining Treatment Paradigm*, 2010 (available at http://www.ohsu.edu/polst/; accessed 8/02/10).

24. Kirchhoff KT, Hammes BJ, Kehl KA, Briggs LA, Brown RL. Effect of a disease-specific planning intervention on surrogate understanding of patient goals for future medical treatment. *J Am Geriatr Soc* 2010;**58**(7):1233–1240.

25. Hickman SE, Nelson CA, Perrin NA, Moss AH, Hammes BJ, Tolle SW. A comparison of methods to communicate treatment preferences in nursing facilities: Traditional practices versus the physician orders for life-sustaining treatment program. *J Am Geriatr Soc* 2010;**58**(7):1241–1248.

26. Hammes BJ, Rooney BL, Gundrum JD. A comparative, retrospective, observational study of the prevalence, availability, and specificity of advance care plans in a county that implemented an advance care planning microsystem. *J Am Geriatr Soc* 2010;**58**(7):1249–1255.

27. Emanuel EJ, Fairclough DL, Slutsman J, Alpert H, Baldwin D, Emanuel LL. Assistance from family members, friends, paid care givers, and volunteers in the care of terminally ill patients. *N Engl J Med* 1999;**341**(13):956–963.

28. Casarett D, Pickard A, Bailey FA, et al. Do palliative consultations improve patient outcomes? *J Am Geriatr Soc* 2008;**56**(4):593–599.

29. Surbone A, Baider L, Weitzman TS, Brames MJ, Rittenberg CN, Johnson J. Psychosocial care for patients and their families is integral to supportive care in cancer: MASCC position statement. *Support Care Cancer* 2010;**18**(2):255–263.

30. Kirkova J, Davis MP, Walsh D, et al. Cancer symptom assessment instruments: A systematic review. *J Clin Oncol* 2006;**24**(9):1459–1473.

31. Bruera E, Kuehn N, Miller MJ, Selmser P, Macmillan K. The Edmonton Symptom Assessment System (ESAS): A simple method for the assessment of palliative care patients. *J Palliat Care* 1991;**7**(2):6–9.

32. Chang VT, Hwang SS, Feuerman M. Validation of the Edmonton Symptom Assessment Scale. *Cancer* 2000;**88**(9):2164–2171.

33. National Cancer Institute. Plans and Priorities for Cancer Research: Spotlight in Research—the Interface of Aging and Cancer 2004, NCI, Washington, DC.

34. Greenberg DB, Sawicka J, Eisenthal S, Ross D. Fatigue syndrome due to localized radiation. *J Pain Symptom Manage* 1992;**7**(1):38–45.

35. Irvine D, Vincent L, Graydon JE, Bubela N, Thompson L. The prevalence and correlates of fatigue in patients receiving treatment with chemotherapy and radiotherapy. A comparison with the fatigue experienced by healthy individuals. *Cancer Nurs* 1994;**17**(5):367–378.

36. Portenoy RK. Cancer-related fatigue: An immense problem. *Oncologist* 2000;**5**(5):350–352.

37. Gutstein HB. The biologic basis of fatigue. *Cancer*. 2001;**92**(6 Suppl): 1678–1683.

38. Rao AV, Cohen HJ. Fatigue in older cancer patients: Etiology, assessment, and treatment. *Semin Oncol* 2008;**35**(6):633–642.

39. Mock V, Atkinson A, Barsevick A, et al. NCCN practice guidelines for cancer-related fatigue. *Oncology* 2000;**14**(11A):151–161.

40. Knols R, Aaronson NK, Uebelhart D, Fransen J, Aufdemkampe G. Physical exercise in cancer patients during and after medical treatment: A systematic review of randomized and controlled clinical trials. *J Clin Oncol* 2005;**23**(16):3830–3842.

41. Courneya KS, Segal RJ, Reid RD, et al. Three independent factors predicted adherence in a randomized controlled trial of resistance exercise training among prostate cancer survivors. *J Clin Epidemiolo* 2004;**57**(6):571–579.

42. Schmitz KH, Holtzman J, Courneya KS, Masse LC, Duval S, Kane R. Controlled physical activity trials in cancer survivors: A systematic review and meta-analysis. *Cancer Epidemiol Biomark Prevent* 2005;**14**(7):1588–1595.

43. Minton O, Richardson A, Sharpe M, Hotopf M, Stone P. Drug therapy for the management of cancer-related fatigue. *Cochrane Database Syst Rev*. 2010, Issue 7, No. CD006704.

44. Jean-Pierre P, Morrow GR, Roscoe JA, et al. A phase 3 randomized, placebo-controlled, double-blind, clinical trial of the effect of modafinil on cancer-related fatigue among 631 patients receiving chemotherapy: A University of Rochester Cancer Center Community Clinical Oncology Program Research base study. *Cancer* 2010;**116**(14):3513–3520.

45. Bruera E, Roca E, Cedaro L, Carraro S, Chacon R. Action of oral methylprednisolone in terminal cancer patients: A prospective randomized double-blind study. *Cancer Treat Rep* 1985;**69**(7–8):751–754.

46. Muers MF, Round CE. Palliation of symptoms in non-small cell lung cancer: A study by the Yorkshire Regional Cancer Organisation Thoracic Group. *Thorax* 1993;**48**(4):339–343.

47. Reuben DB, Mor V. Dyspnea in terminally ill cancer patients. *Chest* 1986;**89**(2):234–236.

48. Dudgeon DJ, Kristjanson L, Sloan JA, Lertzman M, Clement K. Dyspnea in cancer patients: Prevalence and associated factors. *J Pain Symptom Manage* 2001;**21**(2):95–102.

49. Bruera E, Schmitz B, Pither J, Neumann CM, Hanson J. The frequency and correlates of dyspnea in patients with advanced cancer. *J Pain Symptom Manage* 2000;**19**(5):357–362.

50. Mahler DA, Cunningham LN, Curfman GD. Aging and exercise performance. *Clin Geriatr Med* 1986;**2**(2):433–452.

51. Bruera E, de Stoutz N, Velasco-Leiva A, Schoeller T, Hanson J. Effects of oxygen on dyspnoea in hypoxaemic terminal-cancer patients. *Lancet*. 1993;**342**(8862):13–14.

52. Bruera E, Schoeller T, MacEachern T. Symptomatic benefit of supplemental oxygen in hypoxemic patients with terminal cancer: The use of the N of 1 randomized controlled trial. *J Pain Symptom Manage* 1992;**7**(6):365–368.

53. Bruera E, Sweeney C, Willey J, et al. A randomized controlled trial of supplemental oxygen versus air in cancer patients with dyspnea. *Palliat Med* 2003;**17**(8):659–663.

54. Abernethy AP, Currow DC, Frith P, Fazekas BS, McHugh A, Bui C. Randomised, double blind, placebo controlled crossover trial of sustained release morphine for the management of refractory dyspnoea. *Br Med J* 2003;**327**(7414):523–528.

55. Mazzocato C, Buclin T, Rapin CH. The effects of morphine on dyspnea and ventilatory function in elderly patients with advanced cancer: A randomized double-blind controlled trial. *Ann Oncol* 1999;**10**(12):1511–1514.

56. Allard P, Lamontagne C, Bernard P, Tremblay C. How effective are supplementary doses of opioids for dyspnea in terminally ill cancer patients? A randomized continuous sequential clinical trial. *J Pain Symptom Manage* 1999;**17**(4):256–265.

57. Walsh TD. Symptom control in patients with advanced cancer. *Am J Hosp Palliat Care* 1992;**9**(6):32–40.

58. Reuben DB, Mor V. Nausea and vomiting in terminal cancer patients. *Arch Intern Med* 1986;**146**(10):2021–2023.

59. Extermann M, Aapro M. Assessment of the older cancer patient. *Hematol Oncol Clin North Am* 2000;**14**(1):63–77, viii–ix.

60. Burish TG, Tope DM. Psychological techniques for controlling the adverse side effects of cancer chemotherapy: Findings from a decade of research. *J Pain Symptom Manage* 1992;**7**(5):287–301.

61. Vickers AJ. Can acupuncture have specific effects on health? A systematic review of acupuncture antiemesis trials. *J R Soc Med* 1996;**89**(6):303–311.

62. Fallowfield LJ. Behavioural interventions and psychological aspects of care during chemotherapy. *Eur J Cancer* 1992;**28A**(Suppl 1):S39–S41.

63. Stephenson J, Davies A. An assessment of aetiology-based guidelines for the management of nausea and vomiting in patients with advanced cancer. *Support Care Cancer* 2006;**14**(4):348–353.

64. Wickham R. Best practice management of CINV in oncology patients: II. Antiemetic guidelines and rationale for use. *J Support Oncol* 2010;**8**(2 Suppl 1): 10–15.

65. Grunberg SM, Osoba D, Hesketh PJ, et al. Evaluation of new antiemetic agents and definition of antineoplastic agent emetogenicity—an update. *Support Care Cancer* 2005;**13**(2):80–84.

66. National Comprehensive Cancer Network. *Clinical Practice Guidelines in Oncology: Antiemesis*, 2010 (available at `http://www.nccn.org/professionals/physician_gls/PDF/antiemesis.pdf`; accessed 8/04/10).

67. Kris MG, Hesketh PJ, Somerfield MR, et al. American Society of Clinical Oncology guideline for antiemetics in oncology: Update 2006. *J Clin Oncol* 2006;**24**(18):2932–2947.

68. Roila F, Hesketh PJ, Herrstedt J. Prevention of chemotherapy- and radiotherapy-induced emesis: Results of the 2004 Perugia International Antiemetic Consensus Conference. *Ann Oncol* 2006;**17**(1):20–28.

69. Massa E, Astara G, Madeddu C, et al. Palonosetron plus dexamethasone effectively prevents acute and delayed chemotherapy-induced nausea and vomiting following highly or moderately emetogenic chemotherapy in pre-treated patients who have failed to respond to a previous antiemetic treatment: Comparison between elderly and non-elderly patient response. *Crit Rev Oncol Hematol* 2009;**70**(1):83–91.

70. National Hospice and Palliative Care Organization. *Facts and Figures: Hospice Care in America*, 2010 (available at `http://www.nhpco.org/files/public/Statistics_Research/NHPCO_facts_and_figures.pdf`; accessed 8/23/10).

71. Connor SR, Pyenson B, Fitch K, Spence C, Iwasaki K. Comparing hospice and nonhospice patient survival among patients who die within a three-year window. *J Pain Symptom Manage* 2007;**33**(3):238–246.

72. Taylor DH Jr, Ostermann J, Van Houtven CH, Tulsky JA, Steinhauser K. What length of hospice use maximizes reduction in medical expenditures near death in the US Medicare program? *Soc Sci Med* 2007;**65**(7):1466–1478.

73. Earle CC, Neville BA, Landrum MB, Ayanian JZ, Block SD, Weeks JC. Trends in the aggressiveness of cancer care near the end of life. *J Clin Oncol* 2004;**22**(2):315–321.

74. Teno JM, Shu JE, Casarett D, Spence C, Rhodes R, Connor S. Timing of referral to hospice and quality of care: Length of stay and bereaved family members' perceptions of the timing of hospice referral. *J Pain Symptom Manage* 2007;**34**(2):120–125.

75. Christakis NA, Lamont EB. Extent and determinants of error in doctors' prognoses in terminally ill patients: Prospective cohort study. *Br Med J* 2000;**320**(7233):469–472.

76. Weeks JC, Cook EF, O'Day SJ, et al. Relationship between cancer patients' predictions of prognosis and their treatment preferences. *JAMA* 1998;**279**(21):1709–1714.

77. McQuellon RP, Muss HB, Hoffman SL, Russell G, Craven B, Yellen SB. Patient preferences for treatment of metastatic breast cancer: A study of women with early-stage breast cancer. *J Clin Oncol*. 1995;**13**(4):858–868.

78. Smith TJ, Swisher K. Telling the truth about terminal cancer. *JAMA* 1998;**279**(21): 1746–1748.

79. Temel JS, Greer JA, Muzikansky A, et al. Early palliative care for patients with metastatic non-small-cell lung cancer. *N Engl J Med* 2010;**363**(8):733–742.

CHAPTER 27

Pain Management

PAUL GLARE, BEATRIZ KORC-GRODZICKI, NESSA COYLE, and MANPREET BOPARAI

Department of Medicine, Memorial Sloan-Kettering Cancer Center, New York, NY

27.1 INTRODUCTION

In the United States, approximately 60% of new cancer diagnoses and 70% of cancer-related mortality occurs in individuals older than 65 [1–3]. These figures are expected to increase in the coming decades with the progressive expansion of the aging population [4,5]. Older adults with cancer trigger some very unique concerns. Age-related physiologic changes and disease-related changes in organ function affect medication management and response. Frailty and decreased physiologic reserve determine higher susceptibility to adverse outcomes such as institutionalization and/or mortality. Increase in comorbidity may affect survival as well as cancer treatment tolerance. Cancer patients aged 70 years and older have on average three comorbidities, which, in addition to a high incidence of cognitive dysfunction, can affect detection, progression, and treatment of cancer. A diagnosis of dementia is associated with shortened survival [6], and patients who have this diagnosis are likely to be diagnosed with cancer at a more advanced stage and are less likely to receive curative therapy. At the same time cancer therapy may worsen cognitive function in older adults [7]. Symptom management is therefore more complex since cancer may be only one of several coexisting conditions.

27.2 THE IMPORTANCE OF CANCER PAIN MANAGEMENT IN THE ELDERLY

Between 20% to 50% of community-dwelling older persons have important pain problems, and in the nursing home, 70% of residents have pain that is underrecognized and undertreated [8]. Compared with end-stage dementia patients, end-stage cancer patients admitted to New York state nursing homes reported more pain, dyspnea, constipation, and weight loss [9]. An analysis of the data recorded in the Minimum Data Set (MDS) of more than 548,000 nursing home admissions during 2002 revealed that 11.3% of these residents had a diagnosis of cancer on admission [10]. Residents were significantly more likely to be male and older. Compared with other residents at admission,

Cancer and Aging Handbook: Research and Practice, First Edition. Edited by Keith M. Bellizzi and Margot A. Gosney.
© 2012 Wiley-Blackwell. Published 2012 by John Wiley & Sons, Inc.

a significantly larger proportion of these nursing home residents with cancer experienced daily pain, were more dependent in their activities of daily living (ADL) had unstable health patterns, experienced an acute episode or flareup of chronic problems, and were at end stage (with ≤6 months to live). Optimization of pain management is becoming a priority in geriatric oncology. Unmanaged pain is a predictor of loss of function in elders, independent of treatment toxicity or comorbidities [11]. Since older patients have limited reserves, pain can have longlasting and irreversible consequences that compromise cancer therapy, function, and even survival. The possibility that pain may limit movement and induce depression, sleep disturbance, cognitive impairment, malnutrition, and sarcopenia is a special concern among the elderly [11].

27.3   EPIDEMIOLOGY OF PAIN IN CANCER PATIENTS

Although pain is one of the most feared consequences of cancer and its treatment, it is important to remember that pain and cancer are not synonymous. Studies of the prevalence of pain during the timecourse of a cancer illness indicate that approximately one-third of ambulatory patients on chemotherapy have pain [12,13], two-thirds of patients with advanced cancer have pain, and upto 90% of patients with terminal cancer have pain [14]. The prevalence of pain in disease-free cancer survivors also approximates 43% [15].

The incidence of pain varies with the primary site, affecting >80% of patients with primaries of bone, cervix, or head and neck, but <20% patients with leukemia or lymphoma [14]. Cancers of the lung, colon, breast, and prostate are most common in older persons and are frequently associated with significant pain in the advanced stages of disease [16].

It is unclear whether the prevalence and intensity of cancer pain changes with age. Some studies have found that older patients complain of pain 25–50% as often as younger patients, and rate it as severe less often [17]. These clinical findings are consistent with scientific data indicating that pain perception is reduced in the elderly. Nerve conduction appears to be well maintained with age, but the number of nociceptors in the skin and the amount of afferent fibers decrease with age [18], and experimental studies of pain have indicated higher pain thresholds in older patients [19], although there is wide inter-individual variability. The clinical relevance of these scientific data is uncertain, and other clinical studies have failed to find these age-related differences [20]. The inconsistent data may result from variability in cognitive function and the type of pain scales used [11].

It is crucial to understand that cancer pain is not a single entity. Patients with cancer often have multiple concurrent pains. In one survey of patients with advanced cancer, only 20% had only one pain, while 33.3% had four or more pains [21]. There are three dimensions of pain classification in cancer patients, and the type of pain influences the optimal treatment.

27.3.1   First Dimension: Pain Etiology

Not all pain in patients with cancer is due to the tumor. Pain may also be a side effect of cancer treatment, including the newer targeted therapies [22]. Treatment-related

TABLE 27.1   Prevalence of Cancer Pain by Etiology, in Different Settings

Setting	Tumor-Related (%)	Treatment-Related (%)	Debility-Related (%)	Unrelated to Etiology (%)
MSKCC outpatient, 1989 [23]	62	25	—	10
MSKCC outpatient, 2009	67	20	5	10
MSKCC hospitalized, 1989 [23]	78	19	—	3
British inpatient hospice [24]	67	5	6	22

Sources: Data from Foley [23] and Twycross and Fairfield [24].

pain such as chemotherapy-induced peripheral neuropathy is more likely to affect the elderly. Pain may also be due to cancer-related debility or due to unrelated painful co-morbidities, such as degenerative disk disease or osteoporosis which are more common in elderly patients. The prevalence of each depends on the clinical setting (Table 27.1) [23,24].

27.3.2   Second Dimension: Pain Onset and Duration of the Pain

Cancer-related pain may be acute or chronic. Most pain related to the tumor is chronic. Acute pain in the cancer patient is typically secondary to diagnostic procedures (e.g., bone marrow biopsy, post-LP headache), therapeutic interventions (e.g., post-surgical pain, mucositis pain posttransplant), or a sudden cancer-associated complication (e.g., DVT, pulmonary embolus). Most of these acute pains are transient and predictable.

Lists of acute and chronic cancer pain syndromes have been developed and are clinically important since the cornerstone of cancer pain assessment is identification of the underlying pain mechanism. But a simple acute/chronic dichotomy can be problematic in practice, as some cancer-related pain may have an acute onset (e.g., pathological fracture of a vertebra or long bone) but then persist unless effective treatment of the underlying lesion is provided. Many patients with chronic cancer-related pain also experience intermittent, acute flares of pain that can occur even though they are taking analgesic medications on a fixed schedule for pain control. These flares of pain are called *breakthrough pain* (BTP) because the pain "breaks through" the regular pain medication. Approximately 50–67% of patients with chronic cancer-related pain experience episodes of BTP [25,26]. Breakthrough pain is associated with more severe and frequent baseline pain, more pain-related functional impairment, and worse mood. Two types of BTP are described: incident pain and end-of-dosage failure pain. Incident BTP breaks through otherwise-adequate analgesia at any time during the dosing interval. Incident pain can be frequent or rare, and can be predictable or unpredictable. It is usually somatic (e.g., movement-related bone pain), but can also be visceral or neuropathic. End-of-dosage failure BTP emerges toward the end of the dosing interval, usually in a consistent and predictable pattern.

27.3.3 Third Dimension: Pathophysiology of the Pain

Cancer pain shares many of the same neuropathophysiological pathways as non-cancer pain. Traditionally, the pathophysiological classification of pain has recognized nociceptive pain (which features normal transmission of noxious stimuli from somatic tissues or viscera to the brain via an intact nervous system), neuropathic pain (which arises from nerve damage in the absence of a peripheral noxious stimulus), and idiopathic pain (which has no noxious stimulus and an intact nervous system) [27,28]. This simple classification has proved useful in the past with regard to initiating pharmacotherapy, but the paradigm is being challenged by progress in basic science. For example, one study has shown that nociceptive pain due to peripheral inflammation can develop a central neuropathic component due to changes in the dorsal horn of the spinal cord (called *central sensitization*) [29], while animal models of cancer pain reveal unique pain syndromes not seen in nonmalignant pain (e.g., cancer-induced bone pain, chemotherapy-induced peripheral neuropathy) [30–32].

Irrespective of age, a comprehensive assessment of the patient is key to the optimal treatment of cancer pain, aiming to identify the underlying pain mechanism (in effect combining all three classifications mentioned above) and the cognitive (meaning of the pain), emotional (affective and existential), and social (personal history and environmental) factors that are influencing the pain experience. While poor assessment has been identified as the principal barrier to effective pain management [33], it must be emphasized that it may take an extended period of time to determine the precise cause of the pain, as more information about the patient and her/his disease comes to light [34]. Analgesia should not be withheld while the assessment is being made and disease controlling therapies administered. Indeed, it will be much easier to investigate the cause of the pain in a patient who is receiving adequate analgesia. The World Health Organization has provided an eight-item checklist for assessing pain in the cancer patient [35]:

1. Believe the patient's pain complaints.
2. Take a detailed pain history and assess the severity of the pain.
3. Include a substance abuse history.
4. Perform a careful physical examination.
5. Order and personally review any diagnostic tests.
6. Consider pharmacological and nonpharmacological approaches to pain syndromes.
7. Assess the psychological state of the patient.
8. Assess the level of pain control afterward.

27.4 ASSESSMENT OF PAIN IN THE GERIATRIC CANCER PATIENT

The assessment of pain in the older adult presents some unique challenges:

1. Older patients are often reticent to report pain, and are more likely to describe pain as "aching," "soreness," or "discomfort." This may be because they believe pain to be an inevitable part of aging, to be expected and tolerated. Reliable

pain measurements may be obtained from older patients, even if they are mildly or moderately cognitively impaired. While absence of changes in vital signs or behavior should not be used as indicators that the patient's pain reports are not to be believed [36], in patients who are severely demented, behavioral observations become important, such as a decline in their functional status; mood changes leading to depression, increased agitation, and confusion; or an altered appetite.

2. Pain scales should be used in the elderly. There are data that using pain assessment scales with elderly nursing home residents greatly increases the frequency of diagnosing pain, especially among the oldest patients (>85 years of age). When assessing pain severity, some elderly patients may better comprehend a vertical pain thermometer to a horizontal scale, and may prefer verbal descriptors to numbers. In the past, experts recommended a scale utilizing "pain faces" in an elderly patient with aphasia or dementia [37]. However, some cognitively impaired or emotionally disturbed patients appear to incorrectly identify the facial expressions with their feelings rather than the pain.

3. Patients with impaired communication present a challenge for the clinician trying to obtain a comprehensive pain assessment. This may include patients with language barriers, cognitive dysfunction, and mechanical ventilation as well as other nonverbal patients. This will be an increasing issue with the increase in the diversity of the racial/ethnic backgrounds of aging adults. Pain assessment for patients with cognitive impairment should be attempted verbally first. Patients with mild to moderate dementia may still be able to report pain and give verbal descriptors. As dementia progresses, the ability to self-report pain decreases [38]. For this patient population, the practitioner should identify (a) pathologic conditions that are expected to cause pain, (b) behaviors that may indicate pain (facial expression, body movement, labored breathing, and others included in the pain assessment and advanced dementia scale [39], and (c) surrogate reports of pain (nurse, aide, family members).

4. As the "baby boomers" begin to reach retirement age, a history of illicit drug use will become more common in the elderly than what it has been in the past. An affirmative substance abuse history complicates pain assessment and therapy (see text below).

5. The painful area should be carefully examined to determine whether palpation or manipulation of the site produces pain. The neurological aspect of the physical examination is emphasized so that syndromes such as spinal cord compression or base of skull metastases are not overlooked [40]. Common sites of pain referral (e.g., shoulder pain from subdiaphragmatic lesions) should be kept in mind when performing the examination.

6. Appropriate diagnostic tests should be performed to determine the cause of pain and extent of disease, and to correlate this information with the findings on the history and physical exam to ensure that the appropriate areas of the body have been imaged and the abnormalities found do in fact explain the patients' pain. As pain may be the harbinger of tumor progression, imaging may need to be repeated.

7. The clinician needs to be familiar with the common cancer pain syndromes (e.g., epidural disease, plexopathies) in order to facilitate identification of the cause so that treatment can be initiated and morbidity (e.g., paraplegia due to

cord compression) prevented or minimized. As identifying a treatable cause is relevant only in patients amenable to further anti-cancer therapy, investigations may be less appropriate in patients with far-advanced cancer on best supportive care or hospice.

8. Unlike the chronic nonmalignant pain patient, a physical basis for pain can usually be identified in the cancer patient. However, anxiety, depression, and other distress are more common in cancer patients than the general population, so the psychosocial assessment is very important and should emphasize the effect of pain on patients and their families, and should address cognitive, affective, and social aspects of the pain. It is important to identify pathological anxiety or depression that requires specific treatment. Extreme suffering and anguish may present as uncontrollable pain; a "narrative" approach to the cancer pain history will enable the physician to better understand the link between nociception, pain behavior and coping styles, and suffering in the individual patient [34].

9. Subsequent assessment is also required and should evaluate the effectiveness of management. If pain is not controlled, determine whether the cause is related to the progression of disease, a new cause of pain, or the treatment. These eight steps of the "initial" assessment should be repeated with each new report of pain

The assessment of BTP requires specific mention. The characteristics of BTP vary from person to person, including the duration of the breakthrough episode and possible causes. Generally, BTP is transient, lasting seconds to minutes, but may occasionally be present for hours, and often occurs several times a day. BTP can happen unexpectedly for no obvious reason, or it may be triggered by a specific activity, such as coughing, moving, or going to the bathroom. Importantly, the cause of the BTP may not be the same as that of the baseline chronic pain. For all these reasons, BTP needs as thorough a clinical evaluation (proportional to prognosis) as the baseline pain that it relates to: site, radiation, intensity, aggravating/relieving factors, physical exam, and investigations. Pharmacological management is the mainstay of treatment, but as this usually involves taking stronger opioids, often multiple times throughout out the day, the inconvenience and toxicity of extra doses means that treatment of the underlying cause (e.g., radiotherapy, surgery) should be aggressively pursued if treatment is available and the prognosis is appropriate.

A thorough medication assessment is also a key component of the overall pain assessment. Information regarding the medication list, dose, duration of treatment, and reason for discontinuing an agent, if applicable, should be obtained.

27.5 PAIN TREATMENT TIMELINE

27.5.1 Before Initiating Treatment: Medication Management in Older Adults

Pharmacotherapy of the elderly is very complex because of age-related physiologic changes, multiple comorbidities, multiple medications, multiple providers (prescribers and pharmacies), cognitive changes, and caregiver issues. The prescriber's assessment should be multifactorial, including not only clinical but also social, cultural, and economic factors. Older adults with multiple chronic conditions in addition to the cancer diagnosis are at increased risk of toxicity, side effects, and interactions.

Age-related physiologic changes and disease-related changes in organ function affect drug handling (pharmacokinetics) and response (pharmacodynamics). A decrease in lean body mass and total body water and an increase in body fat result in a lower volume of distribution for hydrophilic drugs with higher body concentration and a larger volume of distribution for lipophilic drugs (such as benzodiazepines) with longer times to reach steady state and elimination [41–43]. Drug doses should begin lower and increase more slowly to account for these changes. Decrease in liver bloodflow, size, and mass will result in decreased clearance of drugs metabolized by the liver. Because of reduced enzymatic activity of the cytochrome P450 system, there is increased variability in drug bioavailability. In addition, it is well documented the effects of aging on renal function. Since serum creatinine is not an accurate reflection of renal function in elderly patients, calculation of creatinine clearance is very helpful assisting in determination of the appropriate dose of drugs eliminated through the kidney.

Changes in drug–receptor interactions, homeostatic mechanisms and decreased functional reserves have clinical consequences. Postural and postprandial hypotension are the results of reduced sensitivity of arterial pressure receptors. At the same time, delayed ventilatory response is the result of decreased sensitivity of respiratory centers to hypoxia. Loss of neuronal substance and more ready penetration of drug in the Central Nervous Sytem(CNS) result in higher susceptibility and exaggerated response to drugs with CNS effects

Adverse drug reactions and interactions are very frequent in the geriatric population, and opioids are among the most common drug categories implicated in adverse drug reactions. They can mimic or precipitate geriatric syndromes (such as urinary incontinence, constipation, delirium, functional decline, falls) and, in many cases produce additional unnecessary prescriptions triggering what is called a *prescribing cascade*. It is important to keep in mind that any symptom in an elderly patient may be a drug side effect until proved otherwise.

27.5.2 Initiating Treatment: The WHO Ladder and the Correct Use of Morphine

The American Geriatrics Society has issued guidelines for effective pain management in the older patient [44]. Once the cause of the pain and the psychosocial factors contributing to the pain-related distress and behavior are identified, an individualized multimodal treatment plan can be developed. Ideally, anticancer therapy (surgery, radiation, or chemotherapy) with either curative or palliative intent will be possible that will remove the noxious stimulus and eliminate the cause of the pain. In many cases, however, the pain is due to advanced, progressive disease, and there are no further treatment options available. Provision of analgesia then becomes the main goal of treatment. Furthermore, even if effective anticancer treatment is available, it is necessary to provide analgesia while treatment is being scheduled and taking effect; the use of anti-cancer therapy does not preclude the use of analgesics, and being in pain can interfere with delivering therapy. Nonpharmacologic interventions such as physical therapy, TENS, cognitive behavioral therapies, acupuncture, and other complementary and alternative therapies may also have a role in treating cancer pain and are discussed further below [45].

Analgesics are the cornerstone to management of cancer pain in all age groups, even though the elderly have greater intolerance to NSAIDs, fewer opioid receptors in the CNS, altered ratios of μ- and δ-opioid receptors, and increased sensitivity to opioids [46]. Analgesic drugs fall into three groups: (1) the nonopioids—aspirin, acetaminophen, or nonsteroidal antiinflammatory drugs (NSAIDs); (2) the weak opioids; and (3) the strong opioids. Coanalgesic drugs are often used as opioid sparing agents to reduce toxicity, or when pain does not appears to be completely responsive to single-agent opioids. The sequential use of analgesics of increasing potency according to severity of the pain was proposed in the early 1980s by the World Health Organization (WHO) [35], so is often referred to as the *WHO analgesic ladder*. According to this approach, a trial of opioid therapy should be given to all cancer patients with pain of moderate or greater severity. Some 30 years on, authorities continue to widely endorse the guiding principle behind the ladder, that analgesic selection should be determined primarily by the severity of the pain [47–50], even if the evidence is insufficient for estimation of the efficacy of the ladder [51–53].

The WHO analgesic ladder and cancer pain guidelines recommend that patients with mild pain receive a NSAID or acetaminophen [37,48], but this recommendation conflicts with the current National Comprehensive Cancer Network (NCCN) *Practice Guidelines for Adult Cancer Pain*, which states that the potential side effects of chemotherapy, such as hematologic, renal, hepatic, and cardiovascular toxicities, can be increased by the concomitant prescription of NSAIDs. Patients aged 60 years or older taking NSAIDs or COX II inhibitors plus concomitant nephrotoxic drugs are at higher risk for renal toxicities. NSAIDs also may impair renal function, especially in those who already have compromised renal function due to disease or aging [53]. The WHO recommendation also conflicts with geriatric pain guidelines, which recommended that these agents be avoided whenever possible when treating older patients [54]. A risk/benefit analysis is required for each patient. If they are to be used, a proton pump inhibitor should be coprescribed as NSAID-related gastrointestinal bleeding is common in elderly persons. Absolute contraindications to NSAID use include chronic kidney disease, current active peptic ulcer disease, and heart failure. Relative contraindications and caution include hypertension, *Helicobacter pylori*, history of peptic ulcer disease, and use of corticosteroids or selective serotonin reuptake inhibitors (SSRIs).

27.6 OTHER ANALGESIC AGENTS AND THEIR USE AND POTENTIAL SIDE EFFECTS

Acetaminophen is another step 1 analgesic that is safe and effective for most elderly persons. It lacks many of the toxicities of the NSAIDs but may cause hepatoxicity at doses over 4 g per day, particularly in those with liver disease or a history of alcoholism. Acetaminophen is equally effective as aspirin as an analgesic but will not be as effective for pain that is inflammatory or osseous (from bone) in origin.

Weak opioids currently available in the US include codeine, hydrocodone, tramadol, tapentadol and buprenorphine. These constitute the second step of the WHO analgesic ladder and are recommended for moderately severe pain, or mild cancer pain not responsive to an NSAID or acetaminophen. The need for the second step of the WHO ladder is controversial because low-dose formulations of strong opioids pain have been shown to be more effective than weak opioids for moderate intensity cancer pain [52]. Consequently, many experts now advocate skipping the second step of the ladder and going straight to a strong opioid for all cancer pain of moderate intensity or greater [47,49,55,56]. There has also been controversy about whether weak opioids (alone or in combination with nonopioids) are more effective than nonopioids alone. At therapeutic doses there is no evidence of superiority for one opioid for mild to moderate pain over another [57].

Tramadol is a weak opioid with additional effects on the monaminergic system [58]. At therapeutic doses, its analgesic effect is similar to that of an opioid for mild to moderate pain in combination with a nonopioid [60,61]. The extent to which the dose can be titrated is limited, as at doses just above the normal therapeutic dose, tramadol can cause convulsions and produce serious psychiatric reactions in some patients [58]. Transdermal buprenorphine patches are changed weekly so may be very useful for managing mild-moderate cancer pain in geriatric patients. As buprenorphine is a partial opioid agonist, patients who are currently on a strong opioid need to be tapered off to prevent withdrawal. The initial dose is 5-10 mcg/hr. The dose should not exceed 20 mcg/hr because of the risk of QTc prolongation [59]. For these reasons it appears to offer little advantage over existing opioids for mild to moderate pain in patients with advanced cancer.

Strong opioids are the mainstay of the management of moderate to severe cancer pain. While opioids have been used as analgesics for centuries, it is only quite recently that a systematic review has concluded that oral morphine is effective for cancer pain [62]. Numerous strong opioids are FDA-approved for cancer pain management, but morphine remains the drug of first choice [47], for the following reasons:

- The majority of patients tolerate morphine well, including the elderly.
- It is effective in most cases.
- A wide variety of oral formulations are available, allowing flexibility of dosing intervals.
- It is inexpensive.

Alternative strong opioids to morphine available in the United States include hydromorphone, oxycodone, fentanyl, methadone, oxymorphone, and levorphanol. These should be considered when titration of morphine results in dose limiting side effects. The following 10 principles for the correct use of morphine are based on published guidelines [47,63]:

1. Administer by mouth
2. Administer around the clock, not PRN
3. Start immediate release morphine and titrate up dose
4. Change to sustained release morphine when dose stable
5. Continue immediate release morphine for rescue dosing (BTP)
6. Anticipate and prevent side effects, especially constipation
7. Remember that the oral–parenteral equipotency ratio is 3–1
8. Reduce dose in renal failure because of accumulation of the active metabolite morphine-6-glucuronide
9. Know how and when to use opioid rotation
10. Educate patient and family about morphine

Oral morphine has been shown to be as effective as parenteral morphine, although more drug needs to be given by mouth (approximately triple the IV dose) because oral morphine undergoes extensive first-pass metabolism in the liver. In patients with chronic cancer pain, oral morphine should be given on a regularly scheduled basis, around the clock, to keep the pain under control and prevent the peaks and troughs in blood levels that occur with pro re nata (prn) dosing. The starting dose of oral morphine depends on whether the patient is opioid-naive or is progressing from a weak opioid. Opioid-naive patients should be started on 5 mg of immediate-release (IR) morphine and tolerant patients on 10 mg, given every 4 h (q4h) plus Prn. Even lower starting doses such as 2.5 mg q4h should be considered in the frail elderly. The dose is titrated upward in 50–100% increments every 12–24 h until the pain is controlled. The titration should be on the lower end and slower side of the range in the elderly.

Using this approach, respiratory depression and excessive sedation almost never occur, although the elderly are more prone to side effects such as confusion. Stimulant drugs may be tried to overcome opioid induced sedation, but caution is required in the elderly. It is important to anticipate the side effects of morphine that do occur commonly, especially constipation. Laxatives should be prescribed prophylactically unless the patient has preexisting diarrhea. Nausea is less common than constipation and usually self-limiting, and prophylactic antiemetics are seldom needed.

Once the pain is controlled, the immediate-release (IR) formulation should be converted to one of the sustained-release (SR) morphine formulations to improve adherence. The SR morphine dose is derived by calculating the total daily dose of IR morphine (regularly scheduled plus rescues) and divided by the dosing regimen (1–3 times per day, depending on the formulation). Even though the patient is on SR morphine, a supply of IR needs to be available for rescue dosing in case of BTP. The rescue dose for IR morphine is usually $\frac{1}{12}$th–$\frac{1}{6}$th of the total daily SR dose. The SR morphine dose needs to be reviewed regularly and may require titration upward if there is increasing pain from progression of disease. Transmucosal immediate release fentanyl (TIRF) preparations are also safe and effective for breakthrough pain in opioid tolerant patients. Prescribers of TIRFs and patients using them must enrol in the TIRF Risk Evaluation and Mitigation Strategy (REMS) program before they can be dispensed.

In some patients, the noxious stimulus is eliminated, in which case the dose needs to be reduced [64,65]. A typical tapering regimen is a 25–50% dose reduction every 2–3 days. When tapering, the patient should be educated about possible withdrawal symptoms, and suggestions for abating those symptoms should be given. The dose also needs to be reduced if renal failure occurs, as the active metabolite morphine-6-glucuronide accumulates (presenting with respiratory depression and/or neurotoxicity: drowsiness, confusion, myoclonic twitching) [66,67]. It is recommended that morphine be avoided in renal failure/dialysis patients. In this situation, rotation to an alternative strong opioid is recommended. Fentanyl and methadone are the safest to use [68], although hydromorphone and oxycodone may be used with caution and close monitoring.

Opioid rotation is also required in approximately 25% of patients started on morphine who develop dose-limiting side effects during the titration phase. Rotation may enable the dose to be increased as there is often interindividual variation in side effects for the various opioids. On making the switch, the opioid dose may need to be decreased because cross tolerance between the opioids is limited (see Section 27.6.2). It is important to know the relative potency ratios of the alternatives to morphine; all are more potent, between 1.5 and 100 times (see Table 27.2) [69]. It is important to be sensitive to cost issues for patients when choosing pain medicines as patients may not have insurance coverage for all of them. Methadone is safe to administer in the elderly and

TABLE 27.2 Opioid Equianalgesic Table (Equivalence of Various Opioid Analgesics to 10 mg of IV Morphine)

Drug	Administration Route		Duration (h)	Comment
	IV	PO		
Morphine	10	30–60	3–4	Standard for comparison
Hydromorphone	1.5	7.5	3–4	Multiple routes; available in high potency form (10mg/cc)
Oxycodone	—	30	3–4	Often 5 mg combined with ASA or acetaminophen; longacting form available; shortacting form available as tablet or elixir
Fentanyl[a]	—	—	—	
Methadone[b]	10	20	6–8	May accumulate because of long half-life and result in delayed toxicities; carefully monitor during titration
Oxymorphone	1	10 (PR)	3–4	
Levorphanol[b]	2	4	4–6	May accumulate because of long half-life and result in delayed toxicities during initial dosing or increased dosing
Codeine	130	200	3–4	Metabolized to morphine; often combined with acetaminophen
Hydrocodone	—	30	3–4	Oral formulation only in combination with acetaminophen

[a]Fentanyl at a dose of 100 μ g/h (IV or TD) is equivalent to morphine at 4 mg IV/h or 200 mg/24 h PO.
[b]Because of the long half-life of this drug, much lower doses will be needed for ATC administration. With repeated administration, methadone can be up to 20 times more potent than morphine, and varies inversely with the dose.
[c]Levorphanol also has a long half-life, similar to methadone and lower doses are needed for ATC administration. Levorphanol can be 4 to 8 times more potent than morphine. Wait 72 hours for the patient to reach a new steady-state before a subsequent dose adjustment to avoid excessive sedation due to drug accumulation.

inexpensive, but requires special mention as rotating from other opioids to methadone is not straightforward. While methadone is approximately equipotent with morphine when given short term, with chronic administration, methadone acquires a much greater analgesic effect and becomes 3–20 times more potent than morphine; the ratio is inversely related to the dose [70,71].

In many patients with advanced cancer, parenteral opioids are needed at some stage in the course of their illness either because of a pain crisis or because they become unable to swallow. If patients are hospitalized, the intravenous (IV) route is used; in hospice patients, the subcutaneous (SC) route is used. Intramuscular injections should be avoided. In ≤10% of patients, the spinal route is indicated [72]. Last but not least, when initiating morphine, it is important to educate patients and families on the patient-related barriers to taking strong opioids, including side effects (sedation, respiratory depression), stigma, tolerance, addiction, and fears of approaching death [73].

27.6.1 Parenteral Morphine

Intravenous morphine is usually administered by continuous infusion, with rescue doses administered on demand by clinicians [clinician-activated bolus (CAB)] or self-administered by the patient if using patient-controlled analgesia (PCA). Hospitals will have IV therapy guidelines on how to prescribe and administer IV opioids. Generally, morphine sulfate and hydromorphone can run simultaneously with other solutions, including antibiotics. This is not the case with fentanyl or methadone, for which a separate line is required.

If the patient requires hospitalization because of a pain crisis, IV PCA is preferred. Guidelines suggest a 25% increase in the baseline rate for mild to moderate pain and a 50% increase for moderate to severe pain, but in general the increase should be based on the number of rescues taken. When converting from oral to IV, the IV dose is reduced to one-third of the oral dose, expressed as an hourly rate (e.g., 30 mg oral morphine q4h becomes 2.5 mg IV morphine per hour). Guidelines suggest starting with an IV rescue dose that is half the hourly basal rate q15–20 min or an oral rescue of 10–15% of the total daily opioid dose q1–2h. In managing a pain crisis in an opioid tolerant patient, double that IV dose is administered as a bolus, repeating the same dose in 20 min if there is no relief. If the pain persists at a level >6/10, with no side effects, the IV dose should be increased by 50%, with continued administration of a dose every 20 min until benefit or side effects appear. Once relief is obtained and PCA is to be started, the total amount of morphine that the patient used in the past 24 h is converted into an IV dose equivalent for the past 24 h and converted into an hourly dose for the PCA basal rate, then rescues are ordered. For opioid-naive patients in a pain crisis, morphine sulfate is given in 5–15-mg IV boluses until the pain subsides, and the starting basal rate for PCA is 1–3 mg/h.

When utilizing PCA, staff needs individual instruction on how to assess the readings on the PCA pump and perform other functions. PCA is suitable in cognitively intact elderly provided they have sufficient manual dexterity to press the button, but it is contraindicated in patients who are confused. In those cases, the prn "rescue" button should not be used and can be removed from the pump. Family members should be instructed *not* to push the prn "rescue" button; only the patient should administer the prn rescue dose. Clinician-activated bolus (CAB) is a larger rescue dose (typically double the hourly rate), administered only by a nurse or physician. CABs are useful to assist patients who can not tolerate a recumbent position (lying down) to undergo an MRI or radiation therapy. CABs can also be used for a pain crisis, severe incidental BTP, or other painful episodes. PCA can also be delivered at home with the support of an infusion company.

27.6.2 Opioid Rotation

As previously mentioned, morphine works well in the majority of patients but in ~10–30% of patients, intolerable dose-limiting side effects develop that prevent titration of the morphine dose up to the effective level [74]. In this situation, there are five strategies to consider: (1) continue morphine but treat the side effect with adjuvant medications (e.g., psychostimulants, more aggressive laxatives, antiemetics), (2) continue with morphine but add a coanalgesic drug (e.g., NSAIDs in the case of bone pain or antidepressants or anticonvulsants in the case of neuropathic pain) that will be opioid sparing and allow the morphine dose to be reduced, (3) change the route (e.g., to spinal), (4) try other anesthetic procedures such as a nerve blocks, or (5) change to an alternative strong opioid (referred to as *opioid rotation*).

The underlying premise of opioid rotation is that an alternative opioid will have the same efficacy as morphine but a superior side effect profile, allowing the dose to be increased. Because all strong opioids are μ-opioid agonists, it is unclear exactly how opioid rotation actually works. Possible mechanisms include (1) genetic factors (i.e., differences in drug metabolism), (2) drug factors (i.e., differences in structural formula and opioid binding, binding to μ-opioid receptor subtypes, non-μ-opioid receptor binding, activation of secondary messenger systems, metabolic pathways, and nonopioid activity (e.g., N-methyl-D-aspartate (NMDA) receptors in the case of methadone], or (3) environmental factors (e.g., drug interactions).

There is little high-level evidence for the effectiveness of opioid rotation, and the few well-designed randomized studies of opioid therapy have found no significant difference between agents [75]. However, there is now a large body of anecdotal evidence supporting the effectiveness of rotation, with more than 20 uncontrolled studies involving hundreds of patients indicating that rotation is effective in $\geq 80\%$ of cases [76]. Consequently, opioid rotation is now included in cancer pain guidelines [47], and is commonly utilized in more than 70% patients in one series, with 20% patients having two or more rotations [77]. Not all opioid rotations are made secondary to dose-limiting side effects. Other reasons include comorbidities (e.g., renal failure), availability of formulations and routes, patient preference, and cost. Formulations of the strong opioids currently approved for use in the United States and their dosage strengths are listed in Table 27.3. The principal pharmacokinetic parameters of various weak and strong opioids are summarized in Table 27.4.

27.6.3 Abuse Potential

Abuse of controlled prescription drugs has become a serious problem. In the presence of pain, psychological and physiological factors tend to prevent true addiction from developing, although physical dependence and tolerance will develop with protracted opioid therapy. The experience at MSKCC and elsewhere is that abuse of pain medicines by cancer patients is less common than in general medical populations [78]. However, abuse may potentially afflict the cancer patient, and drug, genetic and environmental factors influence whether an individual will abuse drugs. Opioid administration for pain in cancer patients who have no prior history of substance abuse is rarely associated with significant abuse or addiction [79,80]. Illicit drug abuse had been very uncommon in elders in the past, but as the baby boomer generation reaches retirement age, this is likely to change. Patients in their late 50s and early 60s are now being encountered in the clinic who have a remote history of substance abuse dating from the 1960s and 1970s, and their use of pain medicines should be closely monitored. Older patients without a history of substance abuse also need to be educated about the risks of diversion, especially if they live at home and have school-age children or grandchildren who visit. They should be educated to keep their medicines in a lockbox, and to report the theft of pills or prescriptions to the police.

27.6.4 Coanalgesic Agents

Coanalgesics are agents given to enhance the pain relief provided by an opioid. Some are pain medicines in their own right (e.g., NSAID, acetaminophen, local anesthetics), but most are used primarily for some other purpose. The list of potential co-analgesic drugs is long and may include antidepressants, anticonvulsants, benzodiazepines, skeletal and smooth muscle relaxers, corticosteroids, and antibiotics. The rationale behind

TABLE 27.3   Formulations of Opioids and Dosage Strengths Available in the United States

Morphine
MS Contin	15, 30, 60, 100, 200 mg
MSIR	15, 30 mg
Morphine elixir	20 mg/mL (outside MSK, also available at 1 mg/mL)
Avinza capsule	30, 60, 90, 120 mg
Kadian capsule	20-, 30-, 50-, 60-, 80-, 100-, 200-mg capsules
Suppository	5, 10, 20, 30 mg
Injectable	Multiple strengths available; for PCA, use 1 mg/ml or 10mg/ml.

Hydromorphone
Tablets	2, 4, 8 mg (elixir 1 mg/ml)
Suppository	3, 8, 12 and 16 mg ER tablets now available
Injectable	2, 4 mg/ml; 10 mg/mL for pharmacy use; for PCA, use 1mg/ml or 10 mg/ml concentration

Oxycodone
OxyContin	10, 20, 40, 80 mg
Oxycodone tab	5 mg
Oxycodone elixir	1 or 20 mg/mL

Oxymorphone
Opana	5-, 10-mg tablets
Opana ER	5-, 10-, 20-, 40-mg tablets
Opana injectable	1 mg/mL

Methadone
Tablets	5, 10, 40 mg
Injectable	10 mg/mL; for PCA, use 1mg/ml or 10 mg/ml concentration

Fentanyl
Patch	12, 25, 50, 75, 100 µg/h
Injectable	For PCA, use 50–1 (or 10–1 concentration, if very low basal)
Transmucosal lozenge	200-, 400-, 600-, 800-, 1200-, 1600-µg
Tablet	100, 200, 300, 400, 600, 800 µg

prescribing coanalgesics is that some types of pain appear to be less responsive to opioids than others, and much higher doses of opioids—associated with a higher incidence of side effects—are needed if these pains are managed with single-agent opioids alone. However, prescribing coanalgesic drugs contributes to polypharmacy with its attendant problems of drug interactions, toxicity, inconvenience, and cost, and this is especially so with the elderly. The pharmacokinetics of various NSAIDs, acetaminophen, antidepressants, and anticonvulsants commonly used as co-analgesics are listed in Table 27.5.

Neuropathic pain is the most common example of cancer pain for which co-analgesics are used, and antidepressants or anticonvulsants are the usual agents of choice. Occasionally, coanalgesics are used as first-line options (e.g., for a treatment-related neuropathic pain such as chemotherapy-related peripheral neuropathy), but most neuropathic pain in cancer is due to a tumor mass compressing adjacent neural structures, and an opioid is already being prescribed. The antidepressants and

TABLE 27.4 Principal Pharmacokinetic Parameters of Opioids

Drug	Oral Bioavailability	Protein Binding	Volume of Distribution	Metabolism	Excretion	$t_{1/2}$ (h)
				Strong Opioids		
Morphine	33 (16–68)%	36%	1–5 L	Glucuronidation, active metabolite	Renal, bile	1.5–4.5
Hydromorphone	50%	8–19%	295 L	Glucuronidation	Renal, bile	3
Oxycodone	87%	45%	2.6 L	CYP3A4/2D6	Renal, 19% unchanged	3–4
Fentanyl	Poor	High	60–300 L	CYP3A4	Renal, 10% unchanged	1.5–6 (IV)
Methadone	41–97%	85–90%	Large, variable (140–600 L)	CYP3A4/2D6	Fecal	8–80 h
Levorphanol	—	40%	10–13 L	Glucuronidation	Renal	11–16 h
Oxymorphone	10%	10–12%	3 L	Glucuronidation	Renal, 10% unchanged	1–3 h
Buprenorphine	30–60%; 90% sublingual	High	300 L	CYP3A4	Renal 33%, fecal 66%	4–6 h
Pentazocine	20%	—	—	Glucuronidation	Renal, 5–25% unchanged; bile	2–3 h
				Weak Opioids		
Codeine	12–84%	30%	245 L	glucuronidation; CYP2D6	Renal, 15% unchanged	2.5–4
Hydrocodone	25%	—	3.3–4.7 L	CYP2D6/3A4	Renal, 10–20% unchanged	—
Tramadol	100%	20%	Large	CYP2D6; active metabolite	Renal	—
Tapentadol	—	20%	540 L	glucuronidation; CYP2C9/2C19/2D6	Renal, <5% unchanged	—
Meperidine	Poor	60–70%	300 L	CYP2D6; active metabolite	Renal	3–4; 15–30 (metabolite)

433

TABLE 27.5 Pharmacokinetic Parameters of Selected Coanalgesic Agents

Drug	Bioavailability	Protein Binding	Metabolism	Excretion	$t_{1/2}$ (h)
Acetaminophen and NSAIDs					
Acetaminophen	60–70% oral 30–40% rectal	Negligible at therapeutic doses	80% conjugation; 10% via CYP1A2/2E1	Renal, 5–10% unchanged	2–4
Aspirin	50%, dose-dependent	50–70%	Liver	Renal 5–35%	6, dose-related
Celecoxib	20–40%	97%	CYP2C9/3A4; may inhibit CYP2D6	Renal 25%; fecal 60%	6–12
Diclofenac	50%, dose-dependent	100%	CYP2C9/3A4	Urine 65%; 1% unchanged; 35% bile	1–2
Ibuprofen	100%	99%	CYP2C9	Renal, <1% unchanged	2
Ketorolac	100%	20%	Glucuronidation; <50% metabolized	Renal 90%; bile/feces 5%	3.5–9
Naproxen	90–100%	99%	CYP2C9	Renal 95%; <1% unchanged	12–15
Antidepressants					
Amitriptyline	30–60%	>90%	CYP2D6; also CYP1A2/2C19/3A4; active metabolites	Renal; 20% unchanged	10–50 (average 15)
Nortriptyline	High	—	CYP2D6	Mainly renal: feces	18–44
Venlafaxine	45%	27%	CYP2D6	90% renal, 5% unchanged	5 (metabolite 11)
Duloxetine	50 (35–82)%	95%	CYP2D6/1A2	70% renal, 20% fecal	12
Anticonvulsants					
Gabapentin	33–60%	<5%	Nil	Renal	5–7
Pregabalin	>90%	Nil	Nil	Renal	5–7

anticonvulsants are reasonably effective, with a number needed to treat (NNT) of 3–4, although this figure has been derived from studies of nonmalignant neuropathic pain (diabetic neuropathy and postherpetic neuralgia). The NNT is the number of patients that need to be treated for one to benefit compared with a control in a clinical trial. The higher the NNT, the less effective is the treatment. Most pain medicines have a NNT of 2–6. It was once taught that the neuropathic pain descriptors directed coanalgesic choice—antidepressants for burning, differentiation-type pain, and anticonvulsants for shooting/lancinating (lacerating) neuralgic pain—but this no longer appears to be clinically relevant. Choice of drug will be dictated by toxicity, drug interactions, and coexisting conditions, and this becomes particularly relevant in the elderly.

Among the antidepressants, the tricyclic antidepressants are the most extensively studied and are effective (NNT 2–3), but their anticholinergic side effects are poorly tolerated by elderly cancer patients, and are difficult to recommend as first-line choices in this patient population. Most of the common serotonin reuptake inhibitors, such as escitalopram, are not effective for neuropathic pain, but serotonin–norepinephrine reuptake inhibitors such as venlafaxine and duloxetine are proving to be effective, although less so than TCA (with NNT ~5). Gabapentin and pregabalin are the main two anticonvulsants used nowadays in cancer patients, because of their superior side effect and drug interaction profile when compared to carbamazepine. Carbamazepine is a strong inducer of cytochrome P450 isoenzyme CYP3A4 and causes blood dyscrasias, and so should probably be avoided in cancer patients. Gabapentin and pregabalin may be slightly less effective (NNT 4–5) than the antidepressants but are usually better tolerated; drowsiness, dizziness, and pedal edema are the main side effects. Both work via the same mechanism of action, but pregabalin has some advantages over gabapentin, such as linear pharmacokinetics, faster time to effective dose, and twice-daily dosing. Topical lidocaine 5% patches (applied for ≤12 h per day) are FDA-approved for postherpetic neuralgia and recommended off-label in cancer pain guidelines for malignant neuropathic pain. They are effective (NNT 4–5), have little toxicity other than locally and high acceptability with patients, so they are worth trying if the painful area is not too extensive.

NSAIDs block the cyclooxygenases (COXs), which produce prostaglandin E2 (PGE2) from arachidonic acid. PGE2 is implicated in the production of inflammation and pain, by directly stimulating nociceptors and altering the sensitivity of nociceptors to other pain-producing substances, such as bradykinin, released as part of tissue damage caused by tumor. NSAIDs may also have a role in neuropathic pain as PGE2 has a role in central sensitization of nociception in the dorsal horn of the spinal cord [81]. Two forms of COX exist, and NSAIDS can be classified as to whether they are COX2-selective. COX2-selective agents may cause fewer gastrointestinal (GI) side effects and renal toxicity than the nonselective NSAIDs, but increased risk of thrombotic events has resulted in the recall of all NSAIDs except celecoxib [82].

More than 15 NSAIDs are approved by the FDA, and selection depends on such factors as availability, side effects, contraindications, patient preference, fashion and cost. Unfortunately, NSAIDs are contraindicated in many cancer patients who would otherwise benefit from them because of renal impairment, thrombocytopenia, awaiting an invasive procedure, or being at risk of masking a fever while on chemotherapy. In patients without GI or cardiovascular risk factors, a nonselective NSAID should be used; to reduce toxicity, acidic, short half-life agents such as ibuprofen, diclofenac, or indomethacin are preferred [83]. In patients with GI or cardiovascular risk factors, a selective agent (celecoxib) should be used [83], preferably in low doses.

Acetaminophen is commonly considered together with NSAIDs as a coanalgesic. Although the analgesic potency of acetaminophen and NSAIDs are comparable, their action mechanisms are thought to be different. In the United Kingdom and Australia, acetaminophen is frequently added to strong opioids to improve analgesia, but in the United States it is often used only with weak opioids, in combination. The rationale for adding acetaminophen to a strong opioid regimen is to improve the balance between analgesia and side effects by either increasing analgesia without adding side effects or by maintaining analgesia with fewer side effects from opioids, NSAIDs, or other drugs. Acetaminophen has been shown to provide pain relief without major side effects in cancer patients who have persistent pain even when they are taking strong opioids [84]. Acetaminophen shares none of the subjective side effects of NSAIDs, opioids, or other co-analgesics. It is usually safe and well tolerated in therapeutic doses. Hepatic toxicity is the only serious complication, and the FDA now recommends limiting intake to < 3 gm per day.

27.6.5 Opioid-Induced Constipation

Constipation can be one of the most common and distressing symptoms reported by elderly patients with advanced cancer [85]. Unfortunately, it is often overlooked by the physicians and other healthcare practitioners who are assessing and treating them. Several factors can render constipation prevention and treatment in elderly patients on opioids challenging. These include the additive effects of the underlying terminal illness, especially if there is intraabdominal disease, the patients' limited mobility, and decrease in the intake of food and water and multiple medications with anticholinergic activity. The workup requires an investigation of underlying etiology and should include a digital rectal exam and/or radiological investigation to rule out fecal impaction or bowel obstruction.

The choice of laxatives depends on efficiency, patient preference, cost, and side effect profile. Although a meta-analysis by the Cochrane Collaboration on the treatment of constipation in palliative care patients failed to provide a best option for the management of constipation in palliative patients [86], clinical experience recommends avoiding bulking agents such as fiber in the patient with advanced cancer and instead relying on softeners (e.g., docusate), stimulants (e.g., senna) and osmotic agents [e.g., lactulose or poly(ethylene glycol)]. Suppositories or enemas have a role if there is fecal loading. In patients not responding to these measures, subcutaneous methylnaltrexone is an option that produces laxation in most cases [87].

27.7 COMPLEMENTARY THERAPIES

Nonpharmacologic, noninvasive interventions are important treatment modalities for patients with pain, including the older adult. The NCCN guidelines for management of cancer pain suggest a combination of nonpharmacologic treatment with pharmacological modalities as a standard of care. These nondrug interventions are considered a part of the overall comprehensive pain management plan for adults and are outlined as follows:

1. Physical modalities
    a. Bed, bath, walking supports
    b. Position instructions
    c. Physical therapy
    d. Energy conservation, pacing activities
    e. Massage
    f. Heat and/or ice
    g. Transcutaneous electrical nerve stimulation (TENS)
    h. Acupuncture or acupressure
2. Cognitive modalities
    a. Imagery/hypnosis
    b. Distraction training
    c. Relaxation training
    d. Active coping training
    e. Graded task assignments, setting goals, pacing, and prioritizing
    f. Cognitive behavioral training
    g. Depression/distress consultation
3. Spiritual care
4. Education

Compared to extensive studies that support the use of pharmacological approaches, a strong evidence base supporting the efficacy of many of these techniques is lacking. Evidence specific to the older adult is still to evolve. Patients, however, report finding them helpful in a variety of ways, for example, modifying the pain experience, increasing a sense of control, decreasing anxiety, improving mood, and improving sleep. Some examples of nonpharmacologic approaches that patients may use independent of their clinician's advice are applying heat or cold, pressure, rubbing, meditation, yoga, distraction, and music [88]. Frequently these methods are chosen through word of mouth from family and friends who have found them to be helpful in managing their own chronic pain conditions such as osteoarthritis, osteoporosis, or neuropathies.

The National Center for Complementary and Alternative Medicine (CAM) groups the CAM modalities into five main areas: (1) alternative medical systems (traditional Chinese medicine, ayurvedic medicine, homeopathic medicine, naturopathic medicine, Native American medicine); (2) mind–body interventions (meditation, focused breathing, progressive muscle relaxation, guided imagery, creative visualization, hypnosis, biofeedback, music therapy, art therapy); (3) biologically based therapies, nutrition, and special diets (macrobiotics, megavitamins, metabolic therapies, individual therapies such as shark cartilage, herbal medicine); (4) manipulative and body-based therapies (massage, aromatherapy, reflexology, acupressure, Shiatsu, polarity, chiropractic medicine, yoga, exercise); and (5) energy-based therapies (Reiki, Qi gong, therapeutic touch). Counseling, prayer, and spirituality, which are known to be very helpful to the older cancer patient, are viewed as part of mainstream therapy. Complementary therapies that have the strongest evidence to suggest their role as an adjuvant in the control of pain include acupuncture, massage, hypnosis, relaxation, guided imagery, music therapy, and transcutaneous nerve stimulation (TENS) [45].

As with pain control in general, a variety of factors promote or inhibit the use of these nondrug techniques. Barriers can be clinician-related or patient-related. Physician-related barriers are usually associated with unfamiliarity with the techniques, not knowing who within the team has expertise in the area, lack of interest, greater comfort with pharmacotherapy, and time constraints. Among patient-related barriers are uncertainty about the utility of these techniques and a concern that their introduction suggests that the level of pain being experienced is not believed. Understanding use of nonpharmacological modalities of treatment in different cultures with different traditions regarding healing and health is important as well. It is generally best to introduce these nondrug interventions after some rapport has been established with the patient and when the patient is not in severe pain.

Asking the patient which approaches they have used to manage pain or stress in the past, unrelated to medication, is an important part of the initial assessment. We can learn from the patient what is helpful and what is not. Culture as well as previous experience and trust in the clinician may play a role here. Techniques that have been helpful in the past can be reinforced, and other measures can be introduced according to the characteristics of the new cancer-related pain. When reviewing the nondrug techniques for use in the older adult, it is necessary to consider whether a specific intervention will require high or low levels of patient and caregiver involvement and whether techniques that have been helpful to the patient in the past need to be modified according to their current medical status, fatigue level, mental clarity, continued interest, site of care, and other factors. Assessment is key to developing a realistic plan. The intervention must match the specific problem with an appreciation for the patient's abilities and motivations. In the palliative care setting, especially for end-of-life pain management in the older adult, the inclusion of family, supportive friends, and professional caregivers is essential. These individuals also have important educational needs, and their role in successful pain management cannot be underestimated. A structured pain education program has been shown to improve the QOL outcomes for both elderly patients and their family caregivers [89].

Educating the family on basic nursing care of an older individual with pain can make a significant difference to their overall comfort. For example, if a patient is left in the same position for several hours, this in itself can make existing pain worse or produce new pain, including pressure sores, contractures, frozen joints, and other painful joint conditions. Teaching the family the basic principles of positioning and movement can be helpful in relieving muscular skeletal pain associated with inactivity. Supportive orthotic devices such as a splint, sling, brace, or corset may be useful to immobilize or provide support to painful tissues and to decrease incident or mechanical-type pain for certain patients. Assistive devices such as canes, walkers, and wheelchairs can also be helpful for some patients. These simple measures can make a great deal of difference to an elderly patient's general comfort and quality of life.

Implementing nondrug measures as part of a comprehensive pain management approach in the older adult usually requires expertise of different members of the multidisciplinary team. These include social workers, physical and or occupational therapists, chaplains, psychologists, and nurses. Their use underscores the multidimensional nature of pain and the need for a multimodal approach. The differences in psychosocial factors that influence how older adults adjust to pain may influence how psychological nondrug pain management interventions are implemented in this population.

27.8 CONCLUSIONS

As the population ages and the incidence of cancer increases, pain management in the elderly will become an increasingly prevalent clinical challenge during this twenty-first century. The principles of assessment and management are the same as in the younger adult, but with some specific differences in terms of symptom assessment and pharmacologic management. Basic and translational research is continuously identifying new ways to determine pain intensity in cognitively impaired elders and novel pathways of cancer pain, which is leading to new treatments with an improved side effect profile. But even with these innovative tools, knowledge and attitudinal barriers need to be overcome before pain management in the elderly is significantly improved.

REFERENCES

1. Greenlee RT, Murray T, Bolden S, Wingo PA. Cancer statistics, 2000. *CA Cancer J Clin* 2000;**50**:7–33.
2. Yancik R, Ries LA. Aging and cancer in America. Demographic and epidemiologic perspectives. *Hematol Oncol Clin North Am* 2000;**14**:17–23.
3. Yancik R, Ganz PA, Varricchio CG, Conley B. Perspectives on comorbidity and cancer in older patients: Approaches to expand the knowledge base. *J Clin Oncol* 2001;**19**:1147–1151.
4. Smith BD, Smith GL, Hurria A, Hortobagyi GN, Buchholz TA. Future of cancer incidence in the United States: Burdens upon an aging, changing nation. *J Clin Oncol* 2009;**27**:2758–2765.
5. Erikson C, Salsberg E, Forte G. Future demand and supply of oncologists: Challenges to assuring access to oncology services. *J Oncol Pract* 2007;**3**:79–86.
6. Raji MA, Kuo YF, Freeman JL, Goodwin JS. Effect of a dementia diagnosis on survival of older patients after a diagnosis of breast, colon, or prostate cancer: Implications for cancer care. *Arch Intern Med* 2008;**168**:2033–2040.
7. Hurria A, Rosen C, Hudis C, et al. Cognitive function of older patients receiving adjuvant chemotherapy for breast cancer: A pilot prospective longitudinal study. *J Am Geriatr Soc* 2006;**54**:925–931.
8. Ferrell B. Managing pain and discomfort in older adults near the end of life. *Ann Long Term Care* 2004;**12**:49–55.
9. Mitchell SL, Kiely DK, Hamel MB. Dying with advanced dementia in the nursing home. *Arch Intern Med* 2004;**164**:321–326.
10. Buchanan RJ, Barkley J, Wang S, Kim MS. Analysis of nursing home residents with cancer at admission. *Cancer Nurs* 2005;**28**:406–14.
11. Balducci L. Management of cancer pain in geriatric patients. *J Support Oncol* 2003;**1**:175–191.
12. Jacox A, Carr DB, Payne R. New clinical-practice guidelines for the management of pain in patients with cancer. *N Engl J Med* 1994;**330**:651–655.

13. Cleeland CS, Gonin R, Hatfield AK, et al. Pain and its treatment in outpatients with metastatic cancer. *N Engl J Med* 1994;**330**:592–596.

14. Twycross RG, Lack SA. *Symptom Control in Far Advanced Cancer: Pain Relief*, Pitman, London, 1983.

15. Green CR, Hart-Johnson T, Loeffler DR. Cancer-related chronic pain: examining quality of life in diverse cancer survivors. *Cancer* 2011;**117**(9):1994–2003.

16. Daut RL, Cleeland CS. The prevalence and severity of pain in cancer. *Cancer* 1982;**50**:1913–1918.

17. Caraceni A, Portenoy RK. An international survey of cancer pain characteristics and syndromes. IASP Task Force on Cancer Pain. International Association for the Study of Pain. *Pain* 1999;**82**:263–274.

18. Grove GL. Physiologic changes in older skin. *Clin Geriatr Med* 1989;**5**:115–125.

19. Gibson SJ, Helme RD. Age-related differences in pain perception and report. *Clin Geriatr Med* 2001;**17**:433–456, v–vi.

20. Vigano A, Bruera E, Suarez-Almazor ME. Age, pain intensity, and opioid dose in patients with advanced cancer. *Cancer* 1998;**83**:1244–1250.

21. Twycross RG, Lack SA. *Therapeutics in Terminal Cancer*, Churchill Livingstone, Edinburgh, 1990.

22. Paice JA. Chronic treatment-related pain in cancer survivors. *Pain* 2011;**152** (3Suppl):S84–9.

23. Foley KM. Pain assessment and cancer pain syndromes. In Doyle D, Hanks GWC, MacDonald N, eds. *Oxford Textbook of Palliative Medicine*, Oxford Univ. Press, Oxford, UK, 1993, pp. 148–165.

24. Twycross RG, Fairfield S. Pain in far-advanced cancer. *Pain* 1982;**14**:303–310.

25. Portenoy RK, Hagen NA. Breakthrough pain: Definition, prevalence and characteristics. *Pain* 1990;**41**:273–281.

26. Portenoy RK, Payne D, Jacobsen P. Breakthrough pain: Characteristics and impact in patients with cancer pain. *Pain* 1999;**81**:129–134.

27. Portenoy RK. Cancer pain: pathophysiology and syndromes. *Lancet* 1992;**339**:1026–1031.

28. Besson JM. The neurobiology of pain. *Lancet* 1999;**353**:1610–1615.

29. Dickenson AH. Central acute pain mechanisms. *Ann Med* 1995;**27**:223–227.

30. Honore P, Schwei J, Rogers SD, et al. Cellular and neurochemical remodeling of the spinal cord in bone cancer pain. *Prog Brain Res* 2000;**129**:389–397.

31. Shimoyama M, Tanaka K, Hasue F, Shimoyama N. A mouse model of neuropathic cancer pain. *Pain* 2002;**99**:167–74.

32. Mantyh PW, Clohisy DR, Koltzenburg M, Hunt SP. Molecular mechanisms of cancer pain. *Nat Rev Cancer* 2002;**2**:201–209.

33. Von Roenn JH, Cleeland CS, Gonin R, Hatfield AK, Pandya KJ. Physician attitudes and practice in cancer pain management. A survey from the Eastern Cooperative Oncology Group. *Ann Intern Med* 1993;**119**:121–126.

34. Lickiss JN. Approaching cancer pain relief. *Eur J Pain* 2001;**5**(Suppl A): 5–14.

35. WHO. *Cancer Pain Relief and Palliative Care*. World Health Organization, Geneva, 1990, Technical Report Series 804.

36. Beyer JE, McGrath PJ, Berde CB. Discordance between self-report and behavioral pain measures in children aged 3–7 years after surgery. *J Pain Symptom Manage* 1990;**5**:3506.

37. Jacox AK, Carr DB, Payne R. *Clinical Practice Guideline*. Vol. 9: *Management of Cancer Pain*, Dept Health and Human Services AfHCPaR, Rockville, MD, 1994.

38. Herr K, Coyne PJ, Key T, et al. Pain assessment in the nonverbal patient: Position statement with clinical practice recommendations. *Pain Manage Nurs* 2006;**7**:44–52.

39. Warden V, Hurley AC, Volicer L. Development and psychometric evaluation of the pain assessment in advanced dementia (PAINAD) scale. *J Am Med Dir Assoc* 2003;**4**:9–15.

40. Elliott K, Foley KM. Neurologic pain syndromes in patients with cancer. *Neurol Clin* 1989;**7**:333–360.

41. Cusack BJ. Pharmacokinetics in older persons. *Am J Geriatr Pharmacother* 2004;**2**: 274–302.

42. Montamat SC, Cusack BJ, Vestal RE. Management of drug therapy in the elderly. *N Engl J Med* 1989;**321**:303–309.

43. Avorn J, Gurwitz JH, Rochon P. Principles of pharmacology. In Cassel CK, Leipzig RM, Cohen HJ, Larson EB, Meier DE, Capello CF, eds. *Geriatric Medicine: An Evidence-Based Approach.* Springer-Verlag, New York, 2003, pp. 65–82.

44. American Geriatrics Society (AGS). Pharmacological Management of Persistent Pain in Older Persons. AGS Panel on Chronic Pain in Older Persons. *J Am Geriatr Soc* 2009;**57**:1331–146.

45. Menefee LA, Monti DA. Nonpharmacologic and complementary approaches to cancer pain management. *J Am Osteopath Assoc* 2005;**105**:S15–S20.

46. Fine PG. Opioid analgesic drugs in older people. *Clin Geriatr Med* 2001;**17**:479–487, vi.

47. Hanks GW, Conno F, Cherny N, et al. Morphine and alternative opioids in cancer pain: the EAPC recommendations. *Br J Cancer* 2001;**84**:587–593.

48. Scottish Intercollegiate Guidelines Network (SIGN). *Cancer Pain Guidelines* (SIGN), Edinburgh, 2000.

49. Benedetti C, Brock C, Cleeland C, et al. NCCN Practice Guidelines for Cancer Pain. *Oncology* 2000;**14**:135–50.

50. Hanks G, Cherny NI, Fallon M. Opioid analgesic therapy. In Doyle D, Hanks G, Cherny N, Calman K, eds. *Oxford Textbook of Palliative Medicine*, 3rd ed., Oxford University Press, 2004, pp. 318–321.

51. Jadad AR, Browman GP. The WHO analgesic ladder for cancer pain management. Stepping up the quality of its evaluation. *JAMA* 1995;**274**:1870–1873.

52. Marinangeli F, Ciccozzi A, Leonardis M, et al. Use of strong opioids in advanced cancer pain: a randomized trial. *J Pain Symptom Manage* 2004;**27**:409–416.

53. Whelton A, Hamilton CW. Nonsteroidal anti-inflammatory drugs: Effects on kidney function. *J Clin Pharmacol* 1991;**31**:588–598.

54. Brown JA, Von Roenn JH. Symptom management in the older adult. *Clin Geriatr Med* 2004;**20**:621–640, v–vi.

55. Cleary JF. Cancer pain management. *Cancer Control* 2000;**7**:120–131.

56. Walsh D. Pharmacological management of cancer pain. *Semin Oncol* 2000;**27**:45–63.

57. De Conno F, Ripamonti C, Sbanotto A, et al. A clinical study on the use of codeine, oxycodone, dextropropoxyphene, buprenorphine, and pentazocine in cancer pain. *J Pain Symptom Manage* 1991;**6**:423–427.

58. Anonymous. Tramadol—a new analgesic. *Drug Ther Bull* 1994;**32**:85–87.

59. Pergolizzi J, Boger R, Budd K et al. Opioids and the management of chronic severe pain in the elderly: consensus statement of an international expert panel. *Pain Pract* 2008;**8**(4):287–313.

60. Wilder-Smith CH, Schimke J, Osterwalder B, Senn HJ. Oral tramadol, a mu-opioid agonist and monoamine reuptake-blocker, and morphine for strong cancer-related pain. *Ann Oncol* 1994;**5**:141–146.

61. Leppart W. Analgesic efficacy of oral tramadol and morphine administered orally in the treatment of cancer pain. *Nowotwory* 2001;**51**:257–266.

62. Wiffen PJ, McQuay HJ. Oral morphine for cancer pain. *Cochrane Database Syst Rev*, 2007, Issue 7, No. CD003868.

63. Expert Working Group of the European Association for Palliative Care. Morphine in cancer pain: Modes of administration. *Br Med J* 1996;**312**:823–826.

64. Hanks GW, Twycross RG, Lloyd JW. Unexpected complication of successful nerve block. Morphine induced respiratory depression precipitated by removal of severe pain. *Anaesthesia* 1981;**36**:37–39.

65. Broadbent A, Glare P. Neurotoxicity from chronic opioid therapy after successful palliative treatment for painful bone metastases. *J Pain Symptom Manage* 2005;**29**:520–524.

66. Hagen NA, Foley KM, Cerbone DJ, Portenoy RK, Inturrisi CE. Chronic nausea and morphine-6-glucuronide. *J Pain Symptom Manage* 1991;**6**:125–128.

67. Osborne R, Joel S, Slevin M. Morphine intoxication in renal failure; the role of morphine-6-glucuronide. *Br Med J (Clin Res Ed)* 1986;**293**:1101.

68. Dean M. Opioids in renal failure and dialysis patients. *J Pain Symptom Manage* 2004;**28**:497–504.

69. Indelicato RA, Portenoy RK. Opioid rotation in the management of refractory cancer pain. *J Clin Oncol* 2002;**20**:348–352.

70. Mercadante S, Casuccio A, Fulfaro F, et al. Switching from morphine to methadone to improve analgesia and tolerability in cancer patients: A prospective study. *J Clin Oncol* 2001;**19**:2898–2904.

71. Ayonrinde OT, Bridge DT. The rediscovery of methadone for cancer pain management. *Med J Aust* 2000;**173**:536–40.

72. Smith TJ, Staats PS, Deer T, et al. Randomized clinical trial of an implantable drug delivery system compared with comprehensive medical management for refractory cancer pain: Impact on pain, drug-related toxicity, and survival. *J Clin Oncol* 2002;**20**:4040–4049.

73. Wells N, Johnson RL, Wujcik D. Development of a short version of the Barriers Questionnaire. *J Pain Symptom Manage* 1998;**15**:294–298.

74. Cherny N, Ripamonti C, Pereira J, et al. Strategies to manage the adverse effects of oral morphine: an evidence-based report. *J Clin Oncol* 2001;**19**:2542–2554.

75. Bruera E, Palmer JL, Bosnjak S, et al. Methadone versus morphine as a first-line strong opioid for cancer pain: A randomized, double-blind study. *J Clin Oncol* 2004;**22**:185–192.

76. Hardy JR, Quigley C, Ross Jr. Opioid rotation. In Davis MP, Glare P, Quigley C, Hardy JR, eds. *Opioids in Cancer Pain*, 2nd ed., Oxford Univ. Press, Oxford, UK, 2009, pp. 301–112.

77. Cherny NJ, Chang V, Frager G, et al. Opioid pharmacotherapy in the management of cancer pain: A survey of strategies used by pain physicians for the selection of analgesic drugs and routes of administration. *Cancer* 1995;**76**:1283–1293.

78. Kirsh KL, Casper D, Haley MC, Passik SD. Opioid use in drug and alcohol abuse. In Walsh D, ed. *Palliative Medicine*, Saunders, Philadelphia, 2008, pp. 1416–1421.

79. ASCO. Cancer pain assessment and treatment curriculum guidelines. The Ad Hoc Committee on Cancer Pain of the American Society of Clinical Oncology. *J Clin Oncol* 1992;**10**:1976–1982.

80. Zech DF, Grond S, Lynch J, Hertel D, Lehmann KA. Validation of World Health Organization Guidelines for cancer pain relief: A 10-year prospective study. *Pain* 1995;**63**:65–76.

81. Samad TA, Moore KA, Sapirstein A, et al. Interleukin-1beta-mediated induction of Cox-2 in the CNS contributes to inflammatory pain hypersensitivity. *Nature* 2001;**410**:471–475.

82. Mukherjee D. Selective cyclooxygenase-2 (COX-2) inhibitors and potential risk of cardiovascular events. *Biochem Pharmacol* 2002;**63**:817–821.

83. Brune K, Hinz B. Non-steroidal anti-inflammatory drugs. In Walsh D, ed. *Palliative Medicine*, Saunders, Philadelphia, 2008, pp. 740–745.

84. Stockler M, Vardy J, Pillai A, Warr D. Acetaminophen (paracetamol) improves pain and well-being in people with advanced cancer already receiving a strong opioid regimen: A randomized, double-blind, placebo-controlled cross-over trial. *J Clin Oncol* 2004;**22**:3389–3394.

85. McMillan SC. Presence and severity of constipation in hospice patients with advanced cancer. *Am J Hosp Palliat Care* 2002;**19**:426–430.

86. Miles CL, Fellowes D, Goodman ML, Wilkinson S. Laxatives for the management of constipation in palliative care patients. *Cochrane Database Syst Rev* 2006;**4**: No. CD003448.

87. Thomas J, Karver S, Cooney GA, et al. Methylnaltrexone for opioid-induced constipation in advanced illness. *N Engl J Med* 2008;**358**:2332–2343.

88. Miller MF, Bellizzi KM, Sufian M, Ambs AH, Goldstein MS, Ballard-Barbash R. Dietary supplement use in individuals living with cancer and other chronic conditions: A population-based study. *J Am Diet Assoc* 2008;**108**:483–494.

89. Ferrell BR, Grant M, Chan J, Ahn C, Ferrell BA. The impact of cancer pain education on family caregivers of elderly patients. *Oncol Nurs Forum* 1995;**22**:1211–1218.

PART VIII

EMERGING ISSUES

CHAPTER 28

Caregiver Knowledge and Skills

PAULA R. SHERWOOD

School of Nursing, University of Pittsburgh, Pittsburgh, PA

BARBARA A. GIVEN and CHARLES W. GIVEN

College of Nursing and College of Human Medicine, Michigan State University, East Lansing, MI

28.1 INTRODUCTION

Despite increasing involvement from family members in providing and managing cancer care, the complexity of treatment regimens, changing demands, and deterioration in patients' conditions often lead to high levels of distress that may influence the quality of care provided to patients in the home [1–3]. In addition, providing care has been shown to cause deterioration in the physical health of caregivers, which can have a significant impact on the economic burden of the healthcare system. A MetLife study found that health problems in employed caregivers are estimated to result in $13.4 billion dollars annually [4]. Although the current healthcare system and changes in reimbursement have shifted a significant portion of cancer care to family members, these caregivers often report not knowing how to determine what care is needed, when and how care should be provided, and how to communicate changes and care demands to oncology practitioners [5].

Patient needs for assistance change as the disease trajectory continues, throughout active treatment, remission, recurrence, survivorship, and end of life. The healthcare system expects caregiver duties to automatically change to meet new care demands, and in return, caregivers expect oncology practitioners to impart both the knowledge and skills to enable them to manage patient care in the home while coping with their own often severe levels of distress. Because of the requisite collaboration of both healthcare professionals and family members to provide high quality cancer care, it is vital for healthcare professionals to assist caregivers in prioritizing and guiding care delivery for the home [6]. Consideration of knowledge and skills that family members need should be central to cancer care.

Most literature related to family caregiving focuses on the relationship between care demands and caregivers' psychological distress. The purpose of this chapter, however, is to describe the knowledge and skills required by family caregivers to provide high-quality care to patients undergoing active treatment for cancer. The following topics

Cancer and Aging Handbook: Research and Practice, First Edition. Edited by Keith M. Bellizzi and Margot A. Gosney.
© 2012 Wiley-Blackwell. Published 2012 by John Wiley & Sons, Inc.

are covered in the subsequent sections: (1) how to assess patient and caregiver needs and skills, (2) common needs and skills throughout the care trajectory, (3) ways to integrate caregiver teaching into clinical practice, and (4) recognition and management of caregiver distress to maintain optimal patient care in the home.

28.2   ASSESSING CANCER CARE NEEDS IN THE HOME

A thorough assessment of cancer care needs in the home consists in (1) an appraisal of the family caregivers' current level of knowledge, ability, willingness to learn, and their psychological distress; and (2) recognition and prioritization of patient care needs in the home. Diagnosis, stage of disease, and phase in the treatment and patient status have to be considered. Caregivers who feel prepared to deliver care (i.e., have the knowledge and skills needed) have less burden and improved attitude about the care they provide [7,8]. However, caregiver appraisals often reveal that caregivers feel that they do not have the necessary skills and knowledge to provide care, lack confidence, and generally feel incapable and unprepared [9]. They are seldom familiar with the type and amount of care needed, and when care is needed. As a result, the level of distress caused by caregivers' feelings of inadequacy, or lack of competence, may affect their ability to integrate new information into the care situation and carry out quality home care.

The role of the healthcare practitioner is to first determine whether caregivers are receptive to recommended interventions and can become effective partners for oncology care within the home setting. When caregivers themselves are distressed, burdened, or depressed, they might not attend to cues in the patient situation that require decisionmaking or problem solving. If levels of distress or depressive symptoms are high, family caregivers may also be less able to integrate practitioner recommendations into the patient's care. They may instead benefit from a referral to their own primary care practitioner for pharmacological and psychological therapy [3,10]. Once the feelings of distress return to a manageable level, the healthcare practitioner can begin to assess the needs of the patient and tailor caregiver intervention efforts to meet those patient needs.

Healthcare practitioners should consider additional factors that may interfere with the caregiver's ability to use the knowledge and skills to provide care. Caregivers who are in poor health or have limited financial resources may not be able to provide the level of care that is needed. Relationship to the patient must also be considered, as wives, husbands, daughters, and sons typically have different roles as caregivers and approach care in different ways [11]. Spouses may have stronger established patterns of decisionmaking with the patient, which can facilitate management and care decisions. Patient care by adult children can cause severe disruption in the caregiver's life, due to competing demands (careers, children, and their own spouse) [12]. Being cognizant of caregivers' competing demands and conflicts of family activities and employment is an essential component of the caregiver assessment [13,14]. Adult children caregivers often need extra supportive services in to order become and remain engaged in providing care to a parent.

Caregiver capacity and traits such as mastery have been shown to be important to help the caregiver acquire the necessary knowledge and skills. *Mastery* is the perception of their sense of worth as caregivers and how they perceive their ability to meet the demands of providing care [15–17]. Caregivers with a high sense of mastery have also been reported to use more problem-focused coping strategies to meet patient care demands [8,9,18–20]. The concepts of mastery, preparedness, enhanced confidence, and competence are necessary components for effective decisionmaking and problem solving by family caregivers [9,21–24]. Providers need to consider these factors along with an assessment of patient needs as they seek ways to continue to support the ability of the caregiver to continue to provide the needed cancer care in the home.

Recognition and prioritization of patient care needs in the home are closely related to the care recipient's location in the disease and treatment trajectory. Detailed assessments of the caregiving situation enable healthcare professionals to provide guidance and develop a plan of care with the family, identifying the family's roles in the provision of that care. During treatment, patient needs often include direct care such as symptom management, wound care, dressing changes, managing pumps and other equipment, catheter care, physical care, and medication administration [25].

Assessment areas are as follows:

1. Knowledge about disease and care
2. Self-assessment of capacity, mastery, confidence
3. Attitudes about ability and willingness to provide care
4. Caregiver–care receiver relationships
5. Reciprocity of caregiver to professional recommendations
6. Repertoire of skills based on care needs
   a. Support (social and emotional)
   b. Direct care—physical, symptom management, equipment
   c. Problem solving and decisionmaking
   d. Instrumental care
   e. Communication
   f. Negotiating the healthcare system
   g. Medication management
7. Knowledge of community resources and how to acquire them
8. Competing demands
9. Physical health of caregiver
10. Emotional health of caregiver, stress
11. Sociodemographic characteristics of caregiver

As patients experience multiple and severe symptoms from treatment, including pain, nausea, diarrhea and constipation, fatigue, dyspnea, peripheral neuropathy, and anorexia, symptom management often becomes a primary role for family caregivers [1,25,26,27]. Demands of caregiving become more complex and distressful when the patient has impaired cognition or neuropsychological symptoms [3,11,28,29].

Patients may also require assistance with instrumental activities of daily living (IADLs) such as providing nutrition, housekeeping, handling medical supplies, transportation to diagnostic and clinical appointments, and financial needs, including dealing with medical bills. To improve function and safety for the patient with fatigue, weakness, and peripheral neuropathy, caregivers may need to modify the home environment and acquire equipment and assistive devices, as falls have been documented [3,8,20,30]. Meeting all of these needs requires that caregivers actively navigate the healthcare system and participate in scheduling and attending patients' clinic appointments. Both during active treatment and into survivorship, caregivers may continue to carry out some of these tasks as well as continuing to provide psychological, spiritual, and social support.

Unfortunately, provision of any of these tasks can be more complex than healthcare practitioners may recognize. For example, for patients who require assistance with medication administration, caregivers may be given instructions on dosing and potential side effects. *Medication administration*, however, is a complex task consisting of not only administering the medication but also monitoring side effects or adverse events of medications, new symptoms that might be associated with a complication, and making decisions (e.g., dosing, withholding, discontinuation) based on the effectiveness of the medication [31,32]. If chemotherapy administration utilizes oral agents that vary in dosage and frequency every 2 weeks, then caregivers need to establish reminders and understand potential side effects and how to manage them, particularly in the presence of multiple symptoms. Family members seldom have the knowledge and skills to interpret the meaning or urgency of the sign or the symptom such as increasing fatigue or a temperature that slowly increases that may signal an impending infection. The time and problem solving required for all these tasks can be intense, and the caregiver may not possess the cognitive, financial, or time resources to meet this need.

Cancer care is highlighted by change; family members must have some ability to be aware of the changes in the patient's condition. It is often these changes in condition that are most stressful for family members. For example, changes in the severity and frequency of symptoms or the occurrence of new symptoms are common and can heighten the caregiver's perception of loss of control. Increasing symptom burden may increase the demand for new or changing knowledge and skill but may also require new skills [1,33], as family caregivers attempt to manage a refractory symptom or to decide when or at what level of severity of any given symptom or total symptom burden should be reported to healthcare professionals. Each type of caregiver task and level of involvement demands different caregiver skills and knowledge, judgment, organizational capacities, time, and social and psychological resources [24,34–36].

Healthcare professionals should assess care needs at each phase of the disease and treatment trajectory while concomitantly evaluating the caregiver's willingness, distress, and capacity to meet current and future patient needs. Because of the diversity of healthcare teams in varying treatment centers, this assessment may be done by a nurse, social worker, physician, nurse practitioner, or physician assistant, or may even be part of the paperwork completed by patients while they wait for their appointment and then reviewed with the practitioner. This assessment provides the basis on which to identify new knowledge and skills that will be needed. The predictability and routine nature of the care tasks and demands as well as its duration (weeks or months of care) and quantity (daily hours of care) must be considered when developing and implementing plans of care with the family [28,37,38].

Assessments of the care situation can take several forms. Paper (hardcopy) forms and electronic interface assessments can be completed by the patient and caregiver during wait times for clinic appointments. There are a multitude of assessment tools designed to evaluate the patient's condition and thus identify care needs. Forms such as the SF36, the MD Anderson Symptom Inventory, Economic Hardship, Center for Epidemiologic

Studies-Depression, and Cognistat are examples of tools that may identify areas of need. A more direct approach is to evaluate the patient's current treatment regimen and ask the caregiver what they need assistance with and what will be difficult for them to do. If there are multiple needs in the home, a social work consult may be appropriate, and the caregiver should be asked to prioritize needs. In addition to the assessment of the patient situation it is important to assess the capacity, knowledge, and skills of the family caregiver to meet those needs.

28.3   HELPING CAREGIVERS MEET PATIENT NEEDS

Caregivers can unintentionally cause negative patient outcomes, despite their good intentions, if they lack the knowledge and skills to deliver care. Examples would be nasogastric tube or intravenous catheter displacement or clogging, or lack of attention to an emerging complication such as an infection or dehydration, either of which can threaten the safety of the patient's condition and may result in an unscheduled hospital admission. Helping caregivers meet patient needs, then, should be a top priority for healthcare practitioners.

Working with the caregiver to provide care should take into account the following dimensions: (1) the nature of the tasks; (2) the frequency with which tasks are performed; (3) the hours of care provided each day; (4) the skills, knowledge, judgment, and abilities to perform tasks; (5) ensuring that the tasks are routine enough to be incorporated easily into daily schedules; and (6) the support received from other family members or community resources. As such, family caregivers are "on call" 24 h a day, every day, facing different role demands and utilizing different social and psychological resources [24,39,40]. Demands also vary across the disease trajectory.

The types of intervention that best promote knowledge and skills are

Information
Problem solving
Communication skills
Navigating the healthcare system

Some patient needs require simply the provision of information, while others require problem solving and critical thinking. For those needs that require higher-level cognitive skills (such as critical thinking), interventions that teach problem solving skills are necessary but may be outside the time and personnel resources of healthcare practitioners. For example, a patient whose functional decline necessitates use of a wheelchair will need referral to a community medical supply company, a prescription for reimbursement, and evaluation of the home to ensure that entrances and hallways will accommodate the size of the wheelchair. Managing severe pain in progressive disease requires observation, around the clock medication administration, and monitoring medication effectiveness and adverse effects. Helping a patient deal with clinical depression may require ongoing emotional support, referral to a psychologist, and medication administration.

Healthcare professionals can refer patients to psychologists, social workers, or counselors, who can then intervene using cognitive behavioral interventions to enhance caregivers' sense of mastery, reducing feelings of uncertainty, burden, depressive symptoms, and overall negative responses to care by using cognitive behavioral approaches to provide information to enhance their caregiver knowledge and skill building [16,20,41,42]. The following sections highlight interventions that can be planned once the assessment of patient needs along with caregiver capacity, and existing knowledge and skills is complete. It is important to note that implementing these interventions often requires outside assistance (such as a social worker, visiting nurse, or psychologist) and must be tailored to each individual care situation, considering both patient and caregiver. Also noteworthy is the fact that over a cancer diagnosis, the care situation may change frequently with disease status and treatment approaches.

28.3.1 Providing Information

Caregivers describe lack of information as one of the key areas of unmet needs. Information, however, must be tailored to individual caregiver needs, including literacy level, cultural appropriateness, and mode of delivery, so that caregivers feel more competent and confident as care providers, patients receive safe and effective care, and positive clinical outcomes result [43]. Information needs to be credible and consistent with the patient's plan of care [44]. Providing knowledge that caregivers use to interpret what they see, make decisions, and solve problems provides the foundation for the caregiver's ability to provide quality care. A common area in which caregivers report needing information is the disease state and trajectory and treatment and care regimens. Families also want information about symptoms, medication administration, and possible adverse events. Caregivers want to know how to arrange and provide assistance with daily activities, and on psychomotor and other skills to provide day-to-day care [24]. Other informational needs include available social and emotional support resources and how to access community resources [1,45]. Unless caregivers have the requisite knowledge to make decisions and provide care, poor patient outcomes can result.

It is important that healthcare practitioners recognize that caregivers need information and will seek out that information if it is not provided by the healthcare team. Caregivers commonly use the Internet, family and friends, and support groups as sources of information. Unfortunately, these sources are often unfamiliar with the patient's specific diagnosis and treatment regimen and may provide inadequate, nontailored and incorrect information, forming the basis for poor-quality care. Once this happens, the healthcare practitioner must spend more time correcting misinformation, which takes away from time spent with the patient. Caregivers can be guided to these websites or resources by providers who select the most appropriate sites based on patient and caregiver needs.

Maintaining a list of acceptable web sites in the clinic is a simple way to guide caregivers to credible sources of information. These websites should be reviewed and updated regularly by healthcare professionals. Providing lists of credible websites (such as Family Caregiver Alliance or the National Association of Caregiving) is one method of disseminating information. Obtaining information will lead to increased confidence, and being better informed enables the caregiver to discuss the information with a healthcare professional. Internet applications may successfully support caregivers for the care management as well as provide support [46]. Other informational resource systems, such as voice response, Web-based sites, and printed toolkits, are all available to aid caregivers in providing care [46].

28.3.2 Skill Building

Skills that caregivers use to provide care are based on knowledge and can be classified as psychomotor (such as catheter or wound care, or medication administration), cognitive (such as monitoring, decisionmaking, and problem solving), or psychological (such as offering the patient emotional support) or social, such as resource acquisition. Several interventions have been trialed with the ultimate goal of improving caregiver skills, some of which are general in nature (e.g., problem solving or decisionmaking), while some address specific caregiver and patient needs (e.g., communication). The subsequent sections describe key components of these interventions.

The majority of studies that support caregivers to meet patient needs have utilized a psychoeducational intervention. These interventions emphasize both the provision of information and a psychological/counseling approach that results in improved patient care and decreased caregiver distress [47]. Psychoeducational intervention often involves multiple components that address areas such as symptom management, monitoring patient problems, coordinating resources, communicating with healthcare practitioners, and providing emotional support [48–50]. Pasacreta and McCorkle found that 4 months after attending a psychoeducational caregiver cancer education program that addressed symptom management, psychosocial support, and resource identification, caregivers reported being well informed, and their confidence about caregiving increased [52]. Given and Given [30], in a two-intervention trial using psychoeducational components, documented caregivers' ability to assist patients and symptom management during a course of chemotherapy. Both symptom number and severity improved [30].

28.3.3 Problem Solving

Several types of intervention have been used to assist caregivers to develop problem solving skills (a specific type of cognitive behavioral therapy). Toseland and colleagues [53] and Blanchard and colleagues [54] have successfully implemented such interventions. A problem solving intervention is a specific type of cognitive behavioral therapy that helps caregivers identify problem areas, change misconceptions regarding the source or manageability of those areas, generate and implement strategies to meet patient needs, and evaluate strategy effectiveness. Houts and colleagues [49] describe a prescriptive program that is based on problem solving training and therapy that has been used by others. Designed to empower family members to moderate caregiver stress, the prepared family caregiver model [COPE (Creativity, Optimism, Planning, and Expert information)] teaches caregivers how to design and carry out plans of care that coordinate efforts with healthcare practitioners to meet patient needs.

Family caregivers today are challenged to be care managers and care coordinators for their patients and carry out administrative tasks. Caregivers become advocates for their patients. They include keeping records, seeking needed information, managing insurance claims, paying bills, exercising vigilance for the patient, requesting help from healthcare providers for symptom relief, and encouraging the patient to adhere to treatment regimens. These areas often are difficult for family members, and psychoeducational intervention can provide both skills and knowledge for the patient's care as well as emotional support for the caregivers.

28.3.4 Communication Skills

Communicating with the healthcare team is vital to obtaining information, expressing family preferences, communicating with agencies, and being a general spokesperson for the patient's care. Because they function within the healthcare setting on a daily basis, practitioners may erroneously assume that caregivers have the requisite skills to communicate with healthcare providers. Helping caregivers learn the appropriate terminology and how to communicate with the healthcare team can prevent caregiver–healthcare team conflicts. Numerous assistive devices and interventions are available to help caregivers communicate effectively with family members and healthcare professionals [55]. Interventions, which include role playing, are particularly helpful in teaching the caregiver communication skills on how to communicate with providers in order to be heard.

Communication skills not only are requisite for interactions with the healthcare team but are also vital for interactions with patients and for negotiating with families and friends to enlist and mobilize support. Despite the strength of the caregiver–patient relationship prior to diagnosis, communication after diagnosis can be strained. For example, there is often a lack of congruence between patients and caregivers in reports of symptoms and side effects [56]. Caregivers tend to overestimate the severity of patients' symptoms, particularly when caregivers are distressed. Without an accurate understanding of patient symptom frequency and severity, caregivers will be limited in their ability to support adequate symptom management, and accurate monitoring and interpreting are necessary for caregivers to make decisions and take action [57]. Improving caregiver–patient communication can lead to higher levels of concordance in symptom perception, ultimately leading to more caregiver involvement and better symptom management. As caregivers' communications with patients are more consistent with the patient report, caregivers may be able to better assist them with symptom management. As a result, patients may experience greater relief from symptom severity, number of symptoms, symptom interference, total symptom frequency, and depression.

28.3.5 Navigating the Healthcare System

Learning to communicate with the healthcare team is essential, but can be implemented only when caregivers understand which team member is responsible for specific components of care and how to contact that team member, commonly referred to as *navigating the healthcare system*. One of the most essential aspects of navigating the system is finding home- and community-based services and determining what private and public programs might be available, for which the patient is eligible, and what is useful to complement the abilities of the caregiver. Gaining access to community resources can be extremely complex, depending on various factors, including what is available, what is accessible due to eligibility, what will be covered by insurance, and what is acceptable to both caregiver and patient. Interventions to increase caregivers' knowledge about community services, knowing the eligibility criteria, and how to access them can increase caregiver competence [58]. After the patient needs assessment is complete, healthcare practitioners can suggest potential resources and help caregivers identify exactly what services they should request. For example, respite care is available in many communities and can provide personnel to sit with the patient while the caregiver either runs errands or takes time out. When respite care is not formally available or is financially prohibitive, family and friends can help provide that care.

Caregivers have reported that simply receiving information regarding providing care is not adequate to allow them to provide high-quality care. Family caregivers need a working knowledge, an ability to apply the knowledge to the patients' plan of care through skill building such as medication administration and wound care. The healthcare system's plan of care should be written considering the caregiver, and should be shared and discussed with family members from the onset of cancer care.

28.4 IMPLICATIONS AND CONCLUSIONS

Society depends on family caregivers to provide care for their loved ones, but does little to prepare them for this role. Healthcare practitioners' lack of explicit attention to caregivers is a serious gap in our heathcare delivery system. As a standard of care, healthcare practitioners should perform an assessment of patient needs and caregiver resources, provide specific concrete instructions, and refer them to potential sources of ongoing help. Practice settings need to partner with patients and their families to move from the traditional context of *doing for* clients in the "expert model of service delivery" to more mutuality in provider-caregiver relationships [59]. We need to "enact more empowering partnering approaches" [59]. We can meaningfully change the course of caregiving for both the caregiver and the care recipient by respecting the role that each plays in managing ongoing care beyond the professional care boundaries [60].

In August 2010 NCI released a health professional version of a PDQ on family caregivers in *Cancer Roles and Challenges* (no caregiver version is posted) [61]. This document outlines the caregiver perspective across the illness trajectory and offers suggestions for healthcare practitioners who interact with caregivers. Importantly, the NCI PDQ points out a number of roles for the family caregiver: responding to conflict, convening a family meeting, and dealing with psychological issues. Using the strategies and interventions described in the previous sections can help enable the healthcare professionals to better satisfy the needs of the patients with cancer and their family caregivers as caregivers become more knowledgeable and one their caregiver skills.

To bring about changes in practice, providers need to develop evidence-based standards and guidelines to help families care. These guidelines should cover assessment categories, the types of knowledge and skills that family caregivers need, and the conditions under which information and skills should be evaluated. These standards can be applied and tailored to the patient plans of care. Once the standards are determined, various interventions can be designed and become a part of the practice utilizing a variety of delivery approaches maximizing the use of technology platforms.

REFERENCES

1. Given B, Given CW, Sikorskii A, Jeon S, Sherwood P, Rahbar M. The impact of providing symptom management assistance on caregiver reaction: Results of a randomized trial. *J Pain Symptom Manage* 2006;**32**(5):433–443.

2. Given B, Wyatt G, Given C, et al. Burden and depression among caregivers of patients with cancer at the end of life. *Oncol Nurs Forum* 2004;**31**(6):1105–1115.

3. Sherwood PR, Given CW, Given BA, von Eye A. Caregiver burden and depression: Analysis of common caregiver outcomes. *J Aging Health* 2005;**17**(2):125–147.

4. Metropolitan Life Insurance Company. *MetLife Study of Working Caregivers and Employer Health Care Costs*, MetLife, New York, Feb. 2010 (available at `http://www.metlife.com/mmi/research/index.html?WT.ac=GN_mmi_research`; accessed 12/01/10).

5. Given B, Sherwood P, Given C. What knowledge and skills do caregivers need? *Am J Nurs* 2008;**108**(9 Suppl): 28–34.

6. Weuve JL, Boult C, Morishita L. The effects of outpatient geriatric evaluation and management on caregiver burden. *Gerontologist* 2000;**40**(4):429–436.

7. Ferrell BR, Grant M, Chan J, Ahn C, Ferrell BA. The impact of cancer pain education on family caregivers of elderly patients. *Oncol Nurs Forum* 1995;**22**(8):1211–1218.

8. Scherbring M. Effect of caregiver perception of preparedness on burden in an oncology population. *Oncol Nurs Forum* 2002;**29**(6):E70–E76.

9. Silver HJ, Wellman NS, Galindo-Ciocon D, Johnson P. Family caregivers of older adults on home enteral nutrition have multiple unmet task-related training needs and low overall preparedness for caregiving. *J Am Diet Assoc* 2004;**104**(1):43–50.

10. Del Giudice ME, Grunfeld E, Harvey BJ, Piliotis E, Verma S. Primary care physicians' views of routine follow-up care of cancer survivors. *J Clin Oncol* 2009;**27**(20):3338–3345.

11. Pinquart M, Sörensen S. Associations of caregiver stressors and uplifts with subjective well-being and depressive mood: A meta-analytic comparison. *Aging Ment Health* 2004;**8**(5):438–449.

12. Coristine M, Crooks D, Grunfeld E, Stonebridge C, Christie A. Caregiving for women with advanced breast cancer. *Psychooncology* 2003;**12**(7):709–719.

13. Gaugler JE, Given WC, Linder J, Kataria R, Tucker G, Regine WF. Work, gender, and stress in family cancer caregiving. *Support Care Cancer* 2008;**16**(4):347–357.

14. Sherwood P, Donovan H, Given C, et al. Predictors of employment and lost hours from work in cancer caregivers. *Psychooncology* 2008;**17**(6):598–605.

15. Gaugler J, Hanna N, Linder J, et al. Cancer caregiving and subjective stress: A multi-site, multi-dimensional analysis. *Psychooncology* 2005;**14**(9):771–785.

16. Gitlin L, Belle S, Burgio L, et al. Effect of multicomponent interventions on caregiver burden and depression: The reach multisite initiative at 6-month follow up. *Psychol Aging* 2003;**18**(3):361–374.

17. Kurtz ME, Kurtz JC, Given CW, Given B. (2008). Patient optimism and mastery—do they play a role in cancer patients' management of pain and fatigue? *J Pain Symptom Manage* 2008;**36**(1):1–10.

18. Gitlin LN, Corcoran M, Winter L, Boyce A, Hauck WW. A randomized controlled trial of a home environmental intervention: Effect on efficacy and upset in caregivers and on daily function of persons with dementia. *Gerontologist* 2001;**41**(1):4–14.

19. Li L, Seltzer M, Greenberg J. Change in depressive symptoms among daughter caregivers: An 18-month longitudinal study. *Psychol Aging* 1999;**14**(2):206–219.

20. Sherwood P, Given B, Given C, et al. The influence of caregiver mastery on depressive symptoms. *J Nurs Scholarsh* 2007;**39**(3):249–255.

21. Archbold PG, Stewart BJ, Miller LL, et al. The PREP system of nursing interventions: A pilot test with families caring for older members. Preparedness (PR), enrichment (E) and predictability (P). *Res Nurs Health* 1995;**18**(1):3–16.

22. Farran CJ, Loukissa D, Perraud S, Paun O. Alzheimer's disease caregiving information and skills. Part II: Family caregiver issues and concerns. *Res Nurs Health* 2004;**27**(1):40–51.

23. Gallagher-Thompson D, Coon DW. Evidence-based psychological treatments for distress in family caregivers of older adults. *Psychol Aging* 2007;**22**(1):37–51.

24. Schumacher KL, Stewart BJ, Archbold PG, Dodd MJ, Dibble SL. Family caregiving skill: Development of the concept. *Res Nurs Health* 2000;**23**(3):191–203.

25. Bookman A, Harrington M. Family caregivers: A shadow workforce in the geriatric health care system? *J Health Polit Policy Law* 2007;**32**(6):1005–1041.

26. Gaugler JE, Linder J, Given CW, Kataria R, Tucker G, Regine WF. The proliferation of primary caregiving stress to secondary stress. *Cancer Nurs* 2008;**31**(2):116–123.

27. Given B, Sherwood P. Family care for the older person during cancer care. *Semin Oncol Nurs* 2006;**22**(1):43–50.

28. Sherwood P, Given B, Given C, Schiffman R, Murman D, Lovely M. Caregivers of persons with a brain tumor: A conceptual model. *Nurs Inquire* 2004;**11**(1):43–53.

29. Weinberg DB, Lusenhop RW, Gittell JH, Kautz CM. Coordination between formal providers and informal caregivers. *Health Care Manage Rev* 2007;**32**(2):140–149.

30. Given B, Given CW, Sikorskii A, You M, McCorkle R, Champion V. Analyzing symptom management trials: The value of both intention-to-treat and per-protocol approaches. *Oncol Nurs Forum* 2009;**36**(6):E293–E302.

31. Travis SS, McAuley WJ, Dmochowski J, Bernard MA, Kao HF, Greene R. Factors associated with medication hassles experienced by family caregivers of older adults. *Patient Educ Couns* 2007;**66**(1):51–57.

32. Travis S, Sparks Bethea L, Winn P. Medication administration hassles reported by family caregivers of dependent elderly persons. *J Gerontol A Biol Sci Med Sci* 2000;**55**(7): M412–M417.

33. Kurtz M, Kurtz J, Given CW, Given BA. A randomized, controlled trial of a patient/caregiver symptom control intervention: Effects on depressive symptomatology of caregivers of cancer patients. *J Pain Symptom Manage* 2005;**30**(2):112–122.

34. Breitbart W, Gibson C, Tremblay A. The delirium experience: Delirium recall and delirium-related distress in hospitalized patients with cancer, their spouses/caregivers, and their nurses. *Psychosomatics* 2002;**43**(3):183–194.

35. Pinquart M, Sörensen S. Associations of stressors and uplifts of caregiving with caregiver burden and depressed mood: A meta-analysis. *J Gerontol B Psychol Sci Soc Sci* 2003;**58**(2):P112–P128.

36. Schumacher KL, Stewart BJ, Archbold PG, Caparro M, Mutale F, Agrawal S. Effects of caregiving demand, mutuality, and preparedness on family caregiver outcomes during cancer treatment. *Oncol Nurs Forum* 2008;**35**(1):49–56.

37. Langa KM, Vijan S, Hayward RA, et al. Informal caregiving for diabetes and diabetic complications among elderly Americans. *J Gerontol B Psychol Sci Soc Sci* 2002;**57**(3): S177–S186.

38. Lutgendorf S, Laudenslager M. Care of the caregiver: Stress and dysregulation of inflammatory control in cancer caregivers. *J Clin Oncol* 2009;**27**(18):2894–2895.

39. Barg F, Pasacreta J, Nuamah R, et al. A description of a psychoeducational intervention for family caregivers of cancer patients. *J Family Nurs* 1998;**4**(4):394–413.

40. Stommel M, Given BA, Given CW, Collins, C. The impact of the frequency of care activities on the division of labor between primary caregivers and other care providers. *Res Aging* 1995;**17**(4):412–433.

41. Sherwood P, Given BA, Given CW, et al. A cognitive behavioral intervention for symptom management in patients with advanced cancer. *Oncol Nurs Forum* 2005;**32**(6):1190–1198.

42. Moody L, McMillan S. Dyspnea and quality of life indicators in hospice patients and their caregivers. *Health Qual Life Outcomes* 2003;**1**:1–7.

43. Reinhard SC, Given G, Nirvana H, Bernis A. Supporting family caregivers in providing care. In Hughes RG, ed. *Patient Safety and Quality: An Evidence-Based Handbook for Nurses*, Agency for Healthcare Research and Quality, Rockville, MD, 2008, pp. 14.1–14.64 (available at http://www.ahrq.gov/qual/nurseshdbk/).

44. Eheman CR, Berkowitz Z, Lee J, et al. Information-seeking styles among cancer patients before and after treatment by demographics and use of information sources. *J Health Commun* 2009;**14**(5):487–502.

45. Jansen AP, van Hout HP, van Marwijk HW Sense of competence questionnaire among informal caregivers of older adults with dementia symptoms: A psychometric evaluation. *Clin Pract Epidemol Ment Health* 2007;**3**:11.

46. Kinnane NA, Milne D. The role of the internet in supporting and informing carers of people with cancer: A literature review. *Support Care Cancer* 2010;**18**(9):1123–1136.

47. Pinquart M, Sörensen S. Helping caregivers of persons with dementia: Which interventions work and how large are their effects? *Int Psychogeriatr* 2006;**18**(4):577–595.

48. Given B, Given CW, Jeon S, Sikorskii A. Effect of neutropenia on the impact of a cognitive behavioral intervention for symptom management. *Cancer* 2005;**104**(4):869–878.

49. Houts PS, Nezu AM, Nezu CM, Bucher JA. The prepared family caregiver: A problem-solving approach to family caregiver education. *Patient Educ Couns* 1996;**27**(1):63–73.

50. Kozachik S, Given C, Given B, et al. Improving depressive symptoms among caregivers of patients with cancer: Results of a randomized clinical trial. *Oncol Nurs Forum* 2001;**28**(7):1149–1157.

51. Northouse L, Walker J, Schafenacker A, et al. A family-based program of care for women with recurrent breast cancer and their family members. *Oncol Nurs Forum* 2002;**29**(10):1411–1419.

52. Pasacreta JV, McCorkle R. Cancer care: Impact of interventions on caregiver outcomes. *Annu Rev Nurs Res* 2000;**18**:127–148.

53. Toseland R, Blanchard C, McCallion P. A problem solving intervention for caregivers of cancer patients. *Soc Sci Med* 1995;**40**(4):517–528.

54. Blanchard C, Toseland R, McCallion P. The effects of a problem-solving intervention with spouses of cancer patients. *J Psychosoc Oncol* 1996;**14**(2):1–21.

55. Siminoff LA, Zyzanski SJ, Rose JH, Zhang AY. The cancer communication assessment tool for patients and families (CCAT-PF): A new measure. *Psychooncology* 2008;**17**(12):1216–1224.

56. Silveira MJ, Given CW, Given B, Rosland AM, Piette JD. (2010). Patient-caregiver concordance in symptom assessment and improvement in outcomes for patients undergoing cancer chemotherapy. *Chronic Illness* 2010;**6**(1):46–56.

57. Schumacher KL, Beidler SM, Beeber AS, Gambino P. A transactional model of cancer family caregiving skill. *ANS Adv Nurs Sci* 2006;**29**(3):271–286.

58. Toseland RW, McCallion P, Smith T, Banks, S. Supporting caregivers of frail older adults in an HMO setting. *Am J Orthopsychiatry* 2004;**74**(3):349–364.

59. Brown D, McWilliam C, Ward-Griffin C. Client-centred empowering partnering in nursing. *J Adv Nurs* 2006;**53**(2):160–168.

60. Heinrich M, Neufeld A, Harrison M. Seeking support caregiver strategies for interacting with health personnel. *Can J Res* 2003;**35**(4):38–56.

61. National Cancer Institute. *After Cancer Treatment Ends—the Impact on Caregivers and Families*, report of focus groups with caregivers and oncology social workers. NCI, Bethesda, MD, 2003.

■■■■■ CHAPTER 29

Comprehensive Geriatric Assessment

LAZZARO REPETTO and ANGELA MARIE ABBATECOLA

Italian National Reasearch Center on Aging (INRCA), Rome and Ancona, Italy

29.1 INTRODUCTION

The ability to provide high-quality healthcare to older persons in developed nations is an important concern. The number of individuals over the age of 65 years is projected to double by the year 2030, with a significant rise in the incidence of cancer in older individuals [1]. Cancer incidence is 11-fold higher in persons over the age of 65 years compared to younger adults [1]. Older adults with cancer will require a significantly higher level of functional assistance compared to those without cancer, and such an increase is considered essential for longer survival in these individuals [2]. Indeed, age-related changes impact the tolerance of anticancer therapy and negatively shift the risk benefit ratio in such individuals. With increasing age, physiologic reserve decreases; however, the pace of this decline varies with each individual.

Because they are systematically excluded from randomized clinical trials, older patients are usually treated according to the physician's experience and subjective extrapolations from adult clinical trials rather than on evidence based on controlled "geriatric" trials [3]. Conversely, the benefits and tolerance of commonly approved antineoplastic treatments are expected to differ in this age class. Thus, there is a critical need to develop specific clinical tools to assess the risk of treatment-related toxicity in older cancer patients.

The most important tool used for geriatric assessment of cancer patients is the *comprehensive geriatric assessment* (CGA), designed to identify multiple problems of geriatric patients in order to improve their quality of life and develop interventions. CGA initially starts with a multidimensional approach relevant to medical, functional, mental, nutritional, and social parameters. CGA is also used to recognize those individuals with frailty or at risk for frailty, which represents complex and challenging problems for physicians and healthcare professionals, due to a higher susceptibility for adverse outcomes, such as institutionalization or mortality. In particular, there is evidence showing that cancer patients with the frailty syndrome have a 50% risk for mortality at 2 years [4]. CGA has also been shown to predict other important outcomes, such as morbidity in older patients, especially with regard to drug treatment strategy.

Cancer and Aging Handbook: Research and Practice, First Edition. Edited by Keith M. Bellizzi and Margot A. Gosney.
© 2012 Wiley-Blackwell. Published 2012 by John Wiley & Sons, Inc.

In this chapter, we will highlight the diverse components of the CGA, including functional status, comorbidity, psychological status, social support, cognitive function, polypharmacy, and nutrition and the importance of each CGA domain and the risk of morbidity and mortality in older adults. We will also review current achievements with the use of CGA in cancer patients and discuss the association between geriatric syndromes and multiple adverse clinical outcomes.

29.2 DEFINITION OF COMPREHENSIVE GERIATRIC ASSESSMENT

The comprehensive geriatric assessment (CGA) was originally developed by geriatricians as a multidisciplinary evaluation in order to encompass a important clinical domains, including physical function, psychocognitive status, nutrition, social support, and comorbidity for clinical decisionmaking (Table 29.1). At the moment many physicians are including the evaluation of polypharmacy during CGA; however, data specific to the impact of polypharmacy on tolerance to cancer treatment are still very limited.

29.3 COMPREHENSIVE GERIATRIC ASSESSMENT IN ONCOLOGY

In this context, it is important to underline that different scales are used by geriatricians and oncologists in measuring physical function. In fact, while the oncologist usually measures this domain using subjective scales that estimate the "weight" of functional impairments (e.g., the scale used by the Eastern Cooperative Oncology Group (ECOG) or Karnofski performance status scales), the geriatrician adopts a wider set of instruments that combine subjective and objective evaluations. Besides the "traditional" activities of daily living (ADL) and instrumental ADL (IADL) scales, since the 1980s, physical performance measures, such as walking speed tests, short physical performance battery, muscle strength tests, have become increasingly important. Interestingly, it has been shown that these objective measures of physical function are not only more sensitive to changes than subjective scales but are also associated with major clinical outcomes such as disability, comorbidity, hospitalisation, and mortality [5,6].

29.3.1 Physical Function Assessment

Physical function status is traditionally evaluated using daily living dependence scales, including the Katz index, which has been shown to predict 1-year mortality and hospital readmission in older adults [7]. In particular, researchers have shown that specific geriatric measures of daily dependence, including activities of daily living (ADLs) and instrumental activities of daily living (IADLs), have a greater predictive value on physical function compared to traditional oncology measures of performance [8]. In particular, ADLs are basic self-care skills needed to maintain independence in the home, including the ability to bathe, dress, feed oneself, attend to personal hygiene, transfer from bed to chair and back, and voluntarily control urinary and fecal discharge. IADLs are not necessary for fundamental functioning, but they indicate the ability of an individual to live independently in a community and include the ability to do the following: light housework, prepare meals, take medications, shop for groceries, use the telephone, and manage money.

TABLE 29.1   Diverse Components of Comprehensive Geriatric Assessment and Implications in Elderly Cancer Patients

CGA Component	Test	Implications in Cancer
Key CGA Components		
Functional status	Activities of daily living (ADL) instrumental activities of daily living (IADL)	Disability in the IADLs are associated with decreased survival in non–small cell lung cancer and acute leukemia
Comorbid (coexisting) medical conditions	The cumulative illness rating scale (CIRS)	Increasing extent of comorbidity has been associated with parallel increases in cancer specific and all-cause mortality in patients with breast cancer
Cognition	Mini mental state examination (MMSE)	Presence of dementia may decrease the likelihood of receiving adjuvant systemic therapy in breast and colorectal cancer
Psychological status	Geriatric depression scale Hamiliton depression scale	Distress correlates with poorer physical function in patients with solid tumors
Potential CGA Components		
Social functioning and support	Lubben social network scale	An increase in all-cause and cancer-specific mortality has been observed in older women with breast cancer who are socially isolated
Socioeconomic issues	Socioeconomic assessment	Older patients with limited finances may forgo purchase of supportive care medications in favor of purchasing anticancer therapy, decreasing their ability to tolerate treatment
Polypharmacy	Number of medications	Studies of older adults with cancer suggest an average of up to 9 medications per patient, with limited efforts to assess for drug–drug interactions with chemotherapy

Even though it has been reported that older cancer patients are more likely to present some form of functional dependence compared with older adults without cancer, another study showed different results [9]. In particular this study revealed that performance status was not as predictive as a full CGA, thus underlining the importance of a complete CGA. The presence of dependence in the ADL scales, measured by the Katz index, has been shown to be a good discriminator for 1-year mortality, following hospital admission in individuals over 70 years of age [7]. Additionally, the pretreatment global quality of life using the the European Organization for Research and Treatment of Cancer QLQ-C30 questionnaire and higher IADL scores have been significantly associated with better survival in elderly patients with advanced non–small cell lung cancer treated with chemotherapy [10].

The correlation of ADL dependence and outcome is less established in studies of older patients receiving outpatient oncology care, probably because of the low number of patients requiring ADL assistance and a ceiling effect in detecting dependence using this tool. However, some studies have demonstrated that the presence of impairment in ADL increases the risk of mortality in older hospitalized adults [11].

The use of frailty markers has also been used to detect functional dependency among older cancer patients without any ADL or IADL deficiency [12]. This finding suggests that in addition to the assessment of functional status and in particular the assessment of IADLs and ADLs, the evaluation of frailty markers may be necessary for the recognition of functional disability in those without IADL or ADL dependence.

Approximately 80% of older cancer patients are ADL-independent, and 50% are IADL-independent [8,13]. It has been shown that there was no evidence of any change in ADLs and IADLs scores even in older breast cancer patients experiencing severe toxicity due to chemotherapy [14]. However, the Cardiovascular Health Study (CHS) demonstrated that older persons with three or more frailty markers were at a significantly higher risk of adverse outcomes, such as falls, worsening mobility, ADL dependence, hospitalization, and 3-year mortality [15]. At the moment, the literature lacks similar evidence in older cancer patients. Therefore, the assessment of functional status based on ADL and IADL scores might have a ceiling effect on the recognition of vulnerability in a population of independently functioning elderly cancer patients. Consequently, there is a need to identify different tools, such as frailty markers, that may play a pivotal role in identifying those persons at a significantly higher risk for complications in response to aggressive treatment.

29.3.2 Cognitive and Depression Assessment

Cognitive decline occurs with advancing age and is associated with an increased risk for all-cause mortality [16]. The CGA includes testing for cognitive status and in older patients with cancer. An impairment in cognitive status can result in a significant difficulty in understanding and remembering treatment instructions, which, in turn, could affect compliance with oral cancer therapy and other supportive treatment. In geriatric oncology, cognitive impairment may also be associated with a delay in the diagnosis, due to the patient's inability to recognize and recall signs and symptoms of cancer. The *mini–mental state examination* (MMSE) is considered an easy and validated test for cognitive screening evaluation and is one of the most widely used screening tools in geriatric medicine, as well as geriatric oncology [17]. The MMSE covers the cognitive domains of orientation, memory, attention, calculation, language, and constructional ability. It has a total score of 30 points, and a general cutoff score of <24 is considered abnormal. Performance on this exam also depends on age and education, however, so normative data adjusted for these variables have been reported. Approximately one-third of elderly cancer patients are cognitively impaired using MMSE [8]. However, another test for cognition, the Montreal Cognitive Assessment, detected mild cognitive impairment in cancer patients with a normal MMSE [12]. It has been reported that cancer treatments may worsen cognitive status [18]. These observations confirm the importance of routinely evaluating cognitive status in older cancer patients throughout treatment and survivorship.

Depressive symptoms are common and disabling in older age, particularly in individuals with comorbid physical illness, such as cancer. Up to 50% of older cancer patients have been found to have depressive symptoms [8], and these symptoms are associated with high healthcare and social care costs [19]. Since elderly patients with cancer are at increased risk of depression, the study of the common molecular mechanisms involved in the pathogenesis of both cancer and depression, in association with the physiological changes due to aging, may lead to identification of the interrelation of these diseases and their causal relationships, and therefore provide a valuable tool for new strategy of clinical intervention.

Bernabei and colleagues [20] investigated the relationship between depression and pain in elderly cancer patients and observed that patients with depression were more sensitive to cancer-related pain. These data are consistent with studies on noncancer institutionalized elderly people affected by different medical conditions and underline the importance of appropriate pain management. Notably, the presence of pain increases the prevalence of depression in cancer patients [21] who complain not only of more depressive disorders, but also of anxiety and somatic symptoms, compared to patients without pain [22]. Indeed, it has been argued that anxiety disorders associated with pain in elderly cancer patients are decreased after treatment with analgesics [23] as well as behavioral interventions. The link between pain and depression appears to be bidirectional, and there is strong evidence that pain causes depression in cancer patients [21,24]. At the moment, of the several validated screening instruments for depression, the geriatric depression scale [25] and the Hamilton depression scale [26], are the most widely accepted.

29.3.3 Nutritional Status

There is an association between low body mass index (BMI) and an increased risk for mortality in older community-dwelling adults [27]. Nutritional status is a marker of frailty and a prognostic indicator in patients with cancer. Unintentional weight loss indicates a poor prognosis; similarly, it is important to underline that obesity is also a common problem in cancer patients [2,28]. Early identification of weight loss should alert healthcare providers to recommend an immediate nutritional intervention, as well as to investigate its underlying cause. A study of older cancer survivors demonstrated that a home-based diet and exercise intervention was feasible and can improve nutritional well-being and physical function [28]. Even though several tools have been identified for nutritional screening, one of the most validated in the elderly is the *mini−nutritional assessment* (MNA), which takes into account food intake and weight loss over the last 3 months, anthropometric parameters, self-perceived nutrition and health, mobility, acute disease, and neuropsychological problems [29]. This test is especially important for identifying those patients at risk for malnutrition.

29.3.4 Comorbidy

The incidence and prevalance of comorbid health conditions increase with age, and these conditions have been associated with a higher risk for mortality in older persons with cancer. Comorbidity is frequently measured in terms of an index, scale, or total number of acute and/or chronic conditions. Comorbid medical conditions influence life expectancy, tolerance to cancer therapy, and disease prognosis. Since the risk of comorbid medical conditions may outweigh the risk of the cancer, careful evaluation of comorbidity is strongly recommended in older cancer patients.

Some of the most commonly used scales include the Charlson comorbidity index (CCI) [30], or the cumulative illness rating scale—geriatrics (CIRS-G) [31]. Even though there are many validated comorbidity scales, the ability of these scales to predict clinical outcomes in cancer patients are still under investigation. Further investigations are needed in order to define the best scale for a specific endpoint such as mortality or toxicity. In a study of 7600 cancer patients ≥ 55 years, those aged 55–64 had an average number of comorbid conditions of 2.9 compared with 4.2 comorbid conditions in patients ≥75 years [1]. The prognostic implications of comorbidities were supported in an observational cohort study including 17,712 patients with different cancer types in which the severity of comorbidities affected overall survival (OS) in a dose-dependent fashion, independent of cancer stage [32].

When formulating a treatment plan, oncologists need to estimate the risk of the malignancy with that of comorbid illness on life expectancy. The effect of treatment in decreasing this risk also needs to be weighed. Therefore, indolent cancers may be managed more conservatively in the setting of a substantial comorbid disease that is more likely to have an impact on life expectancy. In contrast, more aggressive malignancies warrant cancer therapy if they are more likely to affect life expectancy than the comorbid illness. The presence and extent of comorbidity appears to impact surgical decisionmaking in oncology, such as the use of axillary clearance, radical prostatectomy, and resection for breast, prostate, and lung cancer, respectively [33–35]. Similarly, comorbidity appears to affect utilization of chemotherapy in colon, breast, and lung cancer [36–38]. Although this trend reflects studies suggesting greater chemotherapy-related toxicity among patients with comorbidity, conflicting data do exist and there is a need to further identify patents at higher risk of treatment-related toxicities in clinical trials and the ability to modify cancer treatment in patients with severe comorbidities.

29.3.5 Polypharmacy

Currently, a standard definition of *polypharmacy* does not exist. Criteria such as taking more than three medications, taking unnecessary or redundant medications, or taking medications that confer a risk for adverse drug events (ADEs) have been proposed. Cancer patients often receive combination chemotherapy, supportive treatment, and drugs to counteract cancer-treatment-related side effects. With aging, comorbidity is more frequent, and it is estimated that four out of five elderly persons present at least one comorbidity, and that 50% of elderly cancer patients take at least five prescribed medications daily [39]. There are little data on the use of *over-the-counter* and *complementary and alternative* medications, even though their use is twofold greater than prescription medication in older patients [40]. One survey showed that >20% of adults take prescription medications concomitantly with nonvitamin dietary supplements [41]. This finding is likely to be higher in older individuals and in those with cancer. Patients prefer these "medications" because they are readily available, widely advertised, often cheaper, and presumed to be safer than prescription drugs. Often patients will not regard such products as "medication."

Thus polypharmacy and its inherent complications are particularly prevalent in the elderly cancer population, and such individuals are at high risk for adverse drug events.

Older patients experience varying degrees of physiological changes that may affect the pharmacokinetic (PK) and pharmacodynamic (PD) properties of a drug; age-associated alterations in PK have not been fully evaluated because of the limited enrollment of older patients in clinical trials. Drug distribution is affected by age-related changes in body composition, hematologic reserves, and nutritional and disease-related decrements in plasma proteins. Also the occurrence of ascites, cachexia, edema, and sarcopenia affect drug distribution.

Most chemotherapy agents similar to other drugs are metabolized by the liver. The cytochrome P450 microsomal enzyme pathway decreases with age. The CYP3A4 enzyme is critical to metabolism of many drugs. Polypharmacy increases competition for enzymatic activity and increases the risk for drug–drug interactions. Kidney function is extremely important in drug excretion. Age-related decrements in the glomerular filtration rate (GFR) may delay the clearance of several drugs. Dose adjustment based on liver function and measured GFR are strongly recommended. Risk factors for polypharmacy include number and classes of drugs, multiple disease processes, disease severity, frailty, nonadherence, medication "hoarding," nondisclosure, and access to multiple healthcare providers. Some interaction examples are as follows:

Interaction	Example
Drug–drug	Warfarin–capecitabine
Drug–disease	Narcotics–chronic constipation
	Dexamethasone–diabetes
Disease–drug	Ascites–various-drug distribution
	Chronic renal insufficiency–various-drug clearance
Drug–food	Bisphosphonates–absorption

When initiating chemotherapy, individual response to toxicity and risk for ADEs should be monitored continuously. Each additional medication, including supportive therapies and growth factors, should be weighed carefully for benefit versus risk of ADEs in the context of the existing regimen. Regular review of all medication for redundancy and interactions and simplification is critical in the oncogeriatric clinical practice.

29.3.6 Social Support

Lack of social support has been associated with increased mortality in the older population [64]. There are no studies that address the prognostic role of social support in elderly cancer patients; thus we lack information to guide interventions in this particular setting. We reported that elderly cancer patients consider family support in clinical communication and coping with the cancer disease to be extremely important [42].

29.3.7 Geriatric Syndrome of Frailty in Older Cancer Patients

The term *geriatric syndrome* is used to capture those clinical conditions in older persons that do not fit into discrete disease categories. Geriatric syndromes (Table 29.2), including delirium, falls, frailty, dizziness, syncope, and urinary incontinence, are among the most common conditions faced by geriatricians on a daily basis [43–45]. Table 29.2

TABLE 29.2   Clinical Descriptions of Commonly Observed Geriatric Syndromes

Geriatric Syndromes	Clinical Description
Delirium	*Delirium* is a transient organic mental syndrome of acute onset, characterized by global impairment of cognitive functions, reduced level of consciousness, attention abnormalities, increased or decreased psychomotor activity and a disordered sleep–wake cycle
Falls	A *fall* is a sudden, unintentional change in position causing an individual to land at a lower level, for example, on an object, floor, or ground, that is not consequence of a sudden onset of paralysis, epileptic seizure, or overwhelming external force
Frailty	According to phenotypic definition, *frailty* is defined as the presence of ≥3 of 5 components: muscle weakness and slow walking speed, exhaustion, low physical activity, and unintentional weight loss; definition of frailty based on frailty index (FI) is based on deficit accumulation using 70 deficits from clinical examination
Dizziness	Painless head discomfort with many causes, including disturbances of vision, brain, balance (vestibular) system of the inner ear, and gastrointestinal system; *dizziness* is a medically indistinct term used to describe a variety of conditions ranging from lightheadedness, unsteadiness to *vertigo*
Urinary incontinence	The inability to control urination or bladder function; severity of *urinary incontinence* ranges from occasionally leaking urine to unpredictable episodes of strong urinary urgency
Syncope	*Syncope* is partial or complete loss of consciousness with a temporary interruption of awareness of oneself and one's surroundings

summarizes these predominately observed clinical conditions even in older cancer patients.

Geriatric syndromes have been regarded as highly prevalent, mostly single-symptom states, caused by diverse impairment in multiple symptoms due to alterations in many pathogenetic pathways. However, one of the most widely studied geriatric syndromes identified today by researchers has a heterogeneous clinical appearance with many symptoms and is called the *frailty syndrome*. Frailty is an important clinical and public health problem. How to define frailty, however, remains controversial. Frailty has been defined as a syndrome of decreased reserve and resistance to stressors characterized by a high degree of vulnerability to negative health outcomes such as disability, comorbidity, and mortality [46].

The term *frailty* is frequently used to describe patients who are in poor overall health, are vulnerable to the ill effects of environmental stressors, and are further at high risk for worsened morbidity, worsened disability, and mortality [47].

In clinical practice, there is an increase in the number of frail patients who require a substantial amounts of medical services. Frailty is associated with alterations of many organs and systems, including the nervous and endocrine systems, the immune function, the respiratory system, and musculoskeletal apparatus. Even biochemical alterations, including increased inflammatory activities, altered carbohydrate metabolism, and intravascular coagulation, have been associated with frailty. Undoubtedly, lifestyle may contribute to frailty with lack of physical activity, smoking, excessive alcohol intake, and an unhealthy diet. The symptoms may be subtle, nonspecific, and even absent. Frailty may be present in apparently healthy persons and become evident following a destabilizing event (e.g., surgical operation, chemotherapy) that exceeds a critical stress threshold.

Kenneth Rockwood et al. [48] compared two approaches to measuring frailty: the specific phenotype and the deficit accumulation. The first defines frailty based on five items (weight loss, low energy expenditure, exhaustion, slowness, weakness), any three of which mark a person as frail. The patients are classified as *frail* if they have three of the five criteria, *prefrail* if they have one or two, and *not frail* if they did not have any of the criteria [48]. Using these criteria, Fried et al. showed that in this older population, 7% were frail, 47% prefrail, and 46% not frail [46]. Frailty is thus defined as the presence of three of five components: muscle weakness and slow walking speed (<75 out of 100 on the RAND-36 physical function scale; counts as two components), exhaustion (<55 out of 100 on the RAND-36 vitality scale), low physical activity (kilocalories of weekly energy expenditure in the lowest quartile, calculated from a detailed physical activity questionnaire), and unintentional weight loss (>5% of body weight in the previous 2 years) [49]. The phenotypic definition of frailty was validated in the Cardiovascular Health Study by showing its predictive value for major health-related outcomes, including disability, falls, hospitalizations, and death over a 3-year period [46].

The second approach does not consider the presence of specific single items (or specific combinations) to define frailty, but rather sums 70 deficits in order to define the frailty index (FI). Frailty is based on a count of accumulated deficits rather than a phenotype [50]. Considerable convergence was found between the two indices. The phenotypic definition of frailty, which readily offers an easy clinical approach, discriminates broad levels of risk. The deficit accumulation approach requires an additional clinical translation that allows for a more precise definition of adverse outcomes, but has a less appealing clinical application [48]. Assessing seven frailty markers (nutrition, mobility, strength, energy, physical activity, mood, and cognition), 88% of older cancer patients (aged >70 years) had at least one altered marker and were considered potentially vulnerable [12]. These findings underline the need for a better definition of frailty and more reliable tools for its assessment, especially in cancer patients. These tools will lead to a better categorization of patients and the ability to predict adverse outcomes. Some basic clinical features associated with the frailty syndrome include the following: (1) mobility, such as lower-extremity performance and gait abnormalities; (2) muscle weakness; (3) poor exercise tolerance; (4) unstable balance; and (5) factors related to body composition, such as malnutrition, sarcopenia, and weight loss (15).

29.4   CGA AND OUTCOMES IN CLINICAL ONCOLOGY

The use of comprehensive geriatric assessment in older cancer patients is strongly recommended [51]. The CGA also evaluates elements of the frailty syndrome, and there is evidence that suggests the use of the CGA has a predictive value on important health outcomes in older cancer patients [12,52].

Despite the paucity of data on frailty assessment in cancer patients, the geriatric assessment may be especially beneficial for frail individuals. Balducci and Extermann proposed frailty criteria in oncologic patients derived from Winograd criteria that includes: age >85 years, ADL impairment, three or more comorbidities, and one or more geriatric syndromes. Using these criteria, Mohile et al. [52] reported that 80% of elderly cancer patients are frail in comparison with 73% of noncancer controls.

Because most of the available treatment for cancer is potentially toxic for patients, selection of the most appropriate treatment is based on patient characteristics. It has been shown that traditional oncology measures of performance status are not adequate in older patients and that specific geriatric measures, such as activities of daily living (ADLs) and instrumental activities of daily living (IADLs) [8] add relevant information in the clinical evaluation of the patient.

It also has been reported that IADL dependence is predictive of decreased survival in cancer patients [53]. Dependence in ADL is more common in metastatic patients in comparison with nonmetastatic [54]. ADLs and IADLs have also been correlated with pain severity and psychological distress [55,56]. In older cancer patients, comorbidity has been associated with both morbidity and mortality [57] and treatment tolerance [58]. Several elements of a geriatric assessment, including need for assistance, as well as depression and polypharmacy, were predictive of severe chemotherapy related toxicity in ovarian cancer patients [59].

According to the available evidence, the prognostic and predictive potentials of CGA have been investigated prospectively to support treatment choices in older cancer patients. To identify risk factors for grade 3–5 chemotoxicity and develop a risk stratification schema, 500 patients aged 65 years and older were recruited from seven institutions, assessed with CGA, and treated with different chemotherapy regimens for different cancer types. Multivariate logistic regression identified seven independent risk factors for grade 3–5 chemotoxicity (age >73 years, cancer type, standard dose, polychemotherapy, falls in the last 6 months, IADL disability, and decreased social activity). This tool, based on the number of risk factors (one to seven), predicts the risk of severe chemotherapy-related toxicity from 23% to 100% [60].

Another study assessed the individual risk of severe toxicity from chemotherapy, defined by Common Toxicity Criteria v. 3.0., as grade 4 hematologic or grade 3/4 nonhematologic toxicity, in older patients with diverse health conditions and functional reserve measured by CGA. Several demographic and clinical variables were analyzed. Chemotherapy-related toxicity (chemotoxicity) was adjusted using the MAX2 score [61]. Using this tool, the CRASH (Chemotherapy Risk Assessment Scale for High-age patients) score, LDH, diastolic BP, and chemotoxicity were the best predictive variables for significant differences in the risk of severe hematological toxicity. ECOG-PS, mini–mental status, mini–nutritional assessment, and chemotoxicity were the best predictive variables for severe nonhematological toxicity. The CRASH score identifies four categories (0–3, 4–6, 7–9, >9) of older patients with different risk of severe toxicity (from 61% to 100%) when starting a new chemotherapy [62].

Although these instruments need further confirmation in the clinical practice, they confirm the strong predictive value of CGA in older cancer patients and provide useful tools to individualize treatment choices on an objective basis. A full CGA was compared with a short 13-item function-based screening instrument, the Vulnerable Elders Survey 13 (VES13) assessment [63,64], in a prospective study conducted in older cancer patients [65]. The differences between the VES13 and the CGA are reported in Table 29.3. In the VES13 scale, patients scoring ≥3 were considered vulnerable; 53% of the cancer patients were vulnerable on VES13, with 30% showing disabilities with

TABLE 29.3   Summary of Vulnerable Elders Survey and Components of Comprehensive Geriatric Assessment

Test	Geriatric Domain	Components Number	Administration (min)	Score Range	Cutoff Point Associated with Adverse Outcomes
VES13	Functionally based screening measure	13	Self-administered (5)	0–10	≥3
ADL	Function	8	Self-administered (5–10)	0–16	≤14
IADL	Function	7	Self-administered (5–10)	0–14	≤12
SPPB	Objective evaluation of function/physical performance	3 separate physical performance tests	Administered by member of research team (10–15)	0–12	<9
CALGB	Comorbidity	18	Self-administered (15)	0–54	>10
Number of medications	Comorbidity/toxicity potential from drug interactions	1	Self-administered (1–5)	0–∞	≥5
Short portable mental status questionnaire	Cognition/risk for dementia	10	Administered by member of research team (10–15)	0–10	>3

Notation: VES13 = Vulnerable Elders Survey 13; ADL = activities of daily living; IADL = instrumental of activities of daily living; SPPB = short physical performance battery; cancer and leukemia group B (CALGB).

CGA. The sensitivity and specificity of VES13 versus CGA were 87% and 62%, respectively. This study shows that VES13 is highly predictive of functional status and can be used as a screening test for the evaluation of older cancer patients. It must be underlined that we lack data on the association between VES13 and chemotherapy-related toxicity, thus this tool cannot be recommended to support the choice of chemotherapy regimens in the older cancer patients.

29.5 CONCLUSIONS

This chapter has outlined the importance of the use of the CGA in older cancer patients. The CGA was designed to identify multiple problems of geriatric patients in order to improve their quality of life and develop interventions. The multidimensional approach of the CGA allows a relevant evaluation of an individual's medical, physical, depression, cognition, nutritional, and social needs. Interestingly, more recent studies have also underlined the importance of the use of frailty markers, especially in older patients with cancer, and especially in those with apparently good physical autonomy. Indeed, the CGA does include some elements of frailty; however, future studies are needed to identify specific frailty markers in order to obtain a complete clinical assessment for older cancer patients. At the moment, the use of the CGA remains pivotal in the choice of specific objectively based treatment options in older persons afflicted with cancer.

REFERENCES

1. Yancik R. (1997) Cancer burden in the aged: An epidemiologic and demographic overview. *Cancer* 1997;**80**:1273–1282.

2. Keating NL, Norredam M, Landrum MB, et al. (2005) Physical and mental health status of older long-term cancer survivors. *J Am Geriatr Soc* 2005;**53**:2145–2152.

3. Levy B, Kosteas J, Slade M, Myers L. Exclusion of elderly persons from health-risk behavior clinical trials. *Prevent Med* 2006;**43**:80–85.

4. Balducci L, Extermann M. Carreca I. Management of breast cancer in the older woman. *Cancer Control* 2001;**8**:431–441.

5. Rozzini R, Frisoni GB, Bianchetti A, Zanetti O, Trabucchi M. Physical performance test and activities of daily living scales in the assessment of health status in elderly people. *J Am Geriatr Soc* 1993;**41**:1109–1113.

6. Cesari M, Kritchevsky SB, Newman AB, et al. Added value of physical performance measures in predicting adverse health-related events: Results from the health, aging and body composition study. *J Am Geriatr Soc* 2009;**57**:251–259.

7. Walter LC, Brand RJ, Counsell SR, Palmer RM, et al. Development and validation of a prognostic index for 1-year mortality in older adults after hospitalization. *JAMA* 2001;**285**(23):2987–2994.

8. Repetto L, Fratino L, Audisio RA, et al. Comprehensive geriatric assessment adds information to Eastern Cooperative Oncology Group performance status in elderly cancer patients: An Italian Group for Geriatric Oncology Study. *J Clin Oncol* 2002;**20**(2):494–502.

9. Repetto L, Venturino A, Vercelli M, Gianni W, Biancardi V, Casella C, Granetto C, Parodi S, Rosso R, Marigliano V Performance status and comorbidity in elderly cancer patients compared to a young neoplastic and an elderly non-neoplastic population. *Cancer* 1998;**82**:760–765.

10. Maione P, Perrone F, Gallo C, et al. Pretreatment quality of life and functional status assessment significantly predict survival of elderly patients with advanced non-small-cell lung cancer receiving chemotherapy: A prognostic analysis of the multicenter Italian lung cancer in the elderly study. *J Clin Oncol* 2005;**23**(28):6865–6872.

11. Ponzetto M, Maero B, Maina P, et al. Risk factors for early and late mortality in hospitalized older patients: The continuing importance of functional status. *J Gerontol A Biol Sci Med Sci* 2003;**58**:1049–1054.

12. Retornaz F, Monette J, Batist G, et al. Usefulness of frailty markers in the assessment of the health and functional status of older cancer patients referred for chemotherapy: A pilot study. *J Gerontol A Biol Sci Med Sci* 2008;**63**(5):518–522.

13. Retornaz F, Seux V, et al. Comparison of the health and functional status between older inpatients with and without cancer admitted to a geriatric/internal medicine unit. *J Gerontol A Biol Sci Med Sci* 2007;**62**(8):917–922.

14. Hurria A, Zuckerman E, Panageas KS, Fornier M, D'Andrea G, et al. A prospective, longitudinal study of the functional status and quality of life of older patients with breast cancer receiving adjuvant chemotherapy. *J Am Geriatr Soc* 2006;**54**(7):1119–1124.

15. Fried LP, Tangen CM, Walston J, et al. Frailty in older adults: Evidence for a phenotype. *J Gerontol Med Sci* 2001;**56A**:M146–M156, 1111–1116.

16. Wolfson C, Wolfson DB, Asgharian M, et al. Clinical Progression of Dementia Study Group: A reevaluation of the duration of survival after the onset of dementia. *N Engl J Med* 2001;**344**(15):1111–1116.

17. Folstein MF, Folstein SE, McHugh PR. "Mini-mental state": a practical method for grading the cognitive state of patients for the clinician. *J Psychiatr Res* 1975;**12**:189–198.

18. Hurria A., Rosen C., Hudis C., et al. Cognitive function of older patients receiving adjuvant chemotherapy for breast cancer: A pilot prospective longitudinal study. *J Am Geriatr Soc* 2006;**54**:925–931.

19. Langa KM, Fendrick AM, Chernew ME, Kabeto MU, Paisley KL, Hayman JA. Out-of-pocket health-care expenditures among older Americans with cancer. *Value Health* 2004;**7**(2):186–194.

20. Bernabei R, Gambassi G, Lapane K, et al. Management of pain in elderly patients with cancer. SAGE Study Group. Systematic assessment of geriatric drug use via epidemiology. *JAMA* 1998;**279**:1877–1882.

21. Spiegel D, Sands S, Koopman C. Pain and depression in patients with cancer. *Cancer* 1994;**74**:2570–2578.

22. Massie MJ, Holland JC. The cancer patient with pain: Psychiatric complications and their management. *Med Clin North Am* 1987;**71**:243–258.

23. Roth AJ, Modi R. Psychiatric issues in older cancer patients. *Crit Rev Oncol Hematol* 2003;**48**:185–197.

24. Spiecker M, Peng HB, Liao JK. (1997) Inhibition of endothelial vascular cell adhesion molecule-1 expression by nitric oxide involves the induction and nuclear translocation of IkappaBalpha. *J Biol Chem* 1997;**272**:30969–30974.

25. Sheikh JI, Yesavage JA. Geriatric depression scale (GDS): Recent evidence and development of a shorter version. In *Clinical Gerontology: A Guide to Assessment and Intervention*, The Haworth Press, New York, 1986, pp. 165–173.

26. Hamilton M. A rating scale for depression. *J Neurol Neurosurg Psychiatry* 1960;**23**:56–62.

27. Rantanen T, Harris T, Leveille SG, Visser M, Foley D, Masaki K, Guralnik JM. Muscle strength and body mass index as long-term predictors of mortality in initially healthy men. *J Gerontol A Biol Sci Med Sci* 2000;**55**(3):M168–173.

28. Demark-Wahnefried W, Clipp EC, Morey MC, et al. Lifestyle intervention development study to improve physical function in older adults with cancer: Outcomes from project LEAD. *J Clin Oncol* 2006;**24**:3465–3473.

29. Guigoz Y, Vellas B, Garry P. Mini nutritional assessment: A practical assessment tool for grading the nutritional state of elderly patients. *Facts Res Gerontol* 1994;**4**(Suppl 2): 15–59.

30. Charlson M, Szatrowski TP, Peterson J, Gold J. Validation of a combined comorbidity index. *J Clin Epidemiol* 1994;**47**(11):1245–1251.

31. Miller MD, Paradis CF, Houck PR (1992) Rating chronic medical illness burden in geropsychiatric practice and research: Application of the cumulative illness rating scale. *Psychiatry Res* 1992;**41**(3):237–248.

32. Piccirillo JF, Tierney RM, Costas I, et al. Prognostic importance of comorbidity in a hospitalbased cancer registry. *JAMA* 2004;**291**:2441–2447.

33. Konety BR, Cowan JE, Carroll PR. (2008) Patterns of primary and secondary therapy for prostate cancer in elderly men: Analysis of data from CaPSURE. *J Urol* 2008;**179**:1797–1803.

34. Smith TJ, Penberthy L, Desch CE, et al. Differences in initial treatment patterns and outcomes of lung cancer in the elderly. *Lung Cancer* 1995;**13**:235–252.

35. Yancik R, Wesley MN, Ries LAG, et al. Effect of age and comorbidity in postmenopausal breast cancer patients aged 55 years and older. *JAMA* 2001;**285**:885–892.

36. Keating NL, Landrum MB, Klabunde CN, et al. Adjuvant chemotherapy for stage III colon cancer: Do physicians agree about the importance of patient age and comorbidity? *J Clin Oncol* 2008;**26**:2532–2537.

37. Hurria A, Wong FL, Villaluna D, et al. Role of age and health in treatment recommendations for older adults with breast cancer: The perspective of oncologists and primary care providers. *J Clin Oncol* 2008;**26**:5386–5392.

38. Blanco JAG, Toste IS, Alvarez RF, et al. Age, comorbidity, treatment decision and prognosis in lung cancer. *Age Ageing* 2008;**37**:715–718.

39. Lichtman S. Pharmacokinetics and pharmacodynamics in the elderly. *Clin Adv Hematol Oncol* 2007;**5**:181–182.

40. Colt HG, Shapiro AP. Drug-induced illness as a cause for admission to a community hospital. *J Am Geriatr Soc* 1989;**37**:323–326.

41. Gardiner P, Graham RE, Legedza ATR, Eiseberg DM, Phillips RS. Factors associated with dietary supplement use among prescription medication users. *Arch Intern Med* 2006;**166**:1968–1974.

42. Repetto L, Piselli P, Raffaele M, Locatelli C, for the GIOGer. Communicating cancer diagnosis and prognosis: When the target is the elderly patient-a GIOGer study. *Eur J Cancer* 2009;**45**:374–383.

43. Landi F, Abbatecola AM, Provinciali M, Corsonello A, Bustacchini S, Manigrasso L, Cherubini A, Bernabei R, Lattanzio F. Moving against frailty: Does physical activity matter? *Biogerontology* 2010;**11**(5):537–545.

44. Inouye SK, Studenski S, Tinetti ME, Kuchel GA. Geriatric syndromes: Clinical, research, and policy implications of a core geriatric concept. *J Am Geriatr Soc* 2007;**55**:780–791.

45. Cicerchia M, Ceci M, Locatelli C, Gianni W, Repetto L. Geriatric syndromes in perioperative elderly cancer patients. *Surg Oncol* 2010;**19**:131–139.

46. Fried LP, Tangen CM, Walston J, et al. Cardiovascular Health Study Collaborative Research Group. Frailty in older adults: Evidence for a phenotype. *J Gerontol Med Sci* 2001;**56A**:M146–M156.

47. Fisher AL. Just what defines frailty? *J Am Geriatr Soc* 2005;**53**:2229–2230.

48. Rockwood K, Andrew M, Mitnitski A. A comparison of two approaches to measuring frailty in elderly people. *J Gerontol A Biol Sci Med Sci* 2007;**62**(7):738–743.

49. Fugate Woods N, LaCroix AZ, Gray SL, et al. Frailty: Emergence and consequences in women aged 65 and older in the Women's Health Initiative Observational Study. *J Am Geriatr Soc* 2005;**53**:1321–1330.

50. Mitnitski A, Mogilner A, Rockwood K. Accumulation of deficits as a proxy measure of aging. *Sci World J* 2001;**1**:323–336.

51. Extermann M, Aapro M, Bernabei R, et al. Use of comprehensive geriatric assessment in older cancer patients: Recommendations from the task force on CGA of the International Society of Geriatric Oncology (SIOG). *Crit Rev Oncol Hematol* 2005;**55**:241–252.

52. Mohile SG, Xian Y, Dale W, Fisher SG, Rodin M, et al. Association of a cancer diagnosis with vulnerability and frailty in older Medicare beneficiaries. *J Natl Cancer Inst* 2009;**101**(17):1206–1215.

53. Fidias P, Supko JG, Martins R, et al. A phase II study of weekly paclitaxel in elderly patients with advanced non-small cell lung cancer. *Clin Cancer Res* 2001;**7**:3942–3949.

54. Gauvin A, Pinguet F, Culine S, et al. Bayesian estimate of vinorelbine pharmacokinetic parameters in elderly patients with advanced metastatic cancer. *Clin Cancer Res* 2000;**6**:2690–2695.

55. Wedding U, Rohrig B, Klippstein A, et al. Age, severe comorbidity and functional impairment independently contribute to poor survival in cancerpatients. *J Cancer Res Clin Oncol* 2007;**133**:945–950.

56. Hurria A, Li D, Hansen K, et al. Distress in older patients with cancer. *J Clin Oncol* 2009;**27**:4346–4351.

57. Satariano WA, Ragland DR. The effect of comorbidity on 3-year survival of women with primary breast cancer. *Ann Intern Med* 1994;**120**:104–110.

58. Kroenke CH, Kubzansky LD, Schernhammer ES, et al. Social networks, social support, and survival after breast cancer diagnosis. *J Clin Oncol* 2006;**24**:1105–1111.

59. Freyer G, Geay J-F, Touzet S, et al. Comprehensive geriatric assessment predicts tolerance to chemotherapy and survival in elderly patients with advanced ovarian carcinoma: A GINECO study. *Ann Oncol* 2005;**16**:1795–1800.

60. Hurria A. Predicting chemotherapy toxicity in older adults with cancer: A prospective 500 patient multicenter study. *Proc. ASCO Annual Meeting*, 2010.

61. Extermann M, et al. MAX2—a convenient index to estimate the average per patient risk for chemotherapy toxicity; validation in ECOG trials. *Eur J Cancer* 2004;**40**(8):1193–1198.

62. Extermann, et al. The Chemotherapy Risk Assessment Scale for High-age patients (CRASH) score: Design and validation. *Proc ASCO Annual Meeting*, 2010.

63. Saliba D, Elliott M, Rubenstein LZ, et al. The vulnerable elders survey: A tool for identifying vulnerable older people in the community. *J Am Geriatr Soc* 2001;**49**:1691–1699.

64. Min LC, Elliott, N, Wenger NS, Saliba D. Higher vulnerable elders survey scores predict death and functional decline in vulnerable older people. *J Am Geriatr Soc* 2006;**5**:507–511.

65. Luciani A, Ascione G, Bertuzzi C, et al. Detecting disabilities in older patients with cancer: Comparison between comprehensive geriatric assessment and Vulnerable Elders Survey-13. *J Clin Oncol* 2010;**28**:2046–2050.

Economic Cost of Treating Older Adults with Cancer

YA-CHEN TINA SHIH

Department of Medicine, University of Chicago, Chicago, IL

BENJAMIN D. SMITH

Department of Radiation Oncology, University of Texas MD Anderson Cancer Center, Houston, TX

30.1 INTRODUCTION

The incidence and prevalence of cancer are much higher among older adults. Persons aged 65 and older accounted for 54.2% of all cancer diagnosed between 2003 and 2007 in the United States [1]. Given current US demographic trends, the number of older adults diagnosed with cancer is expected to increase by 67%, from 1.0 million in 2010 to 1.6 million in 2030 [2]. Worldwide, 22 million people aged 70 and older died of cancer in 2004 [3]. Despite the wealth of information on cancer biology and cancer epidemiology available globally, data on the economic cost of cancer worldwide are quite limited.

Estimating the cost of treating cancer worldwide is difficult because of the many factors that must be considered and the various ways they affect the cost structure in different countries, such as the financing of healthcare, practice patterns, and the state of new technology diffusion. This difficulty was exemplified by a study of the global economic cost of cancer from the American Cancer Society and LIVESTRONG. The study reported a worldwide cost of cancer of $895 billion for 2008 [4]; however, the estimate included costs due to premature death and disability from cancer, but not direct medical costs. Because of the difficulty in estimating the global medical costs associated with cancer treatment, studies of the economic cost of treating cancer published to date have reported country-specific estimates, with a large number of studies based on data in the United States. These US-based cost studies form the basis of the discussions in this chapter.

The purpose of this chapter is to provide an overview of the economic cost of cancer care for older adults so that readers have a basic understanding of the magnitude of the economic burden in this population as well as the associated factors. Factors to consider include tumor characteristics, treatment patterns, treatment phase, reimbursement

Cancer and Aging Handbook: Research and Practice, First Edition. Edited by Keith M. Bellizzi and Margot A. Gosney.
© 2012 Wiley-Blackwell. Published 2012 by John Wiley & Sons, Inc.

mechanisms, and the diffusion of new technologies. The last factor is critical as new technologies are often more costly than conventional technologies. Studies estimating treatment costs for older cancer patients are further complicated by characteristics specific to this population: a higher prevalence of coexisting medical conditions, physiological changes related to aging, and different treatment patterns. All these factors are discussed in greater detail in this chapter, which is organized as follows. Section 30.2 provides an overview of the cost of cancer care in the United States. Section 30.3 describes the medical cost of cancer treatment for the elderly by tumor characteristics and treatment phase or type. Section 30.4 provides information on the unique health concerns in the elderly and their association with cost. Section 30.5 discusses emerging treatment modalities in cancer and projects their potential impact on cancer care costs. To facilitate comparisons of studies published in different time periods, we normalized all costs reported in these studies to 2009 US dollars ($US).

30.2   OVERALL COST OF CANCER CARE

The overall cost of cancer includes three components: direct medical costs, indirect morbidity costs, and indirect mortality costs. *Direct medical costs* are costs related to the prevention, diagnosis, and treatment of cancer. *Indirect morbidity costs* of cancer are productivity losses due to cancer and associated conditions, whereas *indirect mortality costs* refer to productivity losses due to premature death from cancer. The latest estimate from the National Institute of Health reported that the overall cost of cancer in 2006 was $238.9 billion ($284.4 in 2011 dollars), $104.1 billion ($123.9 in 2011 US$) of which was attributed to direct medical costs, and $134 ($160.5 in 2011 US$) to indirect morbidity and mortality costs [5].

The total medical cost of cancer accounts for 5% of the total healthcare expenditures in the United States [6] and accounts for approximately 10% of total Medicare expenditures [7]. The cost of cancer care is rising and was reported to have increased by 75% between 1995 and 2004 [6]. A comparison of the distribution of the overall cost of cancer by the aforementioned cost components shows an increase in the percentage allocated to direct medical costs, rising from 29% in 1990 to 37% in 2004 [8] and reaching close to 40% in 2006. This pattern of an increasing proportion of the overall costs attributed to direct medical costs may be due to two factors: (1) the growing number of citizens reaching their senior years, when they are most affected by cancer; and (2) new technology. The trend of increasing direct medical costs is likely to be more pronounced in the elderly population since the indirect mortality costs would be much lower in this population.

Estimating the economic cost of cancer is a major undertaking because of the wide variations in treatments across cancer types and stages. A number of economic studies have combined all cancers into one disease category and compared persons with cancer to those without. Stafford and Cyr [9] used the 1991 Medicare Current Beneficiary Survey to study the correlation between cancer and Medicare expenditures. They found that while the average annual Medicare expenditure was $2340 ($4927 in 2009 dollars) per beneficiary, it was $3590 ($7559 in 2009 dollars) for beneficiaries with cancer—over 50% higher than that of the general Medicare population [9]. The authors also conducted a multivariate analysis to compare the effect of cancer and other chronic diseases (such as ischemic heart disease and chronic obstructive pulmonary disease) on Medicare expenditures and concluded that a diagnosis of cancer was strongly associated with higher Medicare expenditures [9].

Using data from the 1995 Asset and Health Dynamics Study, Langa and colleagues [10] compared the 2-year out-of-pocket expenses of adults aged ≥70 years without cancer (group A), with those who had a history of cancer but were not currently being treated (group B), as well as with those who currently undergoing cancer treatment (group C) [10]. They found that the out-of-pocket expenditures for the elderly with cancer were much higher than the expenditures for those without cancer. The adjusted annual out-of-pocket expenses for groups A, B, and C were $2061, $2470, and $3203, respectively [10]. The authors then divided the out-of-pocket expenses into four health-care service categories: hospitalization, prescription medications, outpatient visits, and home healthcare. Prescription medications and home healthcare services accounted for a large proportion of the higher costs observed in the cancer groups. When comparing the financial burden of cancer between high- and low-income elderly with cancer, the authors reported that patients in the low-income group spent approximately 27% of their annual income on medical costs, whereas the percentage was only 7% among those in the high-income group; a finding suggesting that cancer imposes a much higher financial burden among elderly patients of lesser economic means [10].

An earlier study showed that the cost of informal caregiving is higher for cancer patients, amounting to ≥3.1 h per week or about $2371 per patient per year [11]. A much higher estimate was reported in a 2009 study [12]. Using data from the Quality of Life Survey for Caregivers collected by the American Cancer Society, Yabroff and Kim estimated the time costs associated with informal caregiving within the first 2 years of cancer diagnosis [12]. Among cancer patients aged ≥65 years, the study reported that the mean total number of hours spent in caregiving in the 2-year duration was 2979 h or over $47,500 if enumerated using the median hourly wage rate in 2009 of $15.95. These two studies estimated the cost of informal caregiving based on the productivity loss associated with time spent on the caregiving activities. It is possible that these studies have underestimated the cost of informal care, as the higher rate of depression and lower self-perceived health status reported by informal caregivers might translate into higher healthcare costs for informal caregiving. Additionally, the higher prevalence of comorbidities in the elderly cancer population is likely to further increase the caregiver's burden.

30.3 COST OF CANCER TREATMENT BY TUMOR AND TREATMENT CHARACTERISTICS

The primary data sources of studies estimating the cost of cancer treatment in the United States are Medicare claims data, the SEER-Medicare data, and administrative claims data from private health insurance plans [13]. The first two databases, in particular the SEER-Medicare data, have been vital to our efforts to understand the economic burden of cancer among the elderly.

The *2007 Update of Cancer Trends Progress Report* summarized the cost associated with medical treatment for the 15 most common cancers based on the cancer prevalence observed in 1998 and cancer-specific costs incurred between 1997 and 1999 [6]. Among these cancers, the medical expenditures associated with the top five most prevalent cancers (lung, breast, colorectal, and prostate cancer, and lymphoma) accounted for more than 50% of all medical expenditures related to cancer treatment ($72.1 billion

TABLE 30.1 Distribution of Cancer Treatment Expenditures and per Capita Medicare Payment (2009 US$) for the 10 Most Prevalent Cancers in the United States in 1999

Cancer	Percentage of All Cancer-Related Medical Expenditures (%)	Average Medicare Payment per Patient within First Year of Diagnosis (US$)
Lung	13.3	29,918
Breast	11.2	13,324
Colorectal	11.7	29,313
Prostate	11.1	13,324
Lymphoma	6.3	26,042
Head and neck	4.4	21,803
Bladder	4.0	14,899
Leukemia	3.7	21,803
Ovary	3.1	44,575
Kidney	2.7	30,645

Source: Cancer Trends Progress Report, 2007 Update [6].

in 2004 $US or $87.3 billion in 2009 $US). The expenditures associated with the 10 most prevalent cancers (see Table 30.1) accounted for over 70% of all cancer treatment expenditures. Table 30.1 reports the proportion of all cancer-related expenditures for each of the 10 most prevalent cancers, as well as the per capita Medicare payment (in 2009 $US) within the first year of diagnosis. As shown, the per capita Medicare payment was highest for beneficiaries with ovarian cancer ($44,575), followed by kidney cancer ($30,645) and lung cancer ($29,918).

Studies estimating the cost of cancer care usually stratify the cost into three phases of care: the initial, continuing, and terminal phases of care. A U-shaped cost curve is often observed, meaning that there are higher costs in the initial and terminal phases of care and lower costs in the continuing phase of care (see Fig. 30.2 for an illustrated example). Two approaches commonly used to estimate the cost of cancer treatment are the attributable cost and the net cost approaches. The attributable cost approach includes all cancer-related medical services in the estimation of cancer care costs, whereas the net cost approach estimates costs in terms of the cost difference between a group of individuals with cancer and a matched noncancer control group [14]. Factors used to construct the matched control group may include age (or age range), gender, and geographic region, among others.

More recent updates of cancer care costs based on cancer cases diagnosed up to December 31, 2002 can be found in Yabroff et al. [15] and Warren et al. [16]; the former study employed the net cost approach, whereas the latter study applied the attributable cost approach. Yabroff and colleagues estimated the cost of cancer care for elderly patients by tumor site, treatment phase, and cancer stage [15]. Table 30.2 summarizes the cost of treating elderly cancer patients by gender and treatment phase for the 10 most prevalent cancers listed in Table 30.1; all costs were updated to 2009 $US using the medical care component of the consumer price index. A U-shaped cost curve was observed across all tumor sites. Among the elderly women diagnosed with 1 of the 10 most prevalent cancers, those with ovarian cancer had the highest costs in the initial phase of care, and those with leukemia had the highest costs in the continuing and terminal phases of care. Among elderly men diagnosed with one of the 10 most prevalent cancers, those with lung cancer had the highest costs in the initial phase of

TABLE 30.2   Cost of Care for the 10 Most Prevalent Cancers in the United States among the Elderly, by Gender and Treatment Phase (2009 US$)

Cancer	Female			Male		
	Initial	Continuing	Terminal	Initial	Continuing	Terminal
Lung	$42,186	$4678	$61,561	$43,208	$4755	$62,690
Breast	$14,206	$1455	$35,368	—	—	—
Colorectal	$36,253	$1932	$40,711	$35,864	$2730	$44,191
Prostate	—	—	—	$12,854	$2585	$40,809
Lymphoma	$33,535	$4837	$55,427	$34,984	$5494	$62,699
Head and neck	$26,706	$3325	$44,796	$26,350	$2562	$39,243
Bladder	$15,894	$2337	$37,148	$15,886	$3407	$38,391
Leukemia	$27,383	$5271	$74,223	$29,156	$6105	$74,922
Ovary	$62,438	$4714	$61,186	—	—	—
Kidney	$33,198	$4288	$44,841	$32,704	$4162	$46,181

Source: Data recalculated from Yabroff et al. [15].

care, and those with leukemia had the highest costs in the continuing and terminal phases of care. Overall, cancer care costs did not differ substantially between males and females.

Another pattern commonly observed is an increase in treatment costs according to cancer stage, as shown in Table 30.3 for the four most prevalent cancers in the United States [15]. The cost of treating some cancer types (e.g., prostate cancer) is associated with only a modest difference when evaluated by tumor stage, whereas the cost of treating other types of cancer (e.g., colorectal cancer) is associated with a twofold increase for elderly patients diagnosed with tumors at an advanced stage compared to those diagnosed with tumors at a local stage. When estimating the cumulative 5-year costs for elderly cancer patients in the United States, using a 3% discount rate, Yabroff and colleagues concluded that the 5-year cancer care cost for men was highest for those with cancer of the brain or other areas of the nervous system ($58,080) [15]. For women, they concluded that the cost was highest among those with ovarian cancer ($67,526). The authors also projected the aggregate 5-year costs of cancer care for Medicare on the basis of an incident cohort of patients diagnosed in 2004, and reported a 5-year aggregate cost of $25.6 billion. Three cancers accounted for more than 45% of the overall cost of cancer care: lung cancer ($5.1 billion), colorectal cancer ($3.8 billion), and prostate cancer ($2.8 billion) [15].

TABLE 30.3   Cost of Initial and Terminal Phases of Care for the Four Most Prevalent Cancers in the United States among the Elderly, by Stage at Diagnosis (2009 US$)

Cancer	Initial Care			Terminal Care		
	Local	Regional	Distant	Local	Regional	Distant
Lung	$37,009	$47,139	$51,882	$47,764	$63,866	$81,117
Breast	$11,820	$22,347	$34,513	$31,992	$37,868	$53,114
Colorectal	$29,338	$43,582	$61,966	$35,076	$41,698	$70,018
Prostate	$12,830		$15,462	$40,413		$45,427

Source: Data derived from Yabroff et al. [15].

It is expected that the cost of cancer care will be notably affected by the type of treatment that patients receive. Therefore, if an increasing proportion of elderly patients receive definitive treatments over time, the cost of treating cancer will rise in this population. This relationship was reported by Warren and colleagues for the elderly diagnosed with breast, lung, colorectal, and prostate cancers between 1991 and 2002 [16]. The costs examined in that study were measured in Medicare payments and included those incurred from 2 months before diagnosis to 12 months afterward. Using the SEER-Medicare database, Warren et al. identified the type of cancer treatment from Medicare claims and classified claims related to cancer treatments into four mutually exclusive categories: cancer-related surgery, chemotherapy, radiation therapy, and other hospitalizations during the 14-month study period. With the exception of prostate cancer, for which the average Medicare payment per patient remained fairly constant over time (around $22,760), the costs of the initial cancer treatments increased substantially over time, from $4189 (1991 $US or $8890 in 2009 $US) in 1991 to $20,929 (2002 $US or $27,525 in 2009 $US) in 2002 for breast cancer; from $7139 to $39,891 (from $15,150 to $52464 in 2009 $US) for lung cancer; and from $5345 to $41,134 (from $11,343 to $54,098 in 2009 $US) for colorectal cancer [16].

Warren et al. also reported the average Medicare payment per patient by the type of treatment. On the basis of the 2002 Medicare claims data, the average Medicare payment for breast, lung, colorectal, and prostate cancers, in 2009 $US, was $26,460, $50,433, $52,004, and $23,087, respectively. The average cost of surgery was highest for colorectal cancer ($37,814) and lowest for breast cancer ($7173), whereas the average cost of chemotherapy was highest for lung cancer ($29,111) and lowest for prostate cancer ($7605), and the average cost of radiation therapy was highest for prostate cancer ($7117) and lowest for lung cancer ($4420). Total Medicare payment for the four cancers combined amounted to $8.43 billion, with the highest total payment observed for the treatment of colorectal cancer ($2.58 billion), followed by lung ($2.53 billion), prostate ($2.00 billion), and breast ($1.34) cancers, respectively [16].

Figure 30.1 depicts the distribution of total Medicare payments according to the treatment type and tumor site. The graph shows a wide variation across tumor sites. The combination of surgery, chemotherapy, radiation, and hospital care accounted for 69%, 82%, and 74% of total costs for breast, colorectal, and lung cancers, respectively,

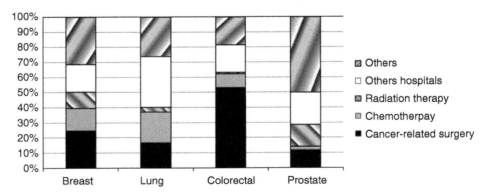

Figure 30.1   Distribution of total Medicare payment by treatment type. (Data derived from Warren et al. [16].)

but accounted for less than 50% of the total cost for prostate cancer, which can be explained by physicians using "watchful waiting" or "active surveillance" for a higher proportion of patients with prostate cancer.

30.4 UNIQUE HEALTHCARE NEEDS IN THE ELDERLY

Clinical management of older cancer patients can be more complex than that for younger patients because of the increase risk for comorbid health conditions and decrease in physiologic reserve that accompanies the aging process. These factors can potentially contribute to a higher rate of treatment-related adverse events among older cancer patients, thus leading to the choice of a more conservative treatment pattern for this population. Aging increases the vulnerability of the hematopoietic and nervous system, heart, mucosa, and other tissues to the side effects of or complications secondary to chemotherapy, surgery, and radiotherapy [17]. In addition, factors such as a higher incidence of depression and anemia, a higher likelihood of polypharmacy, or even the development and response of the cancer itself may further increase the risk of adverse events among the elderly; these events then increase the need (and thus costs) for supportive care products, such as growth factors and erythropoietin.

Figure 30.2 displays breast cancer care cost data divided into phases for women at different age groups, using data from 1990 and 1991 obtained by the Group Health Cooperative [18]. For the initial and terminal phases of care, a negative association was observed between age and the cost of treating breast cancer; the pattern was most pronounced for patients in the terminal phase of care. A similar trend was reported in a more recent study of the economic burden of renal cell cancer. Using data from the MarketScan database, Shih and colleagues estimated the cost of treating renal cell cancer among patients with private insurance in 2007 [19]. Among these patients, the annual medical cost was $43,871 (2009 $US) for the elderly, but was $95,486 for patients younger than 65. These data suggest that elderly cancer patients were being treated less aggressively than younger cancer patients.

Despite the established pattern of higher treatment costs among young cancer patients, several studies have documented a trend of an increasing number of elderly cancer patients receiving more aggressive treatments. Giordano and colleagues reported that the proportion of older women with breast cancer treated with adjuvant

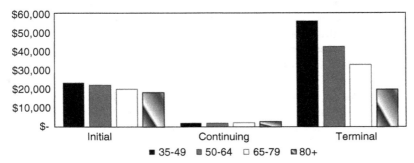

Figure 30.2   Breast cancer cost by age and treatment phase. (Data recalculated from Taplin et al. [18].)

chemotherapy increased from 7.4% in 1991 to 16.3% in 1999 [20]. Earle and colleagues found a trend of increasing aggressiveness in the end-of-life care among elderly patients with lung, breast, colorectal, or other gastrointestinal cancer [21]. Warren and colleagues documented a rising trend in the use of supportive care products, such as erythropoiesis-stimulating agents and granulocyte colony–stimulating factor (G-CSF). The use of erythropoiesis-stimulating agents was found in 1% of elderly patients with breast, lung, colorectal, or prostate cancer in 1991, but the percentage increased to 31.8%, 43.7%, 29.0%, and 14.4%, respectively, in 2002. In terms of G-CSF use, no patients diagnosed with the four cancers discussed above received G-CSF in 1999; however, by 2002 the use of G-CSF was found among 25.4% of breast cancer patients and 19.8% of lung cancer patients [16]. These studies suggest that physicians who treat elderly cancer patients are becoming more willing to offer chemotherapy, provide aggressive end-of-life care, and administer supportive care drugs to this cohort of patients. As these trends continue, it is expected that the cost of treating older cancer patients will markedly increase.

30.5 EMERGING THERAPIES

Many new cancer drugs have emerged in the US market since 2000–2005. Immunotherapy, especially a subset of immunotherapy drugs known as *monoclonal antibodies*, is now considered the fourth modality in cancer care, following the modalities of surgery, chemotherapy, and radiation therapy. These drugs, which fall under a broader category called *targeted therapies*, are priced many times higher than the more commonly used chemotherapy drugs.

In the initial phase of care, the per person cost of providing rituximab (Rituxan) to a patient with non-Hodgkin's lymphoma, providing bevacizumab (Avastin) or cetuximab (Erbitux) to a patient with metastatic colorectal cancer, and providing trastuzumab (Herceptin) to a patient with metastatic breast cancer was approximately $23,700 (2009 $US), $82,500, and $28,800, respectively [19]. The average annual per patient cost for an elderly patient with renal cancer who was treated with targeted therapy (e.g., sorafenib and sunitinib) was $65,827, whereas the per patient cost was $21,956 for those who did not receive targeted therapy drugs [22]. The use of trastuzumab (Herceptin) to treat a patient who has early stage breast cancer costs over $50,000 per year [23]. The utilization of these targeted therapy agents among elderly cancer patients is not well understood. However, a study by Shih and colleagues showed an upward trend in the use of an immunotherapy agent soon after the FDA approved the agent for a specific tumor site. This trend held for patients of all ages who were diagnosed with non-Hodgkin's lymphoma, metastatic colorectal cancer, and metastatic breast cancer, each of which had been approved as an indication for the use of one or more immunotherapy agent [19].

Treatment advances are not limited to targeted therapy drugs. In cancer surgeries, the use of minimally invasive procedures, especially those with robotic assistance, is increasing. Hu and colleagues studied older prostate cancer patients who underwent radical prostatectomy and found that the proportion of patients who received minimally invasive radical prostatectomy increased from 9.2% in 2003 to 43.2% in 2006 and 2007 [24]. Although minimally invasive, these newer, more technology-dependent surgical techniques have been found to have higher hospitalization costs [25,26]. As the use of robotassisted surgery becomes more prevalent among elderly prostate cancer patients who elect surgical treatment, the cost of treatment for older adults with prostate cancer is likely to increase. If surgical treatment of other cancers follows a similar trend in the future, higher costs of cancer care are to be expected.

New technologies are also found in radiation therapy, as exemplified by stereotactic radiosurgery and radiotherapy, high-dose-rate brachytherapy, intensity-modulated radiation therapy (IMRT), and proton therapy. A study comparing different types of radiation modalities in breast cancer showed that the medical costs of radiation for patients treated with high-dose-rate brachytherapy or IMRT were approximately $14,000 higher than those treated with the conventional external beam radiation therapy [27]. Smith and colleagues studied the use of brachytherapy among a cohort of elderly breast cancer patients who had supplemental insurance in addition to Medicare. They reported an increasing utilization from <1% in 2001 to close to 10% in 2006 among those who received radiation therapy following breast conserving surgeries [28]. The same research group examined the use of IMRT and reported a utilization rate that increased from 0.9% in 2001 to 11.2% in 2005 among older breast cancer patients treated with surgery and radiation. This resulted in an overall 33% increase in per patient radiation costs during the study interval [29]. The increasing use of newer techniques in radiation therapy in the treatment of older patients will likely increase the cost of cancer care as well.

Looking to the future, several factors are converging that could precipitously accelerate the growth in cancer care costs for older adults: (1) between 2010 and 2030, the number of older adults diagnosed with cancer is expected to increase by approximately 67% [2]; (2) as outlined above, the cost of new chemotherapy and radiation therapy treatments is ≤4 times that of the older treatment options; and (3) as treatment methods have improved, some diseases, such as metastatic colorectal cancer, have acquired particularly long natural histories that may extend 3–5 years beyond the initial diagnosis. Thus our success in improving long-term patient outcomes is obtained at a hefty price. We will continue to see marked increases in the cost of cancer care as many patients survive a primary cancer but develop metastatic disease that requires ongoing systemic therapy over a prolonged period or will live long enough to be diagnosed with a second primary tumor. Taken together, these factors have the potential to produce exponential growth in the total societal cost of caring for cancer in older adults, and could ultimately undermine the provision of cancer care by rendering the current system financially unsustainable.

30.6   CONCLUSIONS

Given the potential for unsustainable cost growth, a renewed effort is required on the part of clinical researchers and policymakers to encourage the identification of cost-effective treatment strategies in the care of older adults—strategies that could potentially bend the cost growth curve. For example, more recent data on breast cancer have demonstrated that a shorter, less costly course of radiation confers clinical outcomes that are equivalent to those of a longer, more costly course of radiation [30–33]. In addition, given the proliferation of extremely expensive targeted agents, the authors recommend the routine integration of economic analyses into prospective cancer clinical trials to determine whether and under what circumstances the cost of such therapies is clinically justified. Further, with regard to targeted therapy, emerging research seeks to control cost and reduce overtreatment by identifying molecular profiles that predict the likelihood of benefit from specific targeted agents, with the implication that patients without the requisite molecular profile should not receive the targeted agent of interest. For example, more recent investigations have indicated that the benefit of cetuximab in the treatment of metastatic colorectal cancer appears to be limited to individuals with the wildtype K-*ras* gene, implying that patients with a mutant K-*ras* gene should not receive cetuximab [34]. This finding has the potential to markedly improve the cost-effectiveness of cetuximab by limiting its administration to only those patients most likely to benefit.

As cancer care for the elderly moves forward, the prioritization of treatment strategies and translational research efforts that seek to optimize therapy by abbreviating treatment and tailoring it to specific patient subgroups is crucial in the effort to control costs and ensure ongoing access to cancer care.

REFERENCES

1. Altekruse SF, Kosary CL, Krapcho M, et al. *SEER Cancer Statistics Review, 1975–2007*, National Cancer Institute, Bethesda, MD, 2010.

2. Smith BD, Smith GL, Hurria A, et al. Future of cancer incidence in the United States: Burdens upon an aging, changing nation. *J Clin Oncol* 2009;**27**:2758–2765.

3. Boyle P, Levin B. *Word Cancer Report 2008*, WHO, Lyon, France, 2008.

4. Garcia MA, Jemal EM, Ward MM, et al. *Global Cancer Facts & Figures 2007* American Cancer Society, Atlanta, GA, 2007.

5. ACS. *Cancer Facts & Figures 2010*, American Cancer Society, Atlanta, GA, 2010.

6. NCI. *Cancer Trends Progress Report—2007 Update* (available at http://progressreport.cancer.gov; accessed 9/15/10).

7. Reeder CE, Gordon D. Managing oncology costs. *Am J Manage Care* 2006;**12**:S3–S16; quiz S17–S19.

8. Shih YCT. *Proc. Economics of Cancer in the Elderly Population Workshop*, Institute of Medicine, Washington, DC, 2007.

9. Stafford RS, Cyr PL. The impact of cancer on the physical function of the elderly and their utilization of health care. *Cancer* 1997;**80**:1973–1980.

10. Langa KM, Fendrick AM, Chernew ME, et al. Out-of-pocket health-care expenditures among older Americans with cancer. *Value Health* 2004;**7**:186–194.

11. Hayman JA, Langa KM, Kabeto MU, et al. Estimating the cost of informal caregiving for elderly patients with cancer. *J Clin Oncol* 2001;**19**:3219–3225.

12. Yabroff KR, Kim Y. Time costs associated with informal caregiving for cancer survivors. *Cancer* 2009;**115**:4362–4373.

13. Warren JL, Klabunde CN, Schrag D, et al. Overview of the SEER-Medicare data: Content, research applications, and generalizability to the United States elderly population. *Med Care* 2002;**40**:IV-3–IV-18.

14. Barlow WE. Overview of methods to estimate the medical costs of cancer. *Med Care* 2009;**47**:S33–S36.

15. Yabroff KR, Lamont EB, Mariotto A, et al. Cost of care for elderly cancer patients in the United States. *J Natl Cancer Inst* 2008;**100**:630–641.

16. Warren JL, Yabroff KR, Meekins A, et al. Evaluation of trends in the cost of initial cancer treatment. *J Natl Cancer Inst* 2008;**100**:888–897.

17. Carreca I, Balducci L, Extermann M. Cancer in the older person. *Cancer Treat Rev* 2005;**31**:380–402.

18. Taplin SH, Barlow W, Urban N, et al. Stage, age, comorbidity, and direct costs of colon, prostate, and breast cancer care. *J Natl Cancer Inst* 1995;**87**:417–426.

19. Shih YCT, Chien CR, Xu Y, et al. Economic burden of renal cell carcinoma: Part II—an updated analysis. *PharmacoEconomics* 2011;**29**(4):331–41.

20. Giordano SH, Duan Z, Kuo YF, et al. Use and outcomes of adjuvant chemotherapy in older women with breast cancer. *J Clin Oncol* 2006;**24**:2750–2756.

21. Earle CC, Neville BA, Landrum MB, et al. Trends in the aggressiveness of cancer care near the end of life. *J Clin Oncol* 2004;**22**:315–321.

22. Shih YC, Elting LS, Pavluck AL, et al. Immunotherapy in the initial treatment of newly diagnosed cancer patients: Utilization trend and cost projections for non-Hodgkin's lymphoma, metastatic breast cancer, and metastatic colorectal cancer. *Cancer Investig* 2010;**28**(1):46–53.

23. Hillner BE, Smith TJ. Do the large benefits justify the large costs of adjuvant breast cancer trastuzumab? *J Clin Oncol* 2007;**25**:611–613.

24. Hu JC, Gu X, Lipsitz SR, et al. Comparative effectiveness of minimally invasive vs open radical prostatectomy. *JAMA* 2009;**302**:1557–1564.

25. Lotan Y, Cadeddu JA, Gettman MT. The new economics of radical prostatectomy: Cost comparison of open, laparoscopic and robot assisted techniques. *J Urol* 2004;**172**:1431–1435.

26. Mouraviev V, Nosnik I, Sun L, et al. Financial comparative analysis of minimally invasive surgery to open surgery for localized prostate cancer: A single-institution experience. *Urology* 2007;**69**:311–314.

27. Suh WW, Pierce LJ, Vicini FA, et al. A cost comparison analysis of partial versus whole-breast irradiation after breast-conserving surgery for early-stage breast cancer. *Int J Radiat Oncol Biol Phys* 2005;**62**:790–796.

28. Smith GL, Xu Y, Buchholz TA, et al. Brachytherapy for accelerated partial-breast irradiation: a rapidly emerging technology in breast cancer care. *J Clin Oncol* 2011;**29**(2):157–65.

29. Smith BD, Pan IW, Shih YCT, Smith GL, Harris JR, Punglia R, McCormick B, Pierce LJ, Jagsi R, Hayman J, Giordano SH, Buchholz TA. Adoption of Intensity-Modulated Radiation Therapy for Breast Cancer in the United States. *Journal of National Cancer Institute*. 2011;**103**(10):798–809.

30. Bentzen SM, Agrawal RK, Aird EG, et al. The UK Standardisation of Breast Radiotherapy (START) Trial A of radiotherapy hypofractionation for treatment of early breast cancer: A randomised trial. *Lancet Oncol* 2008;**9**:331–341.

31. Bentzen SM, Agrawal RK, Aird EG, et al. The UK Standardisation of Breast Radiotherapy (START) Trial B of radiotherapy hypofractionation for treatment of early breast cancer: A randomised trial. *Lancet* 2008;**371**:1098–1107.

32. Smith BD, Bentzen SM, Correa CR, et al. Fractionation for whole breast irradiation: An American Society for Radiation Oncology (ASTRO) evidence-based guideline. *Int J Radiat Oncol Biol Phys* 2011;**81**(1):59–68.

33. Whelan TJ, Pignol JP, Levine MN, et al. Long-term results of hypofractionated radiation therapy for breast cancer. *N Engl J Med* 2010;**362**:513–520.

34. Au HJ, Karapetis CS, O'Callaghan CJ, et al. Health-related quality of life in patients with advanced colorectal cancer treated with cetuximab: Overall and KRAS-specific results of the NCIC CTG and AGITG CO.17 Trial. *J Clin Oncol* 2009;**27**:1822–1828.

CHAPTER 31

Multidisciplinary Models of Care

KATHLEEN TSCHANTZ UNROE and HARVEY JAY COHEN

Division of Geriatric Medicine and Center for the Study of Aging, Duke University Medical Center, Durham, NC

31.1 INTRODUCTION

A continued increase in the number of people with cancer is expected given the aging of the population. Less than 500 per 100,000 persons under age 50 will develop cancer; in contrast, by age 75 females have a rate of cancer diagnoses of nearly 2000 per 100,000 and males over 3000 per 100,000 [1]. More patients are surviving longer with cancer—in 1971, there were about 3 million cancer survivors in the United States, and by 2001 that increased to nearly 10 million [1]. Worldwide, there are 24 million cancer survivors, more than 60% of whom are over age 65 [2]. Many older patients with cancer have multiple chronic diseases and may take several medications, making their care especially complex. Older patients, including those with cancer, often see several providers. Communication between providers and settings of care is often problematic, and thus various models have been proposed and tried to address these deficiencies that lead to care fragmentation. Many approaches center on multidisciplinary care for these patients. This chapter discusses the rationale for the multidisciplinary care of older cancer patients, the members of the team, including the status of the workforce for various disciplines, and specific models.

31.2 THE IMPORTANCE OF MULTIDISCIPLINARY CARE

When a patient is diagnosed with cancer, the oncologist often assumes most of the responsibility for overall care for the patient. Older patients, however, are likely to have multiple chronic conditions and may have a longstanding relationship with a primary care physician as well as several specialists. The concept of shared care has been advocated, where the oncologist and primary care physician share the care and responsibility for the patient, each assuming a greater role depending on where the patient is along the disease and treatment trajectory [3]. For this to be successful,

Cancer and Aging Handbook: Research and Practice, First Edition. Edited by Keith M. Bellizzi and Margot A. Gosney.
© 2012 Wiley-Blackwell. Published 2012 by John Wiley & Sons, Inc.

transfer of information among providers and clear communication between providers and with patients is imperative [3,4].

A systematic review that examined models designed to provide comprehensive care for older adults with multiple chronic conditions found that multidisciplinary approaches, usually consisting of a team composed of a primary care physician and at least one specialist from other disciplines, such as nurses, social workers, or rehabilitation therapists, performed well. The review found that the multidisciplinary team approach improved primary healthcare and quality of life and functional status in older patients. Some teams reduced use of health services, such as hospitalizations [5].

The concept of multidisciplinary care is particularly relevant to the older cancer patient. Primary care providers or geriatricians must coordinate with oncology providers, including hematologists or oncologists, radiation oncologists, and surgeons. In addition to the primary care and specialist physicians involved, the care of these patients can be improved by incorporating other professionals on the team such as pharmacists or social workers. Patient involvement with the multidisciplinary team encourages patient-centered care and also enhances patient and family understanding of the disease and treatment options [6].

The multidisciplinary case conference model allows for input from multiple professionals on individual cases. In cancer care, teams are typically disease-focused [6]. For example, some institutions have weekly specialty conferences to discuss certain cases. Medical oncologists, radiologists, pathologists, surgical oncologists, and other staff involved in the cases may be present. The treating physicians are able discuss appropriate treatment options together, and tailored treatment recommendations can be made. A potential downside of this model is that the patient's primary care physician is seldom involved.

The multidisciplinary treatment care team is designed to provide ongoing coordinated care and support for the patient. The goal is to ensure open information exchange among providers and to encourage the active involvement of all team members in the development of care plans, including the patient and family. These teams can meet regularly as needed, especially to help smooth transitions between stages of cancer care [6].

The use of multidisciplinary teams has been best studied in heart failure patients. A review that looked at 29 different randomized trials of multidisciplinary management strategies for heart failure patients found that the programs were associated with a 27% reduction in hospitalization rates for heart failure [number needed to treat (NNT) = 11]. Those that included follow-up by a multidisciplinary team reduced all-cause mortality by one-quarter (NNT = 17) [7]. A larger systematic review of multidisciplinary approaches to care for heart failure patients also found reductions in both hospital admission and all-cause mortality [8].

The multidisciplinary approach has been explored for other chronic disease states as well. Practices that enhanced the role of nurses to educate and follow up with patients improved patient outcomes, such as glycemic control, as revealed in a review of approaches to outpatient diabetes management [9]. Group medical clinics, where multiple patients with the same diagnoses meet on a regular basis with a care team, have also been studied. One randomized controlled trial studied diabetes and hypertension outcomes, defined by glycemic control and systolic blood pressure measurements, for Veterans Affairs (previously known as *Veterans Administration*) patients who participated for one year in multidisciplinary group medical clinics involving a physician, a pharmacist, and a nurse. Improved hypertension control was found, but no significant differences in diabetes control were noted [10]. In Belgium, another trial included interdisciplinary treatment teams composed of a nurse educator, an internist, a dietician, and an ophthalmologist, designed to enhance the care of patients with diabetes. They found that diabetes control was improved at 18 months, although there was less patient participation than expected in the intervention [11].

Depression is another chronic condition for which there has been much interest in multidisciplinary care. A review of collaborative care models examined studies that assessed teams of primary care physicians and psychologists or psychiatrists, interventions that focused on care managers, and some that employed nurse specialists. In all three approaches, patients reported more depression-free days compared to control patients [12].

Older patients often have multiple chronic, serious medical conditions. For example, more than one multidisciplinary team might be involved in the care of a patient with congestive heart failure (CHF), diabetes, and cancer. This makes the need to have formal mechanisms, such as shared electronic medical records or patient maintained records, to communicate among providers and teams essential.

31.3 GERIATRIC ASSESSMENT

A comprehensive geriatric assessment (CGA) involves a multifaceted assessment of factors that contribute to the health and well-being of an older patient using standardized tools. In addition to a full medical assessment and review of medications, a cognitive and affective evaluation is needed as well. Particular attention is paid to geriatric syndromes such as dementia, falls, and incontinence. A nutritional evaluation is performed. A detailed functional assessment is a key component. Evaluation of the patient's social support, economic resources, and environment provides further helpful information. The goals of these detailed assessments are to aid in prediction of outcomes, including likelihood of toxicity of therapies, improve patient selection for various interventions, enhance patient management during treatment, and strengthen the development of survivorship plans. The application of CGA to the older cancer patient was discussed in Chapter 29.

31.4 MULTIDISCIPLINARY APPROACHES

31.4.1 Case Conferences

Multidisciplinary case conferences for cancer patients, sometimes called *tumor boards*, are used by many institutions to prospectively discuss diagnosis and treatment options for patients. There is some evidence that the use of these multidisciplinary case conferences improves patient care and outcome. In a study at a Veterans Affairs hospital, patients who had rectal cancer were more likely to receive therapy concordant with National Cancer Institute guidelines if their case had been discussed at a multidisciplinary conference [13]. These conferences have also been found to have other benefits, including ongoing education for participants and improved professional relationships among colleagues [14].

As cancer care has become increasingly multidisciplinary in nature, these conferences have increased in acceptance as an appropriate forum to gain input from various providers and debate the merits of approaches to treatment for a given patient. They are typically held on a monthly basis. The patient and family are rarely present [6]. Multidisciplinary case conferences for cancer patients have been integrated into healthcare systems internationally, including Australia, Europe, the United Kingdom, Asia, and the United States [14,15]. Geriatricians or primary care providers might be a valuable addition to such conferences, as the involvement of these professionals throughout the course of treatment of the older patient has been advocated by some [3,16].

31.4.2 Treatment Teams

For cancer patients, multidisciplinary treatment teams are used in inpatient and outpatient settings. Teams that include attending physicians, nurse practitioners or physician assistants, registered nurses, pharmacists, and other staff, such as social workers, may round on hospitalized cancer patients. Multiple disciplines may also be represented in outpatient settings.

Multidisciplinary treatment or care teams who meet regularly to discuss patients have evolved from traditional case conferences or tumor boards. These teams allow consultants to work collaboratively as the patient progresses along a care pathway. Elements that distinguish teams from conferences include patient involvement and an interactive team structure [6].

There are many points along the cancer continuum where multidisciplinary treatment teams can be beneficial to patients. At diagnosis, when there are changes in major treatment modality (i.e., surgery, radiation, chemotherapy), development of survivorship care plans, and when end-of-life care is being discussed (Fig. 31.1) are all appropriate times for treatment teams to meet. There has not been much research on how the patient experience differs with respect to different characteristics of the multidisciplinary team, such as involvement of various specialties [6]. Depending on the issues identified for specific patients, different team members may need to be involved for older patients, such as increased involvement from social workers, rehabilitation specialists, or geriatricians. It has been suggested that rehabilitation specialists can also

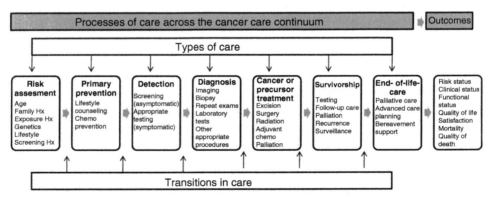

Figure 31.1 Care across the cancer continuum encompasses different types of care, including risk assessment, detection, diagnosis, primary treatment, survivorship and surveillance, and end-of-life care [20].

play an important role on the team for many cancer patients, especially since cancer patients and survivors have higher rates of disability [17].

31.4.3 Coordination between Primary Care and Specialty Care: Shared Care

Shared care has been defined as the joint participation of primary care and specialty physicians in the delivery of care for patients with a chronic condition. It requires information exchange that goes beyond routine care [18]. Shared care can be delivered in various ways, including the following [19]:

1. *Community clinics*—specialists run a clinic in a primary care setting; communication between primary care providers and specialists is informal.
2. *Basic model*—a regular communication system is established between primary care and specialty providers, perhaps facilitated by an administrator.
3. *Liaison*—meetings are held where primary care and specialist providers discuss management of patients.
4. *Shared care record*—formal arrangement to share information where agreed-on data are entered into a record, usually held by the patient.
5. *Health information systems*—agreed-on data are collected by both primary care and specialty providers and circulated among them.

For oncology patients, primary care providers are involved in patient care mostly at the beginning and end of the cancer continuum. Diagnosis and treatment are largely handled by specialists [20]. While patients are undergoing active treatment for cancer, oncologists report that they are providing the majority of their care. About one-third stated that it was rare for their patients to see a primary care provider while they were receiving active cancer treatment [1]. Following active treatment, care may shift between primary care and specialty oncology care depending on the needs of the patient. Thus, information and responsibility must be transferrable easily and seamlessly among providers such as through a shared electronic medical record. As the care plan changes or new providers or organizations become involved, these transfers are especially critical [20]. In the United States, multiple independent practitioners render communication and coordination challenging, which can lead to fragmentation. By default, patients may be placed in the role of coordinating most of their own care.

Primary care providers are usually involved in the initial stages of cancer diagnosis, either by ordering a screening test or performing a diagnostic workup based on new signs or symptoms. Patients are then referred to oncology specialists, who then take the lead in terms of further testing and evaluation. The oncologist may assume most responsibility for care of the patient at this point, including the development of a treatment plan, but input from the primary care provider is often valued by the patient [3]. The oncologist will care for the patient during the active treatment phase, and the level of involvement of the primary care provider may vary, but the primary care provider may be useful in addressing issues associated with other comorbidities and age-related disabilities [3] (Fig. 31.2).

Problems that occur at the interfaces of primary care and oncology specialty care lead to role confusion among providers and poor information exchange, as well as potential for missed referrals and inefficient treatment of the disease [20]. A randomized trial of

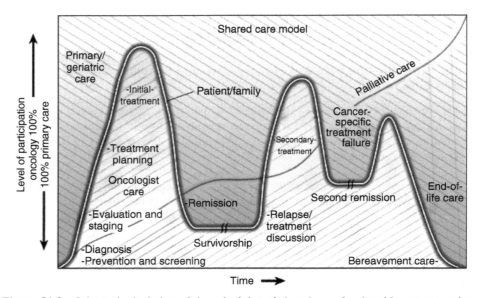

Figure 31.2   Schematic depiction of the principles of shared care for the older cancer patient. Over time, the contribution and responsibility of each specialty will vary according to the disease stage and needs of the patient [3].

shared care that tested the effects of a communication intervention among oncologists and primary care providers was conducted in Denmark. They found that the number of primary care visits increased and there was greater patient satisfaction, but there were no differences in the technical quality of care delivered [21].

It is not clear how often primary care providers or geriatricians participate on oncology multidisciplinary teams; however, some have stated that these providers are important participants on the team [16]. Primary care providers are important for post-treatment care, as well as in a consultative role during treatment to manage other illnesses and conditions. Large size of the multidisciplinary team could limit effectiveness, and this may argue against having nonspecialists present [6]. Involvement of these providers, however, is worth considering, given the importance of developing overall goals of care and the need for expertise in the management of comorbidities.

As patients move from active treatment into a survivorship phase, they are sometimes confused as to the best way to receive ongoing care. Moreover, primary care providers may not understand the follow-up care that the patient needs for the particular cancer, and the oncologist may not understand the patient's other medical needs [4,22]. For many patients, the oncologist assumes the role of primary care provider. However, this may not be the most appropriate use of oncologists' time, especially given concerns about adequate workforce in oncology. There is evidence that both providers are needed to provide ongoing high-quality care. A study of elderly breast cancer survivors found that those who continued to have follow-up with oncologists were more likely to receive appropriate follow-up mammography. However, those who were followed by primary care providers were more likely to receive all other non-cancer preventive services. Those women who saw both providers were more likely to receive more of both types of service [23]. Another study found that patients with advanced colon cancer were more likely to receive an influenza vaccination from a primary care provider rather than an oncologist, and those that did showed a trend for increased survival, although detailed cause of death information was not available [24].

Transitioning to survivorship changes the focus from active cancer treatment to longer-term follow-up, including recognizing recurring and new primary tumors, managing late effects of the cancer and treatment, rehabilitation, preventive health services, and management of other health conditions [22]. Studies have shown that primary care providers, when provided with guidelines, are able to provide follow-up care for cancer survivors with outcomes equivalent to those effected by oncologists. A trial that compared outcomes of breast cancer survivors followed by either oncologists or family practitioners found no differences in serious clinical cancer-recurrence-related events or in patient reported health related quality of life [25].

The creation of a survivorship plan, developed with the patient, oncologist, and primary care provider, and often completed by nurses, can help with this transition along the cancer continuum and serve as an effective guide and communication tool. The Institute of Medicine recommends that all patients completing primary treatment be provided with a follow-up plan or "survivorship care plan" as well as a treatment summary [22]. However, for older cancer patients a more tailored survivorship plan may be needed, especially including guidance in the setting of multiple comorbidities [26].

31.4.4 Workforce

Many disciplines are needed to care for older cancer patients; however, there are concerns that the workforce will be inadequate to meet projected needs. Given the large numbers of older people with cancer and the projected growth of this population, there are not enough oncologists or geriatricians to care for this population. Specific efforts, funded in part by private foundations, to train physicians dually in oncology and geriatrics has led to a small professional group with particular expertise. This is especially important in terms of the development and design of research studies that are inclusive of and sensitive to the needs of the older cancer patient [27,28].

Even relatively conservative projections show that the demand for oncologists will outstrip the supply. It is predicted that by 2020, there will be a shortage of several thousand medical oncologists in the United States [1].

There are also predicted shortages for primary care physicians in general [29] and geriatricians in particular. According to a 2008 report, there were an estimated 7100 geriatricians in the United States: a ratio of one geriatrician to over 2500 people over age 65. It is predicted that by 2030, there will be about 7750 geriatricians, falling far short of a predicted need for 36,000. There are only about 1600 geriatric psychiatrists. Unfortunately, only about half of the available fellowship slots for geriatric medicine training and even fewer geriatric psychiatry slots fill each year [30].

Many oncologists work with nurse practitioners (NPs) and/or physician assistants (PAs). In a 2006 survey, 56% of oncologists reported the use of these professions in their practice; 30% of all oncologists reported having NPs/PAs manage patients during visits, do patient education and counseling, as well as pain and symptom management. About 25% of respondents indicated that NPs/PAs were involved in more advanced procedures and practices, including ordering chemotherapy, assisting with new patient consults, or performing invasive procedures. Of those who use NPs/PAs, over two-thirds believe that it improves efficiency, improves patient care, and contributes to physicians' professional satisfaction [1].

The PA workforce is growing—between 1999 and 2005 the number of PAs increased by 55%, and a similar increase is expected between 2005 and 2014. However, in 2005, only 10% of PAs practiced in an internal medicine subspecialty. The NP workforce is also expanding, with a 60% increase in the number of NPs between 1999 and 2005. In 2004, 1% of NPs specialized in oncology [1].

According to a 2008 report, about 2.6% of NPs were certified in geriatrics in the United States; about 300 graduate annually with geriatrics training. Fewer than 1% of PAs specialize in geriatrics. Accreditation for PA programs requires "exposure" to geriatrics, but there is no minimum time required for this subject area. There are no advanced training programs available in geriatrics for PAs [30].

Fewer than 1% of nurses receive additional specialization in geriatrics. In 2005, one-third of baccalaureate nursing programs required a course focused on geriatrics [30].

The National Institute on Aging estimated in 1987 that there would be a need for 70,000 geriatric social workers by 2020. Only 4% of social workers specialize in geriatrics, which represents about one-third of the estimated need. Between 1996 and 2001, the number of social work students specializing in geriatrics decreased by >15%. About 80% of social work baccalaureate programs have no coursework in aging [30]. Other healthcare professionals critical to the care of older cancer patients lack geriatrics training as well. For example, fewer than 1% of pharmacists specialize in geriatrics, and only 22% of undergraduate programs in dietetics and nutrition offer courses in aging [30].

Addressing the workforce shortages will require a multifaceted approach. Developing incentives for postgraduate medical trainees to choose fellowships, such as loan forgiveness, have been discussed. But likely the most key APPROACH is increasing student exposure to geriatrics and oncology, through patient experiences and seeing role models in the field, at earlier stages in their education. Later in training it may be difficult to influence the choice of specialties that students make.

31.5 CONCLUSIONS

The case for multidisciplinary care of the older cancer patient is compelling. Caring for older cancer patients across the continuum of their disease requires collaboration and communication among providers. There is evidence that multidisciplinary care for patients with chronic disease is beneficial, including cancer patients. Primary care and geriatrics expertise is important in the care for these often complicated patients. Geriatric assessment is an important tool that can help with diagnostic and therapeutic decisionmaking.

Formal arrangements for coordinating care for older cancer patients, such as multidisciplinary teams and shared care arrangements, are essential, given the complexities of patient needs and the fragmentation of healthcare systems. Multiple quality-of-care issues have been documented due to lack of coordination, including inadequate or delayed communication between primary care providers and specialists [29].

There are challenges to using multidisciplinary teams. Administrative time and costs can be burdensome. This can be addressed by standardizing protocols, ensuring sufficient volume to justify the logistic requirements, and sharing personnel and space. Standards of care could vary, which requires the development of clinical guidelines.

Differing cultures between geriatrics, primary care, and oncology could lead to turf wars. Solutions for this include consensus decisionmaking and multidisciplinary executive management. This approach can also be inconvenient for the patient, so it is important to hold meetings in a location familiar to the patient and to issue uniform recommendations. Reimbursement for the time spent on these activities may be an issue for providers, so careful documentation is required; further changes in current reimbursement policies should be made to support multidisciplinary approaches [31]. More sophisticated health information technology (HIT) systems, including electronic health records, have the potential to improve communication among providers and across settings of care. HIT, if designed carefully, has the potential to increase coordination of care for cancer patients [32].

The model of shared care can be realized through the different approaches described earlier. The most important elements of this model are open communication and collaboration between the specialist and the primary care physician or geriatrician. The proportion of care provided by any one physician is based on the disease stage, and the needs of the patient and should vary over time (Fig. 31.2).

The professional workforce is insufficient to meet the demands of this population. Incentives to encourage students to enter these fields are needed, as are more extensive educational opportunities and exposure to these important issues.

Multidisciplinary care leverages the expertise of team members with different perspectives and skills in order to provide evidence-based care for patients that is tailored to meet their needs and goals. As studies in multiple countries continue to show the benefit of this approach, healthcare systems will need to evolve in order to support these models.

REFERENCES

1. ASCO. *Forecasting the Supply of and Demand for Oncologists*, a report to the American Society of Clinical Oncology (ASCO) from the AAMC Center for Workforce Studies, Center for Workforce Studies, 2007.

2. The President's Cancer Panel. *Living beyond Cancer: Finding a New Balance* (prepared by Reuben SH), National Cancer Institute, National Institutes of Health, US Dept. Health and Human Services, 2004.

3. Cohen HJ. A model for the shared care of elderly patients with cancer. *J Am Geriatr Soc* 2009;**57**:S300–S302.

4. Taplin SH, Clauser S, Rodgers AB, Breslau E, Rayson D. Interfaces across the cancer continuum offer opportunities to improve the process of care. *J Natl Cancer Inst Monogr* 2010;**40**:104–110.

5. Boult C, Green AF, Boult LB, Pacala JT, Snyder C, Leff B. Successful models of comprehensive care for older adults with chronic conditions: Evidence for the Institute of Medicine's "Retooling for an Aging America" report. *J Am Geriatr Soc* 2009;**57**:2328–2337.

6. Fennell ML, Prabhu Das I, Clauser S, Petrelli N, Salner A. The organization of multidisciplinary care teams: Modeling internal and external influences on cancer care quality. *J Natl Cancer Inst Monogr* 2010;**40**:72–80.

7. McAlister FA, Stewart S, Ferrua S, McMurray JJJV. Multidisciplinary strategies for the management of heart failure patients at high risk of admission: A systematic review of randomized trials. *J Am Coll Cardiol* 2004;**44**(4):810–9.

8. Holland R, Battersby J, Harvey I, et al. Systematic review of multidisciplinary interventions in heart failure. *Heart* 2005;**91**:899–906.

9. Renders CM, Valk GD, Griffin SJ, et al. Interventions to improve the management of diabetes in primary care, outpatient, and community settings: A systematic review. *Diabetes Care* 2001;**24**:1821–1833.

10. Edelman D, Fredrickson SK, Melnyk SD, et al. Medical clinics versus usual care for patients with both diabetes and hypertension: A randomized trial. *Ann Intern Med* 2010;**152**(11):689–696.

11. Borgermans L, Goderis G, Van Den Broeke C, et al. Interdisciplinary diabetes care teams operating on the interface between primary and specialty care are associated with improved outcomes of care: Findings from the Leuven Diabetes Project. *BMC Health Serv Res* 2009;**9**:179.

12. van Steenbergen-Weijenburg KM, van der Feltz-Cornelis CM, Horn EK, et al. Cost-effectiveness of collaborative care for the treatment of major depressive disorder in primary care. A systematic review. *BMC Health Serv Res* 2010;**10**:19.

13. Abraham NS, Gossey JT, Davila JA, Al-Oudat S, Kramer JK. Receipt of recommended therapy by patients with advanced colorectal cancer. *Am J Gastroenterol* 2006;**101**:1320–1328.

14. Hong NJL, Gagliardi AR, Bronskill SE, Paszat LF, Wright FC. Multidisciplinary cancer conferences: Exploring obstacles and facilitators to their implementation. *J Oncolo Pract* 2010;**6**(2):61–68.

15. Wright FC, Lookhong N, Urbach D, et al. Multidisciplinary cancer conferences: Identifying opportunities to promote implementation. *Ann Surg Oncol* 2009;**16**:2731–2737.

16. Wright FC, DeVito C, Langer B, Hunter A. Multidisciplinary cancer conferences: A systematic review and development of practice standards. *Eur J Cancer* 2007;**43**:1002–1010.

17. Vargo MM. The oncology-rehabilitation interface: Better systems needed. *J Clin Oncol* 2008;**26**(16):2610–2611.

18. Hickman M, Drummond N, Grimshaw J. A taxonomy of shared care of chronic disease. *J Public Health Med* 1994;**16**(4):447–454.

19. Smith SM, Allwright S, O'Dowd T. Effectiveness of shared care across the interface between primary and specialty care in chronic disease management. *Cochrane Database of Systematic Reviews* 2007. Issue 3. Art. No.: CD004910. DOI:10.1002/14651858.CD004910.pub2

20. Taplin SH, Rodgers AB. Toward improving the quality of cancer care: Addressing the interfaces of primary and oncology-related subspecialty care. *J Natl Cancer Inst Monogr* 2010;**40**:3–10.

21. Nielson JD, Palshof R, Mainz J, et al. Randomised controlled trial of a shared care programme for newly referred cancer patients: bridging the gap between general practice and hospital. *Qual Safety Health Care* 2003;**12**:263–272.

22. Grunfeld E, Earle C. The interface between primary and oncology specialty care: Treatment through survivorship. *J Natl Cancer Inst Monogr* 2010;**40**:25–30.

23. Earle CC, Burstein HJ, Winer EP, Weeks JC. Quality of non-breast cancer health maintenance among elderly breast cancer survivors. *J Clin Oncol* 2003;**21**:1447–1451.

24. Earle CC. Influenza vaccination in elderly patients with advanced colorectal cancer. *J Clin Oncol* 2003;**21**:1161–1166.

25. Grunfeld E, Levine MN, Julian JA, Coyle D, et al. Randomized trial of long-term follow-up for early-stage breast cancer: A comparison of family physician versus specialist care. *J Clin Oncol* 2006;**24**(6):848–855.

26. Cohen HJ. Keynote comment: Cancer survivorship and ageing—a double whammy. *Lancet Oncol* 2006;**7**:882–883.

27. Hurria A, Balducci L, Naeim A, et al. Mentoring junior faculty in geriatric oncology: Report from the Cancer and Aging Research Group. *J Clin Oncol* 2008;**26**(19):3125–3127.

28. Bennett JM, Hall WJ, Sahasrabudhe D, Balducci L. Enhancing geriatric oncology training to care for elders: A clinical initiative for long term follow-up. *J Geriatr Oncol* 2010;**1**:4–12.

29. Bodenheimer T. Coordinating care—a perilous journey through the health care system. *N Engl J Med* 2008;**358**(10):1064–1071.

30. Institute of Medicine. *Retooling for an Aging America: Building the Health Care Workforce*, released: April 11, 2008.

31. Tripathy D. Multidisciplinary care for breast cancer: Barriers and solutions. *Breast J* 2003;**9**(1):60–63.

32. Hesse BW, Hanna C, Massett HA, Hesse NK. Outside the box: Will information technology be a viable intervention to improve the quality of cancer care? *J Natl Cancer Inst Monogr* 2010;**40**:81–89.

Cancer and Aging Handbook: Research and Practice, First Edition. Edited by Keith M. Bellizzi and Margot A. Gosney.
© 2012 Wiley-Blackwell. Published 2012 by John Wiley & Sons, Inc.